Foundations of physical education

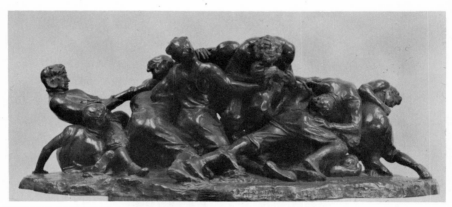

WORK OF R. TAIT MCKENZIE. COURTESY JOSEPH BROWN, SCHOOL OF ARCHITECTURE, PRINCETON UNIVERSITY.

SIXTH EDITION

Foundations of physical education

Charles A. Bucher, A.B., M.A., Ed.D.

Director of Physical Education and Professor of Education,
New York University, New York, N. Y.

With 287 illustrations

The C. V. Mosby Company

SAINT LOUIS 1972

Sixth edition

Previous editions copyrighted 1952, 1956, 1960, 1964, 1968
Printed in the United States of America

International Standard Book Number 0-8016-0865-1
Library of Congress Catalog Card Number 70-182043

Distributed in Great Britain by Henry Kimpton, London

To

OUR PHYSICAL EDUCATION COLLEAGUES IN OTHER LANDS

Preface

The world and conditions under which human beings live are changing rapidly. Education, if it is to serve humanity, must also change. Schools, colleges, and youth-serving agencies should strive to have programs that meet the needs of today's populace. Black studies, student activism, teacher accountability, peace demonstrations, women's liberation, and ecology are developments that need to be thoughtfully considered in light of our changing world and the role that education can play in helping to develop a better place in which to live.

A textbook such as *Foundations of Physical Education,* in order to render its greatest service to readers and members of the profession, must reflect the changes taking place in society and in education. It must describe these new developments clearly and give direction to the manner in which physical education relates to them and how it can contribute most to all human beings in today's world.

The role of physical education in a changing world is the primary thrust of the sixth edition of this text. Each chapter has been completely reorganized and rewritten in light of the changes taking place today in our society and in education. Particular stress has been placed on bringing up to date the historical, international, biological, psychological, and sociological chapters. At the same time, new developments and changes taking place in such areas as movement education, employment opportunities, preparation of teachers, health education, and services that physical educators render have also been incorporated into this text.

I am often asked why this book is somewhat larger than the usual textbook. There are many reasons. The task of writing a text for the many professional students and leaders in the field requires many hours of research, writing, editing, rewriting, and typing. The easiest way to perform such a task would be to cover the material superficially and have a smaller book. However, if I produced such a book I would render a disservice to students and to the profession. Furthermore, I have been told by many college faculty members and other professionals utilizing this text that they would rather have an in-depth treatment of the various subjects rather than a superficial coverage. These professors and other persons go on to say that such in-depth treatment serves many useful purposes. *First,* such coverage provides for flexibility in the selection of topics to be covered in the course. All topics in education and physical education are not considered in the same priority order by each instructor. Therefore, a broad range of topics and an in-depth coverage enables each instructor to select those chapters and topics that he considers most important. *A second advantage,* they point out, is that such a book eliminates the need to have students utilize many additional references in the library. The text has such extensive coverage of many different topics that the basic subject matter of physical education is incorporated within the covers of this one book. *A third reason* why these professionals like the extensive coverage of this book is that, although the entire text may not be assigned to be read by students, the more highly motivated and interested students have the opportunity to voluntarily read on their own the important information covered in this book. I am told that many students take advantage of this opportunity and thus become better informed about their field of endeavor.

As a result of the laborious task of bringing this text abreast of a changing society the student and reader are provided with a book that is *relevant*—relevant *to today's world*—relevant *to today's student*—relevant *to today's society*—relevant *to today's educational programs*—and relevant *to today's physical education programs*.

I would like to pay particular thanks to the many persons who read and critically evaluated parts of the manuscript. I am particularly indebted to my wife Jacqueline who spent many hours reading, editing, and typing the manuscript. Much credit is also due Mark Schaffel who helped in the research of many of the new materials found in this text and who attended to many of the details that are a part of writing a book.

Charles A. Bucher

Contents

PART ONE

Nature and scope of physical education

1   Physical education—its meaning and professional status, 3
2   Services rendered by physical educators, 30
3   Settings for physical education activities, 62
4   Projecting physical education into the future—forecast for the 70's, 90

PART TWO

Philosophy of physical education as part of general education

5   Philosophy of education, 117
6   Objectives of physical education, 143
7   Role of physical education in general education, 174

PART THREE

Relationship of physical education to health, recreation, camping, and outdoor education

    Introduction, 199
8   School health program, 203
9   Recreation, 237
10   Camping and outdoor education, 261

PART FOUR

Changing concepts of physical education

11   Changing concepts from early times to modern European period, 275
12   Changing concepts from beginning of modern European period to present, 298
13   Movement education—a developing concept in physical education, 342
14   International physical education in our contemporary world, 357

PART FIVE

Scientific foundations of physical education

15 Biological makeup of man, 403
16 Biological fitness, 428
17 Psychological interpretations of physical education, 477
18 Sociological interpretations of physical education, 520

PART SIX

Leadership in physical education

19 The teaching profession and physical education, 553
20 Duties of physical education personnel, 573
21 Preparation of the physical education teacher, 588

PART SEVEN

The profession

22 Professional organizations, 615
23 Certification requirements for employment in physical education, 639
24 Employment opportunities, 649
25 Challenges facing physical education, 666

PART ONE

Nature and scope
of physical education

1/Physical education—its meaning and professional status
2/Services rendered by physical educators
3/Settings for physical education activities
4/Projecting physical education into the future—forecast for the 70's

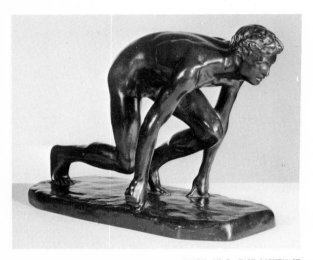

WORK OF R. TAIT MCKENZIE.
COURTESY JOSEPH BROWN, SCHOOL OF ARCHITECTURE,
PRINCETON UNIVERSITY.

1/Physical education—its meaning and professional status

The word *physical* refers to the body. It is often used in reference to various bodily characteristics such as physical strength, physical development, physical prowess, physical health, and physical appearance. It refers to the body as contrasted to the mind. Therefore, when you add the word *education* to the word *physical* and use the words *physical education,* you are referring to the process of education that concerns activities that develop and maintain the human body. When an individual is playing a game, swimming, marching, working out on the parallel bars, skating, or performing in any one of the gamut of physical education activities that aid in the development and maintenance of his body, education is taking place at the same time. This education may be conducive to the enrichment of the individual's life or it may be detrimental. It may be a satisfying experience or it may be an unhappy one. It may help in the building of a strong and cohesive society or it may have antisocial outcomes for the participant. Whether or not physical education helps or inhibits the attainment of educational objectives will depend to a great extent upon the leadership responsible for its direction.

Physical education is a very important part of the educational process. It is not a "frill" or an "ornament" tacked on to the school program as a means of keeping children busy. It is, instead, a vital part of education. Through a well-directed physical education program, children develop skills for the worthy use of leisure time, engage in activities conducive to healthful living, develop socially, and contribute to their physical and mental health.

A study of history reveals that other civilizations have recognized the important place of physical education in the training of their youth. In ancient Athens, for example, three main studies were followed by every Athenian: gymnastics, grammar, and music. Here in America the contributions of physical education in the educational program have been recognized for many years. In 1918 the National Educational Association set forth its well-known *Cardinal Principles of Secondary Education,* which listed seven objectives of education: health, command of fundamental processes, worthy home membership, vocation, citizenship, worthy use of leisure time, and ethical character. Physical education is playing a very important part in achieving these objectives. Through such contributions as the benefits of exercise to physical health, the fundamental physical skills that make for a more interesting, efficient, and vigorous life, and the social education that contributes to the development of character and good human relations, these cardinal principles are brought nearer to realization.

TERMINOLOGY

The multiplicity of terms that are sometimes used synonymously for physical education makes it imperative that the meaning of these various terms be clarified.

HYGIENE. Hygiene comes from the Greek word *hygieinos,* meaning healthful. It refers to the science of preserving one's health. It

3

often refers to rules or principles prescribed for the purpose of developing and maintaining health. In past years many school physical education departments were known as departments of hygiene; a few still use this term. It appears that the term became popular as a result of legislation in various states that sought to have the effects of tobacco and alcohol brought to the attention of all students through a course often known by the name of hygiene. There are still many laws on the statute books prescribing such instruction. Since World War I the term *hygiene* has become more or less obsolete. Newer terminology is being used, such as health education and personal and community health.

PHYSICAL CULTURE. The term *physical culture* is obsolete in education. It was used in the late nineteenth century to parallel names of other courses such as religious culture, social culture, and intellectual culture. This term is still used by some faddists in commercial ventures to popularize the beneficial effects of exercise. Such men as the late Bernarr Macfadden have, through their publications and business enterprises, done a great deal to spread the use of such terminology. Physical culture has been used synonymously for physical training. It implies that health may be promoted through various physical activities. It is a term, however, that is not in use today in our institutions of learning.

GYMNASTICS. The word *gymnastics* refers to exercises that are adaptable to or are performed in a gymnasium. It is the art of performing various types of physical exercises and feats of skill. The term has been and still is used extensively in the

A sixth-grade student on overhead ladder.

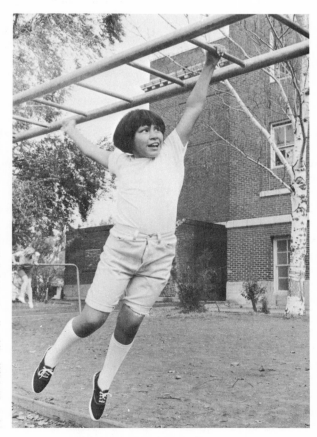

BROADFRONT PROGRAM, ELLENSBURG PUBLIC SCHOOLS, ELLENSBURG, WASH.

various physical education programs in Europe. Anyone trained in physical education has heard mention of such programs as the German and Swedish systems of gymnastics. Formal drills such as calisthenics were until recently utilized extensively in many physical education programs in the United States. Today, when one thinks of gymnastics, what comes to mind is formal drills conducted either with or without the use of apparatus. Americans do not use the term synonymously with physical education but, instead, with just that phase of the physical education program concerned with formal drills. Physical education programs today are more concerned with allowing the individual to express himself in various types of games rather than just through formal drill. This is believed to be more in keeping with the democratic way of life.

PHYSICAL TRAINING. The term *physical training* has a military tinge to many individuals. It is a term that has been used in school programs of physical activity and also in the armed forces. Hetherington used the term to connote big-muscle activity in the school program of physical education. On the other hand, both during World War II and at the present time, its use refers to the entire program of physical conditioning that the armed forces require men to go through as preparation for their rigorous duties. Most individuals agree that because of the military connection the term is used to imply training. This term has become rather outmoded for the modern-day physical education programs found in the public schools. Today, physical education programs realize outcomes other than just those concerned with the physical aspects. For example, there are sociological outcomes that result in an individual's better adaptation to group living. The term *physical education* also implies that physical activity serves the field of education in a much broader sense than physical training does.

FITNESS AND PHYSICAL FITNESS. A group of members of the American Association for Health, Physical Education, and Recreation approved the following definition of fitness: "That state which characterizes the degree to which the person is able to function." In other words, it represents the individual's capacity to live most vigorously and effectively with his own resources. Physical fitness refers primarily to bodily

Calisthenics demonstration by cadet academy students at Asian games.

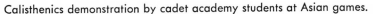

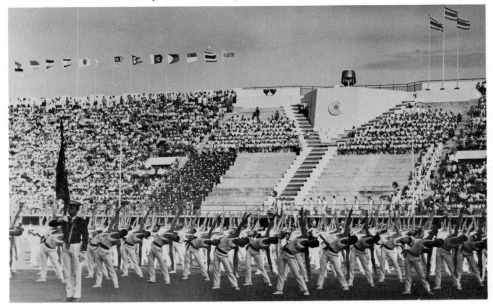

aspects of fitness. It implies such abilities as that of resisting fatigue, performing with an acceptable degree of motor ability, and being able to adapt to muscular stress.

HEALTH. Health, according to the World Health Organization, refers to such qualities as physical, mental, emotional, and social health. It is not limited to the mere absence of disease and infirmity. It means total fitness.

RECREATION. Recreation is concerned with those activities performed by an individual during hours not at work. It is frequently referred to as leisure-time activity. Recreation education is aimed at teaching people to utilize their leisure hours in a constructive manner. This implies a careful selection of activities.

ATHLETICS. The term *athletics* refers to the games or sports that are usually engaged in by individuals who are strong, robust, skilled, and able to participate in vigorous exertions. The interest in athletics in the United States has been largely inherited from Great Britain. With the introduction of athletics into colleges and universities, there has been a rapid growth in all sports engaged in on an intercollegiate basis. The first intercollegiate meet was a boat race in 1852 between the crews of Harvard University and Yale University. The first intercollegiate football game is believed to have been played between Rutgers University and Princeton University in 1869. These rivalries still exist today.

Many lay persons frequently think of athletics and physical education as being similar in meaning. However, most physical education personnel think of athletics as one phase of a broad physical education program—that division of the program concerned with interscholastic or intercollegiate sports competition. A director of athletics in a school has as his primary responsibility the direction of this competitive program.

SPORTS MEDICINE. Dr. Neal Tremble* of

---

*Tremble, Neal: What is sports medicine? Iowa Journal of Health, Physical Education, and Recreation **1:**11, 1969.

Drake University, a Fellow in the American College of Sports Medicine, points out that the meaning of sports medicine involves the interprofessional and interdisciplinary implications of the following components:

Athletic medicine
Accident prevention
Athletic training
Evaluation and management of injuries
Traumatology
Biomechanics
Anatomic analysis of movement
Kinetic analysis of movement
Clinical medicine
Clinical consequences of physical activity
Health appraisal of physical activity
Pharmacology
Physical activity and health
Prescriptions of activity for patients
Therapy and rehabilitation
Growth and development
Maturation and aging
Physical anthropology
Tissue changes
Physiology
Biochemistry of exercise
Environmental influences
Human performance
Nutritional considerations
Pathophysiological conditions and exercise
Psychology and sociology
Behavior
Cybernetics
Group dynamics
Motor learning
Perception

PHYSICAL EDUCATION. The term *physical education* is much broader and much more meaningful for day-to-day living than many of those terms discussed previously. It is more closely allied to the larger area of education, of which it is a vital part. It implies that its program consists of something other than mere exercises done at command. A physical education program under qualified leadership aids in the enrichment of an individual's life.

Before formulating a definition of physical education, it is interesting to note how three former leaders in the field of physical education defined this term.

Hetherington listed two things with which

physical education is concerned. First, physical education is concerned with big-muscle activity and the benefits that may be derived therefrom and, second, with its contribution to the health and growth of the child so that he may realize as much as possible from the educational process without having growth handicaps.

Nash pointed out that physical education is one phase of the total education process and that it utilizes activity drives inherent in each individual to develop a person organically, neuromuscularly, intellectually, and emotionally. These outcomes are realized whenever physical education activities are conducted in such places as the playground, gymnasium, and swimming pool.

Sharman pointed out that physical education is that part of education that takes place through activities involving the motor mechanism of the human body and resulting in the individual's formulating behavior patterns.

From these various definitions of physical education, it can be seen that any definition of the term should incorporate such concepts as selected physical activities and related learnings realized through participation in these activities, and it should show that this is a part of the educational process.

I propose the following as a definition of physical education: *Physical education, an integral part of the total education process, is a field of endeavor that has as its aim the development of physically, mentally, emotionally, and socially fit citizens through the medium of physical activities that have been selected with a view to realizing these outcomes.*

In a larger sense, this definition of physical education means that the leaders in this field must develop a program of activities in which participants will realize results beneficial to their growth and development; that they will develop, through participation, such physical characteristics as endurance,

Physical education class at West High School, Davenport, Iowa. Physical educators should offer a program of activities in which participants will realize results beneficial to their growth and development.

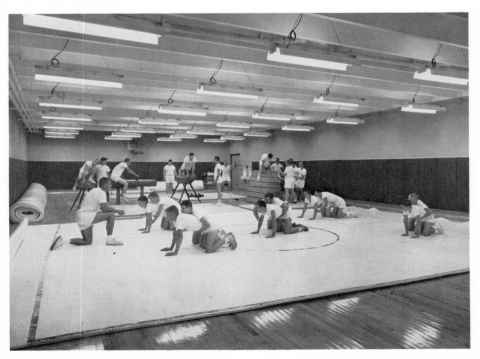

LOUIS C. KINGSCOTT AND ASSOCIATES, INC.

strength, and the ability to resist and recover from fatigue; that neuromuscular skill will become a part of their motor mechanism so that they may have proficiency in performing physical acts; that socially they will become educated to play an effective part in democratic group living; and that they will be better able to interpret new situations in a more meaningful and purposeful manner as a result of these physical education experiences.

NEED FOR UNDERSTANDING TRUE MEANING OF PHYSICAL EDUCATION

Indications that the public does not appreciate the value of physical education include lack of facilities, insufficient time allotted to physical education in the schools, failure to give credit for physical education in school programs, frequent emphasis on a few gifted athletes at the expense of all the students, haphazard scheduling of classes, indifference on the part of many administrators, poor financial backing, poorly planned programs, and inadequate training programs in many teacher-education institutions. If the true meaning of physical education were understood by all, these conditions would not exist, and instead of encountering opposition to the establishment of acceptable physical education programs, they would be welcomed with open arms because their values and contributions to enriched living would be recognized.

PHYSICAL EDUCATION AS A CAREER

Physical education as a career offers many opportunities to the young person who likes to work with children and adults, who likes a large variety of games and sports, who enjoys working in the out-of-doors, the gymnasium, or the swimming pool, and who is interested in rendering a service to mankind and in leading a vigorous and interesting life. Each potential and active member of the physical education profession should understand clearly such

things as the meaning of the name given to this field of endeavor, the activities comprising this field, the qualifications necessary for an individual performing this type of work, the opportunities available, the preparation required, and the responsibilities involved. Such information will help the individual to become more fully aware of the part he can play in physical education.

PROFESSIONAL STATUS OF PHYSICAL EDUCATION

Many occupations, trades, crafts, and other fields of endeavor constantly strive to achieve professional status. Library workers, pharmacy specialists, social workers, business management people, and physical educators, to name a few, hope to eventually receive the accolade of the status of a profession. At the present time these fields of endeavor are not members of the family of professions in the same sense that medicine and law are, but they are constantly working toward that goal.

Although some vocations call themselves professions, this does not mean it is necessarily true. They may have satisfied some of the requirements but have failed to achieve full-fledged professional status. Physical education is at times labeled a profession by some of its practitioners and leaders. Most of us use the term rather loosely and, in so doing, mean that we who perform this valuable service are bound together by close ties that have been developed through training and experience. We are dedicated to our work and contribute to the good of society, and therefore we feel we rate the status of a profession. In fact, the reader will find physical education referred to as a profession in this light throughout this book. However, in a strict interpretation of the term *profession,* it can be stated more accurately that physical education is emerging as a profession rather than having achieved the professional status of medicine, law, or theology.

We who associate ourselves with the field of physical education want to see it become a strong profession and be widely accepted by educators and the public in general. We feel strongly about the importance of our work and the service it renders to education and humanity. At the same time we recognize that we must earn the right to the professional label, and therefore we are working hard to see that this becomes a reality. We recognize there are certain benefits associated with being called a profession. As physical educators, we want to achieve these benefits for ourselves and our colleagues.

PHYSICAL EDUCATION–AN EMERGING PROFESSION*

Eero Saarinen's majestic work of art, the 630-foot Gateway Arch in St. Louis, symbolizes man's desire to surmount his obstacles, to reach greater heights, to achieve his destiny. Our aspiration as physical educators is to become a mature and respected profession. We desire to be respected for our expertise in physical education in the way doctors and lawyers are respected for their skill, training, and experience. The Gateway Arch reflects the spirit to which each of us should be committed if we are to gain this professional goal. In the days and months ahead we need to explore, to reach, and to achieve.

The word *profession* is a common term in our language, as characteristic of our world today as was the term *craft* in ancient times. In the language of the man on the street, many fields of endeavor—for example, selling, insurance management, or banking—are labeled "professions." To the more knowledgeable person the term is limited to such fields of specialization as medicine, law, the ministry, architecture, psychiatry, and social work. Those who have traced the origin of the term *profession* cite the fact that the three classic professions were theology, law, and medicine.

---

*This section is based on a speech the author delivered at the Physical Education Division meeting during the 1968 American Association of Health, Physical Education, and Recreation convention in St. Louis.

What is a profession?

Alfred North Whitehead in his book, *Adventures of Ideas,* distinguishes between a craft and a profession. A craft is based, he says, on "customary activities and modified by trial and error." A profession "is subject to theoretical analysis and modified by theoretical conclusions derived from that analysis."

Everett C. Hughes, professor of sociology at Brandeis University and former president of the American Sociological Association, cites the role of the profession in society: "A profession considers itself the proper body to set the terms in which some aspect of society, life, or nature is to be thought of and to define the general lines or even the details of public policy concerning it." Lawyers, he points out, not only give advice to clients and plead their cases for them but also develop a philosophy of law, of its nature and functions, and of the proper way to administer justice. "Physicians consider it their prerogative to define the nature of disease and of health, and to determine how medical services ought to be distributed and paid for."

Myron Lieberman, in *Education as a Profession,* explains the roles of the "physical" and the "intellectual" as they apply to professional status. "Proficiency in physical techniques may or may not be required," he points out. For example, in legal work the physical is minimal, but in surgery the exercise of skill and dexterity is very important. The important point to remember is that the physical activities of professional workers are guided by a high level of intellectual control: it is not just physical activity without rationale, it is not just arms and legs and good intentions. Instead, a body of knowledge undergirds how the physical activity is best performed, under what conditions and when it is best performed, and the results achieved when it is performed correctly.

Criteria for professional status

One way to better understand what constitutes the requirements for professional status is to look at what the experts say constitute the criteria for a profession. Many respected persons have written on this subject, including Abraham Flexner, Bernard Barber, and Myron Lieberman. After studying the list of some twenty authorities, I came to the conclusion that the criteria could be stated under four headings. In order to achieve full professional status, a field of endeavor must:

1. Render a unique and essential social service
2. Establish high standards for the selection of members
3. Provide a rigorous training program to prepare its practitioners
4. Achieve self-regulatory status for both the group and the individual

Many of the illustrious physical education leaders of the past referred to their field of endeavor as a profession. Luther Halsey Gulick, who contributed so much to Springfield College and to the Playground Association of America, to mention only two items, wrote an article in 1890 entitled "Physical Education—A New Profession."

George L. Meylan, president of our national association from 1907 to 1911, referred in a presidential address to the physical education profession. James Edward Rogers, who gave the initial impetus to the Society of State Directors of Health, Physical Education, and Recreation, wrote an article published in the *American Physical Education Review* entitled "Physical Education—A Profession." William Gilbert Anderson, who provided the spark for the founding of our association, writing in our national journal, entitled his article "The Founding of the American Physical Education Profession."

These early leaders used the term *profession* because of reasons advanced at that time: the philosophical and psychological foundations upon which physical education rests and the general cultural and specialized education that characterized professional preparation programs.

Is physical education considered a profession today? This is a question that should concern each person who is interested in becoming a physical educator.

What difference does it make?

One way to answer the question, "What difference does it make whether physical education is labeled as a profession?" is to think back to the time of World War II and ask the question: "Who were the persons selected to head our national Armed Services programs designed to physically train the country's manhood?" Do you recall such names as Hank Greenberg (a baseball player), who was head of the Air Force program, and Gene Tunney (a boxer), who was head of the Navy program? Do you recall the time in the middle 1950's when President Dwight D. Eisenhower was concerned with the fitness of American youth and called together a group of persons for consultation purposes, thinking he had the nation's experts on physical fitness? Among those present were Joe Louis (a boxer), George Mikan (a basketball player), Willie Mays (a baseball player), and Sammy Lee (a diver). Why were these sports heroes selected rather than physical educators? Would this have happened if physical education had been labeled a profession in the public's thinking and in the mind of the President of the United States?

It makes a great difference whether or not physical education is labeled a profession. There are many reasons, but I list only three:

1. *It means public recognition.* The doctor and lawyer, members of recognized professions, are highly respected. The public trusts their judgment and skill and seeks their advice.
2. *In an occupational sense, the professional person is placed above the rank and file of workers who do not possess specialized knowledge and skill.* The true professional, according to traditional thinking, is not hired; instead, the doctor is consulted, the lawyer is retained.
3. *It identifies an individual as a member of a group with such special qualifi-*

cations as knowledge, skill, and intellectual competency for rendering a particular specialized service. It yields a feeling of self-respect, of achievement. It separates the fit from the unfit, the qualified from the unqualified, the respected practitioner from the quack.

If physical education can lay claim to professional status, perhaps it falls into the classification of an emerging profession. An emerging profession is one in which leaders who are dedicated to the field of endeavor try to upgrade standards, gain public recognition, develop strong professional associations, strengthen professional schools, and undertake other responsibilities, that will move the field into the ranks of a mature profession. Many of the practitioners in an emerging profession, however, are apathetic and do not seek to improve themselves or their service in the same way the leaders do.

What must physical education do?

The question that must now be answered is: In light of the four criteria, what are some things physical education must do in order to become a mature and full-fledged profession?

1. *If physical education desires full-fledged professional status, it must render a unique and essential social service.* What is a unique and essential social service? Webster's dictionary says the word *unique* means something without a like or equal; it is matchless. The term *unique* also implies that the nature and scope of the service is clear in the minds of the group and in the minds of the public. The public clearly understands the function of the group and the group is recognized for this service. For example, in respect to medicine and law, for all practical purposes it can be said that only medical doctors perform surgery or prescribe drugs for persons who are sick and only lawyers practice law.

What then is physical education's unique and essential social service? Are physical educators the only persons who perform this service in the scientific manner that sets them apart from the rank and file? Students of history, like VanDalen and Bennett in their book, *A World History of Physical Education,* trace the services rendered by physical educators since early times. They point out: "Physical education . . . has been utilized for worthwhile and ennobling aims and conversely it has been employed for brutal and degrading purposes." They cite the fact that since the time of primitive man physical educators have rendered such services as developing physical efficiency, providing recreation, and encouraging participation in physical activities.

History also tells us that the service we render has been increasingly based on scientific grounds. Scientific advances in physiology, for example, started us on the road to placing physical education in a more respected position. This made it possible to render our service on a much sounder educational basis and provided us with a basis for training our practitioners in a way that would enable them to render their service in a more scientific manner, as contrasted with those persons who were untrained. Other scientific advances have also made it possible for us to better adapt exercise to age and sex and to have a better understanding of such things as motor learning, body mechanics, tests and measurements, and movement education.

Our field of endeavor has advanced until today, as VanDalen and Bennett point out: "Physical education is both a science and an art—the laws of movement, the reaction of the organs of the body to exercise, and the effects of motor response make it a science; the skillful execution of movement in sport, dance, or gymnastics makes it an art."

As the public looks at physical education programs today, what does it see? Does the public view physical education as a science and an art capable of being rendered only by persons trained in the foundational sciences? Physical education classes too often follow this pattern: a tall, muscular-looking young man takes roll, has the students snap

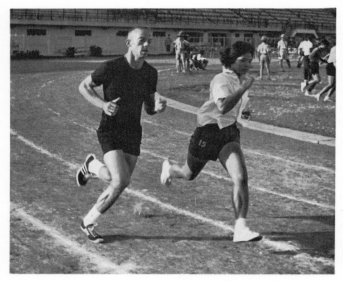

PHYSICAL EDUCATION
MUST RENDER A
UNIQUE AND ESSENTIAL
SOCIAL SERVICE.

A Peace Corps volunteer teaching
the Thailand National Girls'
Track Team.

PEACE CORPS PICTURES.

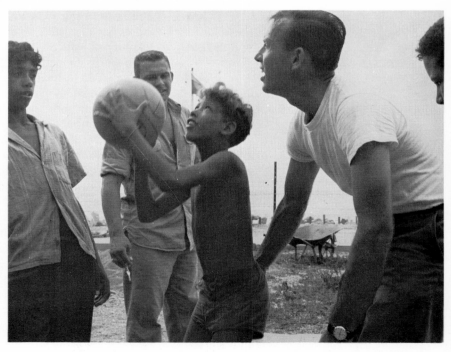

COURTESY PHIL HARDBERGER, PEACE CORPS.

A Peace Corps volunteer in Caracas, Venezuela, in his job as recreational
director at one of the YMCA playgrounds.

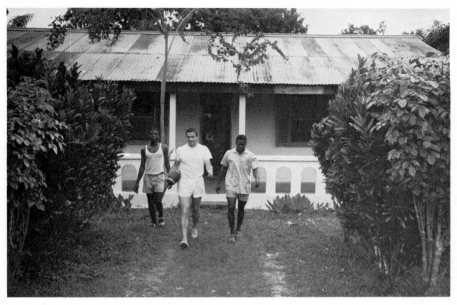

JOHN AND BINI MOSS FROM BLACK STAR.

A Peace Corps volunteer who teaches in Ghana is on the way to a
football match with some of his students.

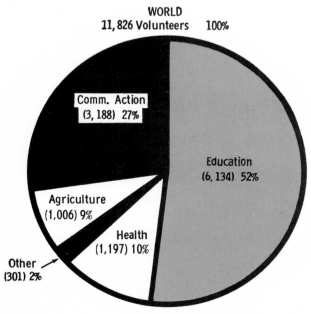

WORLD
11,826 Volunteers   100%

Comm. Action
(3,188) 27%

Education
(6,134) 52%

Agriculture
(1,006) 9%

Health
(1,197) 10%

Other
(301) 2%

SATURDAY REVIEW, APRIL 23, 1966.

Activity categories of Peace Corps volunteers. More than half
of them teach, half of these for the first time.

to attention, marches them around the gymnasium a couple of times, leads a series of warm-up exercises, and then runs them through an obstacle course. The pupils choose up sides and play racehorse basketball the rest of the period with the teacher acting as referee. Finally, the boys go dripping with perspiration to the showers. This is the service rendered in the ninth grade. And, unfortunately, it is sometimes also the service rendered in the tenth, eleventh, and twelfth grades. Confusingly enough, it often seems to be the same thing: exercise, basketball, perspiration. *Is this our unique and essential social service?*

There are, of course, examples of another kind. The best teachers of physical education are providing sound educational experiences for their students, teaching motor skills in a scientific manner, providing for progression in their activities from grade to grade, and providing for theory as well as physical activity in their classes. *This is the physical education that is both a science and an art.*

If the service physical educators render is unique with us, we who are trained in the foundational sciences of physiology and anatomy, the behavioral sciences of psychology and sociology, and various learning theories, especially as they relate to motor learning, how does our service differ from that performed by Debbie Drake, who poses seductively in her leotard on television, or Jack LaLanne or Ed Allen, who tell their audiences to smile and kick? Is our service the same as theirs, or is ours unique with us? If unique with us, how do we make this clear in the public's mind? How do we become recognized for our expertise? How do we separate ourselves from the untrained and the services rendered by the shapely ladies, muscle men, and drill sergeants?

Perhaps in order to become a more mature profession we must be more concerned than we have in the past with the intellectual controls that provide the rationale, understanding, and scientific foundations for what we do and the intellectual controls that make it possible for us to teach and utilize physi-

cal activity in a most effective manner. Perhaps we need to be more concerned with the participant than with the spectator. Perhaps we should go beyond physical activity and try to get our students to do some thinking—to get at the "why" of the activity as well as the activity itself.

2. If physical education desires full-fledged professional status, it must be very selective about whom it permits to perform this service. The profession of medicine is highly selective about those whom it permits to enter its ranks. It is very difficult to be admitted, to be tapped on the shoulder and told you can be one of the select group. One person describes it as the "inner fraternity" of medicine—a profession that uses potent mechanisms to repel the intruder. The minute the young man files an application with a medical school the selective machinery begins to work, with the medical hierarchy standing guard at the controls. The unfit are cast aside without fear.

Myron Lieberman, an astute observer of what constitutes professional status, has said: "A profession cannot in good conscience or in good faith with the public gain respect and have full-fledged status unless it is *willing* and is *able* to undertake the onerous task of weeding out the unethical and incompetent practitioners who, in some numbers, get admitted to practice."

Writer Arthur Corey's words still haunt us: "To the teaching profession, the most devastating canard ever invented is the oft-repeated assertion, 'He who can does, and he who can't teaches.' " Our goal as physical educators should be to try to change this phrase and to direct our organized efforts toward the end that those who *can* teach physical education *will* teach.

Historically, it seems, we in physical education have attempted to become more selective, primarily by upgrading our professional preparation programs in institutions of higher learning. In 1861, the first class of teachers graduated from the Normal Institute of Physical Education founded by Dio Lewis; they had only a 10-week course at this institution. We have made outstanding progress over the years; the length of training has been increased, degrees are now awarded, affiliation with colleges and universities of distinction has taken place, more general education is required, and there is now more stress on graduate study and research. But does this mean we are really selective about whom we permit to render this service?

Are we selective in respect to the quality of intellect and academic achievement of our practitioners? Certainly we have made progress since the Peik and Fitzgerald study, reported in the December, 1934, *Research Quarterly,* which indicated that physical education majors stood at the bottom of all teaching fields studied in the range and depth of their general academic training. We have come a long way, but we still need to stretch, to recruit the scholar into our ranks, to appeal to the brain power of our youth: young people who rank high on College Board scores, National Merit Scholarship Honor winners, and the valedictorians and salutatorians of their high school senior classes.

Are we selective in regard to licensure? Certification requirements for teaching physical education vary from state to state, ranging anywhere from as little as 16 semester hours to 40 credit hours. There are few if any requirements for coaches in many states other than a teaching certificate. Private schools and colleges to a large degree establish their own standards for faculty members (governed somewhat by the standards or criteria of the accrediting bodies to which they belong) but, unfortunately, they are frequently very lenient in the area of physical education.

Emergency certificates are quite common in physical education, but there are no emergency certificates for medical students. None of us would want a surgeon with an emergency certificate to operate on us. A question can be raised as to whether there should be any emergency certificates in physical education.

Are we selective in regard to members who make a full-time commitment to physi-cal education? Everett Hughes points out that once the medical schools select their students, they watch over them carefully and are very much disturbed if a sheep is lost from the fold. The medical profession wonders what it has done wrong. As Professor Hughes states: "The medical profession and schools make it clear to the professional recruit that he owes it to himself, the profession, and the school to stick with his choice. The theme is mutual commitment—one owes allegiance for life to the profession."

How about the full-time commitment of physical educators to their field of endeavor? Why is it so many have changed into the fields of administration and guidance?

3. *If physical education desires full-fledged professional status, it must provide rigorous training programs for those who are to perform this unique and essential social service.* Elbert Hubbard once said: "Education is a conquest, not a bequest. It cannot be given, it must be achieved. The value of education lies not in its possession but in the struggle to secure it."

There are very few worthwhile accomplishments in this world that are possible except through much toil and effort. The best things in life are *not* free. There is no substitute for hard work, and this goes for students who desire to major in physical education.

At an Eastern university recently I noticed the following motto over a student's bed: "Do not let your studies interfere with your college education." This is a humorous way of expressing the pleasant philosophy that the play of the side shows in college is more important than the work that goes on in the main tent. A college is, or at least should be, first and foremost an institution for education, and the departments, divisions, and schools that make it up should be likewise. This should be particularly true of physical education, where sometimes the play of the side shows seems to take over.

In respect to quality of training, John W. Gardner captured the idea in his book,

Excellence: Excellence implies more than competence; it implies striving for the highest standards." Can we achieve this excellence and quality of training by following such practices as dual majors and minors in physical education; students working on their degrees who seek just to get by, with some professors helping to pave an easy road for them; master degree students whom we call "coupon snatchers" in New York State because they can get their permanent teaching certificate not by taking work to make them more competent in their special field but instead by taking a variety of courses that may or may not have any relationship to improving their performance or service and that are frequently taken because they are "snap" courses?

We should insist upon our students stretching a little rather than just being satisfied with getting by, with receiving a gentlemanly "C." We should expose our students to the best minds on the faculty—to general sociologists, general psychologists, as well as to educationists. We need to follow an interdisciplinary approach. We need to do away with much of the inbreeding of faculty, a practice that seems to have infested some institutions of higher learning.

In training our practitioners, we need a longer period of formal education. The student of medicine follows a 7-year course, the student of theology 7 years, and students in law and dentistry 6 years. The period of preparation at the undergraduate level should be increased for our students. Although many of our practitioners take graduate work, there is a need for an extended period of preparation before any teaching is done. As one observer has said: "There is a world of tragedy for all of us bound in the fact that it takes six years of college training for a veterinarian to work on a sick pig, while a very large percentage of our teachers can work on a child's mind and body with less than four years of training."

4. *If physical education desires full-fledged professional status, the individual and the group must be self-regulatory in nature.* Lawyers have the power to decide such things as the requirements for admission to the bar, rules in regard to the suspension or exclusion of a member from practice, and the standards for ethical and unethical conduct. Physical educators should also be self-regulatory.

In achieving this autonomy, the profession must have some recognized organization that can and will speak for it with an authority that springs from and is granted to it by its membership. According to sociologists, the recognized organization must have a quality called "completeness." This means the organization must be representative of the members in the field, provide for two-way communication, and have sufficient consensus to be able to speak authoritatively in behalf of the profession.

Since the American Association for Health, Physical Education, and Recreation (AAHPER) is probably our most representative organization, let's examine it for a moment. The AAHPER has grown until today it has more than 50,000 members. But more important than size, from a professional viewpoint, the question must be asked as to whether this organization speaks for all the physical educators in this country. Does it speak for elementary school, high school, and college teachers; coaches; physical educators in YMCA's and other organizations and agencies; and young people who are majors in physical education in our colleges and universities? Does this organization have "completeness"? Does this organization speak out authoritatively on the great issues of the day in a manner comparable to the way the medical profession speaks out on Medicare? Has this organization taken effective steps to cast out the intruders, the charlatans, the unfit? And does this organization speak for our young people? Students represent nearly one-fourth of AAHPER membership. These young people want a respected profession, a recognized profession. I would suggest to those of us who are older that we should listen to them very attentively. Our young people have the courage and the fortitude to be standard-bearers for their convictions. Along with many of you, I have admired and have been greatly impressed with the great outpouring of youth and their efforts in political campaigns. Youth represents a significant and potent force throughout the world today and also in our field of endeavor. The young should play an active role in determining what officers should lead them and what issues the Association should speak out about authoritatively and convincingly. The young person has much at stake—his destiny, his hopes, his self-respect, his future.

In addition to having an organization with "completeness," to achieve autonomy the individual practitioner himself has to assume some responsibility. The professional worker is confronted with a wide variety of problems that require the application of a high degree of intelligence and specialized training. Therefore, he must be free to exercise his own best judgment. But in order to have this freedom he must accept responsibility for acting in an informed and intelligent manner.

Do we, the practitioners of physical education, accept the responsibility that goes with such autonomy, for judgments made and for acts performed within the scope of professional autonomy? For example, do we keep up with the latest trends, read the latest professional literature, keep abreast of what is new in such areas as learning theory, and understand the scientific foundations underlying our field of work?

Do we, the practitioners of physical education, accept the responsibility for our professional behavior? We need to police ourselves. This is essential in light of our obligations to our clients and to society. To guide our behavior, there must be a code of ethics that has been clarified and interpreted at ambiguous and doubtful points by concrete cases. Does physical education have a code of ethics? If so, are we, the practitioners, familiar with it? Has it been clarified? Has machinery been established to enforce high standards of professional conduct? What penalties can the group levy against an offending member? Is the power of expulsion available, if necessary? What

happens to the coach like the one, for example, just outside New York City, who told one of his basketball players who fouled out of the game to go down in the locker room and switch jerseys with different numerals with another player and go back into the game under an assumed name? The answer in this case—*nothing* happened. What happens if one of our researchers manipulates data in order to get what he considers to be desired results? The answer—*nothing* happens. What happens to the teacher who breaks a contract? The answer—usually *nothing* happens. What happens to the physical educator turned faddist who advertises in newspapers and magazines advocating some miracle way for removing fat from human bodies, charging a fabulous price, and thereby bilking the public out of thousands of dollars? The answer—*nothing* happens.

A full-fledged profession?

We would all agree, I suspect, in light of this discussion, that physical education at this time is not yet clearly established or fully accepted as a mature profession. We have not yet arrived. We are emerging as a profession, and there are many difficult tasks that lie ahead. Down deep in our hearts, however, we yearn for the day that we will have full-fledged status as a profession.

We yearn for this day because it will enable us to better exercise our powers—powers that we have spent years developing in the form of knowledge, understanding, and skill. We yearn for this day because it will enable us to render a greater service to our fellow human beings. We yearn for this day because we will be able to live more abundantly in loyalty to a growing brotherhood. Being a member of a profession means that each of us no longer is merely an individual person but instead belongs to a group. As a group, we possess a common stock of knowledge, common purpose, and common standards, which are continually growing and to which each member of the group contributes. Knowledge of our science and art accumulates from generation to generation and furnishes the common stock from which we all grow. To have this day arrive for which we all yearn we need a dynamic quest for truth and excellence among our membership.

The great threat to our future is apathy. We need more persons who will stand up and be counted, more persons who do not accept the status quo, more vigorous stands by our Association on issues where we provide the expertise, more satirists, and more critical abrasiveness among our students and colleagues to test our ideas and thoughts.

Unfortunately, we have too many members among us who are noninvolved, nonparticipating, and, most devastating of all, noncommittal. The ambition of this group, our enemy within, is a quiet life, a regular paycheck, freedom from controversy, and an absence of stress and unpleasantries. Such issues as determining our unique and essential social service, gaining greater selectivity in our ranks, providing for more rigorous training programs, and becoming more self-regulatory are not important as far as they are concerned. Such members contribute to a dying field of endeavor that never will achieve its destiny, make progress, be a mature profession—a field of endeavor no longer nourished by perspectives and values of informed judgment. Rather, it will starve to death in its own aimlessness and inertia.

To gain the professional label is not an easy road. It is a rough journey. It is full of bumps, pressures, and uncertainties. But one thing is certain. Full-fledged professional status cannot be bought, forced, or legislated. *It must be earned.* It is up to physical educators themselves whether their occupation is ever recognized as a profession. As Lieberman has pointed out, it is the physicians who have created the profession of medicine by constantly advancing its standards; it is the lawyers who have converted practice of law into a profession by continually striving for excellence. So must it be the physical educators who establish their vocation upon a strong professional footing.

To gain full professional status is physical education's priority for progress. This is what Eero Saarinen's Gateway Arch symbolizes for us—our desire to reach, to explore, and to achieve full-fledged professional status.

CURRENT ATTITUDE TOWARD PHYSICAL EDUCATION

The attitude that human beings have toward physical education plays a major role in determining the support that physical educators and physical education programs receive, the roles such persons and programs play in schools, colleges, and other organizations, and the status that physical education has in today's world. For example, the public attitude toward the medical, legal, and theological professions has raised their stature in the eyes of the American people to a place of great respect, importance, and recognition of their need for the society in which we live. In the same context, what is the attitude toward physical education? Some surveys and research studies provide some indication of this attitude.

Attitude of students

My surveys of the thinking of many students in elementary, secondary schools, and colleges provide these findings.

SOME STUDENTS FEEL THAT PHYSICAL EDUCATION HAS GREAT VALUE FOR THEM. Young people list such values as the help it provides in learning physical skills; the exercise it supplies for becoming physically fit; the social contributions such as the development of sportsmanship qualities, learning how to get along with others, teamwork; the psychological benefits in the form of self-confidence, an outlet for mental frustration, improvement of personality, and development of qualities of courage and self-discipline; and the knowledge learned in respect to the role of sports in the cultures of the world, rules of games and sports, and some of the physiological and other benefits of exercise to health.

SOME STUDENTS FEEL THAT PHYSICAL EDUCATION HAS LITTLE VALUE FOR THEM. Students cite such deficiencies in physical

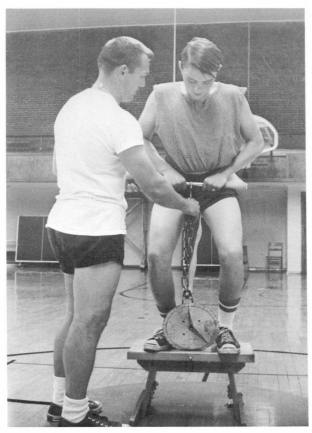

Some students feel that physical education has great value for them. Junior high school teacher readies a student for a leg-lift test, which is part of the testing program in the Ellensburg Public Schools, Ellensburg, Washington.

education programs that resulted in the experience having little value for them, such as poor instruction, lack of planning and organization, crowded classes, lack of motivation, program not adapted to the individual, and too much stress on competition.

SOME STUDENTS FEEL THAT PHYSICAL EDUCATION HAS GREATEST VALUE FOR THEM WHEN CERTAIN CONDITIONS ARE MET. The conditions that make physical education a dynamic part of the educational program in the eyes of students include good instruction in skills, a variety of activities, excellent facilities, well-organized program, vigorous exercise, and many interesting after-school activities.

SOME STUDENTS ARE CONFUSED AS TO THE MEANING OF PHYSICAL EDUCATION. In a study conducted by Wilson,* an attempt was made to determine the meaning of physical education as perceived by students and teachers involved in physical education. Some 283 high school students and 119 college physical education major students were surveyed. This study showed that students have six basic orientations to physical education: (1) physical fitness, (2) sports and games, (3) development of physical, social, mental, and emotional well-being, (4) social adjustment, (5) recreation, and (6) enjoyment and fun. Most high school students (80%) had a physical fitness and sports-games direction with little awareness

---

*Wilson, Clifford: Diversities in meanings of physical education, Research Quarterly **40:**211, 1969.

of the other values. As part of the study, extraneous comments by students were recorded. Some of these are very revealing:

> The student shouldn't be forced to take exercise.
> Physical education is when you go into a room and are supposed to be able to do the same things as the teacher, who spent years learning to do it himself.
> The basic purpose of gym class is to fill the law. The gym classes I have experienced gave little or no help to the physical condition of the student's body.
> I feel that physical education is not as strenuous as it should be.
> Physical education is a criminal waste of time. Grading is entirely ridiculous.
> Physical education should be an elective course.
> We should be able to participate in games instead of doing dumb drills all year.
> A gym class is waiting 15 minutes for you to put up a volleyball net and play volleyball for 5 minutes.
> Physical education means going to gym classes and throwing a basketball around.
> Supposedly, we are in gym for the purpose of keeping physically fit. If this is so, then a poor job is being done by the teachers.
> The attitude about gym is bad. If gym was made more enjoyable, kids would like it more.
> Unless the student desires instruction there should be none given.
> In this school all the teachers (gym) do is talk and stand around watching.
> Physical education is for people who don't exercise and have to be made to do it.

Beter,* in a study that involved gifted, average, and below average twelfth-grade girls, found that all groups had favorable attitudes toward physical education. Beter used the Wear Attitude Scale and also an opinion questionnaire to determine the attitudes of students who were gifted (score on intelligence test of 115 or above), average (100 to 110 score), and below average (scores on intelligence test below 100). The conclusions from the study were:

1. All three groups of students felt the greatest contribution to physical edu-

cation was in the area of physical development.
2. The gifted group had a higher percentage who participated voluntarily in gymnastics.
3. A higher percentage of the gifted group as compared to the other two groups felt that archery and softball should be offered in high school programs.
4. The gifted enjoyed individual sports, spent more of their leisure time reading than exercising, and engaged less in intramurals than did the average and below-average groups.

Attitude of educators, parents, and general public

I conducted a survey of 100 teachers, professors, parents, representatives of the general public, superintendents and principals of schools, and directors of physical education to determine what role physical activity had in their own lives and what they believed its role should be in education. Some general concepts derived from this survey include the following.

THERE IS A NEED FOR PHYSICAL ACTIVITY IN ONE'S DAILY ROUTINE. A majority of the persons interviewed (87%) spent more than one-half hour per day in some type of physical activity. Educators were the only group surveyed where the majority indicated that they spent less than one-half hour per day in physical activity outside of work hours; the other groups surveyed indicated that they spent more than one-half hour in physical activity outside of working hours. Of the persons surveyed, 97% felt that at least one-half hour of physical activity should be engaged in each day; 63% participated in some form of individual sports, 11% participated in team sports, and 49% engaged in some type of calisthenic exercise during out-of-work hours. Most of the adults surveyed indicated that physical activity was beneficial to their work. They listed such factors as the following: they felt better, they were more alert, they could work longer without fatigue, they obtained relief from nervous tension, they did not

---

*Beter, Thais R.: Attitudes of intellectually gifted twelfth grade girls toward physical education, and interest in physical activities and leisure time preferences, The Physical Educator **27:**30, 1970.

tire so easily, and their appearance improved. All persons surveyed indicated they felt there was a positive correlation between physical activity and general health. Reasons they listed to support this belief included: improvement of weight control, waste elimination, muscle tonus, relaxation, and cardio-respiratory development.

VIEWING PROFESSIONAL SPORTS ON TELEVISION DOES NOT ENHANCE THE HUMAN DESIRE FOR PARTICIPATION IN PHYSICAL ACTIVITY. The majority of the persons surveyed felt that it could possibly have some effect on the nation's physical activity participation, but most persons surveyed had grave doubts. Some of their comments included: "It might help in certain sports such as tennis, golf, and bowling." "Small children might idolize the professionals and this could motivate them to participate." "Watching sports will only make the person more adept at watching and will not aid in getting him to participate." "Watching will make the person more passive toward physical activity."

PHYSICAL EDUCATION IS AN IMPORTANT PART OF THE EDUCATIONAL PROGRAM. Overwhelming support for physical education as a part of the educational program was indicated by 89% of the persons surveyed. The exact role that physical education should play in general education is not clear in their minds, but the need for such a program was recognized by most of those persons surveyed. In general, the persons surveyed (59%) felt there was a positive correlation between what physical education is trying to do and what other aspects of the program are attempting to accomplish. A question that was raised by many of those persons surveyed was whether physical education should be concerned with a mental objective in the same way as mathematics, history, English, and other subjects. Some persons surveyed felt that physical education should be concerned only with education relating to the development of the physical aspects of the body.

PHYSICAL EDUCATION IS VERY BROAD IN ITS SCOPE AND SHOULD BE SCHEDULED SEVERAL TIMES EACH WEEK IN THE SCHOOL PROGRAM. When asked which of the following terms best defines physical education—athletics, calisthenics, movement, physical fitness, and skill development—the majority of persons surveyed (52%) indicated that all the terms cited should be included in a definition of physical education. The term *physical fitness* was thought by many (27%) to be the term that characterized physical education most completely. Furthermore, when these same persons were asked how much time should be devoted to physical education in the school program, 61% felt that physical education should be scheduled once a day. Only two groups, the professors and the parents, indicated they might possibly be more in favor of three times a week. One principal made an interesting comment: "Physical education should be conducted at the close of school and [be] required for all students. Those on athletic teams would practice at this time and the others would have regular physical education classes."

PHYSICAL EDUCATION PROGRAMS SHOULD PROVIDE MANY DIFFERENT TYPES OF ACTIVITIES. Most of the persons surveyed felt that all types of activities including team sports, carry-over activities, individual sports, general exercises, and recreational activities should be part of the physical education program. However, there was some feeling that recreational activities should not be a part of physical education. Some persons stressed that the type of program would depend upon the student's needs and age, facilities, and teachers available.

When asked what should be the average size of the physical education class, the principals and superintendents felt that the physical education class should be larger than the size of classes for the academic subjects. However, many of the other persons surveyed felt that the size of the school, activity involved, facilities, and number of teachers available would determine the size of classes.

In respect to what should be the basis for grading in physical education classes, the majority of the persons surveyed felt that physical education grades should be on a report separated from the other educational offerings. School administrators and professors were the only groups who felt that it should correspond with the marking in other subjects. Some comments made by the persons surveyed included: "It should be based upon the improvement the student makes in class." "Unsatisfactory and satisfactory are sufficient grades for students in physical education." "It depends upon the objectives of the school." "Marking in physical education is so subjective that it cannot be done properly."

PHYSICAL EDUCATORS BELIEVE CERTAIN BASIC CONCEPTS CHARACTERIZE THE PURPOSES OF THE MODERN PROGRAM OF PHYSICAL EDUCATION. Pelton,* in his study entitled "A Critical Analysis of Current Practices and Beliefs Underlying General Physical Education Programs in Higher Education," cites six basic concepts of physical education that were considered very important or important by three groups of physical educators (a group of physical educators in college physical education programs considered to be experts, a jury of physical educators who were considered experts in the overall field of physical education, and a group composed of deans of instruction). The six concepts are as follows:

1. The development of "strength and endurance" as an aspect of biological fitness.
2. The achievement of a personally satisfying level of motor skills involving "fundamentals of movement."
3. The development of an esthetic appreciation for the role of "sports as a cultural force" in the modern world.
4. The acquisition of knowledge concerning "agencies and resources useful in solving personal health problems."
5. The "clarification of self-image" and

6. The acquisition of "facility in the combined use of physical skills and mental interpretation."

The current attitude of students, educators, parents, and the public in general toward physical education and the questions raised when the four criteria for professional status are applied to physical education practices today indicates that steps must be taken if physical education is to move ahead professionally. In this regard, it may be of help to see what some selected occupations are doing to achieve professional status.

PROBLEMS AND STEPS BEING TAKEN BY OCCUPATIONS TO ACHIEVE PROFESSIONAL STATUS

Occupations desiring to become professions follow many steps in order to achieve the coveted status. For example, they try to find an intellectual base for their work. The YMCA secretary wants to be recognized for more than the help he gives to young people looking for the right path to a meaningful life. Therefore, he points out, there is an intellectual base to his work. This consists of a knowledge of human growth and development, of human behavior, and of the nature of life in the community. The school administrator is busy trying to develop a science of administration, as is the specialist in business management. The librarian is trying to be recognized as an expert on the effects of reading on human beings and also in certain areas of communications. Therefore, it can be seen that occupations desiring to become professions establish a rationale, a system of knowledge, which forms the intellectual foundation of the field of endeavor. Furthermore, since members of the special group are not uniformly inculcated with this knowledge, the group attempts to see that the selection and training of the members make such a goal possible. The leaders in the group take the initiative in encouraging such achievement.

Occupations desiring to become professions try to show that they are rendering a

*Clifton: A critical analysis of current beliefs underlying general programs in higher education, 38:678, 1967.

service rather than working entirely for profit. This is why insurance agents say they are not selling but that they are instead rendering a service by giving people expert, specialized advice on risks they face from day to day in their lives and by telling them how to protect themselves from these risks. There is a concerted effort on the part of the group seeking professional status to establish the fact that the profit motive is not the basis for their operation; rather, it is a concern for the welfare of society and the need for human betterment.

Occupations desiring to become professions have courses established in undergraduate and graduate schools for training in their fields of work. In so doing, they show that an extended period of preparation is needed to effectively perform their service. Furthermore, since more special knowledge is needed for the more elite positions in their occupational structures, the advanced work frequently related to a master's or doctorate degree is an indication that the individual has mastered the advanced knowledge and is thereby eligible for a higher position.

Occupations desiring to become professions seek more independence, more recognition, and a clear delineation of their service, as related to other outside groups that perform similar services. This step requires a careful delineation of the training required and service performed by the occupational group in order to clarify and show how their membership differs from others who claim to perform similar services for society. The problem is not only establishing the rationale involved for such reasoning but also communicating effectively this line of reasoning to the public in general.

Occupations desiring to become professions seek to establish requirements for entry into their professions. Furthermore, they try to police the profession, with the result that in some cases charlatans and quacks are expelled from the organizations. There is keen competition on the part of the group to attract to its fold the most qualified trainees possible. Once they have

in their ranks the most eligible candidates, they shepherd them with great care, impressing upon them their commitment to their field of endeavor.

Occupations desiring to become professions become more sensitive to public opinion, and therefore public relations becomes a necessity in conveying to outsiders the esoteric service being rendered by this important group of individuals.

Occupations desiring to become professions construct codes of ethics to guide the behavior of the members of the group. However, in many cases, the members find that these codes are too general in nature and quite difficult to identify with. Very often the machinery for enforcement of the codes is inadequate and ineffective.

Finally, the leaders and intellectuals in the occupational group recognize the weaknesses and inadequacies of their membership and the difficulties in striving for the status of a profession. In justifying this problem, however, they point to the fact that many of the traditional professions experienced the same growing difficulties and problems that they are experiencing, and that with time they will erase these weaknesses. Thus, as one leader of the American Management Association pointed out: "It's something like medicine years ago, when the doctors came to the realization that working in a drugstore was not sufficient training for their profession. Now management is going through a similar transition."*

Physical education as an emerging profession is facing problems that many occupational groups have faced in trying to achieve their goals. A field of endeavor does not receive the status of a profession in one quick step or in a short period of time. This takes many years to accomplish and requires outstanding leadership, sound thinking, a great deal of research, and a dedicated membership. Physical education as we know it today is comparatively young. The American Association for Health, Physical Education, and Recreation (AAHPER) was

---

*The New York Times, December 27, 1957.

established in 1885. We have come a long way. We are emerging as a profession. We should stride forward with great vigor to ensure that we become a strong profession.

THE CHALLENGE

If physical education is to become a strong profession, changes are needed. The "old," traditional type of physical education must be scrapped and a "new" physical education must replace it. Some essentials in a strong profession are discussed in the following sections.

A new physical education must emerge

A new physical education must develop that relates more to the latter part of the term, namely, *education*. A new physical education must relate to such concepts as academic achievement, learning, and knowledge, as well as to skill and physical well-being. Physical education must be identified as an important part of the education of each student. Academicians, parents, and the public in general must clearly understand and identify the values and contributions physical education can make to boys and girls, and human beings in general, that are closely linked with the educational process and that are essential to becoming an educated person prepared to meet life's challenge.

PHYSICAL EDUCATION MUST FORMULATE A BODY OF KNOWLEDGE THAT CLEARLY ESTABLISHES THE FACT THAT THIS FIELD OF ENDEAVOR INVOLVES A HIGHLY SPECIALIZED INTELLECTUAL TECHNIQUE. Physical education needs a well-defined intellectual foundation. A theory and body of knowledge that show that we are engaged in physical education, not just physical training, must be clearly stated. Research in physical education must be directed toward the identification of basic concepts that serve as threads of knowledge common to physical education work. Abernathy* identifies six

*Abernathy, Ruth: The search for significant persistent themes in physical education, Journal of Health, Physical Education, and Recreation **36:** 26, 1965.

points that perhaps offer clues to the theory and body of knowledge underlying physical education. These include the empirical study of successful and unsuccessful experience, a study of methodology, the kinesiological approach aimed at the anatomical basis of activities, human behavior and action systems, motor learning, perception, motivation, and a mathematical approach where accurate models and formulas exist to describe the field of endeavor.

Several leaders in the profession have advocated human movement as the basis for the intellectual orientation, providing knowledge as to its nature, determinants, and role in the growth, development, and education of human beings.

There should be considerable thought, research, and discussion on the intellectual basis for physical education. Physical education cannot achieve professional status without such a rationale.

PHYSICAL EDUCATION MUST CLEARLY SHOW THAT THE SERVICE IT RENDERS IS UNIQUE TO THIS FIELD AND CAPABLE OF BEING EFFECTIVELY PERFORMED ONLY BY ITS QUALIFIED MEMBERS. There are many imposters who claim to render a service similar to that with which physical education is identified. The physical fitness movement has attracted hundreds of quacks and charlatans who claim to build strength, take off weight, and make women beautiful. These impostors are using the term *physical education* and many times claiming to be physical educators themselves. Such inroads by misfits act as a strong deterrent to the achievement of professional status and result in loss of public confidence. The persons who are not trained do not belong and should be expelled. Stringent regulations must be adopted for membership and strong disciplinary action taken when professional standards are swept aside.

A new physical educator must emerge

A new physical educator is needed if physical education is to become a strong profession. The new physical educator will have an opportunity to select a role within the broad field of physical education suitable to his abilities and interest. These roles include teaching, administration, research, coaching, and working with the handicapped.

The new physical educator needs to be a scholarly individual who understands thoroughly the principles of learning theory involved in teaching skills, the implications of the behavioral sciences for his field of endeavor, and the scientific research that has been conducted and can be applied to his work and profession. In addition, the new physical educator must meet the following requirements.

1. *Physical education must have members within its ranks who are well prepared for their work.* Physical educators must have a liberal education. There needs to be a recognition that they are educators first and specialists second. This means being well versed in such subject matter areas as English, history, science, mathematics, foreign language, art, and music. Physical educators must have intensive training in psychology, philosophy, teaching methods, values, tests and measurements, and other disciplines that are frequently called educational theory and applied techniques. Finally, physical educators need sound preparation in their own specialty—the scientific foundations and the tools of their trade. They must be specialists to whom the public looks for guidance, help, and professional direction in the fields of sports, physical fitness, and allied areas. As the public looks to the lawyer for guidance in matters concerning litigation and law, so they should look to physical educators for direction in matters concerning physical activities. Physical educators should stand out above the rank and file of the general population as being expertly equipped, trained, and prepared in their specialized area. Such preparation is essential to being recognized as one who belongs to a profession.

2. *Physical education must have members within its ranks who wish to render a service to mankind.* The idea of service must be predominant in the minds of physical education practitioners. The consuming idea must not be what the profession can do for them but rather what they can do for the profession—the services they can render to human beings in helping them to live happier, healthier, and more vigorous and interesting lives. Physical education, as well as all subjects that comprise the educational program, must be designed and constituted so that it educates and prepares people to become all that they are capable of becoming. Such qualities as physical fitness and good human relations are worthy goals of accomplishment and will make for a better world. A member of any profession who is concerned with human beings and who is determined to leave this earth a little better for his having been here is the kind of individual who will contribute to making his profession a dynamic and important one.

3. *Physical education must have members within its ranks who believe in and practice excellent performance.* Whether it is preparing for class, developing a skill, gaining knowledge of an effective teaching technique, planning a lesson, teaching a class, coaching a team, or engaging in any other activity that is a part of the physical education profession, the performance should be characterized by excellence. Each practitioner should strive at all times to do his best. Since the principle of individual differences will operate, the quality of performance will vary from individual to individual; nevertheless, each one strives to do the best within his own abilities. Members giving their best for their profession will bring rich dividends to themselves as well as to their chosen field of endeavor.

4. *Physical education must have members within its ranks who have formulated a sound philosophy of physical education and who are articulate in communicating this philosophy to others.* It has been my experience that some physical educators have not given careful thought to the worth of their subject within the broad field of education.

Consequently, they find it difficult to interpret meaningfully the importance and place of their field of work in schools, colleges, and youth-serving agencies. A person without a clear-cut, soundly based philosophy is like a ship without a rudder. Vacillation, indifference, indirection, and ineffective performance will be reflected in his actions. Physical educators should study carefully such disciplines as biology, psychology, and sociology, from which physical education derives its scientific foundations, and then they should formulate what they believe to be a sound philosophy that has worth and that can be clearly communicated to colleagues, parents, students, and the public in general. A person who is going to devote a lifetime to a career should want to be able to clearly interpret the value of his chosen field to others.

5. *Physical education must have members within its ranks who have high standards of ethical conduct.* It is common knowledge that most people would "rather see a sermon than hear one any day." Members of outstanding professions attempt to translate their sermons into action. The members are living examples of that which they proclaim to be good for others. Most of us would not be impressed if a minister had the habit of swearing, a banker spent his money foolishly, or a businessman cheated his clients. Neither will the public be impressed by the physical education profession unless the members themselves believe in it to the extent that they feel that what they advocate for others is also good for themselves. This means that they will be in good physical condition, practice good health habits, have wholesome attitudes, set a good example for students, and be active in professional associations. The American Association for Health, Physical Education, and Recreation has a *Code of Ethics* for its membership. It might be useful for each member to review this code once each year.

6. *Physical education must have members within its ranks who play an active part in professional organizations.* Professions prosper and contribute only as their members band together to improve themselves, upgrade their services, solve knotty problems, enhance working conditions, and in general make their fields continually better vocations with which to be associated. Such professional endeavors require much time and effort on the part of members. Time and effort must be given unselfishly, without pay and personal gain and primarily for the purpose of improving and contributing to a better society. Unfortunately, too few members are professionally active in their associations at the present time. Members are not assuming their rightful responsibility. Some persons are living off the efforts, enjoying the privileges, and benefiting from the work expended by a few dedicated members. In a sense these people are parasites. Members of a profession should be professionally active from the time they are students in a college or university to the time they are separated from the profession.

Some professional leaders believe a member has his first loyalty to his local and state associations and then to the district and the national associations. This is a question that each person will have to answer for himself.

Physical education must be relevant to today's world

Times have changed and physical education must change with the times. New problems face our society and the world. Such words and terms as "the black athlete," "peace marches," "black studies," "ecology," "overpopulation," "drugs," "race," "student unrest," "inner city," and "ghetto" characterize some of the issues with which we are faced today. As a result, if education is to be relevant to the needs of the times it must do something about these problems. Consequently we are experiencing such things as "open admissions," "environmental teach-ins," "student strikes," "gloved fists," and "flower power."

Physical education must also be concerned with the problems of the times.

Thought must be given to how to contribute most to the black athlete; how our programs can make the greatest contribution to the culturally disadvantaged, physically handicapped, mentally retarded, emotionally disturbed, and poorly coordinated; what part physical education can play in helping to solve problems associated with drugs and student unrest; and what can be done by physical educators to improve our environment.

Physical education must be relevant to at least three important aspects of our culture if it is to contribute to the problems of present-day society.

PHYSICAL EDUCATION MUST BE RELEVANT TO THE INDIVIDUAL. The blanket type of physical education program is obsolete. Modern-day physical education programs must relate to all types of individuals whether they be handicapped or normal, whether they be female or male, whether they are dubs or skilled, and whether they live in the inner city or suburbia. Years ago, students in schools and colleges were willing to adapt themselves to required physical education programs. Today, they want a say in what type of program exists and want to be able to identify with the contributions it can make to them as individuals. They must be allowed a voice in present-day programs, and modern-day programs of physical education must relate to them.

PHYSICAL EDUCATION MUST BE RELEVANT TO THE ENVIRONMENT. The term *environment* as used here refers to the changing structure of communities and the problems they face. It refers to the tax rebellion against the high costs of running our schools as well as to the problems generated by pollution and crowded conditions. Neighborhood groups in many large cities are currently seeking a greater voice in managing the affairs of their schools, especially those aspects related to curriculum and administration. In many suburbs, recent referendums to increase tax limits to gain money needed to run the schools have been defeated. Ten years ago most taxpayers fully supported their schools, but many now feel that the schools are not adequate to modern needs and they are unwilling to pay higher taxes without the guarantee of educational reform. Furthermore, we find a move to suburbia, a rising civic interest in education, and a deep concern in determining the priorities in education.

Physical education is being challenged. Physical education personnel have been dropped, swimming pools and other facilities have been voted down by irate taxpayers, athletic programs are having trouble with crowd control as well as budgets, and programs are being questioned. The community environmental character determines the educational support available, and the physical education program depends on the community's educational outlook.

If physical education is to be relevant to the environment it must prove its worth to the taxpayers. Expensive facilities must be well cared for and used to their capacity. The interest the public is showing in their schools should be used to advantage to clarify to them the true meaning and worth of physical education. Programs must be constructed so that all individuals readily see the contributions they make to the total school and to the community.

PHYSICAL EDUCATION MUST BE RELEVANT TO EDUCATION. Physical education can no longer be merely exercise, games, and fun. It must relate more directly to the goals of general education and the primary goals of schools and colleges. There must be a sound rationale for the need of physical education programs. There must be a scientific foundation and intellectual base for physical education programs that show clearly the need for these programs in institutions designed primarily for the purpose of developing "brain power." There must be progression and an orderliness to our programs that evolve and produce the physically *educated* person. There must be an imparting of knowledge as well as the development of physical skills. There must be evidence that the physical education experience actually and definitely changes the behavior of individuals for the better.

The motives that prompt human beings to participate in physical education must be better understood*

If physical educators are to have greater support and make a more complete contribution to the human beings they serve, then the motives for participation must be more clearly identified and programs changed to reflect these motives. Max Cogan, in a presentation before the 1968 meeting of the National College Physical Education Association for Men, gave motives for participating in physical education. As he pointed out, Goodwin Watson's statement that "The clue to personality and its needs is usually found less in what people do, and more in why they do it" has implications for physical educators.

Some of the positive motives that Cogan identified after a very extensive evaluation of the psychological literature are:

Maintenance and improvement of health and fitness

Development of physique and general appearance

Social approval

Competition, self-evaluation, and social control

Satisfaction of mastering particular skills and its relation to self-esteem

Desire for creative experience

Integration of personality

QUESTIONS AND EXERCISES

1. What are some of the essential facts that every member of the physical education field should know in regard to his specialty?
2. What are some of the erroneous conceptions of physical education that exist in the minds of many individuals?
3. Do you feel that John Dewey would be in favor of physical education? Why?
4. Define the term *education*. What in your own thinking would be an acceptable definition of an educated person? What are the advantages of being an educated person in light of your definition? Why do you feel that you are or are not an educated person?
5. Why would an individual who had training

only in the accumulation of facts not be an educated person?
6. What is meant by each of the following terms: hygiene, physical culture, gymnastics, physical fitness, health, recreation, physical training, and athletics? What is the relation of each to physical education?
7. What is an acceptable definition of physical education? From your personal observations and experiences, why do you feel that members of this field of endeavor are or are not interpreting physical education correctly?
8. Why is physical education an integral part of any educational program?
9. To what extent did the physical education program in which you participated in elementary and high school contribute to your physical, social, mental, and emotional welfare? Where and how do you feel that it could have made a greater contribution?
10. Why is there a great need for understanding the true meaning of physical education? What are your responsibilities as a member of the physical education specialty to interpret your work correctly?

Reading assignment

Bucher, Charles A., and Goldman, Myra: Dimensions of physical education, St. Louis, 1969, The C. V. Mosby Co., Reading selections 2, 5, 6, and 7.

SELECTED REFERENCES

American Academy of Physical Education: The academy papers no. 3, Tucson, Arizona, based on program for the Fortieth Annual Meeting, April 9-10, 1969. Topics: The nation's physical fitness, Student activism of the university campus, Health education and the ghetto, Needed curriculum reform.

American Association for Health, Physical Education, and Recreation: This is physical education, Washington, D. C., 1965, The Association.

Bucher, Charles A.: Administration of health and physical education programs including athletics, St. Louis, 1971, The C. V. Mosby Co.

Bucher, Charles A.: Administrative dimensions of health and physical education programs, including athletics, St. Louis, 1971, The C. V. Mosby Co.

Bucher, Charles A.: Fitness and health (editorial), Educational Leadership 20:356, 1963.

Bucher, Charles A., editor: Methods and materials in physical education and recreation, St. Louis, 1954, The C. V. Mosby Co.

Bucher, Charles A., and Goldman, Myra: Dimensions of physical education, St. Louis, 1969, The C. V. Mosby Co.

Bucher, Charles A., Koenig, Constance, and Barn-

---

*For fuller discussion of motives, see Chapter 17.

hard, Milton: Methods and materials for secondary school physical education, St. Louis, 1970, The C. V. Mosby Co.

Bucher, Charles A., and Reade, Evelyn M.: Physical education and health in the elementary school, New York, 1971, The Macmillan Co.

Hetherington, Clark W.: School program in physical education, New York, 1922, World Book Co., part III.

Journal of the American Academy of Arts and Sciences, Daedalus **92:**647, 1963.

Kaufman, Earl: A critical evaluation of the components basic to certain selected professions with a view to establishing recreation as a profession, Doctoral thesis, 1949, New York University.

Lieberman, Myron: Education as a profession, Englewood Cliffs, N. J., 1956, Prentice-Hall, Inc.

Morris, Van Cleve, and others: Becoming an educator, New York, 1963, Houghton Mifflin Company.

Stinnett, T. M.: The profession of teaching, New York, 1962, Library of Education, The Center for Applied Research in Education, Inc.

VanDalen, Deobold B., and Bennett, B. L.: World history of physical education, New York, 1971, Prentice-Hall, Inc.

Weston, Arthur: The making of American physical education, New York, 1962, Appleton-Century-Crofts.

2/Services rendered by physical educators

In Chapter 1, the criteria by which physical education can become a full-fledged profession were listed. One of the four criteria stated that physical education must render a service to humanity that is needed and recognized by the public in general. The practitioner regards the rendering of this service as being more important than the economic gain derived and renders it in a manner that will benefit the entire populace, whether young or old, male or female, rich or poor. This chapter is concerned with identifying the services that physical educators perform in utilizing physical activity as a medium for contributing to the physical, mental, and social well-being of human beings.

Physical education is a rapidly expanding field of endeavor. There are more than 700 institutions training personnel for some phase of this specialized field. It has been estimated that there are over 200,000 men and women in the United States who perform physical education duties related to the field of education. There are more than 50,000 members in the American Association for Health, Physical Education, and Recreation, an organization that is very active in furthering physical education. The different games and sports played in our society are innumerable. These and other physical education activities are conducted in the smallest hamlet and in the largest city; in back yards and in public sports palaces; in public school classrooms, gymnasiums, and swimming pools and in the YMCA, YWCA, YMHA, and YWHA; in industrial plants and in athletic clubs; in settlement houses and in public playgrounds; in boys' and girls' clubs and in adult recreation centers; in hospitals and in penal institutions.

The nature and scope of physical education include not only the teaching and coaching of games and sports but also much activities as dancing, rehabilitation, and camping. The picture of physical education may be portrayed to the prospective teacher by describing the nature and scope of physical education, first, as services provided by physical educators, which will be considered in this chapter, and second, as settings where these services are rendered (Chapter 3).

The services performed by three physical education teachers, as shown on p. 31, provide a picture of some of the responsibilities and contributions made by physical educators in two schools and one university. One can readily see that a physical educator is busy from morning until night rendering services to students and to the community and public in general.

The services rendered by physical education personnel may be divided into the following for purposes of convenience:

Teaching
    Movement experiences
    Games and other selected physical education
       activities
    Dance
    Teachers (professional preparation programs)
    Teacher Corps
    Health
    Recreation programs
    Camping and outdoor education programs
Coaching
Counseling

Services rendered by Mrs. Jones, teacher of physical education in Midwest	Services rendered by Mr. Smith, teacher of physical education in East
Teaches six classes of games and other physical education activities each day Gives tests over subject matter pertaining to rules, courts, and skill tests Engages in individual work with students on rhythm activities Teaches activities before school from 7:50 to 8:25 A.M., including tap dancing, soft-shoe dancing, and attending committee meetings with special dance groups and gymnasium leaders Supervises after-school activities, including Can-Can dance class, modern dance group, as well as giving advice to Future Nurses' Club Engages in after-dinner activities, including chaperoning school dances, ushering at football and basketball games, helping with such special programs or events as homecoming, Christmas plays, and dance rehearsals for school variety show	Teaches six classes of physical education each day Supervises the noon lunch period in the gymnasium Prepares equipment list for physical education classes, six interscholastic sports, and all intramural activities Arranges transportation for after-school sports activities Secures officials for athletic activities Serves on various community and school committees, including buildings and grounds committee, Boosters' Club, curriculum committee Conducts coaching and staff meetings Attends all athletic contests at home and away Chaperons school functions such as dances Inspects and determines what equipment should be reconditioned and discarded Attends league athletic meetings Arranges for all details in respect to game and athletic management

Services rendered by Professor Brown, Division of Physical Education, Health, and Recreation, in a large state university in the Far West	
Teaches a course in the history and principles of physical education to undergraduate students 3 hours per week Teaches activity courses in team sports and also gymnastics twice a week to nonmajor freshman students Attends faculty meeting or committee meeting 2 hours per week Teaches course in methods and materials for teaching games of low organization to major students three times per week	Chaperons one undergraduate function, such as a dance or a club activity, once every 2 weeks Keeps office hours for students and sees students 4 hours per week Spends 2 hours in preparation for each class taught each week Works regularly on proposal to obtain research grant Spends 10 hours per week on research project Teaches administration of physical education course three times per week

Administration
Conducting safety and driver education programs
Conducting research
World service
Changing human behavior
Working with handicapped and exceptional persons
Interpreting the worth of physical education

TEACHING

Teaching represents one of the most essential services that physical educators render to mankind. Each new generation must be taught motor skills and the importance of physical activity in developing a healthy human mechanism. Physical education is concerned not only with teaching about the physical aspects of the body but also utilizing the physical aspect as a medium of developing mental, emotional, and social qualities essential to effective living. Physical educators teach a variety of activities and in a variety of programs.

Movement experiences

A service that represents the heart of physical education is that of providing meaningful movement experiences. Movement relates to developing body awareness as well as the experiences provided in games, skills, gymnastics, dance, and other activities taught in this field of endeavor. The factors of time, space, force, and flow are explored as the student engaging in the physical education experience learns to understand how his body relates to these various factors. The individual learns about his body and how it functions under various conditions where physical activity is involved. The teacher acts as a guide in helping the student to better understand his body and its performance capabilities. The student develops understanding about and appreciation for human movement. He learns about the important place of movement in all of life's activities. He gains an awareness of his body.

A significant group of professional physical educators feels that movement is an educational discipline. It is a science. It has a subject matter, a body of knowledge. There are principles and laws involved in the efficient performance of movement.

When the knowledge, principles, and laws are brought into play, contributions can be made to the physical, mental, social, and emotional growth of the individual.

There are different schools of thought and approaches to movement within the field of physical education. Some leaders subscribe to definite units or courses devoted to movement, whereas others feel that movement education constitutes the whole, encompassing physical education (see Chapter 13 for a fuller discussion of movement). There are those persons who advocate movement as an academic discipline and those who advocate it as an educational process.

Regardless of the school of thought to which a physical educator subscribes, a valuable service can be rendered by physical educators through the application of principles underlying movement. It represents an attempt to enrich the total life of the individual through selected experiences that relate to physical activity.

Furthermore, it is apparent that movement education as such is only in its embryo

Teaching games and sports is one of the services rendered by physical educators.

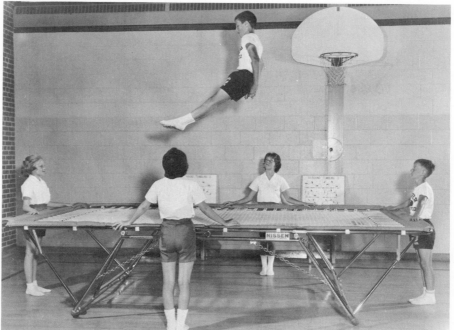

stage and that as our knowledge and understanding of this phenomenon increase and our thinking is clarified, the service that we will be able to render to human beings will be increased. It is up to each physical educator to study the various theories being advocated in regard to movement and to investigate on his own what form movement should play in his program. In so doing, he will better understand its possibilities for improving his physical education program and the contributions it can make to human beings.

Games and other selected physical education activities

Games are a popular pastime for the young and the old, for boys and girls, and for men and women. They offer an opportunity for all to obtain exercise, fun, and relaxation. They can play an important part in developing physical fitness and developing skills for use in leisure time, now and, perhaps more important, in later years. Many of the skills developed through games may be used in years to come to help keep physically fit. Older people who believe in the value of exercising to keep active and healthy participate in some activity—tennis, skating, swimming—that they learned at an early age.

The teaching of games represents one of the main components of any physical education program; therefore, the physical educator must be familiar with many of them in order to render this service. He should know the essential features of the various games, rules, methods of organization, values received from participation, equipment and facilities needed, and ways of motivating the participants. He should also have motor skill in as many of these activities as possible. The ability to demonstrate a particular skill aids greatly in the teaching process and also increases the prestige of the teacher in the eyes of the students.

Some of the games and other related physical education activities with which every person in physical education should be familiar are listed:

Team games
1. Softball
2. Baseball
3. Basketball
4. Football (men only)
5. Touch football
6. Volleyball
7. Soccer
8. Speedball
9. Field hockey
10. Water polo
11. Ice hockey (men only)

Dual and individual sports
1. Track
2. Deck tennis
3. Table tennis
4. Shuffleboard
5. Bowling
6. Wrestling (men only)
7. Golf
8. Squash
9. Darts
10. Badminton
11. Horseshoes
12. Handball
13. Archery
14. Fencing
15. Tennis

Formal activities
1. Calisthenics
2. Marching

Aquatics
1. Swimming
2. Diving
3. Lifesaving
4. Canoeing
5. Rowing
6. Water games

Outdoor winter activities
1. Skating
2. Snow games
3. Skiing
4. Tobogganing
5. Hiking

Self-testing activities
1. Running
2. Jumping
3. Climbing
4. Hanging
5. Chinning
6. Sit-up
7. Forward roll
8. Stunts
9. Knee dip
10. Push-up

Games of low organization
1. Dodge ball
2. Hopscotch
3. Rope jumping
4. Two deep
5. Under leg
6. Ring games
7. "Tag" and "It" games

Gymnastic activities
1. Tumbling
2. Pyramid building
3. Apparatus
4. Acrobatics
5. Obstacle course
6. Rope climb

Relays
1. Potato relay
2. Over and under relay
3. Jump the stick relay
4. Sack relay
5. Hopping relay

Dance

Dancing is one of the oldest arts and should be an important part of every physical education program from the primary grades through college. As far back as one can go into history, popular dancing was a pastime in the lives of all peoples. The members of early tribal groups danced as part of their religious festivals, in preparing for combat, and for entertainment. Dance has come down through the ages, bringing with it an account of the way people lived in other lands and other times. It is a means of communication. Through dance one may creatively express how he feels about people, forces of nature, and other phases of our culture. It provides enjoyment, a means of emotional release, and expression of desires in action. It results in beneficial physiological effects by stimulating the various organic systems of the body. It helps to develop balance, control, and poise and provides the opportunity to respond to music through movement.

The dance program consists of *fundamental rhythms,* such as running, walking, skipping, jumping, hopping, and the imitation of real and imaginary characters through rhythmic activities; *folk dances* and *singing games,* such as "Farmer in the Dell," "Csebogar," "Pop Goes the Weasel," "Norwegian Mountain March," and "Schottische"; *athletic* or *gymnastic dancing,* which is dancing done with vigor and which includes such acts as cartwheels, rolls, running, and skipping; *social* or *ballroom dancing,* which is rapidly being included in many physical education programs for its social value; and *modern dancing,* which is a medium of expressing oneself creatively and esthetically through movement.

The elementary school program in rhythms and dance includes such forms of dance as fundamental rhythms, pantomimic and dramatic dances, dramatic and singing games, folk dances, and character dances. Dance may constitute as much as 20% to 40% of the entire physical education program.

In junior and senior high school, the more popular phases of the dance program include social, folk, square, and modern dancing.

At the college and university level, folk, square, ballroom, and modern dancing are frequently included in the curriculum. In addition, such courses as the history and philosophy of dance, methods of teaching various forms of dance, dance production, and cultural concepts of dance are offered.

Dance is becoming a popular and rewarding career for those physical educators who wish to render a service by helping young persons to better understand their bodies and to express themselves through rhythmical activity. Although many opportunities present themselves in elementary and secondary schools and also in dance studios and community agencies and recreation programs, the college and university levels (where more often than not dance teachers work in departments, divisions, or schools of physical education) also offer many opportunities to serve. There has been considerable expansion of dance programs in recent years in institutions of higher learning. Liberal arts colleges are offering expanded programs of dance experiences for their students, professional preparation programs are training teachers of physical education with an emphasis in the area of the dance, and other institutions are providing instruction in modern, ballroom, and folk dancing for the general student body.

As the dancing program in schools and colleges becomes increasingly popular, there is a demand for teachers of physical education who are specialists in the various phases of dance. Prospective teachers interested in dance will find more positions available if they prepare themselves to teach the other activities in the physical education program as well. The opportunities for teaching dance alone are limited.

In addition to schools and colleges, dance personnel are needed in such other places as the theater, private studios, recreation centers, armed forces, summer camps, and hospital therapy. Roles that dance personnel play include that of teacher, performer, choreographer, notator, and director in a concert group and in television, movie, and theater productions. To render the service of teaching dance effectively requires a study of such areas as the scientific principles of body movement; an understanding of dance forms, dance composition, and technique; skills of notation; theories relating to costuming, staging, and lighting; and also a good grounding in the scientific foundations of physical education and a sound general education.

Teachers (professional preparation programs)

For those physical educators who aspire to the college and university level and who are interested in helping to shape the future of their field of endeavor by contributing to the preparation of future leaders of their field, there are many opportunities to render this valuable service in the more than 700 institutions that have such programs.

The qualifications for teaching in professional preparation programs include advanced degrees, a high academic record, an interest in and understanding of college students, a broad view of educational problems, and, many times, previous experience at elementary or secondary school levels. The college teacher must be particularly well versed and competent in his field and have desirable personality and nonacademic traits, such as good character. The sought-after teacher is one who can be characterized as truth seeking, humble, steadfast, and possessing a sympathetic understanding for human beings.

A professor in a professional preparation program might render a variety of services, including teaching such courses as history and philosophy of physical education, tests and measurements, methods, skills, organization and administration, programs for the atypical individual, and health observation. In addition, there might be research activities, committee service, advice and counsel of students, writing, community service, consulting, and participating in the work of professional associations.

A college or university staff usually includes various instructional ranks, including that of instructor, assistant professor, associate professor, and professor. In some cases there are distinguished professors. Furthermore, there is usually a head or chairman of the department, division, and, in some cases, a dean of a school or college of physical education, health, and recreation.

The services rendered by physical educators in professional preparation programs can be very rewarding. By providing experiences that will help to develop those qualities, competencies, and attributes in students preparing to become leaders in the field and by doing an outstanding job in this training experience, a teacher's work will live on forever in the lives of his students and other leaders of future generations.

Teacher Corps

The Teacher Corps was established by the Higher Education Act of 1965. It enrolls college graduates who had not previously intended to teach and provides them with an orientation and an internship for 2 years in schools in poverty areas. During the internship program they are provided with educational experiences that enable them to meet certification standards for teaching and also confer upon them a master's degree. The Teacher Corps program has proved to be an imaginative type of experience and has resulted in outstanding services to education in ghetto communities.

Health

Surveys indicate that many physical educators teach concentrated health courses in the nation's schools. In some cases physical education personnel have been qualified to assume this responsibility and in other cases they have not. The teaching of health* as a subject-matter area should be done by a person who has training and experience to do the job effectively. However, there are many areas of health teaching not involved in a concentrated health course where all physical educators should be active. Physical educators should be concerned with emphasizing good health practices in their various activities; in stressing proper sanitary procedures conducive to a healthful environ-

---

*Sometimes referred to as health instruction or health science.

ment; in pointing out to students the importance of such things as nutrition, rest, sleep, and medical examinations to physical fitness; in showing the need to abstain from using tobacco, alcohol, and drugs; and in capitalizing on many other opportunities to impart knowledge and help in the development of wholesome health attitudes and practices in the physical education program. In these various ways physical educators can render a valuable service.

Health within the school structure consists of health education,* health services, and healthful school living. In the area of health education, scientific knowledge is imparted and experiences are provided so that students may better understand the importance of developing good attitudes and health practices. Information concerning such topics as nutrition, communicable disease, rest, exercise, sanitation, first aid, and safety is presented. On the elementary level the responsibility for such health education rests on the shoulders of the classroom teacher, although in some school systems trained specialists are provided as resource persons. On the secondary level it is recommended that individuals who have had special training in health education be responsible for concentrated health instruction. This is not always the case. Sometimes in the absence of a trained specialist the teacher of physical education, home economics, science, or some other subject is given the responsibility. It should be reiterated that if a physical educator teaches health, he should be qualified to perform this service.

Other phases of the school health program include health services and healthful school living. The health services include health appraisal, health counseling, correction of defects, provision for the exceptional child, prevention and control of communicable disease, and emergency care of injuries. Healthful school living refers to the physical and emotional environment in which the child lives while at school.

*See also Chapter 8.

A significant study in the field of health education conducted in recent years is the School Health Education Study. This study has included a synthesis of research in selected areas of health instruction, a national study of health instruction in the public schools, and the development of a concept approach to the teaching of health, which identifies the key concepts to be taught, conceptual statements for organizing the curriculum, and substantive elements that delineate the subject matter content. All of these concepts are directed at certain behavioral outcomes deemed desirable for the student. This study has determined the nature and scope of health education in the public schools of the United States, the kind of instruction students receive, how much boys and girls know about health matters, who teaches these pupils, how the subject is organized and scheduled in the school program, the health content areas that are emphasized, and many other factors of importance to all educators and persons interested in health. The study also gives special concern to curriculum materials.

All physical educators should have some preparation in the field of health. A physical educator who is well grounded in the health sciences will be a better physical educator, since physical education has many health outcomes. Therefore, the physical educator cannot isolate himself from the field of health; instead, he should be well informed in this area of specialization since it is so closely related to his own specialized field.

Some physical educators are interested in and want to be prepared to teach health science courses in schools and colleges. To render the greatest service in this area, these persons should prepare themselves by taking considerable work in such areas as chemistry, nutrition, the behavioral sciences, and specialized health courses. The specialization that the physical educator pursues in his undergraduate training, such as anatomy and physiology, will be of great help. However, this alone is not sufficient because of the many areas that health courses cover today, such as personality development, ecology, drugs, mental health, nutrition, and protective and preventive health measures.

Recreation programs*

Recreation programs in schools, communities, youth-serving agencies, industry, hospitals, and other organizations are growing rapidly. These programs are designed to provide young and old alike with profitable activities in which they can engage during their leisure hours. Special skills are needed for physical educators working in such programs. Such activities as games, sports, dance, and rhythms play an important role in many communities. It is a common practice for physical educators in our schools to find supplementary work in the recreation programs of their communities.

Various personal attributes are important for the physical educator desiring to perform services in recreation programs. These include such characteristics as integrity,

friendly personality, enthusiasm, initiative, organizing ability, and other qualifications that will aid in the achievement of recreation objectives. It is especially important that the person working in recreation understand and appreciate human beings. He must have respect for the human personality; a broad social viewpoint; the desire to inculcate a high standard of moral and spiritual values; a recognition of the needs, interests, and desires of individuals; an appreciation of the part that recreation can play in meeting these needs and interests; and a desire to serve humanity. There is also a special need for recreators to have an understanding and appreciation of community structure and the place of recreation at the "grass roots" level of this structure.

Camping and outdoor education programs*

Many physical educators render services in camping and outdoor education pro-

*See also Chapter 9.

*See also Chapter 10.

Recreation programs provide young and old alike with activities in which they can engage during their leisure hours.

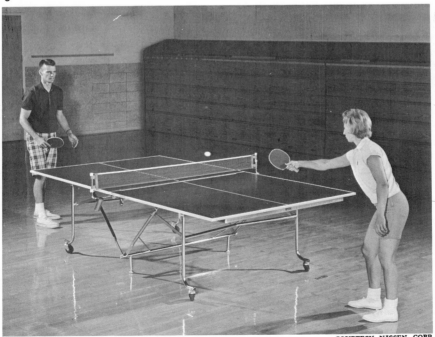

COURTESY NISSEN CORP.

grams. These programs are recognized as having an educational value that should be experienced by every boy and girl. Some camps throughout the United States are associated with school systems, and camping is a part of the educational experience. Outdoor education programs in camps and other settings are also becoming popular.

Outside the field of education, camps are sponsored by state, county, and municipal governments and by such organizations as churches, Boy Scouts and Girl Scouts, YMCA, YWCA, YMHA, and YWHA groups, 4-H clubs, and private corporations.

Many educational institutions preparing teachers of physical education recognize the value of camping and its importance in education. In some training programs, prospective teachers of physical education are required to spend one or more sessions at a camp. This experience orients the student in camp living and in the organization and administration of a camp, and it emphasizes the value of outdoor education.

Camping should be included in the educational experience of every boy and girl because of the many values that it offers. In the camp situation individuals learn how to live together cooperatively and democratically. Regardless of whether a camper comes from a rich or a poor home, is white or Negro, is Jewish or Protestant, he shares camp responsibilities and lives peacefully with others. Campers live in the fresh air 24 hours a day and engage in activities that are conducive to both mental and physical health. In the camp situation they are free from the tensions caused by irritating noises, bright lights, and crowded conditions of urban life. They develop an appreciation of nature. They experience adventure. They learn skills.

The program in most camps consists of such sports activities as swimming, boating, fishing, horseback riding, tennis, badminton, hiking, horseshoes, basketball, and softball; such social activities as campfires, frankfurter and marshmallow roasts, dancing, mixers, and cookouts; and opportunities to develop skills and an appreciation in arts and crafts, photography, Indian lore, drama, music, and nature study.

Any individual trained in physical education may play a major part in the organization and administration of any school camp. Through his training in education, through his specialized skills that make up a great part of the program of any camp, and through his experiences in working with others in a camp situation, he is in a most important position to play a major role in this trend back to nature.

Outdoor education is not the same as camping, although it may and frequently does take place in a camp setting. Outdoor education refers to the use of nature's classroom as a learning situation. This does not necessarily have to be a camp setting. It can take place on a hike, an overnight trip, a visit to the museum or zoo, or anywhere that the wonders of the out-of-doors are utilized. In this setting it is possible to do such things as discover how plants grow, study the stars, use a map and compass, discover the meaning of "contour," collect native craft materials, build outdoor shelters, experience the beauty of nature, engage in conservation projects, plant trees, care for animals and pets, and learn safe use of simple hand tools. Science, art, social studies, and other student groups will find many materials that they can study and experiences that will broaden their knowledge.

COACHING

One of the most popular services that physical educators perform is that of coaching. A great many students who show exceptional skill in some interscholastic sport such as basketball, baseball, or football feel that they would like to become members of the physical education profession so that they may coach. They feel that since they have proved themselves athletes in high school they will be successful in coaching. This, however, is not necessarily true. It may seem paradoxical to the layman, but there is insufficient evidence to show that exceptional skill in any activity necessarily guarantees that one can be a good teacher of that activity. Many other factors such as personality, interest in youth, psychology of learning, intelligence, integrity, leadership, character, and a sympathetic attitude carry as much or more weight in coaching success.

Coaching should be recognized as teaching. Because of the nature of his position, a coach may be in a more favorable position to teach concepts that make for effective daily living than any other member of a school faculty, YMCA staff, or community center staff. Youth, with an inherent drive for activity, action, and quest of excitement and competition found in sports, look up to the coach and in many cases feel that he is the type of individual to be emulated. Therefore, the prospective coach should recognize the influence he has over youth and see the value of such attributes as character, personality, and integrity. Although a coach must know thoroughly the game he is coaching, these other characteristics are of equal importance. The coach of an athletic team has within him the power to build future citizens with traits that are desirable and acceptable to society or citizens who have a false concept as to what is right and proper. Incidents that occur at many sports events throughout the country show that some of the leadership provided in athletics today is working to the detriment of acceptable character and moral outcomes. The coach is often tempted—because of the insecurity of his position, the emphasis on winning teams, student and alumni pressure, the desire for lucrative gate receipts, and the publicity that goes with winning teams— to seek outcomes not educational in nature. Unless the coach is an individual of strong character and is willing to follow an unswerving course in the direction of what he knows to be right, many evils will enter the picture. As a result the outcomes derived from competition in athletic events will inhibit rather than contribute to the building of good citizenship in youth.

The question is often raised as to whether it is necessary for a coach to have skill in the activity he coaches. There are many coaches today who sat on the bench for 4 years during their college football, basketball, baseball, tennis, or swimming days. There are many who excelled in the particular sport they are now coaching. There are others who never competed in the activity. Although exceptional skill in an activity is definitely desirable, it would be a fallacy to say that it should be a requirement for coaching. Through study and as a result of interest in an activity, many individuals have developed themselves to a point where they have been able to do a superior job in this area.

Any student of physical education planning to enter the coaching profession should recognize the uncertainty of tenure associated with this work. Pressure from alumni, sports writers, students, and the public can cause him to lose his job when the number of games in the "won" column does not meet with their approval. Many coaches have done commendable work and yet have been forced to leave their jobs because the material with which they had to work was not of championship caliber. Hughes and Williams have pointed out some significant facts in respect to this malady associated with coaching:

> Whereas no Professor of English is judged by the number of Miltons, Stevensons, Shakespeares or Howells he graduates from his courses, the coach is judged by his team's scores. Regardless of whether or not his team plays well, knows the game, conducts itself as gentlemen, is alert, reliable, and resourceful, the measure of winning still remains the sole criterion of success.*

Coaching on the secondary school level can sometimes prove just as insecure as on the college level—much depends upon the school, community, and the school administration. Coaching offers an interesting and profitable career to many individuals. However, a coach should recognize the possibility of becoming located in a school where the pressure may be so great as to cause unhappiness, insecurity, and even the loss of a job.

---

*Hughes, William Leonard, and Williams, Jesse Feiring: Sports, their organization and administration, New York, 1944, A. S. Barnes & Co., p. 76.

It should be understood very clearly that coaching is only one phase of the physical education profession and that coaching is teaching. Because of this close relationship with physical education and the education field in general, it should be recognized that a prospective coach should be qualified in certain phases of physical education. He should have a background in physical and biological science, skills, social sciences, education, humanities, and certain physical education subject matter. Only in this way will it be possible for the coach to best serve the youth of this country.

A recent development in respect to coaching and directing athletics is the National Council of Secondary School Athletic Directors (NCSSAD), which was formed by the American Association for Health, Physical Education, and Recreation to render services to those personnel involved in athletic programs in the schools. Members of the first Executive Committee of the NCSSAD were elected in January, 1969, when a national conference was held. Membership in this organization is open to members of the AAHPER who have responsibilities for directing, administering, or coordinating athletic programs in secondary schools.

Another movement is the increase in college professional preparation to provide specialized programs for coaching. These programs are appearing in many parts of the country and include such courses as problems related to sports psychology, health aspects of athletics, athletic administration, the sociology of sports, and philosophy of athletics as part of the physical education program.

The increased professional interest in preparing coaches for their responsibilities is also leading to the certification of coaches in several states in order to ensure they have at least the minimum necessary preparation for conducting athletics in our schools.

COUNSELING

The teacher of physical education plays a unique role in the life of each student with whom he comes in contact. One of the greatest services that can be rendered is that of counseling boys and girls concerning matters that affect their physical selves and the development of their personalities. Boys and girls are concerned with their body image, how to build physical fitness, the way to gain strength, how to become skilled in their favorite physical activities, suggestions for developing poise, how to maintain weight control, finding the path to a beautiful body, and a host of other desires and interests. They want to sit down and discuss face to face some of the physical changes that are taking place in their bodies, what they mean, and what they should do about them. Young people desire accurate and objective information in regard to the role of sex in their lives. They want to know what it means if they smoke, drink, or use drugs. They want to have information on why they are required to attend physical education class, learn skills, and know certain physiological facts.

In order to be an effective counselor, the physical education teacher must have a sincere desire to help young people. He must recognize that this is an important service to render if he is to be worthy of membership in his specialty. He must want to render this service and be prepared to render it most effectively. Furthermore, he needs to provide the time in his schedule when students and other persons will have the opportunity to utilize this service.

In order to be an effective counselor, the physical education teacher must be acquainted with how boys and girls grow and develop, their developmental tasks, and the problems they experience. He must be able to clarify their problems, give encouragement, offer friendship, and provide a feeling of belonging.

The effective counselor will get as much information as possible about the person needing advice. In so doing, he will talk with parents, use school records, and know other sources of help when referral becomes necessary. He will work closely in a school situation with the guidance officer and the personnel in this area.

The physical educator can render a valuable counseling service to all persons who are interested in and have problems that relate to his specialty. This service can go beyond the students in the school, to men and women in the community who want accurate information that will help them solve some of their physical problems.

Cassidy,* in discussing counseling in physical education, points out that teachers should function in six areas: (1) set climate, (2) locate needs, (3) provide goal-centered instruction, (4) change the situation by changing relationships, (5) make referrals to other school or community personnel, and (6) keep records. Cassidy graphically presents this guidance process in the diagram on p. 42.

ADMINISTRATION

A valuable service is rendered by those physical educators who administer programs in schools, colleges, governmental agencies, and other agencies, wherever they exist. Such work requires special qualifications if one is to perform the service well. Such qualifications would include a knowledge of the theory of administration, integrity, administrative mind, ability to instill good human relations, ability to make decisions, health and fitness for the job, willingness to accept responsibility, understanding of work, command of administrative technique, and intellectual capacity.

It is being recognized increasingly that administration is not a matter of hit or miss, trial and error, or expediency. Instead, a theory of administration is emerging. It is further recognized that from a study of this administrative theory one will gain insights into how to administer and how human beings work most effectively. Administrative theory will also help in the identification of problems that need to be solved if an effective working organization is to exist. Although some educators oppose

the idea that a framework of theory can be established, it seems assured that administration is rapidly becoming a science and is thereby characterized by more objectivity, reliability, and a systematic structure of substance. Such theory is explaining what administration is and is providing guides to administrative action.

Those students who aspire to administrative positions in physical education, in addition to mastering the theory of administration, should also recognize that one of the most important services they render is to human beings. Although some functions and areas can be somewhat mechanical—such as office management, budget making and financial accounting, purchase and care of supplies and equipment, legal liability, insurance management, curriculum planning, public relations, teacher and program evaluation, and facility management—relations with staff, colleagues, and the public in general can never become mechanical and routine. The administrator must always be sympathetic and understanding, friendly and considerate, honest and fair. In other words, he must be an expert in the area of human relations.

One further point should be mentioned. There is a trend for both men and women to be hired as administrators. In the past, when an administrative opportunity opened, the man was always the first to be considered. Although the odds in most situations are still in favor of the man, they have been reduced considerably. Sex is no longer the important factor it was years ago in the selection of an administrator. Many outstanding women administrators have proved they are competent to perform such a service.

Several types of administrative positions exist for the physical educator who desires to render this type of service.

Most schools and colleges have physical education, including athletic programs. In addition, many youth-serving and other types of agencies also have these programs for their members. As a result, physical educators are frequently hired to administer

*Cassidy, Rosalind: Counseling in the physical education program, New York, 1959, Appleton-Century-Crofts, pp. 5-6.

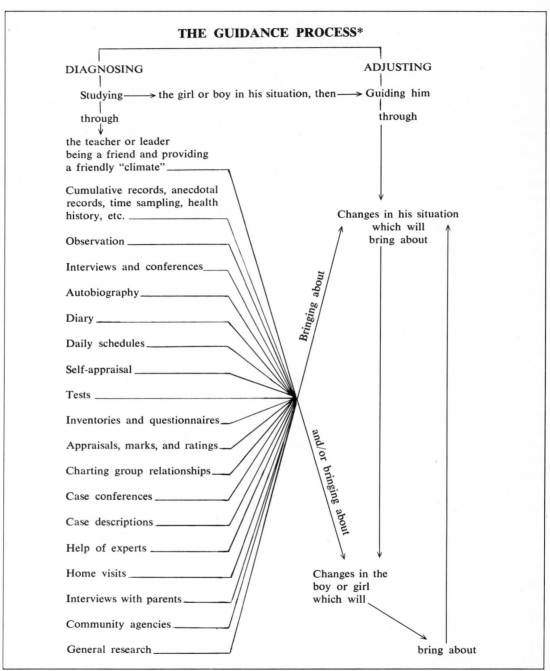

THE GUIDANCE PROCESS*

DIAGNOSING   ADJUSTING

Studying⟶ the girl or boy in his situation, then⟶ Guiding him

through   through

the teacher or leader
being a friend and providing
a friendly "climate"

Cumulative records, anecdotal
records, time sampling, health
history, etc.

Changes in his situation
which will
bring about

Observation

Interviews and conferences

Autobiography

Diary

Daily schedules

Self-appraisal

Tests

Inventories and questionnaires

Appraisals, marks, and ratings

Charting group relationships

Case conferences

Case descriptions

Help of experts

Home visits

Interviews with parents

Community agencies

General research

Bringing about

and/or bringing about

Changes in the
boy or girl
which will

bring about

*From Cassidy, Rosalind, and Kozman, Hilda: Counseling girls on a changing society, New York, 1947, McGraw-Hill Book Co.

these specialized offerings. In some cases one person is designated to administer the physical education instructional program, the intramural and extramural, the adapted and the interscholastic or intercollegiate athletic program. In other situations these programs are separated, with personnel in charge of administering each of the programs. In some states, a director's certificate is issued after specialized training has been pursued. It certifies those persons who are qualified to direct programs in these specialized areas.

In addition to interscholastic, intercollegiate, and intramural athletics and other programs, clubs, such as boosters' clubs, cheer-leading clubs, varsity clubs, and physical fitness clubs, sometimes need special administrative services for which the physical educator qualifies. In the administration of such programs, duties must be performed that relate to fiscal management, public relations, personnel management, facility management, insurance management, curriculum planning, and other responsibilities that go with such a position.

To render the administrative service effectively requires good human relations, personal qualities that relate to the group that composes the organization one is administering, a reasonable degree of intelligence, initiative, persistence, creativity, and an understanding of the job that needs to be done.

CONDUCTING SAFETY AND DRIVER EDUCATION PROGRAMS

Closely allied with health is the program of safety and driver education. This important field of work gained divisional status in the American Association for Health, Physical Education, and Recreation on March 31, 1959. It is concerned with promoting active and effective programs in all forms of safety and driver education including recreational safety, home and community safety, driver and traffic safety, safety in physical education and athletics, and safety throughout the school environment. Schools are being urged to hire qualified personnel to conduct and supervise the safety and driver education program. Where such programs have been initiated, the safety record has been considerably improved.

Many physical educators are being assigned duties and responsibilities in safety and driver-education programs. It is recommended that those physical educators who desire to participate in such programs should qualify themselves accordingly.

For persons trained in safety education, opportunities are available in the schools as supervisors of safety education and as teachers of driver education, in industry and government as safety supervisors and safety directors, in communities as supervisors and consultants in community safety and as safety education officers, and in colleges and universities as teachers of safety and driver education and directors of college campus safety activities.

Qualifications for safety positions include being able to work with people, having a knowledge of the field of safety, demonstrating effectiveness in group dynamics, possessing intellectual curiosity, and possessing desirable safety skills and attitudes.

CONDUCTING RESEARCH

The purpose of research in any field is to push back the frontiers of knowledge. Physical education has lagged behind other fields in both its production and its use of research. Physical education has tended to rely heavily on research done in related fields. This may be one of the reasons why physical education is not considered an academic subject with academic status.

The major physical education research publication, *Research Quarterly,* has made a concerted effort in recent years to improve and stimulate the quality of research. Considerable physical education research is being done by graduate students who publish their theses and dissertations in *Research Quarterly.*

Recently, funds for research in physical education have been made available by the United States Office of Education, the National Institutes of Health, and the Department of Defense. Many leading colleges and universities have built, or are building, research laboratories. Most graduate programs on the master's and doctoral level require the completion of a course in research design and also a research project, but some schools do not require the writing of a scholarly paper for advanced degrees.

The tools of research in physical education include both the tried and tested and the newer, more sophisticated devices. Dynamometers, ergometers, treadmills, tensiometers, goniometers, fleximeters, silhouettographs, reaction timers, and the techniques of slow- and stop-motion cameras, special projection devices, and other means are used to measure the range of the body's abilities and reactions. Various attitude and personality tests are frequently correlated with the results of physical tests. The results of these tests are converted to statistics, charts, and tables. A recent criticism of research in physical education was that it depended too heavily on statistical analysis and disguised the true meaning and the possible applications of the results.

Considerable physical education research has been in the area of physical fitness, although the mechanics of movement in various sports skills have also been intensively scrutinized. In spite of the recent advances, much research remains to be done in the areas of motor learning, movement education, skill testing, physical fitness and physical ability, teaching methods, and curriculum.

Any occupation that desires to achieve the status of a profession must continually be pioneering, on the cutting edge of new developments, uncovering new knowledge, supporting hypotheses that have been formulated, and determining new truths pertinent to its field. Therefore, physical educators recognize the importance of conducting research in order to achieve this status and accomplish these objectives. Some of the research that has been conducted by physical educators in the past has not been significant and has not been conducted according to sound scientific procedures. However, with the renewed emphasis upon

this service, the increased recognition of its significance and value in advancing physical education, and the various services that physical educators perform, more scholarly research is gradually being accomplished.

Physical educators who desire to render a service in the field of research should become well grounded in such areas as the sciences, research methodology, quantitative methods of treating data, understanding of laboratory testing, and organization and conduct of research studies. These competencies take considerable time to develop and usually require many years of graduate work, including pursuing programs leading to masters' and doctoral degrees. For those persons who have the interest and develop the competencies, however, there are many opportunities for rendering a valuable professional service. Approximately thirty colleges and universities engaged in physical education work now have research laboratories where research experimentation is carried on. There are job opportunities open to the qualified physical educator for conducting research on a full-time basis, carrying on research in addition to his teaching responsibilities, and serving as a laboratory and research assistant. In addition, there are research opportunities available in voluntary agencies, industry, and other settings.

There is a trend today toward interdisciplinary research, with a team approach being utilized. In such cases, the physical educator–researcher and a psychologist or sociologist, for example, work together, combining their knowledge and skills on problems that cut across both their fields of endeavor.

Most of the research being conducted today in physical education appears to be in the area of exercise physiology. However, there is an increasing number of studies being devoted to the relation of physical activity to psychological and sociological development of human beings.

Although research is stressed in most graduate programs, the undergraduate should become familiar with the research experience. This can be accomplished by becoming familiar with the various sources of research findings, achieving competence in the ability to interpret findings of studies, developing skill in the formulation of a research study, and actually working on a research project. In our more sophisticated professional preparation institutions, the research process is integrated into many courses. Students from the very beginning of their professional preparation think in terms of what facts concerning and what claims for physical education can be supported. These students thus begin to understand the true worth of physical education and its scientific basis for being included in educational offerings. These students become valuable members of their field of endeavor and bring prestige and respect to their work.

Every physical educator should be acquainted with the Educational Research Information Center, commonly called ERIC. This is a nationwide service designed to provide the results of new educational research to teachers, administrators, researchers, and others who need it. ERIC consists of a headquarters office in Washington, D. C., and a network of clearinghouses in universities and other institutions throughout the United States. Each of the designated clearinghouses is responsible for information in a particular area of education. The staff of each clearinghouse selects and abstracts all relevant documents on the particular subject to which they have been assigned. Central ERIC then coordinates the efforts of all clearinghouses, records the research on microfilm and in pamphlet form, and makes it available to educators at a very nominal cost. Therefore, if an educator desires to have information on the disadvantaged, motor learning, personnel services, junior colleges, or reading, the researched information available on these subjects can be secured.

Ten significant lines of educational research

Ten of the most significant lines of educational research dating from 1957 were outlined by Daniel E. Griffiths* in a speech delivered to the convention of the American Association of School Administrators. These research findings are presented here in adapted form.

The first study† was concerned with an analysis of the rate of growth and the changes in certain human characteristics over a specified length of time. The characteristics studied included height, general intelligence, male aggressiveness, female dependence, male and female intellectuality, and general school achievement. The researcher developed two hypotheses: (1) environment affects the changes in human characteristics and has its strongest effect when the change is taking place most rapidly, and (2) the relevant factors in the environment are highly correlated with the changes that take place. The implications of the study for general education include the following: that primary education is extremely important and deserves more consideration in regard to highly qualified teaching personnel, smaller class size, inservice teacher training, increased budget allocations, diagnostic services for pupils, and increased use of psychologists and specialists in testing, evaluation, reading, and languages.

The second study‡ was concerned with the analysis of human intelligence. Primary intellectual abilities were classified by the use of special tests and placed into three groups. The first group, basic processes, included five factors: cognition, memory, convergent thinking, divergent thinking, and evaluation. The second group, content, included four factors: figural, symbolic,

---

*Griffiths, Daniel E.: The ten most significant educational research findings in the past ten years, Executive Action Letter **6:**10, 1967. Publication of the Croft Educational Services, New London, Conn.

†Bloom, Benjamin S.: Stability and change in human characteristics, New York, 1964, John Wiley & Sons, Inc.

‡Guilford, J. P.: Three faces of intellect, American Psychologist **14:**469, 1959.

semantic, and social. The third classification, products, included six factors: units, classes, relations, systems, transformations, and implications. The researcher concluded that one of the many implications of his study dealt directly with education. In regard to education, he said that the concept of the learner and the learning process is subject to change and that "learning is the discovery of information, not merely the formation of associations." This particular implication has influenced the new curriculums in many academic areas.

The third study* discussed the use of computer technology in studying theories of learning. The use of computers in a learning laboratory allows researchers to study and analyze more effectively the rate of learning of each individual and differences in learning rates between individuals. Computers can also help, according to the findings of this study, to reinforce correct responses immediately or correct wrong responses; facilitate the transfer of learning concepts from subject to subject; and aid in the determination of the best way to present and organize material to be learned.

The fourth study† was concerned with the effect of the environment on individual development. The results indicated that for the first- and fifth-grade students in this study, the more disadvantaged children were significantly lower generally in verbal and conceptual measures than were more advantaged youngsters. The researchers pointed out that the disadvantaged tend to decrease in intellectual performance unless they are exposed to specialized programs.

The fifth study‡ also dealt with individual development and is based largely on the theory and work of the Swiss psychologist Jean Piaget. This study pointed out that the individual develops by sequential stages, but the appearance of each developmental stage varies with the individual and among individuals. Nervous maturation, experience, social transmission, and autoregulation help to control individual development. This study implied that the individual must determine his own readiness to learn and is best suited to guide his own learning.

The sixth study* was concerned with the characteristics of administrators and their styles of administering. The activities and styles of 232 elementary school principals were scored and analyzed in a simulated school created for this study. Eight different administrative methods and personalities were identified and their relationship shown to basic mental ability, basic personality factors, interests, job performance values, group instruction, superior's ratings, teacher ratings, professional and general knowledge, and biographical data.

The seventh study† discussed Project Talent, which was developed to investigate interests, career plans, and the relationship of high school courses to the life objectives of approximately 440,000 students in public and private high schools. Their responses to a battery of tests were analyzed, along with other data. Follow-up studies will be conducted on these same students at intervals of 1, 5, 10, and 20 years after they complete high school. The hoped-for outcomes include a comprehensive youth-talent inventory, improved standards of measurement and evaluation, an understanding of career choice, and evaluation of the relationship of education to career.

*Suppes, Patrick: Modern learning theory and the elementary school curriculum, American Educational Research Journal 1:2, 1964.

†Annual Report 1965, Institute for Developmental Studies, School of Education, New York University.

‡Ripple, Richard E., and Rockcastle, Verne N., editors: Piaget rediscovered, New York, 1964, School of Education, Cornell University.

*Hemphill, John, Griffiths, Daniel E., and Frederiksen, Norman: Administrative performance and personality, New York, 1962, Teachers College Press.

†Flanagan, John C.: Maximizing human talents, The Journal of Teacher Education 13:209, 1962; Flanagan, John C., and others: The identification, development, and utilization of human talents: the American high school student, Cooperative Research Project No. 635, 1964, University of Pittsburgh.

The eighth line of research* was devoted to the results of curriculum revision projects, such as the "new math," and their influence on modern learning concepts, the structuring of knowledge, and emphasis on laboratory methods in the teaching of sciences.

The ninth line of research† discussed the Conant reports on various phases of American education and pointed out the significance of Conant's recommendations for education.

The final line of research‡ discussed the biological bases for memory and learning and the role of deoxyribonucleic acid and ribonucleic acid in such processes.

The study discussed by Griffiths indicated that while no positive conclusions can be drawn from the research to date, important findings would probably be evidenced within the succeeding 10-year period.

WORLD SERVICE

The shrinking world and the space age have brought about a vast interchange of specialists in all forms of endeavor. Physical educators, because of their special services, have been able to render a valuable service in many parts of the world. Operation Crossroads, the Peace Corps, the American Specialist Program, and other programs carried on by the U. S. State Department and others have resulted in physical educators rendering services in such countries as Japan, Taiwan, Nepal, Nigeria, Pakistan, Peru, Senegal, Thailand, Turkey, Venezuela, Korea, the Philippines, and many other nations. These specialists have taught basketball, football, dodgeball, dance, and other sport and activity skills; coached athletic teams; organized recreation programs; lectured to civic groups and college students; attended and participated in conferences; and performed other outstanding services wherever they have gone.

Sports and physical education activities have great appeal for people in all countries. Since the United States has succeeded in many types of international sports competitions and developed physical education programs in its schools and colleges that have achieved prominence in world circles, the physical education specialist has been in increasing demand by other governments and professional groups as a consultant, organizer, and teacher.

During an age when international strife is prevalent in many parts of the globe, when peace is a constant goal of humanity, when better understanding among the peoples of the world is a desperate need, when international education is an urgent necessity, and when emerging nations need assistance, physical educators can render a valuable service in utilizing their skills to help those in need. This service can be rendered here at home as well as abroad.

CHANGING HUMAN BEHAVIOR

Physical educators render their greatest service to mankind when they change behavior for the better. The worth of physical education depends upon rendering this social service effectively. Through excellent programs of physical education man's behavior can be changed so that he lives a daily regimen that contributes to his biological, mental-emotional, and social development.

Changing human behavior in regard to biological development

During the last decade there has been much emphasis upon physical fitness. Ever since tests revealed that American children and youth were physically inept compared to the young people in other countries, there has been much concern in school, college, agency, and community programs to upgrade

---

*Ripple, Richard E., and Rockcastle, Verne N., editors: Piaget rediscovered, New York, 1964, School of Education, Cornell University.

†Conant, James Bryant: The American high school today, New York, 1959, McGraw-Hill Book Co.; Education in the junior high school years, Princeton, 1959, Educational Testing Service; Slums and suburbs, New York, 1961, McGraw-Hill Book Co.; The education of American teachers, New York, 1963, McGraw-Hill Book Co.

‡Gaito, John: DNA and RNA as memory molecules, Psychological Review **70:**471, 1963.

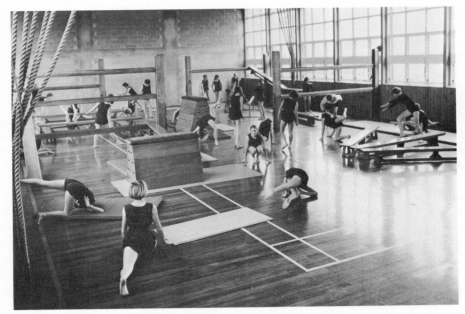

Secondary school girls in New Zealand working at educational gymnastics lession using equipment.

the physical fitness of the American population.

Physical educators recognize the necessity of developing physical fitness in human beings and organize their programs to accomplish this objective and to render this service to their constituency (see also Chapters 15 and 16).

The building of physical fitness involves many essentials other than physical activity; these include nutrition, rest, sleep, relaxation, and proper medical care. However, research has indicated that physical exercise is an important ingredient. Therefore, physical educators can render a valuable service by organizing programs that include opportunities for individuals to engage in physical activity and also to learn something about the scientific foundations underlying the development and maintenance of physical fitness. Such programs should motivate students to apply during their school years, and also throughout life, not only the physical skills they have learned but also the knowledge and understanding that have provided insights into the importance of being physically fit.

Changing human behavior in regard to mental-emotional development

Physical education cannot be content merely with building such qualities · as strength, endurance, and agility. It must also be concerned with providing scientific knowledge in regard to the contribution that physical activity can make to human development and with shaping desirable attitudes toward the need for physical activity and physical education programs in our schools and colleges. It must help educators, parents, and the public in general to understand the contribution that physical education can make to special classes of students who need perceptual-motor development and who have atypical conditions that can be helped by proper motor development. It must be concerned with providing a laboratory in which emotions can be properly channeled in constructive physical activity. Physical education does not only contribute to physical development but to mental-emotional development as well. This is a valuable service when physical educators have the knowledge and skill and render it effectively.

Physical education must also recognize

that body image has a direct relation to self-concept. The mental image a person has of his physical self is important in how he feels about himself. Perception of self, body image, and physical self-image are all important sources of knowledge that lead to full self-actualization. (For further discussion of this service see Chapter 17.)

Changing human behavior in regard to social development

Physical education has the potential for changing the social aspects of human behavior. Motor skill development contributes to peer group approval. It results in recognition, status, and achievement. In addition, human values develop in games and in the game situation. The rules of the game are the rules of the democratic way of life. This is democracy in action. Valuable social qualities such as respect for the other fellow, courage, and fair play are developed in game and sport situations. (For further discussion of this service, see Chapter 18.)

WORKING WITH HANDICAPPED AND EXCEPTIONAL PERSONS

A valuable service that can be rendered by physical educators is the individualization of the program to fit the needs of each person. Blanket programs of physical education are not suitable. There are many students who have some atypical physical condition, and physical educators should try to alleviate or eliminate these conditions. Physical educators sometimes do a fine job helping the healthy and gifted student to become healthier and more skilled but do a poor job in helping the unhealthy or handicapped person to develop to his optimum capacity. A valuable service can and should be performed by physical educators in the adapted physical education program. Physical education programs that help the handicapped person are frequently referred to by such terms as *corrective physical education, individual physical education, posture training, developmental physical education, reconstructive physical education, physical education for the atypical child,* and *body building.*

Since there is considerable emphasis today on educating the handicapped individual, this subject is treated at length in this chapter.

Defining the handicapped and exceptional student

The handicapped or exceptional student is so classified because of many factors. These may be physical, mental, emotional, or social in nature. Included under the heading of physical deviations are those of postural nature, heart malfunction, nutritional deficiencies, locomotive problems, speech impediments, and vision and hearing defects. Also, there is the problem of the physically gifted and the creative student.

Emotional deviations include many maladjustments, such as aggressiveness, antisocial behavior, withdrawal, or depression. These maladjustments will not be helped by programs that are not adapted to the physical and mental abilities of the child and that fail to ensure his satisfactory emotional and social development.

The mentally handicapped or exceptional student may be either gifted, possibly to the point of genius, or retarded. Socially handicapped or exceptional students include those who have specific deviations in their human relations, who are culturally disadvantaged, or who exhibit disruptive behavior.

The services rendered by physical educators in teaching the handicapped or exceptional student will be discussed in the following sections.

Mentally retarded students

Mentally retarded children need physical education, and a valuable service can be rendered by providing programs for these students. Yet in many schools throughout the United States, there is no provision made for meeting this need. It has been estimated that there are now about 7 million mentally retarded children and adults in the United States. Approximately 126,000 mentally retarded babies are born in this country each year.

Mental retardation is a major problem and

one to which the field of physical education needs to give more attention. There has been little research conducted in the area of mental retardation by physical educators. Although federal funds have been made available for research concerned with mentally retarded persons, only small amounts have been requested by physical educators. At present, there are only a few professional preparation programs in physical education that train teachers of the mentally retarded, although there is a great need for physical educators trained in this area.

The Joseph P. Kennedy Jr. Foundation is an organization concerned with all phases of research on, and education for, the mentally retarded. In 1964, the Kennedy Foundation was the only group providing summer camp experiences and recreation programs for the mentally retarded. In 1966, the Kennedy Foundation sponsored a series of regional seminars for physical educators to acquaint them with the physical education needs of the retarded.

The mentally retarded boys and girls that attend public schools benefit from a program of physical activity carefully tailored to their needs. These children show a wide range of intellectual ability and, in general, are below average in physical performance and capacity. While some mentally retarded boys and girls are sufficiently skilled to participate in a regular program of physical education, the vast majority are physically 2 to 4 years behind normal youngsters of the same age. The mentally retarded are not as physically strong, lack endurance, and tend to be overweight. While their physical development is slower, they seem to mature physically at an earlier age than do most boys and girls. In general, the retarded have poor motor coordination, lack physical and organic fitness, and have poor posture. Some mentally retarded children have physical handicaps, and some also have personality disturbances.

Recent research reports published in England and the United States have drawn similar conclusions concerning the effect of a well-balanced program of physical education. The researchers have pointed out that while normal boys and girls attain high scores on physical performance tests, the mentally retarded received scores almost as high following exposure to a physical education program designed to meet their specific needs. One of the measures that researchers

Teaching the handicapped represents a valuable service. A Central Washington State College student helps a special education handicapped student get used to the water. Swimming is an important part of the physical education program for the handicapped.

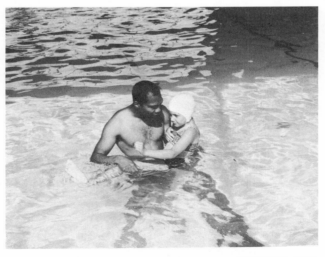

BROADFRONT PROGRAM, ELLENSBURG PUBLIC SCHOOLS, ELLENSBURG, WASH.

have used most consistently has been the AAHPER Youth Fitness Test. Other researchers have said that the difference in motor performance between the mentally retarded and the normal is based on the differences in mental ability rather than on any significant difference in natural motor ability.

Still other researchers have pointed out that the mentally retarded have been denied planned programs in physical education. Often, they are placed in regular physical education classes without regard to their unique needs. Surveys have indicated that most of the mentally retarded spend their leisure time in sedentary pursuits, have little interest in hobbies, and have not been encouraged to be active. Also, they are given little opportunity to participate in organized, leisure-time physical education or recreation programs. Because they have not had a strong background of play experience, the mentally retarded must be taught how to play.

The physical education teacher who is responsible for teaching a group of mentally retarded children cannot proceed as he would with a group of normal children. The mentally retarded need to be successful, they need to achieve. Thus, any goals that are set must be reachable ones. The mentally retarded often lack confidence and pride. They need a patient teacher who will praise the smallest effort or improvement. Continued frustration at failure to reach a skill level that is too high and lack of recognition often lead to aggressive or asocial behavior. The mentally retarded make slow progress in skill development and have great difficulty in abstract thinking. Their program of physical education must be a varied and interesting one. Skills must be taught by demonstration. Because the attention span of a mentally retarded child is short and because he tires easily, the program must be designed to maintain his interest and involve him personally.

Those who have extensively taught the mentally retarded find that they enjoy swimming, tumbling, rhythmics, climbing over obstacles, lead-up games, and trampolining. They point out that the concept of team play is too abstract and that the retarded at times have difficulty in following directions. Thus, lead-up games present the needed challenge and competition and prevent the frustration encountered in the more highly organized team sports. Movement education seems almost ideally suited to programs for the mentally retarded.

Physical education is essential to the mental and physical development of the retarded. A well-planned program will help these youngsters to develop the fitness and endurance they need. Physical education adds to their physical and mental well-being and gives them an opportunity to experience success and achievement.

Culturally disadvantaged students

The culturally disadvantaged are of many races and colors. Physical educators can render a valuable service by organizing programs adapted to their needs and interests. The culturally disadvantaged live in the slums of the large cities or in rural poverty pockets in all areas of the country. Their numbers are constantly on the increase, particularly in the large cities. Estimates made by the Ford Foundation classify 50% of the children who live in large cities as culturally disadvantaged.

The culturally disadvantaged child does not resemble his middle- or upper-class peers in home and neighborhood environment, economic level, scholastic achievement, motivation, or aspiration level. These differences set the culturally disadvantaged child apart and are, in fact, the causes of his deprivation and resulting scholastic and personal adjustment problems.

The culturally disadvantaged child often reflects the negative influences of his home and neighborhood environment in a school situation. The cultural standards of these environments are frequently inconsistent. Because the home is often neither a place where conversation is stimulated nor reading encouraged, the child enters school ill-equipped to communicate easily or to adapt

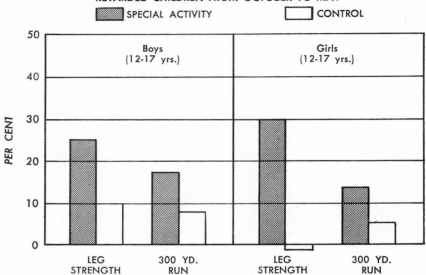

AVERAGE PER CENT IMPROVEMENT IN THE STRENGTH AND ENDURANCE OF RETARDED CHILDREN FROM OCTOBER TO MAY*

*These are examples of measured improvements produced by an intensive organic fitness program. The special activity consisted of running activities engaged in twice weekly.

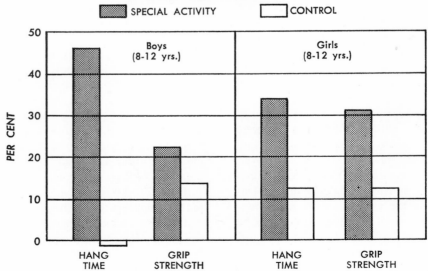

AVERAGE PER CENT IMPROVEMENT IN THE MUSCULAR FITNESS OF RETARDED CHILDREN FROM OCTOBER TO MAY*

*These are examples of measured improvements produced by intensive muscular activity involving the arms and shoulders. The special activity consisted of medicine ball games, engaged in twice weekly.

FROM HAYDEN, FRANK J.: PHYSICAL FITNESS FOR THE MENTALLY RETARDED, LONDON, ONTARIO, CANADA, 1964. COPYRIGHT BY FRANK HAYDEN.

to the learning environment as readily as does the more advantaged child. Furthermore, the disadvantaged family is frequently a transient one, moving from city to city in search of better-paying jobs or other advantages. The culturally disadvantaged child thus moves from school to school, making adjustment more difficult with each change.

The culturally disadvantaged often resent the school, the teachers, and its administrators because each represents the unattainable middle-class image of society at large. Education is viewed as valuable, but the values are quite different in context from those sought or defined by the advantaged segment of society.

The culturally disadvantaged child does not feel that he is a part of the society in which he lives. In a classroom situation, he is unable to compete. He is unstable emotionally, and his excitability and restlessness contribute to a short attention span. He cannot think in the abstract, form concepts, use logic, or communicate well verbally. Thus, he falls behind grade level in achievement and attains low scores on intelligence and standardized tests. These failures contribute to a lack of motivation, a low level of aspiration, and lack of ambition. The final result of years of failure is a negative self-image expressed by hostile, aggressive, and nonconforming behavior.

Education must be adapted to the specific needs of the culturally disadvantaged child. What motivation he does possess, what creativity he has, what abilities he shows must be fostered and encouraged rather than suppressed. Understanding teachers and a classroom climate geared to the specific needs of this child are of the utmost importance. This child needs an opportunity to change his negative image of himself to a positive one. A chance to succeed on his own level, rather than on imposed levels, will aid not

The mean percentile scores on the AAHPER Youth Fitness Test of 270 educable mentally retarded boys and girls, ages 10 to 17, in the St. Louis County (Missouri) Special School District for the Education and Training of Handicapped Children.

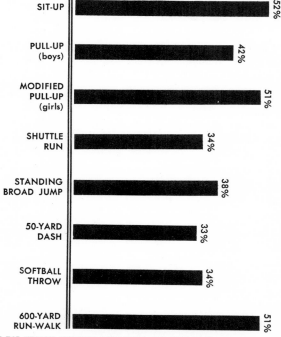

SIT-UP	52%
PULL-UP (boys)	42%
MODIFIED PULL-UP (girls)	51%
SHUTTLE RUN	34%
STANDING BROAD JUMP	38%
50-YARD DASH	33%
SOFTBALL THROW	34%
600-YARD RUN-WALK	51%

only in building a more positive image but also in increasing his self-respect, his poise, and his confidence.

Physical education can contribute to the culturally disadvantaged in a very positive manner. Often, the disadvantaged child has no recreational facility available to him. He must use streets or littered lots, and his games and sports are unsupervised. Within the environment of the school, the disadvantaged child can be given a worthwhile physical education experience geared to him. A small class size will allow the instructor to give each student the attention, help, encouragement, and praise he needs. Within a relaxed, low-pressure, and informal environment, discipline will be easier to learn and maintain. Skill learnings will accrue more readily. Careful progressions in the skills that are offered will increase the opportunities to achieve success and give a measure of personal satisfaction. The instructor must strive to develop rapport with these students, and he must be able to understand and respect them. He must provide the experiences and learnings that they need to cope with their immediate and future recreational pursuits.

The physical education program for the culturally disadvantaged must be designed to allow for the release of tension, to foster creativity, to answer the need to exert leadership, to instill knowledge of hygiene, to allow for social interaction, to provide competition of a worthwhile nature, and to give a background of lifetime sports. Above all, the physical education program must be an *activity* program that stresses and values the individual.

Team, dual, and individual sports all have their place in a physical education program for the culturally disadvantaged. On the elementary school level, movement education and its jumping, running, throwing, and other activities natural to childhood will help encourage creativity and the ability to abstract and will provide the child with needed self-expression and activity. For the older child, such activities as bowling, skating, swimming, archery, rhythmics, and self-

testing activities not only provide constant activity but also offer a broad exposure to those skills from which the individual can gain confidence as he achieves higher skill levels. Team sports provide an invaluable opportunity to compete, to let off steam in an acceptable manner, and to learn the give-and-take that these sports help to teach. After school hours, the physical education program can do invaluable service to the culturally disadvantaged by organizing intramurals and providing supervision for leagues in various sports.

Physically handicapped students

Physical handicaps may stem from congenital or hereditary causes or may develop later in life from environmental factors such as malnutrition or from disease or accident. Sometimes negative psychological and social traits develop because of the limitations imposed on the individual by a severe physical handicap.

The physically handicapped student may have a temporary disability, such as a broken arm, or he may be in a postoperative stage of recovery. Other physically handicapped students suffer from more permanent disabilities such as blindness, deafness, or irremediable orthopedic conditions. The range of physical handicaps extends from minor to major in severity and directly affects the kinds and amounts of participation in physical activity.

There are about 3 million children and youth between the ages of 4 and 19 years in the United States who are physically handicapped in varying degrees, according to estimates made by the Bureau of Census through its ongoing National Health Survey. Many of the more severely handicapped school children attend special schools where their unique needs can be met by highly trained staff members. The remainder are enrolled in the public schools. It is this latter group with which the physical educator must be especially concerned.

Whatever the disability, a physical education program should be provided. Some handicapped students will be able to participate in a regular program of physical education with certain minor modifications. A separate, adapted program should be provided for those students who cannot participate in the basic instructional program of the school. The physically handicapped stu-

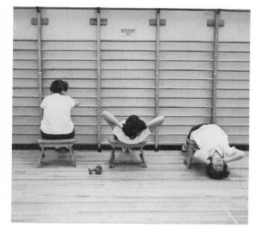

NATHAN HALE HIGH SCHOOL,
SEATTLE PUBLIC SCHOOLS, SEATTLE, WASH.

dent cannot be permitted to sit on the sidelines and become only a spectator. He needs to have the opportunity to develop and maintain adequate skill abilities and fitness levels.

The blind or deaf student or the student with a severe speech impairment has different problems from the orthopedically handicapped student. The student who is partially sighted, blind, or deaf or who has a speech impairment cannot communicate with great facility. The orthopedically handicapped student is limited in the physical education class but not necessarily in the academic classroom. The student with vision, hearing, or speech problems may be limited in both the physical education classroom and the academic classroom.

There is a lack of physical educators specifically trained to teach the physically handicapped. School systems find that the cost of providing special classes taught by specially trained physical educators is prohibitive. Where there are no special classes,

A class in body mechanics.

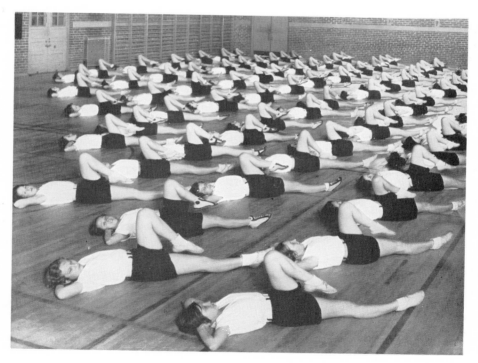

LOS ANGELES PUBLIC SCHOOLS, LOS ANGELES, CALIF.

the physical educator must provide, within the regular instructional program, those activities which will meet the needs of the handicapped student. Further, placing the physically handicapped student in a regular physical education class will help to give him a feeling of belonging. This advantage is not always possible where separate, adapted classes are provided.

To be able to provide an adequate program for physically handicapped students, the physical educator needs special training. Advanced courses in anatomy, physiology, physiology of activity, and kinesiology are essential, along with special work in psychology and adapted physical education. The professional preparation curriculum should also include courses in movement education and body mechanics.

The physical educator must have an understanding of the physical disability of each handicapped student and must be aware of any psychological, social, or behavioral problems that may accompany the disability. The physical educator must know the capacities of each handicapped student so that he can provide him with an individualized program. Some handicapped students will be able to participate in almost all the activities that nonhandicapped students enjoy. Blind students, for example, have successfully engaged in team sports where they can receive aural cues from their sighted classmates. Some athletic equipment manufacturers have placed bells inside game balls, and the blind student is then able to rely on this sound as well as on the supplementary aural cues. Ropes or covered wires acting as hand guides also enable the blind student to participate in track and field events. Still other activities, such as swimming, dance, calisthenics, and tumbling, require little adaptation or none at all, except in regard to heightened safety precautions.

In general, deaf students will not be restricted in any way from participating in a full physical education program. Some deaf students experience difficulty in activities requiring precise balance, such as balance-beam walking, and may require some re-medial work in this area. The physical educator should be prepared to offer any extra help that is needed.

Other physically handicapped students will have a variety of limitations and a variety of skill abilities. Appropriate program adaptations and modifications must be made in order to meet this range of individual needs.

Poorly coordinated students

The student with low motor ability is often ignored by the physical educator. He may be unpopular with his classmates because he is poor in team sports. He may be undesirable as a partner in dual sports and therefore is paired with equally uncoordinated and awkward partners. The student with low motor ability needs special attention so that he can improve his physical skill performances, derive pleasure from success in physical activity, and gain a background in lifetime sports.

Physical education makes special arrangements for the physically handicapped, the mentally retarded, and the athlete. Too little is done for the poorly coordinated student. This is where physical educators can render a valuable service.

The poorly coordinated student exhibits a measurable lack of physical ability. Less often considered is the psychological effect of the student's physical inabilities. The poorly coordinated student who is not given special help in the school often becomes the adult who abhors any physical activity and who is reluctant to participate in adult recreational activities.

The poorly coordinated student may resist learning new activities because the challenge this presents offers little chance for success. The challenge of a new skill or activity to be learned may create such tension within the student that he becomes physically ill. In other instances this tension may result in negative behavior.

Poor coordination may be the result of several factors. The student may not be physically fit, he may have poor reflexes, or he may not have the ability to use mental imagery. For some reason, such as a lengthy childhood illness, the poorly coordinated student may not have been normally physically active. Other poorly coordinated students, for example, will enter a secondary school physical education program from an elementary school that lacked a trained physical educator, had no facilities for physical education, or had a poor program of physical education. A single factor or a combination of any of them will help to retard motor skill development.

The physical education program can frequently motivate students with specific problems to perform better in the academic classroom by offering an opportunity for success in physical activity. This process may work in reverse with the poorly coordinated student. A student's dread of his physical education class may have a detrimental effect on his ability to perform well in the classroom. Both his behavior and his academic achievement may be adversely affected.

In working with poorly coordinated students, the physical educator must exercise utmost patience. He must know why the student is poorly coordinated and be able to devise an individual program for him that will help him to move and perform more effectively. The physical educator must be sure that the student understands the need for special help and should try to motivate him to succeed. When a skill is performed with even a modicum of improvement, the effort must be praised and the achievement reinforced.

With a large class and only one instructor, there can be relatively little time spent with each individual. The buddy system, in which a poorly coordinated student is paired with a well-coordinated partner, if properly done, may enable both students to progress faster. Immediate success will not be forthcoming for the poorly coordinated student, and the physical educator must be careful not to push the student beyond his limits. An overly difficult challenge, coupled with the fatigue that results from trying too hard, may result in retarding rather than accelerating improvement. Any goal set for the poorly coordinated student must be a reachable goal.

The physical educator has a very definite responsibility to the poorly coordinated student. Poor attitudes concerning physical activity can too easily be carried over into adult life. If these negative attitudes can be reversed by the physical educator early in the student's school career, the student may find that he will be motivated to develop abilities in several of the lifetime sports.

Physically gifted or creative students

Gifted and creative students in physical education are atypical because they also need a specially tailored physical education experience. We are concerned here with the student who is exceptional because of his motor skill abilities. The physically gifted student has superior motor skill abilities in many activities and maintains a high level of physical fitness. He may be a star athlete, but in general he is simply a good all-around performer. In a game situation, he always seems to be in the right place at the right time.

The physically gifted student learns quickly and requires a minimum of individual instruction. He is usually enthusiastic about physical activity and practices his skills of his own volition. Any individual instruction he does require is in the form of coaching rather than remedial correction. The physically gifted student has a strong sense of kinesthetic awareness and understands the principles of human movement. The student may not be able to articulate these two qualities, but observation by the physical educator will reveal that the student has discovered how to exploit his body as a tool for movement.

The physically gifted student may also have special problems. He may be impatient, even to the point of causing class disturbance, during instructional periods. He already knows how to perform the skill or play the game; he does not enjoy standing and listening but instead wants action and participation. The gifted student may become bored and lose interest in physical education if the program does not constantly stimulate him.

The physically creative student also has a well-developed sense of kinesthetic awareness and knows how to use his body properly. This student is the girl who dances with ease and grace or who is highly skilled in free exercise. It is the boy who is the lithe tumbler or gymnast. These students develop their own sophisticated routines in dance, tumbling, gymnastics, apparatus, and synchronized swimming. They may or may not be extraordinarily adept in other physical education activities but are as highly teachable as are the physically gifted.

The beginning physical educator may find it especially difficult to teach a student who seems to possess many more physical abilities than he does. However, there is no student in a school who knows all there is to know about an activity. Students' knowledge is limited by what they have been taught or have learned on their own. Many experiences will still be new to them.

The physically gifted or the physically creative student may not have attempted a wide range of activities—he may have experienced only those activities offered in the school physical education program. Both the physically gifted and the physically creative student, as well as the average student, will be stimulated and challenged by the introduction of new activities. The creative student in dance may be introduced to a new kind of music, or the boy who is skilled on apparatus may enjoy adding new moves to his routines. The athlete may be a good performer, but he may need to become a better team player. He may rely on his superior skills rather than on a complete knowledge of the rules and strategies of sports and games.

The physical educator has a contribution to make to each student in the physical education program. The challenges presented by students of exceptional ability will help to keep the physical educator alert, stimulated, and enthusiastic about his teaching. Some ways in which the physically gifted and creative student may be helped in physical education include using them in the leaders' program, providing special challenges in the form of research and reading on various aspects of physical education, using them in the buddy system (working with and helping a poorly coordinated student), requesting them to design a new dance or game strategy, assigning students to coaching responsibilities, and using them to demonstrate skills during instructional periods.

Emotionally disturbed students

Emotionally disturbed students have difficulty in maintaining good relationships with their classmates and teachers. Some of their abnormal behavior patterns stem from a need and craving for attention. Sometimes the disruptive student exhibits gross patterns of aggressiveness and destructiveness. Other emotionally unstable students may be so withdrawn from the group that they refuse to participate in the activities of the class, even to the extent of refusing to report for class. In the class of physical education, the disruptive student may refuse to dress for the activity when he does report. These measures draw both student and teacher reaction, focusing the desired attention on the nonconforming student.

Emotionally disturbed students are often restless and unable to pay attention. In a physical education class they may poke and prod other students, refuse to line up with the rest of the class, or insist on bouncing a game ball while a lesson is in progress. These are also ploys to gain attention; the student behaves similarly in the academic classroom for the same reason.

Some disruptive students may have physical or mental handicaps that contribute to their behavior. Others may be concerned about what they consider to be poor personal appearance, such as extremes of height or weight or physical maturity not in keeping with their chronological age. Still other disruptive students may simply be in the process of growing up and finding it difficult to handle their adolescence.

According to a recent study more than 60% of students in a county of a large eastern state were emotionally disturbed. These students are in need of guidance and counseling. The school cannot impose discipline on the disruptive student before the causes for his behavior have been ascertained. The school has many services available to it through which it can help the emotionally disturbed student. School psychologists can test the student, and social welfare agencies can assist by working with both the student and his family. Case studies of the student and conferences with all the student's teachers can be invaluable in determining his needs. It is also important that the records of these students follow them from grade to grade and school to school. Teachers can more effectively help such students if they are aware at the beginning of the school year that a problem exists. The school health team will also have pertinent information to contribute, as will the student's guidance counselors. Conferences with the student also help to open the doors to understanding.

If the physical educator is faced with many disruptive students in a single class, he must first examine himself and his relationship to that class. The physical educator's rapport with the entire class, his relationships with individual students, his disciplinary standards, and his program will all affect student behavior to some degree.

If negative student behavior stems from some aspect of a student's personality, then the physical educator must take positive steps to resolve the problem so that teaching can take place. The physical educator must deal with each behavioral problem on an individual basis and seek help from the school personnel best equipped to give aid. The student's guidance counselor will have information that will be of help to the physical educator. A conference with the counselor may reveal methods that have proved effective with the student in the past. Further, the observations made by the physical educator will be of value to the guidance counselor's continuing study of the student.

The physical educator will find that not all emotionally disturbed students are continual and serious behavior problems. As do teachers, students have their good and bad days. The physical educator should have a private conference with the student whose behavior suddenly becomes negative and try to understand why the student has reacted in a way unusual for him. Such a conference will lead to mutual understanding and often help to allay future problems with the same student.

Much of the physical educator's task is student guidance. In individual cases of disruptive behavior, the physical educator should exhaust all his personal resources in order to alleviate the problem. Sometimes the solution may be in a deviation from normal—being more strict or more lenient with these students than with other students. More praise, lower achievement standards, and assigning them special jobs (coaching, scorekeeping, setting up equipment) whereby they obtain personal recognition may also help the disruptive student. Any case of disruptive behavior demands immediate action on the part of the physical educator to prevent minor problems from becoming major ones.

A majority of pupils enjoy physical activity and physical education. They look forward to the physical education class as one part of the school day in which they can express themselves and gain a release of tension in an atmosphere that encourages it. For this reason, the student who is emotionally disturbed is often one of the best citizens in the physical education class.

INTERPRETING THE WORTH OF PHYSICAL EDUCATION

Physical educators can and should render the service of interpreting the values that physical activity has to human welfare. When the scientific values to each individual become known by students, educators, parents, and the public in general, they will be more likely to make physical activity a regular part of their personal regimen and thereby contribute to their health and well-being. Unfortunately, too many people do not recognize the need for making physical activity a regular part of their routines. Consequently, they may be less productive, healthy, and active and unable to obtain the most that life has to offer. A service can be rendered to humanity by interpreting in lay terms—terms that each boy and girl, mother and father, businessman and others will understand and be able to identify with. Interpretation must be relevant to their needs, their health, their welfare, their future, and their well-being. Accurate and significant facts need to be presented regarding the biological, psychological, and sociological advantages of physical education. Physical educators who are well-trained themselves in the scientific foundations of their field will render the greatest service in interpreting the program to others. They will provide scientific, accurate information that can be supported through research as to the worth of their field. They will have outstanding programs in their school, agency, or college, knowing that this is a strong medium of interpreting the worth of their field. They will symbolize through their appearance and health habits the values that physical education provides. They will exploit every opportunity to speak to their academic colleagues, the community, and civic and other groups about their field of endeavor.

QUESTIONS AND EXERCISES

1. In approximately 250 words describe the nature and scope of the services performed by physical educators.
2. List as many games and other related physical education activities as possible with which every person in physical education should be familiar.
3. What are the advantages and disadvantages of coaching?
4. Describe what you would consider to be the ideal coach.
5. What part does dance play in the physical education program? Why should men as well as women physical educators be trained in the field of the dance?
6. Discuss the contributions of camping and outdoor education to child growth and development.

7. What values can be derived from a camp experience that could not be gained from a formal classroom environment?
8. Describe a camping or outdoor educational experience in which you have engaged. What values did you receive from such an experience?
9. What are the essentials of good posture?
10. What are the advantages of observing good body mechanics?
11. What evidence is available to support the premise that good body mechanics should be stressed by parents and the school?
12. Describe the meaning inherent in the slogan: "Out of Bed Into Action."
13. What are qualifications needed to be an administrator? Researcher? Teacher of health?

Reading assignment

Bucher, Charles A., and Goldman, Myra: Dimensions of physical education, St. Louis, 1969, The C. V. Mosby Co., Reading selections 1, 8, and 9.

SELECTED REFERENCES

American Association for Health, Physical Education, and Recreation: Activity programs for the mentally retarded, Journal of Health, Physical Education, and Recreation **37**:23, 1966.

American Association for Health, Physical Education, and Recreation: Promising practices in elementary school physical education, Washington, D. C., 1969, The Association.

Arnheim, Daniel D., and others: Principles and methods of adapted physical education, St. Louis, 1969, The C. V. Mosby Co.

A Symposium by Selected Physical Educators: Dance as an art form in physical education, Journal of Health, Physical Education, and Recreation **35**:19, 1964.

Bucher, Charles A.: Health, physical education, and academic achievement, NEA Journal **54**: 5, 1965.

Bucher, Charles A.: Administration of health and physical education programs including athletics, St. Louis, 1971, The C. V. Mosby Co.

Bucher, Charles A.: Administrative dimensions of health and physical education, including athletics, St. Louis, 1971, The C. V. Mosby Co.

Bucher, Charles A., Koening, Constance, and Barnhard, Milton: Methods and materials for secondary school physical education, St. Louis, 1970, The C. V. Mosby Co.

Bucher, Charles A., and Reade, Evelyn M.: Physical education and health in the elementary school, New York, 1971, The Macmillan Co.

Carlton, Lessie, and Moore, Robert H.: Culturally disadvantaged children can be helped, NEA Journal **55**:13, 1966.

Cassidy, Rosalind: Counseling in the physical education program, New York, 1959, Appleton-Century-Crofts.

Christensen, Dagney: Creativity in teaching physical education to the physically handicapped child, Journal of Health, Physical Education, and Recreation 41:73, 1970.

Conant, James B.: Slums and suburbs, New York, 1964, New American Library.

Cureton, Thomas K.: What is physical education research? Journal of Health, Physical Education, and Recreation 39:96, 1968.

Daniels, Arthur S., and Davies, Evelyn A.: Adapted physical education, New York, 1965, Harper and Row, Publishers.

Four Dance Pioneers (feature), Journal of Health, Physical Education, and Recreation 41:23, 1970.

Fantini, Mario D., and Weinstein, Gerald: The disadvantaged, New York, 1968, Harper and Row, Publishers.

Felsin, Jan: Sport and modes of meaning, Journal of Health, Physical Education, and Recreation 40:43, 1969.

Godfrey, Barbara B., and Kephart, Newell C.: Movement patterns and motor education, New York, 1969, Appleton-Century-Crofts.

Hanson, Carl H.: Teaching the handicapped child, Today's Education 58:46, 1969.

Hayden, Frank J.: Physical fitness for the mentally retarded, Toronto, Canada, 1964, Rotary Clubs.

It's up to you to do something about public relations (special feature), Journal of Health, Physical Education, and Recreation 39:39, 1968.

Jones, George W.: Compensatory education for the disadvantaged, NEA Journal 56:21, 1967.

Kleinman, Seymour: What future for dance in physical education? Journal of Health, Physical Education, and Recreation 40:101, 1969.

Kraus, Richard: Recreation today program planning and leadership, New York, 1966, Appleton-Century-Crofts.

Mudra, Darrell: The coach and the learning process, Journal of Health, Physical Education, and Recreation 41:26, 1970.

Oberteuffer, Delbert, and Beyrer, Mary K.: School health education, New York, 1966, Harper and Row, Publishers.

Oliver, James N.: Physical education for the visually handicapped, Journal of Health, Physical Education, and Recreation 41:37, 1970.

Riessman, Frank: The culturally deprived child, New York, 1962, Harper and Row, Publishers.

Shriver, Eunice Kennedy: A new day for the mentally retarded, The Physical Educator 25:99, 1968.

Stein, Julian U.: A practical guide to adapted physical education for the educable mentally handicapped, Journal of Health, Physical Education, and Recreation 33:30, 1962.

Stier, William F., Jr.: The coaching intern, Journal of Health, Physical Education, and Recreation 41:27, 1970.

Wienke, Phoebe: Blind children in an integrated physical education program, The New Outlook for the Blind 60:3, 1966.

3/Settings for physical education activities

The services that physical educators render to children, youth, and adults are an important consideration for young people who are preparing for a professional career in physical education and also for those individuals who are already on the job in communities throughout the country. However, services cannot be considered in a meaningful manner by themselves. They must be considered in relation to the settings in which they are performed.

CONSIDERATIONS FOR PHYSICAL EDUCATORS IN SELECTING A SETTING IN WHICH TO WORK

In this chapter many settings in which physical education activities are administered, supervised, taught, coached, performed, and carried out as parts of school and other organizational programs will be discussed. Physical educators will be interested in seeking job opportunities and in performing services in one of these settings, depending on pertinent factors relating to their qualifications for the job and their ability to perform effectively. A few considerations in selecting the setting are professional preparation, abilities, interests, and job availability.

Professional preparation

The preparation an individual has had in respect to general education and such courses and experiences as psychology, methodology, skills, student teaching, and other aspects of training programs will play a part in the selection of a setting.

A person who has prepared for elementary school teaching will obviously be interested in teaching at that educational level, just as the person who has prepared for college teaching wants to be situated in an institution of higher learning. Such preparation has oriented the individual to a particular setting and provided knowledge, understanding, and skill to do an effective job in that location. Therefore, professional preparation plays an important part in determining the setting in which the individual will work.

Abilities

It is important to match personal abilities with the job and setting. At an early age Einstein showed an uncanny aptitude with figures, and Henry Ford showed superior ability working with machines and gadgets. These great leaders had abilities that helped them to be successful in their work. Some people have greater ability than others in the area of research, which might better qualify them for college work. Others may demonstrate ability in working with children, which might better qualify them for elementary school work, or exceptional skill in golf, which might better qualify them for a professional job in a country club. Each person should match his abilities against several settings as a means of arriving at the right decision for a successful career. Strong preference should be given to those settings where there is tangible evidence that the individual possesses outstanding ability for success in those areas.

Interests

Other things being equal, the setting where there is greatest interest should offer a better chance for success because the person will be doing what he wants to do. However, if other factors such as abilities are not taken into consideration, it may mean that the job will not be done well. There are people with exceptional interest in engineering who are poor in mathematics, which would jeopardize their chances for success.

Since interests may change, it is also important to carefully evaluate them in order to cement realistic desires and rule out passing fancies.

Job availability

Professional preparation, abilities, and interests are important, but at the same time there is a practical consideration—job availability. After a person spends 4 or 5 years preparing for a career, he naturally wants to find a job in his field. It may be that the chances of obtaining employment in one setting may be brighter than in another. Therefore, availability of work is a consideration that cannot be overlooked.

SETTINGS

Physical education activities are conducted in many and varied settings. The most popular and prominent settings at the present time are as follows:

1. Public and private schools and colleges
2. Service organizations
3. Industrial concerns
4. Youth organizations
5. Recreational areas
6. Athletic clubs and other sport organizations
7. Professional and commercial areas
8. Camps
9. Governmental and welfare agencies
10. Churches
11. Hospitals
12. Penal institutions
13. Other countries

Public and private schools and colleges

Physical education activities play an important part in schools and colleges. The nation's schools and colleges may be categorized as nursery schools, kindergarten, primary grades, upper elementary grades, middle school, junior high school, senior high school, junior college, college, and university.

The nation's schools and colleges in the years to come will continue to be the settings where most physical educators will find work. The reason for this is the growth of the school and college population and the continued demand for teachers in these institutions.

Nearly 65 million people in the United States—students, teachers, and administrators—are participating full-time in the nation's educational enterprise. The vast educational establishment consists of approximately 88,000 elementary schools, 31,000 secondary schools, and 2,500 universities, colleges, and junior colleges. The nation is committing between $75 and $100 billion each year to education—public and non-public—at all levels.

Today, the public and private school enrollment in all institutions from kindergarten to graduate school is approximately 60 million, with over 7 million in higher education alone. Fifteen years ago school and college enrollments were under 40 million. The U. S. Office of Education foresees enrollments of more than 62 million by the middle 1970's. Two-year college enrollments have jumped from less than 300,000 students in 1954 to more than 1 million, and they are growing at the rate of 20% each year. About fifty new community colleges are being opened each September.

More men are entering the teaching profession. Fifteen years ago the men made up approximately 26% of the nation's teaching staff. Today, the figure is approximately 32% (men make up about 15.4% of the elementary school faculty and 53.5% of the secondary school faculties). Some facts about teachers in the schools follow.

AVERAGE AGE. The average is 39 years of age; women teachers on the average are almost 8 years older than men teachers. Aver-

The Magnitude of the American Educational Establishment (1969-70)

More than sixty-one million Americans are engaged full-time as students, teachers, or administrators in the nation's educational enterprise. Another 132,000 make education a time-consuming avocation as trustees of local school systems, state boards of education, or institutions of higher learning. The breakdown is given here:

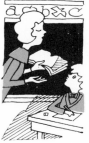

Teachers

Elementary School Teachers	
Public	1,099,000
Nonpublic	152,000
Secondary School Teachers	
Public	904,000
Nonpublic	88,000
College and University Teachers	
Public	344,000
Nonpublic	188,000
Total	2,775,000

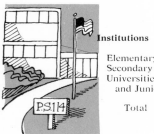

Institutions

Elementary	88,556
Secondary	31,203
Universities, Colleges, and Junior Colleges	2,483
Total	122,242

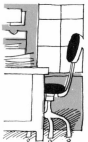

Administrators and Supervisors

Superintendents of Schools	13,106
Principals and Supervisors	119,365
College and University Presidents	2,483
Other College Administrative and Service Staff	82,000
Total	216,954

School Districts 20,440

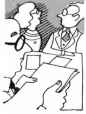

Board Members

Local School Board Members	106,806
State Board Members	500
College and University Trustees	25,000
Total	132,306

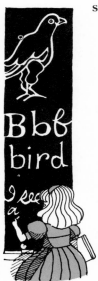

Students

Pupils in Elementary Schools (Kindergarten through eighth grade)	
Public Schools	32,600,000
Nonpublic (Private and Parochial)	4,300,000
Total	36,900,000
Secondary School Students	
Public High Schools	13,200,000
Nonpublic	1,400,000
Total	14,600,000
College and University full- and part-time students enrolled for credit toward degrees	
Public Institutions	5,100,000
Nonpublic	2,000,000
Total	7,100,000
Total Students Enrolled	58,600,000

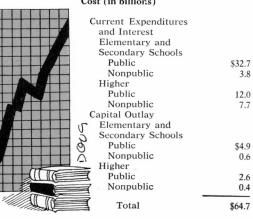

Cost (in billions)

Current Expenditures and Interest	
Elementary and Secondary Schools	
Public	$32.7
Nonpublic	3.8
Higher	
Public	12.0
Nonpublic	7.7
Capital Outlay	
Elementary and Secondary Schools	
Public	$4.9
Nonpublic	0.6
Higher	
Public	2.6
Nonpublic	0.4
Total	$64.7

Figures are based on latest available estimates from the U.S. Office of Education and the National Education Association.

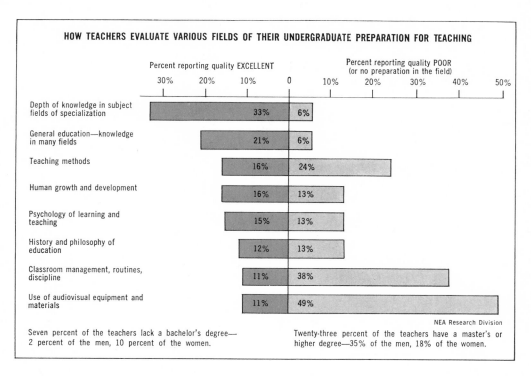

HOW TEACHERS EVALUATE VARIOUS FIELDS OF THEIR UNDERGRADUATE PREPARATION FOR TEACHING

Percent reporting quality EXCELLENT | Percent reporting quality POOR (or no preparation in the field)

Field	Excellent	Poor
Depth of knowledge in subject fields of specialization	33%	6%
General education—knowledge in many fields	21%	6%
Teaching methods	16%	24%
Human growth and development	16%	13%
Psychology of learning and teaching	15%	13%
History and philosophy of education	12%	13%
Classroom management, routines, discipline	11%	38%
Use of audiovisual equipment and materials	11%	49%

NEA Research Division

Seven percent of the teachers lack a bachelor's degree—2 percent of the men, 10 percent of the women.

Twenty-three percent of the teachers have a master's or higher degree—35% of the men, 18% of the women.

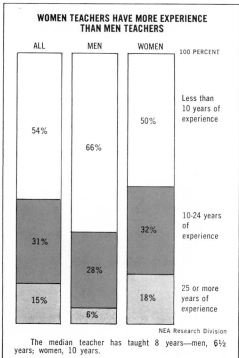

WOMEN TEACHERS HAVE MORE EXPERIENCE THAN MEN TEACHERS

NEA Research Division

The median teacher has taught 8 years—men, 6½ years; women, 10 years.

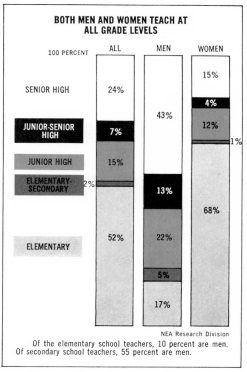

BOTH MEN AND WOMEN TEACH AT ALL GRADE LEVELS

NEA Research Division

Of the elementary school teachers, 10 percent are men. Of secondary school teachers, 55 percent are men.

FROM DAVIS, HAZEL: PROFILE OF THE AMERICAN PUBLIC SCHOOL TEACHER, 1966, NEA JOURNAL 56:11, 1967.

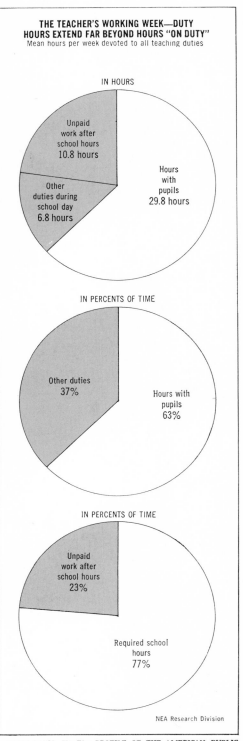

FROM DAVIS, HAZEL: PROFILE OF THE AMERICAN PUBLIC
SCHOOL TEACHER, 1966, NEA JOURNAL **56**:11, 1967.

age age of elementary school teachers is 41 years, of secondary school teachers, 37 years.

MARITAL STATUS. About 82% of public school teachers are or have been married (84% of men and 81% of women).

EXPERIENCE. The median teacher has 12 years of teaching experience. Women teachers on the average have been teaching twice as long as men.

DEGREES. Over 95% of all public school teachers have a bachelor's degree and over 30% have a master's or higher degree.

ELEMENTARY SCHOOL

The objectives of elementary school education have been well stated by a group of teachers in Winnetka, Illinois.* These objectives are presented here in adapted form. The elementary schools should be designed to (1) encourage intellectual growth, (2) develop basic skills, (3) give consideration to the child as a total human being, (4) help children develop attitudes, habits, values, appreciations, and understandings that will ensure a constructive adult life, (5) discover and meet the special talents and needs of all children, (6) develop habits of rational thinking and problem solving, (7) foster physical and mental health, (8) establish a setting that furthers social and esthetic development, (9) inculcate an appreciation of hard work, and (10) stress moral and spiritual values.

The 1970's show an increased interest in elementary school physical education as evidenced by such happenings as the hiring of more physical education specialists in elementary schools, the increased interest in motor activity particularly at the preschool level, the interest shown by psychologists and other disciplines in our field of work, and a recognition of the contributions physical education can make to scholastic achievement.

Some reasons given by physical educators

---

*Beliefs and objectives of the Winnetka public schools, Winnetka, Illinois, 1961, The Board of Education.

as to why they like teaching in the elementary schools include the following:

1. It offers a combination of opportunity, reward, challenge, and deep gratification for services performed.
2. Pupils are motivated, eager, and enthusiastic and take pride in their progress.
3. The child has a natural craving for activity that makes work a pleasure.
4. At the elementary level it is possible to witness rapid, visible advancement of pupils.
5. It is a joy to work with happy youngsters.
6. There is a great challenge in working with a child during his most impressionable and formative years.
7. There are more job openings at the elementary level.
8. The personal satisfaction is great when a small hand slips into yours and a voice says, "I like you."

In elementary schools the program consists mainly of movement experiences (see Chapter 13), including rhythmical activities, story plays, creative activities, self-testing activities, relays, hunting games, aquatics, and winter sports. These activities are largely conducted by the classroom teacher. Many educators feel that since the elementary school teacher teaches a variety of school activities to children all day, he should also teach physical education. At the same time, however, many educators feel that the physical education program in the elementary school should be directed by specialized personnel because it is recognized that physical education at this level is one of the most important subjects because of the need to develop body awareness, the activity drive in children, the necessity for "big-muscle" activity, and the need for developing a broad foundation of motor ability for future use. A sound foundation of physical education in the early years will help to guarantee the pursuit of physical activity in the later years and will motivate individuals into activity on their own initiative.

To provide qualified leadership in physical education on the elementary level, different procedures are followed. More persons trained in physical education are being hired to teach in the elementary schools.

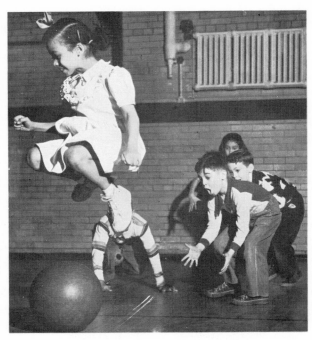

DETROIT PUBLIC SCHOOLS, DETROIT, MICH.

Supervisors of physical education are provided in many school systems to aid the classroom teachers in developing a sound program. Some systems have "demonstration" teachers who are on call, and any classroom teacher may request their services if they are interested in having some particular game, rhythmical activity, or relay demonstrated or discussed. There is also what is known as a "resource" teacher in physical education on the elementary level. This individual is a specialist in physical education and is relieved of many routine classroom duties to coordinate the physical education program in a particular elementary school. Some teacher-training institutions are certifying teachers with a double major, one in physical education and one in elementary education. This enables the prospective teacher to accept a position in the elementary school where part of the time will be utilized to coordinate the physical education program. With stress being placed on physical education in the elementary school, it is hoped that more personnel qualified in physical education will be added to school faculties throughout the country.

MIDDLE SCHOOL

The middle school, a new movement in American education, is designed to provide an educational program for preadolescents and early adolescents that begins where the school for earlier childhood ends and continues to the school for adolescents. Pupils usually range in age from 9 to 14 years, with ages 10 to 13 being most common. Middle schools usually house grades five through eight, although several other administrative patterns exist. Some of the characteristics of the middle school are that it tries to combine the best features of the self-contained classroom of the elementary school with the departmentalized pattern of the secondary school, it emphasizes self-understanding with programs that aim at the problems of young adolescents, and it stresses self-direction for learning.

The physical education program in the middle school should be part of a developmental program that builds upon the movement experiences of earlier grades. Such a program must be based on the child's growth and development characteristics and the physical activities that meet his needs at his particular stage of development.

Eichhorn* has pointed out another important point of emphasis in what he calls the *physical-cultural curriculum* for the middle school. He indicates that research scholars say that the physical growth that takes place during this period of transition represents a most vital educational concern and cannot be ignored. The physical-cultural curriculum provides for an interrelation in the areas of the fine arts, physical education, social studies, and practical arts. Eichhorn illustrates this by showing how a physical-cultural unit could focus on the culture of Japan, for example. The unit would include art and music (fine arts); an acquaintance with Japanese foods, crafts, clothing, and hobbies (practical arts); participation in games, sports, and other activities (physical education); and a study of Japanese government and social institutions (social studies). The purpose of the unit is to have the totality of the culture permeate all content areas.

Eichhorn stresses the point that the physical-cultural curriculum can render a valuable contribution in "freeing youngsters from intellectual disequilibrium" through social interaction. Physical education can provide the child with a medium for obtaining peer group approval, gaining self-confidence, understanding the personal growth process, and developing qualities of health. The physical education experience is a very valuable part of this curriculum and can render an invaluable contribution to the total education of the child, according to Eichhorn.

SECONDARY SCHOOL

The secondary school level refers to those grades that follow elementary school, start-

ing with grade seven and continuing to the college years. Secondary schools are organized according to various administrative patterns. Some of the more prevalent patterns are: the traditional high school or 8-4 system, the combined junior and senior high school or 6-6 or 7-5 plan, the 6-3-3 system where the junior high school is grouped separately, the 4-4-4 plan with the middle school, and the 6-2-4 system with the 4-year high school.

The purposes of the secondary school have been stated by many educational groups (see Chapter 7 for a discussion of such objectives). The primary functions allocated to the secondary school include promoting the total development of the pupil, including his intellectual powers, a basic knowledge of major fields of study, and his unique talents, whatever they may be. A second purpose is to help the pupil achieve a better understanding of his abilities, interests, and potentialities. A third purpose is to orient the pupil in various fields of work so that he may learn how his abilities and interests relate to these areas of endeavor. A fourth purpose is to help each student develop a sound system of values. A fifth purpose is to help the pupil develop a philosophy of life together with the skills, health, interests, appreciations, and social attributes essential to a good life. A final purpose is to develop an understanding of the democratic process and the role of the student in furthering this way of life.

Some reasons given by physical educators as to why they like teaching at the secondary school level include the following:

1. Love of team sports
2. Excitement of and interest in coaching sports
3. The compartmentalization of subject matter
4. An interesting group of students with whom to work
5. Satisfaction derived in seeing students transfer skills from physical education class to after-school intramurals and recreation
6. The challenge of guiding students through the awkward, transitional period of unrest and uncertainty of the junior high school years

---

*Eichhorn, Donald H.: The middle school, New York, 1966, Library of Education, The Center for Applied Research in Education, Inc., p. 67.

7. The inspiration derived in working on a staff with other professional colleagues
8. Love of more highly organized games and activities

JUNIOR HIGH SCHOOL. In junior high schools the physical education program includes aquatics, posture work, dual and individual sports, self-testing activities, formal activities, games and relays, sports of higher organization, rhythmics and dancing, contests, apparatus, and tumbling and stunts. Many of the activities for both boys and girls are very similar at this level, but it is desirable that they be separated for a large part of their work. The activities must be selected with care because of the anatomical and physiological nature of this age group. Pupils at this level are susceptible to fatigue, are in a period of rapid growth, and find it difficult to coordinate their actions, which results in awkwardness. There must be careful supervision by qualified personnel of all physical education activities in order that the student may experience optimum development. In some school systems the physical education programs in the junior high school grades (seventh, eighth, and ninth) are administered in much the same way as the first six grades. The classroom teachers handle the physical education programs for their respective grades. In other school systems the junior high school is separate from the elementary and the senior high schools. In this particular type of setup it is common to find trained physical education men and women handling the classes in physical education. In still other school systems, one or more grades of the junior high school are included in the senior high school building, where trained physical education personnel usually handle the classes. The teachers on the junior high school level should be specialists in physical education. They should be sympathetic to the problems of boys and girls and should be able to guide children successfully during this formative period. They should understand the needs of chil-

dren and their interests and capacities and should realize that they may be of exceptional service to the student during this time when he is planning his future.

SENIOR HIGH SCHOOL. The senior high school physical education program should be the responsibility of specialized persons. During high school more stress is placed on the team games of higher organization and on dual and individual games. It is also during this period that the student should develop sufficient skill so that when he leaves school he will have the necessary fundamental skill, the desire, and the knowledge to participate successfully and enjoyably. Because many students do not go on to college, it is essential that they acquire this skill, knowledge, and interest before they leave school. The competitive element is very prominent in high school students; and the more highly organized games, intramural and interscholastic sports, and field and play days offer an opportunity for the students to give vent to this instinct. However, the physical education teacher, through careful supervision and guidance, must ensure that the activity is not too strenuous and that excessive demands are not placed on the participant. Girls are frequently as interested in sports as boys, and many activities may be modified in order to provide a corecreational program.

The program of activities in the high school should include a core and an elective program both for boys and for girls. The program includes such activities as basketball, formal activities, field hockey, advanced rhythms, volleyball, tumbling, track and field, touch football, swimming, softball, soccer, archery, badminton, bowling, tennis, dance, winter activities, handball, golf, camping, and corrective activities.

Because of the differences in strength, interests, and skill, the boys' and girls' physical education programs are usually separate on the senior high school level. This necessitates at least one specialist for the girls and one for the boys. Furthermore, in larger schools there are frequently

Table 3-1. Time and grade requirements for physical education in elementary and secondary schools—states and possessions*

State	Required by law or regulation	Time requirement	Grade requirement
Alabama	Yes	1-6—30 minutes/day; 7-8—daily; 9-12—1 credit	1 through 12
Alaska	Yes	1-8—required but no time specified; 9-12—1 credit	1 through 12; secondary—1 credit required
Arizona	No	Recommended only; 1-3—10% of day; 4-8—14% of day; 9-12—not specified	None
Arkansas	Yes	1-8—required but no time specified; 9-12—1 credit	1 through 12; secondary—1 credit required
California	Yes	1-6—200 minutes/2 weeks; 7-12—400 minutes/2 weeks	1 through 12
Colorado	No	None	Nonregulatory state
		(Physical education in grades 1 through 12 is required for state accreditation.)	
Connecticut	Yes	Not specified	Required by law in elementary and secondary schools; grade level optional
Delaware	Yes	1-6—suggested 200-250 minutes/week; 7-8—2 periods/week; 9-10—2 periods/week one semester, 3 periods/week adjacent semester; 11-12—elective	1 through 10; 11-12—elective (effective April, 1970)
District of Columbia	Yes	Grade 1—150 minutes/week; 2-6—125 minutes/week (combined with health); 7-9—90 minutes/week; 10-11—3 periods/week; 12—elective	1 through 12
Florida	Yes	1-6—daily period; 7-8—90 periods/year (2 55-minute periods/week); 9-12—2 credits	1 through 8; 9-12—2 credits
Georgia	Yes	1-8—30 minutes/day (combined HE & PE)	1 through 8
Hawaii	Yes	K-6—90 minutes/week; 7-10—½ credit/year	K through 10
Idaho	Yes	1-8—not required; 9-12—1 credit	9-12—1 credit
Illinois	Yes	1-12—daily period equal in length to other subject periods	1 through 12
Indiana	Yes	1-6—10% of day recommended; 7-8—15% of day recommended; 9-12—1 credit	9 through 12—1 credit required
Iowa	Yes	50 minutes/week minimum	1 through 12

*From Grieve, Andrew: State legal requirements for physical education, Journal of Health, Physical Education, and Recreation **42**:20-22, 1971.

Table 3-1. Time and grade requirements for physical education in elementary
and secondary schools—states and possessions—cont'd

State	Required by law or regulation	Time requirement	Grade requirement
Kansas	Yes	9-12—55 minutes/day	1 through 8—recommended only; 9-12—required
Kentucky	Yes	1-8—120 minutes/week; 9-12—1 semester (suggested in 9 or 10)	1 through 8; 9 through 12—1 semester or ½ credit for graduation
Louisiana	Yes	1-8—120 minutes/week; 9-12—150 minutes/week minimum, 300 minutes/week maximum	1 through 12
Maine	Yes	1-11—2 periods/week for all pupils in public schools	1 through 11
Maryland	Yes	1-6—required but no time specified; 7-8—daily period; 9—daily where possible, 9-12—1 credit	1 through 12; 9-12—1 credit
Massachusetts	Yes	1-6—90 minutes/week; 7-12—120 minutes/week	1 through 12
Michigan	Yes	Not specified	Not specified
Minnesota	Yes	1-6—30 minutes/day; 7-10—2 55-minute periods/week	1 through 10
Mississippi	Yes	1-6—20 to 30 minutes/day	1 through 6
Missouri	Yes (use voluntary classification plan)	1-6—2 30-minute periods/week; 7-12—required but no time specified	1 through 12
Montana	Yes	1-3—15 minutes/day; 4-6—20 minutes/day; 7-8—30 minutes/day; 9-10—3 periods/week	1 through 10
Nebraska	No	None by law; for accreditation: elementary—150 minutes/week; secondary 2 55-minute periods/week	Can get accreditation for meeting indicated requirements
Nevada	Yes	1-8—not specified; 9-12—3 years of 5 daily periods/week	9 through 12—3 years required
New Hampshire	No	None	New law in 1972 will require PE at all levels
New Jersey	Yes	1-12—150 minutes/week	1 through 12 (includes some health education)
New Mexico	Yes	1-3—125 minutes/week; 4-6—150 minutes/week; 7-8—equivalent of 1 period/day for 1 year; 9-12—equivalent of 1 period/day for 1 year	1 through 6; 7-8—equivalent of 1 period/day for 1 year; 9-12—equivalent of 1 period/day for 1 year
New York	Yes	1-6—120 minutes/week; 7-12—300 minutes/week	1 through 12

Table 3-1. Time and grade requirements for physical education in elementary and secondary schools—states and possessions—cont'd

State	Required by law or regulation	Time requirement	Grade requirement
North Carolina	Yes	1-8—150 minutes/week; 9—daily period (combined with health)	1 through 9
North Dakota	Yes	Daily instruction for all	1 through 12
Ohio	Yes	1-8—100 minutes/week; 9-12—2 periods/week for 2 years	1 through 12 (dependent upon fulfillment of 2-year requirement)
Oklahoma	No	None	None
Oregon	Yes	K-3—10% of school day; 4-6—15% of school day; 7-8—35-45 minutes/day; 9-10—45-60 minutes/day; 11-12—optional	K through 10; 11-12—optional but strongly recommended
Pennsylvania	Yes	1-6—daily but no time specified; 7-12—2 periods/week but no time specified	1 through 12
Rhode Island	Yes	1-12—average of 20 minutes/day (combined with health)	1 through 12
South Carolina	Yes	1-6—daily period; 7-8—2 or 3 periods/week; 9-12—1 credit	1 through 8; 9 through 12—1 credit required for graduation (may apply 2 credits toward graduation)
South Dakota	Yes	1-9—90 minutes/week	1 through 9
Tennessee	Yes	1-6—30 minutes/day; 7-8—1 hour twice weekly or 45 minutes alternate days or 30 minutes/day; 9-12—1 credit	1 through 12; 9 through 12—1 credit required
Texas	Yes	1-6—required but no time specified; 7-8—130 clock hours/year (minimum); 9-12—1½ credits (240 clock hours)	1 through 12; 9 through 12—1½ credits required
Utah	Yes	1-6—30 minutes/day recommended; 7-9—1 semester; 10-12—1 semester in 2 of 3 grades	7 through 12 (time requirements indicated
Vermont	Yes	1-8—no time specified; 9-12—1 credit	1 through 12
Virginia	Yes	1-8—no time specified; 9-12—3 credits required of combined health and physical education	1 through 12
Washington	Yes	1-8—20 minutes/day; 9-12—90 minutes/week	1 through 12
West Virginia	Yes	1-6—30 minutes/day; 7-8—1 period/day; 9-12—minimum of 2 periods/week	1 through 12

Table 3-1. Time and grade requirements for physical education in elementary and secondary schools—states and possessions—cont'd

State	Required by law or regulation	Time requirement	Grade requirement
Wisconsin	Yes	1-6—daily period; 7-12—3 periods/week	1 through 12
Wyoming	Yes	1-8—required but no time specified	1 through 8
		POSSESSIONS	
Canal Zone	Yes	1-6—30 minutes/day; 7-12—55 minutes/day	1 through 12
Guam	Yes	1-6—no time specified; 7 to 9—1 period/day; 10 and 11—1 period/day	1 through 6; 7 to 9; 10 and 11
Puerto Rico	Yes	1-6—80 minutes/week; 7-9—50 minutes/week; 10-12—250 minutes/week elective	1 through 9; 10 through 12 elective
Virgin Islands	Yes	1-6—45 minutes/week; 7-10—180 minutes week	1 through 10

additional personnel for such phases of the program as coaching and work with the handicapped. It has been recommended that classes in physical education be limited in number of students to not more than thirty-five to forty. If this becomes standard practice, more physical educators will be needed. As it is, the senior high school level is one of the most popular and important settings for physical education personnel in the national education setup.

The preparatory school and private school have much the same type of program as is found in the senior high school. In many of these schools, however, the advantages for a well-rounded and successful physical education program are much greater. Because of small enrollments, beautiful athletic fields, spacious gymnasiums, and swimming pools, these schools may offer a program that is in many ways superior to those found in many public schools, colleges, and universities.

COLLEGE AND UNIVERSITY

There are many types of colleges including public and private; large and small; resident and nonresident; urban and rural; secular or sectarian; liberal, technical, or professional; 2-year or 4-year; coeducational or for a single sex; or a combination of these.

Colleges and universities take their goals and direction from many sources. The founders, faculty, trustees, donors, alumni, or administration of a college or university might indicate that it is to devote its endeavors to agriculture or to the liberal arts, to training teachers or to preparing architects, to ensuring social competence or to promoting intellectual growth, to preparing for a profession or to getting a general education, or to a combination of these purposes. In other words, the purposes of colleges are varied—all do not have the same goals.

Some reasons given by physical educators as to why they like teaching at the college level include the following:

1. Students are more mature.
2. The instructor and professor have more freedom.
3. Professional preparation programs offer opportunities to train future professional leaders.

4. Campus living is satisfying, as is college life in general.
5. There is more prestige in teaching at the college level.
6. There are more opportunities to participate in work of professional associations.
7. Opportunities to improve one's own educational background by taking graduate work are greater.

The status of required physical education programs in colleges and universities throughout the United States was determined by Oxendine,* who surveyed 1,046 institutions of higher learning. Some 723, or 69%, of the institutions returned completed questionnaires. The information gained from this survey showed that:

Eighty-seven percent of reporting institutions have physical education programs for all students.
Of those institutions having a physical education requirement, two-thirds require physical education for a period of 2 years.
Large and public institutions place physical education on a sounder academic basis than small and private institutions.
Programs have shown recent gains in "recreational" and "fitness" activities.
Team sports are not offered as frequently as they were in the past.
Coeducational classes are on the increase among most institutions of learning.

Ruffer,† in his study of college physical education requirements, found that 86% of 714 institutions studied require physical education for all undergraduates. However, his research did not completely concur with Oxendine's study in respect to offerings in large and small institutions. For example, his findings were contrary to Oxendine's study, which concluded that large institutions schedule physical education as a regular academic course more often than small colleges.

---

*Oxendine, Joseph B.: Status of required physical education programs in colleges and universities, Journal of Health, Physical Education, and Recreation **40**:32, 1969.
†Ruffer, William A.: A study of required physical education for men in United States colleges and universities, The Physical Educator **27**:79, 1970.

Kelly,* in her study of thirty-seven colleges and universities (twenty-five returned questionnaires) regarding current trends in women's required physical education, had these findings:

Twenty-three institutions had required physical education programs for women.
Twenty-two institutions had intramural programs.
Thirteen of the institutions had a 2-year requirement; the rest had less.
Sixteen colleges and universities gave credit for physical education.
Twenty-one colleges and universities had either two or three periods of physical education per week.

Some of the new and different features that characterized women's physical education programs, according to Kelly's study, were:

Tap dancing
Complete elective system
Movement foundations courses
Personal defense
Field archery
Modified program to meet the needs of all skill levels
Scuba diving
Perceptual motor movement, problem-solving approach
Saturday morning institute that gives students the opportunity to work with exceptional children
Work with physical therapist for handicapped (several)

Some of the new developments in college physical education not completely identified in these studies include independent study in physical education where, with faculty guidance, students pursue a special project as opposed to attending and participating in the conventional physical education class. Examples of projects are competing in a bowling tournament, attending a conference on sports, or participating in a dance program. Another new development worthy of mention is the foundation

---

*Kelly, Susan E.: Current trends of women's required physical education in coeducational, urban colleges and universities in the northern and eastern United States, independent study conducted at New York University, 1969.

or theory course where students get at the "why" of physical education. Foundation courses cover such topics and items as an evaluation of a person's health and fitness, body mechanics, health concepts, cardiovascular fitness, values of physical education, principles of exercise, training techniques, and kinesiological principles. Another new development is the addition of many new activities to the college curriculum such as scuba diving, judo, cross-country skiing, jogging, rock climbing, and sport parachuting. These activities may be offered in the required physical education program or on a club basis.

THE 2-YEAR COLLEGE. There are nearly 900 2-year colleges in the United States, and it is predicted that there will be 1,000 by 1975. Approximately one-third of these colleges are private, with two-thirds being public. Enrollment in 2-year colleges is approximately 1.5 million, with more male than female students. The average enrollment for a junior college is approximately 1,600 to 2,000 students. Most of the 2-year colleges require physical education for approximately 2 hours a week for each of the 2 years. In a few colleges physical education is required the first year and is made elective the second year. The activities offered in the first year are predominantly team sports. The activities offered in the second year include individual, dual, and carry-over sports, along with team sports. The most common activities offered in the 2-year colleges include basketball, gymnastics, track and field, volleyball, tennis, touch football, soccer, golf, archery, bowling, weight lifting, wrestling, swimming, field hockey, badminton, and dancing.

Some colleges require a textbook as part of the physical education experience. Many 2-year colleges require health courses for their students, and these are frequently taught by physical education professors. A majority of the 2-year colleges has a director of physical education who frequently is also the athletic director.

Since the 2-year college is comparatively new on the American scene, programs are varied from state to state and college to college. In the future it would appear that physical education programs would become more purposive and provide initial preparation for those students desiring to make physical education a career, offer 2 years of basic instruction in physical education activities, meet the needs of the atypical student, provide college credit for courses taken, develop a broad intramural and intercollegiate program, engage in research activities, and help college students in the development of lifetime skills and understanding and appreciation of the importance of physical activity throughout life for their physical, mental, and social betterment.

The 2-year college is an institution that is progressing with great rapidity in our country. This is the institutional level where probably the greatest expansion will take place in our educational system during the next decade. California and New York are two of many states that have instituted extensive systems of junior and community colleges. These colleges are being developed so that students may live at home or will not have to travel very far and still continue their education beyond high school. For some students these colleges may provide terminal formal education, and for others they may provide the first 2 years of a 4-year college course. These schools recognize the value of regular physical education classes as well as a broad athletic program for their students.

THE 4-YEAR COLLEGE AND UNIVERSITY. The college and university physical education program is designed for providing opportunities for physical conditioning, developing skills in recreational and leisure-time activities, and participating in intramural and intercollegiate athletic competition. In the basic instructional or service physical education programs, college students usually participate for 2 years in various team sports, dual and individual activities, rhythmical activities, and recreational sports for the purpose of maintaining good physical condition. At the same

Table 3-2. Physical education in 2-year colleges*

	PCC†	PJC‡	BSU§	STC‖
Specific programs available in 2-year colleges				
Physical education service program	283 (86%)	44 (66%)	31 (94%)	7 (58%)
Physical education majors program	185 (56%)	12 (18%)	12 (36%)	0 (0%)
Intramural program	291 (88%)	65 (97%)	33 (100%)	8 (67%)
Median full-time enrollment	1,069.43	454.09	930.63	799.00
Median salary of athletic directors				
Working 9-10 months	$12,968.53	$ 7,998.50	$ 9,747.65	$11,499.00
Working 11-12 months	$14,718.78	$10,568.93	$11,998.50	$13,249.25
Colleges in which the physical education service program is required				
Required	261 (92%)	42 (95%)	25 (81%)	6 (86%)
Not required	22 (8%)	2 (5%)	6 (19%)	1 (14%)
Semesters required in physical education service program				
2 semesters	103 (37%)	15 (34%)	10 (32%)	5 (71%)
4 semesters	132 (47%)	22 (50%)	11 (35%)	1 (14%)
Colleges in which the physical education service program carries academic credit				
Credit	268 (95%)	38 (86%)	24 (77%)	5 (71%)
Noncredit	15 (5%)	6 (14%)	6 (19%)	2 (29%)
Colleges which count quality points of the physical education service program in the GPA				
Count quality points	260 (92%)	34 (80%)	23 (74%)	4 (57%)
Do not count quality points	23 (18%)	9 (20%)	5 (16%)	3 (43%)

*From Yarnall, Douglas: A survey of physical education in two-year colleges, Journal of Health, Physical Education, and Recreation **42**:81, 1971.

†Public community colleges.

‡Public junior colleges.

§Branches of state universities.

‖State technical colleges.

time there are many other beneficial results, such as the alleviation of tensions. Probably the most beneficial result from participation is the development of physical skills, making it possible for students to continue physical activity after leaving college. Most college programs offer some freedom in the choice of activities, so that the student may further develop his skill in a sport in which he has particular interest. The intramural and intercollegiate sports program plays an important part in college and university physical education programs as well as in 2-year colleges. Intramural athletics offer an opportunity for all students, regardless of degree of skill, to participate. Leagues are usually formed according to some method of homogeneous grouping and in such a manner as to add flavor and interest to the competition. In many colleges, fraternities, sororities, and other organizations enter teams. This usually adds additional vigor and interest to the rivalry. Participants in intercollegiate sports are for the more skilled players in various sports such as basketball, football, baseball, track, swimming, soccer, and tennis. Teams in these various sports vie with teams from other schools. The National Collegiate Athletic Association and the National Association for Intercollegiate Athletics are set up to govern, regulate, and establish standards for this competition. In many colleges field and play days take the place of intercollegiate athletic competition for the girls.

In addition to the teaching of service courses for college students, there is also a need for teachers of physical education in the many teacher-education institutions throughout the country. As the demand for more physical education personnel grows, there will be an equal demand for teachers to train this personnel. Personnel who work in teacher-training institutions teach such courses as anatomy, physiology, methods and materials, tests and measurements, remedial physical education, principles of physical education, and organization and administration of the physical education

program. They also teach various skill courses in the activities and provide other necessary experiences such as camping and outdoor education.

SPECIAL SCHOOLS

In addition to the nation's public and private schools that serve many of the nation's children and youth, there are also special schools in which other pupils are enrolled. These include trade and vocational schools; schools for atypical persons such as the blind, retarded, and crippled; and schools for men and women who are primarily interested in adult education.

TRADE AND VOCATIONAL SCHOOLS. Many schools exist to prepare for careers in certain trades, crafts, and other vocations. The privately operated schools of commerce, technical institutes, and schools for dental assistants are a mere sampling of the types of schools one sees constantly advertised in newspapers, magazines, subways, or buses. Most of these schools offer some type of physical education program for their students. Such a program is usually similar to those discussed under secondary education and exist in the junior and senior high schools of the nation.

SCHOOLS FOR ATYPICAL INDIVIDUALS. Opportunities exist for teaching individuals who have special physical afflictions such as blindness, deafness, or hearing difficulties; who are crippled; or who find they can obtain greater benefits by pursuing an education with individuals who have similar handicaps. In recent years, particularly with the emphasis on providing education for all persons in our society, such schools have multiplied. As a result, there have been directors of special education appointed in state departments of education, and colleges and universities have introduced courses for the professional preparation of teachers specializing in the education of exceptional children. School, college, and university programs where the handicapped are taught have been established. Foundations and agencies, such as the American Foundation for the Blind,

Inc., have been established. In addition to teachers and counselors being needed to work with handicapped children, they are also needed to work with handicapped adults.

Wherever possible, the disabled are taught in regular school and college classes along with the able-bodied. Nevertheless, in many instances where the affliction warrants, education has proved to be more satisfactory in special schools and colleges especially adapted for such purposes.

SCHOOLS FOR ADULTS. Adult education is thriving throughout the country. Programs are being established in most communities that provide experiences for men and women who desire to enrich their lives. These experiences cover the gamut of educational activities including English, music, Spanish, art, and typewriting. They also provide opportunities to develop physical fitness, skill in some sport or dance, or other area of competency associated with physical education.

Service organizations

There are many service organizations such as the YMCA, American Red Cross, settlement houses, and the armed forces that provide employment for physical educators.

YOUNG MEN'S CHRISTIAN ASSOCIATION, YOUNG WOMEN'S CHRISTIAN ASSOCIATION, YOUNG'S MEN'S HEBREW ASSOCIATION, AND YOUNG WOMEN'S HEBREW ASSOCIATION

The YMCA, YWCA, YMHA, YWHA, and similar service organizations serve many groups of people. They serve the people of various communities where they have been established, both the young and adult population. Religious training was the main purpose in forming many of these organizations. However, activities directed at the physical are an important part of their programs. Classes in various physical activities; athletic leagues and contests for industries, churches, young people's groups,

and boys' and girls' groups; and camping programs are a few of the activities organized and administered by these voluntary agencies. The cost of financing such organizations is usually met through membership dues, community chest drives, and contributions of private individuals.

These organizations are designed to improve our society physically, morally, mentally, and spiritually through their programs of physical activity. An example of the extent to which these organizations render services in this country and throughout the world can be seen in the Young Men's Christian Association. There are more than 1,700 YMCA's in the United States and 121 in Canada. The YMCA operates in seventy-eight countries of the world. In the United States there are approximately 5.5 million members in the YMCA and over 2 million members in the YWCA.

Usually these agencies have directors for the physical activities who have received specialized training in their field. Many organizations have complete staffs of trained physical education personnel who aid in the organization and administration of the programs.

A typical physical activity schedule of a YMCA is shown in Table 3-3.

AMERICAN RED CROSS

The American Red Cross in its various program offerings provides a setting for physical education activities, especially along institutional lines. These activities are mainly concerned with some phase of aquatics, water safety, first aid, and hospital recreation. Through this organization many qualified persons in physical education help to demonstrate proper techniques and procedures in these activities to interested persons throughout the country and help to provide for the needs of individuals who have been hospitalized.

SETTLEMENT AND NEIGHBORHOOD HOUSES

Settlement and neighborhood houses are largely confined to cities. In many communities they are also known as com-

Table 3-3. YMCA physical activity schedule

Activities	Mon.	Tues.	Wed.	Thurs.	Fri.	Sat.
Basketball	4:15-5:30 6:00-7:30	4:15-8:00	4:15-5:30 6:00-8:00	4:15-8:00	4:15-5:30 6:00-7:30	3:30-9:00
Boxing (furnish own speed bag)	10:00-10:00	10:00-10:00	10:00-10:00	10:00-10:00	10:00-10:00	9:00-9:00
Boys' swimming class						9:00-1:00
Calisthenics	12:15-12:45 5:30-6:00	12:15-12:45 6:00-6:30	12:15-12:45 5:30-6:00	12:15-12:45 6:00-6:30	12:15-12:45 5:30-6:00	
Father and son swim					7:00-10:00	1:00-9:00
Fencing	8:00-10:00				8:00-10:00	
Gymnastics		8:00-10:00		8:00-10:00		
Handball (reservation required)	10:00-10:00	10:00-10:00	10:00-10:00	10:00-10:00	10:00-10:00	9:00-9:00
Lifesaving (as scheduled)		8:00-10:00		8:00-10:00		
Swimming—beginners (1st Mon. each month)	7:00-7:45		7:00-7:45			
Swimming—intermediate and advanced (1st Mon. each month)	7:45-8:30		7:45-8:30			
Scuba (as scheduled)			Pool 8:00-10:00	Class room 8:00-10:00		
Special programs —gym			8:00-10:00			
Squash (reservations required)	10:00-10:00	10:00-10:00	10:00-10:00	10:00-10:00	10:00-10:00	9:00-9:00
Track	9:00-10:00	9:00-10:00	9:00-10:00	9:00-10:00	9:00-10:00	9:00-9:00
Volleyball	12:45-2:00 6:00-8:00		Advanced 12:45-2:00 6:00-8:00		12:45-2:00 6:00-8:00	
Weight lifting and body building	9:00-10:00	9:00-10:00	9:00-10:00	9:00-10:00	9:00-10:00	9:00-9:00
Wrestling	8:00-10:00				8:00-10:00	

munity centers or community houses. They are usually organized and administered by a religious or social welfare group in the low-income or ethnic neighborhoods of cities. Their aim is to establish a higher standard of living by improving the spiritual, mental, and cultural welfare of the people. They work with all types of people regardless of age, sex, and national or racial origin. However, they give special attention to children. They offer varied programs of activities, which include arts and crafts, athletics, games, singing, dancing, photography, music, dramatics, and discussion forums. Physical education activities play an important role in many of these centers where they have gymnasiums, playgrounds, summer camps, swimming pools, and game rooms. Physical directors and staff occupy prominent positions in many of these social enterprises. Physical activity offers many of these people the opportunity for self-expression and helps them gain a better outlook on life in the midst of poverty and poor living conditions.

ARMED FORCES AND UNITED SERVICE ORGANIZATIONS

The Army, Navy, Marines, Coast Guard, National Guard, and Air Force have extensive physical activity programs that aid in keeping service personnel in good mental and physical condition. Furthermore, the United Service Organizations (USO), an appendage to these various branches of the armed forces, also utilize such programs of activity. The United Service Organizations consist of such agencies as the Young Men's Christian Association, Young Women's Christian Association, Travelers' Aid, Salvation Army, Catholic Charities Organization, Jewish Welfare Board, and Camp Shows, Incorporated.

The armed forces utilize thousands of acres of land, hundreds of gymnasiums and other buildings, hundreds of swimming pools, and thousands of qualified persons in physical education to organize and administer a physical training program. These programs are designed to keep military and naval forces in good physical and mental

Physical education program at United States Military Academy, West Point, New York.

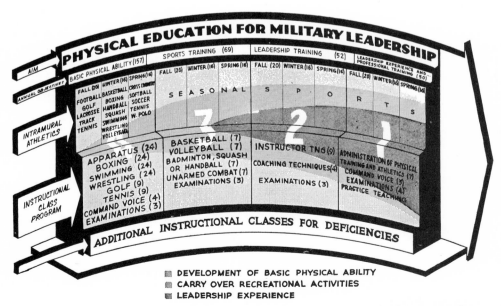

OFFICE OF PHYSICAL EDUCATION—
U. S. CORPS OF CADETS.

condition at all times, to develop skills so that officers and men will have the foundational equipment to spend leisure hours in a worthwhile manner, and to help build morale through a broad sports program. The armed forces have long known that a strong America means a healthy and physically fit America.

In one year one Army installation had many team and individual sports in its program. Tables 3-4 and 3-5 give a report on sports participation.

Table 3-4. Team sports participation at one Army installation*

Sport	No. of teams	No. of competitions
Football	241	1,501
Baseball	1,197	9,137
Softball	6,205	38,347
Basketball	3,716	95,800
Volleyball	6,958	84,875
6-Man volleyball	47	672
Touch football	2,350	10,450
Handball	4	25
Soccer	245	3,580
Field hockey	1	31
Water polo	6	15

*Personal communication.

Industrial concerns

Both labor and management recognize the importance of physical education activities as part of the industrial recreational program that pays mental and physical dividends to all participants. It further results in better health, more efficiency, greater production, and more happiness for employer and employee. Recreational programs in which physical activities play an important part have been organized in industrial plants and in various commercial agencies, such as insurance companies, banks, and department stores. These programs are financed in various ways: by the company, by the employees, or jointly by management and labor. Skating rinks, dance halls, swimming pools, gymnasiums, bowling alleys, and outdoor areas are some of the facilities provided; activities include bowling, tennis, horseshoes, volleyball, basketball, softball, golf, fishing, outings, table tennis, and baseball. Some companies have developed playgrounds in those sections of a community where their employees live, whereas others have leased large buildings where sports can be held and camps where men and women employees, as well as children of employees, have an opportunity to relax and enjoy the out-of-doors.

Table 3-5. Sports participation at one Army installation*

Sport	No. of participants		Sport	No. of participants
Boxing	244,517		Skeet	210,858
Bowling	17,282,040	(Lines bowled)	Horseshoes	326,958
Swimming	489,036		Gymnastics	89,603
Tennis	172,982		Roller skating	44,840
Badminton	243,589		Judo	19,380
Track	85,594		Archery	12,440
Golf	602,902		Wrestling	41,987
Equestrian	4,200		Curling	120
Basketball	20,168		Trampoline	8,355
Fishing	143,833		Shuffleboard	260
Handball	183,622		Skiing	11,580
Weight lifting	269,463		Soccer	16,030
Volleyball	12,544		Boating	1,623
Table tennis	1,690,014		Hunting	400
Squash	15,239		Surfing	117,280
Fencing	1,830			

*Personal communication.

A typical company recreation program frequently offers more than one-half of its activities in athletic or sports activities. The popularity of these activities among the workers is usually the factor that creates this situation. These activities are offered on an individual participation basis; in family groups; in the form of intramural-type leagues, interdepartmental teams and leagues, varsity teams, club groups; and on a class instruction basis.

Also, many different types of physical fitness programs are being developed in the nation's industries. These include fitness programs for workers, and recently there has been much emphasis aimed at fitness for executives. For example, Stromberg Carlson in Rochester, New York, has developed a health service area, steam room, private exercise room, shower, and locker rooms for their chief executives. Industry is increasingly recognizing that it has considerable money invested in key men (one company pointed out that when a young executive died from a heart attack it cost them $250,000 to replace him). Physical fitness programs are aimed at helping these executives and other members of the staffs of industry to maintain their health and well-being.

Youth organizations

There are many clubs and organizations for boys and girls that provide a setting for many physical education activities. Some of the organizations that fall in this group are the Boy Scouts of America, Boys' Brigades of America, Girl Scouts, Camp Fire Girls, Big Brother and Big Sister Federation, 4-H Clubs, Boys' Clubs of America, Boy Rangers of America, Hi-Y, Y-Teens, Red Shield Clubs, Future Farmers of America, and Pioneer Youth of America. Some of these organizations are international as well as national in scope. The extent of their membership is very great. For example, the Boys' Clubs of America have 870 clubs in more than 560 cities and towns in forty-seven states with over 800,000 boys as members. Girls' Clubs of America have 100,000 members. The Girl Scouts of the United States of America has 369 Girl Scout Councils; 163,000 Girl Scout troops; 672,000 adult members; and over 3 million girl members. In addition, girl scouting in the United States is affiliated with the World Association of Girl Guides and Girl Scouts. This association links together more than 5.5 million members in over sixty-five countries around the world. The Boy Scouts of America have approximately 147,000 units; 4.144 million registered scouts; and 1.59 million volunteer adult leaders. Big Brothers of America have 30,000 members and 135 member agencies. There are 600,000 members of Campfire Girls, Inc. The 4-H Program includes over 2.381 million members in 94,700 local clubs.

The American Youth Hostels, Inc., with 35,000 members in twenty-five councils, is an agency that provides overnight housing facilities for individuals who are anxious to travel, see, and study conditions in various parts of the United States and other countries. The mode of transportation in most cases is either hiking or bicycling. Every year many groups of young people, under trained leaders, set out for some distant point. The educational benefits derived from such an experience have proved very valuable. Personnel are needed to provide the necessary leadership, and physical educators are qualified, by reason of their training, to play an important part in this movement.

The purpose of these organizations is to serve youth in a manner that will prepare them for adulthood and make them better citizens. They are interested in developing in each boy and girl such characteristics as self-reliance, courage, and patriotism. They encourage the development of skills for the worthy use of leisure time. They promote projects that result in better health, better mental hygiene, stronger character, and a sounder physical condition. For example, the four "H's" of the 4-H Club stand for "Head, Heart, Hand, and Health" development.

Physical education activities play a major part in the program of activities for these various clubs and organizations. Out-of-door activities on the playground and in the camp are as important as indoor activities in the gymnasium and in the swimming pool. Sports and other physical education activities strongly appeal to boys and girls, and as long as this interest exists, physical activity will be an essential phase of the total program.

Recreational areas

Most communities have playgrounds. In small towns the playground functions during the summer months; in larger towns they function in the spring, summer, and fall; and in many large cities they are organized and administered on a year-round basis. Playgrounds are established mainly for children and young people, although adults frequently participate in many of the activities offered. The playground is a place where children may develop skills, enjoy themselves in wholesome physical activity, develop healthy bodies, and develop good citizenship traits under competent leadership. The type of facilities and equipment varies from playground to playground,

depending upon the amount of money available for such a purpose and the value placed on such an enterprise by the community concerned. On well-equipped playgrounds, facilities and equipment may be found for all types of games, athletics, dancing, swimming, self-testing activities, and arts and crafts. The number of staff members varies with the size of the playground. Both men and women may be found supervising and directing playgrounds and the special activities within a single playground.

In addition to playgrounds, communities and apartment dwellings are including recreation areas where swimming pools, paddle tennis courts, and other activity areas exist. This is particularly true where new housing developments are coming into being and the developers are making it a practice to include facilities for physical activities for the occupants.

Many parks and green spaces have also been developed, and they utilize the services of physical educators. These may be located in a community, city, county, park, or other place where recreational facilities

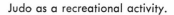
Judo as a recreational activity.

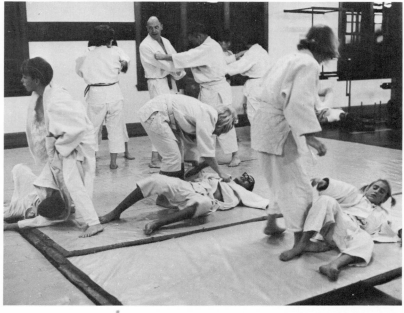

FROM MICHAELSON, MIKE: JUDO: NOW IT'S A SAFE FAMILY SPORT,
TODAY'S HEALTH, FEBRUARY, 1969.

have been created for the use of the populace.

Athletic clubs and other sport organizations

Because of the increased popularity of sports and physical activity in the United States during the late 1800's and early 1900's, many athletic clubs were organized. The membership at that time was usually composed of young adults who wanted a place where they might engage in some form of wholesome physical activity. The idea has gradually grown, until today we find numerous athletic clubs and other sports organizations mushrooming all over the nation. The membership in these organizations is great. Some clubs cater to the wealthy, whereas others serve persons in various income brackets. At first these athletic clubs offered many sports, but today many clubs also cater to individuals who are interested mainly in one sport or, at the most, a very few. Thus can be found such organizations as archery clubs, fencing clubs, golf clubs, tennis clubs, fishing clubs, rod and gun clubs, bowling clubs, yachting clubs, and polo clubs. Also, many country clubs stress social life as well as such sports as golf, tennis, and swimming.

Many of these clubs are staffed with professionals who are experts in some particular sport as well as other individuals trained in various physical education activities.

In addition to the organizations that have been mentioned, there are Turnvereins and Sokol organizations that are designed to provide a place for physical activities primarily of a gymnastic variety and also a place for social activities. (See Chapter 12 for more information on Turnvereins.)

Professional and commercial areas

The area of professional sports and other physical education activities offers a setting for many highly skilled individuals. Professional football, basketball, baseball, hockey, golf, soccer, and tennis are a few of these areas, and, in addition, there are other physical education activities that have professional possibilities, such as gymnastic acts, aquatics, and dancing. In the commercial area can be found dance studios, theaters, radio and television programs, roller rinks, golf courses, swimming pools, bowling alleys, sports equipment stores, resort areas, reducing and exercise clubs, beauty spas, and many places of amusement

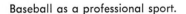
Baseball as a professional sport.

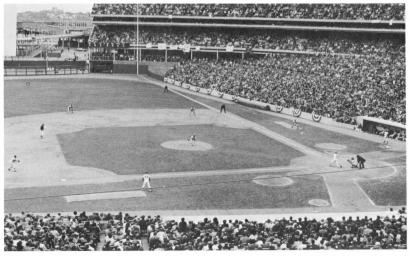

COURTESY AMERICAN BROADCASTING CO.

that utilize physical education activities as a means of entertainment. As a rule, the public wants to be entertained, and physical educators have capitalized on this desire.

Camps

Camping has grown in popularity until today there are numerous camps located in nearly every section of the country. There are over 20,000 camps throughout the nation. These are operated by cities, counties, and states; by such social agencies as churches, schools, and settlements; by such youth-serving agencies as YMCA, YWCA, YMHA, YWHA, Boy Scouts, Girl Scouts, Camp Fire Girls, 4-H Clubs, and Boys' Clubs Federations; by employer and labor organizations; and by private individuals and corporations. Some camps are operated for profit, whereas others work on a nonprofit basis. Some are open only during the summer months, others during the spring, summer, and fall, and others all year round. Some are for children, others for adults, and still others for adults and children. Some are day camps, whereas others operate on a seasonal basis. Some are for just one sex, and others operate on a corecreational basis. In recent years, tennis, football, basketball, baseball, horseback riding, and other activity camps have been opened to provide a place for the young person interested in developing further skill in a particular sports activity.

Regardless of the type of camp, most utilize physical education activities as one of the main features in their program. They stress outdoor living and utilize such activities as sailing, swimming, canoeing, all types of athletics, horseback riding, archery, and dancing.

Government and welfare agencies

Several governmental agencies such as state departments of education, city boards of education, U. S. Office of Education, President's Council on Physical Fitness and Sports, and other such agencies utilize physical education personnel to direct, adminis-

ter, and supervise programs. In addition, they act in a consulting capacity to the schools, industry, and other groups that have need for their services.

Village, county, city, state, and national governmental units have provided settings for physical education activities as well as privately supported welfare agencies. Some of these settings are orphanages, homes for the aged, wildlife preserves, and Job Corps and Head Start centers. The last two programs should receive special attention because of their place in modern times.

Job Corps

The Job Corps program was established as part of the Economic Opportunity Act of 1964. The Job Corps is a voluntary program that provides programs of education, vocational training, or conservation work for young people. Many of the underprivileged young men who participate in the Job Corps program are school dropouts, job applicants, or those who failed tests for the armed forces.

The training that Job Corps trainees follow is designed to give them an opportunity to assume responsibility and prepare them for useful work. It provides intensive education in basic skills at the same time it gives work experience.

In many Job Corps programs opportunities are provided for participation in sports and other physical activities where physical educators are needed.

Head Start

The objective of Head Start, another phase of the government's antipoverty program and administered by the U. S. Office of Economic Opportunity, is to take children from disadvantaged neighborhoods and provide 8 weeks of preschool experience, plus physical care, during the summer prior to their entering either kindergarten or first grade. In other words, it is preschool education for deprived children. It is now realized that it is during the earliest years of a child's life that his capacity for learning is largely developed; if this opportunity is lost, it can never be fully retrieved.

In its first summer of operation in 1965, Project Head Start enrolled some 560,000 children in 13,400 child development centers in 2,400 communities. It was so successful that it has been continued on a permanent basis with programs running throughout the year as well as in the summer. The government appropriates up to 90% of the cost.

Several million children have taken part in the Head Start program. Many questions have been raised about the program: for example, what are the long-range effects of the program on the child after he leaves Head Start? Such questions indicate that much more research needs to be done as to the worth of the program.

Any community is permitted to initiate its own Head Start program. However, it must comply with such requirements as that of seeing that classes are small and that they are taught by a professional teacher assisted by two other adults. The program is nonstructured and consists of many activities such as painting, reading, listening to music, modeling, playing with all sorts of toys, and engaging in various games.

Each child receives a medical and dental examination, something that many of them have never experienced. Medical and dental problems are referred to the public health department in the local community.

The Head Start program has claimed to be successful in showing that pupils have a significant gain in verbal intelligence equivalent to a rise of 8 to 10 points in IQ scores, better social relations as evidenced by the ability to engage in group play, and improved self-confidence.

Thousands of parents are serving as volunteers in the program, including both men and women. Many physical educators who are parents volunteer to make toys and instruct pupils in games. There are many opportunities in this setting to serve youngsters and make sure that they get off on the right foot toward a meaningful, physically healthy, educational existence. Physi-

cal educators should recognize the opportunities that are present for them to render this special service.

Churches

Protestant, Catholic, Jewish, and other religious leaders recognize that the religious life of man is closely tied in with his physical, mental, and social life. They are beginning to see that all are essential to living a "good" life. Furthermore, the old Puritan idea that play is sinful and something that should not be associated with the church is rapidly becoming a thing of the past. The church is concerned with how it can help people to spend their leisure hours in a more profitable manner and how it can further promote fellowship and social and physical well-being among its members.

Many churches are providing leadership and facilities so that physical education activities may become a vital part of their programs. Frequently gymnasiums, bowling alleys, tennis courts, and various items of apparatus are part of a church's physical plant. Churches are organizing programs of physical activity around various age groups. They are finding that it aids considerably in helping to attract youth to the church.

The Catholic Youth Organization, for example, has a program that is church sponsored and carries on a vigorous and interesting sports program. This organization serves not only boys and girls under high school age but also youth not attending school.

Hospitals

The utilization of physical education activities in hospitals is rather new. Federal hospitals utilize various physical education activities to some extent, as do the Veterans Administration Hospitals. In federal hospitals the American Red Cross is largely responsible for such a program, whereas the Veterans Administration has its own specialized staff located in central and regional offices and in each hospital. The entire program of physical activity in these hospitals is under the close supervision of the medical staff. The activities offered vary according to the condition of the patient and the facilities available. It is individual work to a great degree, and the activity must be adapted to the needs of the patient. A person suffering from a cardiac ailment might need restricted exercise, whereas, according to many doctors, a neuropsychiatric patient would need to engage in active sports to alleviate his mental condition. Therefore it can be seen that sports and other types of physical activity are a form of therapy for individuals who are hospitalized and as such are becoming recognized as a part of the total hospital program.

Penal institutions

The method of treating criminals, delinquents, and individuals who have displayed antisocial conduct has changed greatly during recent years. The repercussions of the Attica prison riot will make it change much more. Formerly it was thought that the inmate of a penal institution should be regimented, disciplined, and forced to pay for his crime or misdoing by suffering the rigid routine of prison life. It was believed that he should not enjoy his existence, nor should he be allowed to participate in any activities from which he might receive some satisfaction. Today, however, prison and reform-school authorities realize that the inmate may be rehabilitated. Through a planned program of reeducation, the criminal or delinquent may learn to develop social responsibility to the extent that when he is freed he may become a useful and responsible citizen.

Jackson Prison in Jackson, Michigan, is an example of a penal institution where athletics are used as a medium to help in the rehabilitation of inmates. The program includes weight lifting, baseball, tennis, volleyball, touch football, handball, basketball, and miniature golf. Nearly all the prisoners participate in some activity and part of the program, which includes intramurals and varsity competition.

In any program of rehabilitation and reeducation, sports can play and are playing a valuable and important part. They aid in contributing to the physical and mental health of the participants and also aid in demonstrating the need for cooperation, fair play, and other desirable traits.

There are over a million people in the United States in institutions for the delinquent, defective, and dependent. With such a large group of the population in these institutions, physical education activities have much to offer in helping to rehabilitate individuals so that they may serve society in constructive action rather than inhibit society's progress through antisocial conduct. The inmates in such institutions as reformatories, prisons, workhouses, penitentiaries, jails, prison farms, and detention homes should have the benefits of what a physical education program under qualified leadership has to offer.

Other countries

For a discussion of physical education activities in other countries, see Chapter 14.

QUESTIONS AND EXERCISES

1. List the various settings in which physical education activities are conducted. Which one do you feel is best adapted to your abilities, needs, and interests? Why?
2. To what extent do the nation's schools offer a prospective employment setting for the physical educator?
3. What are the responsibilities of physical education personnel at the elementary, junior high, senior high, and college levels?
4. How do the physical education programs differ at the various school levels?
5. Describe the physical education program in a Young Men's Christian Association or a Young Women's Christian Association with which you are familiar.
6. Make a survey of your home town to determine the various settings where physical education is being used or could be utilized effectively.
7. What are the objectives of settlement and neighborhood houses? How do physical education activities help in the achievement of these objectives?
8. What is the American Youth Hostels, Inc.? How does it help to satisfy the needs of American youth?

9. List as many boys' and girls' organizations as possible that utilize physical education activities.
10. Compare the attitude of the early church with the attitude of the church today in respect to physical activity.
11. To what extent are the playgrounds of your community helping to make your town a better place in which to live?
12. What is the importance of physical education to both labor and management?
13. What part do the following play as settings for physical education activities: athletic clubs and other sports organizations, hospitals, camps, penal institutions, professional and commercial areas, and the American Red Cross?
14. How can physical education contribute to the welfare of the armed forces?

Reading assignment

Bucher, Charles A., and Goldman, Myra: Dimensions of physical education. St. Louis, 1969, The C. V. Mosby Co., Reading selections 4 and 6.

SELECTED REFERENCES

American Council on Education: College teaching as a career, Washington, D. C., 1965, Publications Division, American Council on Education.

Brickman, William W.: Educational systems in the United States, New York, 1964, The Library of Education, The Center for Applied Research in Education, Inc.

Bucher, Charles A.: Administration of health and physical education programs including athletics, St. Louis, 1971, The C. V. Mosby Co.

Bucher, Charles A.: Administrative dimensions of health and physical education, including athletics, St. Louis, 1971, The C. V. Mosby Co.

Bucher, Charles A.: Health and physical education in other lands, Journal of Health, Physical Education, and Recreation **33**:14, 1962.

Bucher, Charles A., Koening, Constance, and Barnhard, Milton: Methods and materials for secondary school physical education, St. Louis, 1970, The C. V. Mosby Co.

Bucher, Charles A., and Reade, Evelyn M.: Physi-cal education and health in the elementary school, New York, 1971, The Macmillan Co.

Chevrette, John M., and Tolson, Homer: Individual prescription, Journal of Health, Physical Education, and Recreation **41**:38, 1970.

Ciszek, Raymond A.: A new dimension in international relations for the profession, Journal of Health, Physical Education, and Recreation **33**:17, 1962.

Eichhorn, Donald H.: The middle school, New York, 1966, The Library of Education, The Center for Applied Research in Education, Inc.

Kessel, J. Bertram: Trends in college physical education, The Physical Educator **25**:3, 1968.

Moore, Clarence A.: Building a junior college program, The Physical Educator **25**:78, 1968.

Morris, Van Cleve, and others: Becoming an educator, Boston, 1963, Houghton Mifflin Co.

Oxendine, Joseph B.: Status of required physical education programs in colleges and universities, Journal of Health, Physical Education, and Recreation **40**:32, 1969.

Rosewarren, Leonard: The YMCA physical directorship, Journal of Physical Education **63**:70, 1966.

Ross, Irwin: Head start is a banner project, The PTA Magazine **60**:20, 1966.

Ruffer, William A.: A study of required physical education for men in the United States colleges and universities, The Physical Educator **27**:79, 1970.

Shriver, Sargent: Five years with the Peace Corps, Saturday Review, p. 14, April, 1966.

Trump, J. Lloyd: An image of a future secondary school health, physical education, and recreation program, Journal of Health, Physical Education, and Recreation **32**:15, 1961.

U. S. Department of Health, Education and Welfare, Office of Education: Digest of educational statistics, Washington, D. C., 1965, U. S. Government Printing Office.

Vaughn, Jack: The Peace Corps, now we are seven, Saturday Review, January 6, 1968, p. 21.

Watkins, Angeline: Physical education activity requirement for women in selected colleges and universities in the South, Journal of Health, Physical Education, and Recreation **37**:71, 1966.

4/Projecting physical education into the future—forecast for the 70's

The space age offers a new and exciting way of life that has implications for physical education. Here are some of the conditions that will exist in A.D. 2000.

Three hundred and fifty million people will inhabit the United States, as contrasted with today's more than 200 million. Three out of four persons will reside in cities— elongated strips of land dotted with thousands of home and other buildings. The cliff dwellers will include many of the younger set, since one out of every five persons in the country will be between 15 and 24 years of age. College will be a reality for four out of five high school graduates, most of whom will later go into the ranks of the professional and white-collar workers. The added years of education will pay off handsomely; the college graduates are destined to earn a higher salary and, coupled with this increased income, they will work fewer hours of work per week—32 on the average.

High income and more leisure will change the lives of most people. Some persons will continue to drink space cocktails, operate their 50-inch wall television screens, and read about life on the moon. But many will forsake the lazy life for more physically active pursuits. The total population will spend $10 billion a year on sporting goods alone, to play all types of games, many of which will be imported from abroad by some of the 4 million Americans who go overseas annually.

In the future, homes will be equipped electronically with thermoelectric refrigerators, electroluminescent lights, ultrasonic washing machines, controls on windows to close them when storms develop, picture phones, self-cleaning kitchen floors, microwave ovens, and garbage disposal units built into dishwashers. Clothes and bed sheets will be made of disposable material, eliminating the need for laundry. There will not be locks on doors since special computer arrangements will react to a person's voice, and in this way the door will open on command.

The future will find science developing pills to control the mind. There is much research going on to discover how man's brain works and to discover drugs to influence its operation. It appears probable that the day will come when pills can be purchased to help you to think better, improve your ability to concentrate, and help the memory processes. Much research is being done in connection with the production of a key chemical, ribonucleic acid or RNA, and its influence on the brain cells. There is some evidence to show that this chemical influences learning, and therefore science is trying to find a chemical compound that could be introduced into the brain to increase the production of RNA and thus influence learning.

The future will find that the health of man can be vitally improved for the better. Life expectancy will be increased as a result of a better understanding of medical science. Interchangeable human parts will help to ensure longer life. Other conditions and new techniques that are predicted for the years ahead are: cameras and miniature broadcasting systems that can be swallowed to take pictures inside the stomach and give a

Supersonic transport of the future.

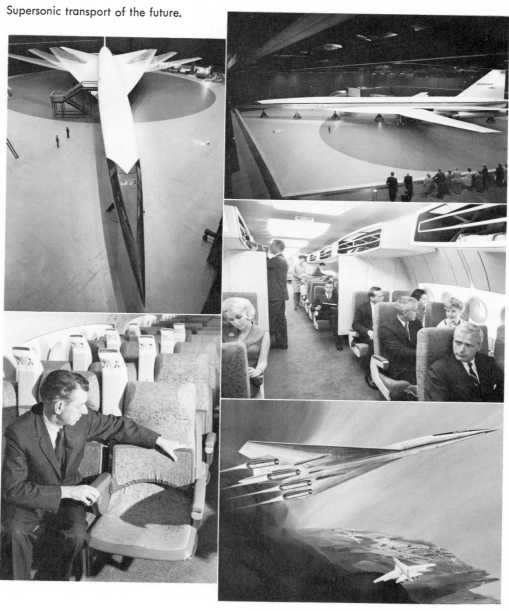

The promise of the seventies*

- At a real growth rate of 4% for the whole economy, and inflation curbed to 2½%, the whole economy may *double* in the next 10 years.

- At least 225 million Americans—22 million more than in 1969. Eleven million—45%—more between the ages of 25 and 34.

- 10.3 million new primary families, for a total of 61.5 million.

- In 1979, a third of U. S. households will have incomes of over $20,000.

- The typical consumer in 1979 will have at least 32% more to spend—in today's buying power—than he does now.

- Twenty million new living units—homes and apartments.

- 70% increase in plant and equipment spending—to $172 billion.

- 80% of high school graduates will go on to college in 1975 compared to 70% now.

- There will be almost 10 million college students by 1976-77.

- Value of production to *double*—to nearly $2 trillion by 1980.

Ten solid reasons for faith in the promise of the seventies.

---

*Adapted from The Putnam Management Company, Inc., 265 Franklin Street, Boston, Mass. 02110, investment adviser to The Putnam Group of Mutual Funds. Copyright 1969 by The Putnam Management Company, Inc.

listening doctor vital information; transistorized gadgets to stimulate damaged muscles; pocket radars to help the blind to see and the deaf to hear; and drug control of personality.

An article by Harold G. Shane and June Grant Shane* in *Today's Education,* the journal of the National Education Association, identifies, as a result of perusal of recent publications in the physical, natural, and social sciences, changes that are taking place in our society. These changes involving the people and cultures of the world have implications for education in general and also for physical education. They are summarized here in adapted form. In the years ahead, according to this report:

Individuals throughout the United States and the world will increasingly have more freedom, but this freedom will mean that their responsibility for this freedom will increase.

The IQ of the average boy and girl will be in the 125 to 135 range.

There will be a greater standardization of the cultures of the world as a result of the impact of mass media and greater mobility of people.

There will be greater consensus as to what constitutes desirable standards for the cultures of the world as a result of easier access to more information by all concerned. There will be greater consensus of desirable standards particularly in such areas as family life, art, recreation, education, diet, economic policies, and government.

Cruelty and inhuman treatment will be gradually eliminated.

Leadership roles will be played by persons who are the most able, regardless of ethnic origin, religious belief, and economic condition.

The role of women will change radically, giving females more worldwide status and influence.

The economic differences between the wealthy and the poor will diminish.

The better identification of trends will assist society in providing for the welfare of future generations of mankind.

IMPACT OF THE COMPUTER ON EDUCATION

Electronic information retrieval will make it possible to store in computers the contents of books and other information that can be instantly obtainable.

*Shane, Harold G., and Shane, June Grant: Forecast for the 70's, Today's Education **58:**29, 1969.

Computer centers will be established on a regional basis throughout the United States. Each will link many colleges and research institutions together in a high-speed computer network. Small institutions as well as large ones will benefit from these high-level computer services that will enable simultaneous computer use by many persons. The heart of each center will be large, high-speed computers capable of doing more than 1 million information manipulations a second. Through the utilization of typewriter-to-computer connections, involving regular telephone lines at many remote stations, the colleges will have round-the-clock access to this stored information.

Eventually, there will be extensive computer hookups to homes to help adults or children in solving advanced mathematics problems or obtaining valuable research information on health or other matters. By 1990, Professor Kemeny of Dartmouth College predicts, computer terminals will be as commonplace and as important a part of the American home as television or telephones are today. Professor Kemeny goes on to predict that each household will be connected to a central computer that can be used by thousands of people at the same time through the medium of teletype consoles connected through an ordinary telephone line. If a person wants some information he will dial the computer as he would use a telephone today. In addition to getting valuable knowledge about academic studies, the computer will prove useful to housewives in preparing balanced menus, placing orders for groceries, or doing their banking. For the education-minded housewife it will also provide an opportunity to work for an advanced degree at a university without leaving her living room. Children will also use the computer to do their homework for school.

It has been suggested that the computer may even be used in coaching. By feeding the computer information about football, for example, such as certain plays, the role that each player is assigned to play, the capabilities of the opponent, and as much other information as possible, the computer could then help to plan game strategy and also furnish valuable material for postgame critiques. It has been predicted that a coach on the bench might even feed into the computer the down and yards to go, time left in the game, the score, the playing conditions, the physical condition of each player, wind velocity, and other factors and find the best plays that will work against the opponents.

Another feature of the automated era of the future will make it possible for persons to engage in many dual sports by themselves. Computer mechanical arms will be developed so that a person can play such dual games as tennis or badminton, for example, between himself and a robot.

Furthermore, the accuracy of the official will be enhanced in such sports as baseball, for example, where an umpire with a photographic electronic eye will accurately record whether it is a strike or ball, fair or foul.

FORECAST FOR THE 70's—
GENERAL EDUCATION

Education in general during the 1970's will undergo many changes. Changes will have implications for the students who attend our schools and colleges, the teachers who make up the faculties of these institutions, the administration responsible for the vast educational undertaking, and the educational programs offered.

Students

Students will begin their education much earlier, in most cases at ages 3 and 4. More of the educational budget will be spent in the earlier years of education, which will be designed to increase the sensory imput from which young children develop their intelligence.

Education will become more individualized, with greater stress on the needs of each student, including the handicapped, mentally retarded, emotionally disturbed, gifted, and others. These atypical conditions will be identified earlier in the educational process, provided for from the earliest educational levels, and continued as long as necessary throughout the school years. More effective diagnostic tools will be used to indicate what students can benefit most from what types of educational programs.

Until the educational program of the ghetto and inner city can be improved to a more acceptable level, children will be transported to outlying areas where they will have the opportunity to experience better educational programs and more extensive contact with children from other social groups.

There will be more emphasis placed on student involvement in the learning process. Students will play an active part in determining at what rate they will proceed and in what projects and experiences they will participate.

All students who are so motivated and have the ability will be able to go to college and receive financial aid if necessary. All ethnic groups will be adequately served by the educational establishment. Educational opportunity centers will be established on a wide scale. They will provide study space, tutorial work, and advice, help in clarifying vocational and educational goals, conduct testing programs to determine abilities and interests, and provide information about financing educational careers.

Elementary, middle, and secondary schools will continue to attract students to their doors regardless of level of intelligence, emotional stability, desire for education, and socioeconomic levels. The type of education offered to the student who has the intellectual ability will differ from that for the student who is lower on the intellectual scale and must therefore pursue a slower academic pace. The student who is a fast learner, for example, will have much source material and equipment made readily available to him and have many opportunities for independent study and research. The student who is lower on the intellectual scale will have educational hardware and other techniques available to him in order to reinforce and ensure his mastery of at least certain basic concepts in basic subject matter

areas. There will also be a great expansion in vocational schools in order to furnish this type of education to those who so desire.

Students will move at an academic pace during their elementary, middle, and secondary school years in accordance with their ability and degree of motivation. Placement in classes will not be done according to age but instead by intellectual and scholastic ability.

At the college and university level students will fall into two classes. On the one hand will be the most promising students with outstanding mental capabilities who will go to the university where they will have the finest facilities and many opportunities to learn. The professors will arrange their time and attention to motivate and inspire the intellectually gifted and creative students so that they may develop their talents to the utmost. At the other end of the ability scale will be the average or subpar student who does not possess exceptional intellectual promise. These students will go to the 2-year colleges and state-college systems where standards will be lower than those in the universities.

The growth in the number of college-age men and women has slowed and will begin to decline after 1978. With nearly three-fourths of the high school graduates now going on to higher education, it is unlikely that there will be any further increase in the percentage of high school graduates continuing their education. Even a major influx of nonwhites, who have been underrepresented in college in the past, will not affect the total numbers significantly. The major influx of students will be into the graduate schools, where they will work on advanced degrees.

Teachers

Teachers will prepare for specialized roles where they feel they can make the greatest contribution to education. There will be researchers, scientists, artists, writers, media specialists, game theory specialists, and evaluation experts, for example.

The role of the teacher will be more of a "learning clinician" whose responsibility is to provide meaningful psychosocial treatment for students. The teacher will be especially concerned with such things as the environment, learning styles of students, and interpersonal relations.

Teachers will play a more important role in the administration and decision-making process of schools and colleges. The autocratic administrations will gradually disappear, with faculties and students playing a more active role in policy and decision making.

The profession of teaching will become more attractive, particularly to men, and consequently more males will enter this profession. However, according to the Bureau of Labor Statistics, so many young women are entering the teaching profession that by 1980 is it expected there will be an oversupply of 75% in elementary, middle, and secondary schools.

The beginning teacher will be given more time to orient to the task of a full-time teacher. Furthermore, the relationship with professional preparation institutions will be extended, with followup to help and advise the beginning teacher regarding problems encountered during the first years on the job.

Local Teacher Corps will be established to service ghetto, poverty, and other educationally deprived areas.

There will be many more paraprofessionals—teacher aides who will assist regular teachers. These assistants will assume clerical work, noon-hour supervision, and other details that do not require the attention of trained teachers. Consequently, the teacher will be free to spend more time on teaching, helping students, and doing those things where his training indicates the greatest service can be rendered. The teacher will also have more time for planning and thinking about the tasks to be performed.

Professional associations of teachers will play a more important role in seeing that proper ethical standards are maintained by the teaching profession and also will partici-

Airshelters. The city of the future.

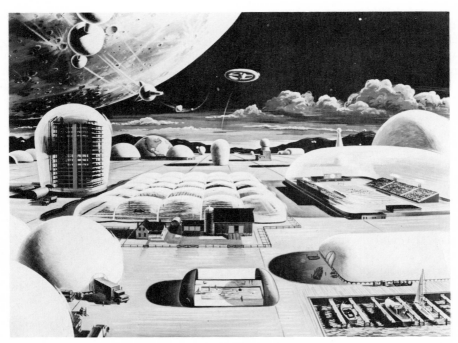

DIVISION OF BIRDAIR STRUCTURES, INC., BUFFALO, N.Y.

pate more in the certification and standard establishment processes for determining who is or is not eligible to teach in schools.

The status of the teaching profession will be upgraded slowly in the years ahead as education becomes a more important consideration in our society. Elementary, middle, and secondary school teachers, at least through the 1970's, will continue to be recruited from backgrounds that stress lower-middle-class values and conventional means of obtaining economic security. Most teacher-training institutions will be slow to change because of the conservatism of the educational establishment.

Teachers will become more militant. Labor unions will infiltrate into the schools and colleges on a wide scale. The unions, utilizing strikes and other labor union techniques, will be effective in securing teacher demands. A survey by the National Education Association shows the number of teachers approving of strikes has jumped 40% since 1965. It finds that 73% of them now think strikes are justified.

The teacher of the future will not have to repeat himself, since taped classroom discussions will be kept on file to facilitate makeup work for students who have missed class for some reason or who failed to get material that has already been presented. Videotapes will also assist the teacher in critically evaluating his own presentation, and in this way teaching will become more of an art.

Salaries for teachers will continue to increase in the years ahead, particularly for those persons who become master teachers and research scholars. The single-salary schedule will eventually give way to a merit plan that pays salaries to outstanding teachers on a scale comparable to the business and industrial executive class. The great number of the nation's teachers who are compelled to take a second job will eventually disappear. For college professors, the compensation of senior members of the faculty will be much greater than that of their junior associates.

Teachers in schools will be given more released time from teaching duties to pursue research studies and conduct experiments in their local research and development centers. Sabbatical leaves will be common to all schools and colleges. There will be a leveling off of the decline in teaching loads of college professors. This leveling off is the result of such factors as the scarcity of positions available and public dissatisfaction with professors making teaching a small part of their total load.

The shortage of Ph.D.'s is at an end. By the end of the 70's only a quarter or less of new doctorates will enter college teaching, compared to 50% or more of new Ph.D.'s employed by the colleges and universities over the last 10 years.

Other changes at the college level will find the retirement age of faculty members being lowered, an increase in the sense of faculty stability and institutional identification, more selective tenure decisions, and a greater faculty involvement in the decision-making process.

Administration

Those individuals desiring to be school administrators will be required to serve internships after graduating from college (much like doctors do today) and pursue graduate study that will include an extensive study of administrative theory, particularly as it relates to the behavioral sciences.

School administration will be much more democratic, with faculties and students working with administrators in shaping policies and making decisions.

Administrators and boards of education will be required to justify the amount of money that they spend on education in terms of more tangible results. For example, how much more effectively does a student learn mathematics under one system of teaching as compared to another, or how effectively does the physical education program teach skills to all its students?

School administration will be decentralized, particularly in the large cities, with more and more control being vested in the inhabitants of a particular community.

Federal and state involvement in the educational process will increase. Many new demands will be made upon educational programs by federal and state authorities to ensure that all children receive an acceptable standard of education.

In addition to the local contributions, more and more money invested in education will come from federal and state levels as well as business sources.

At the college level, there will be a decentralization of administration and social control, through a division of the student body into "houses" or "colleges." Each of these units will be self-sustaining with its own cafeterias, dormitories, classrooms, educational facilities, gymnasiums, and recreational facilities.

At the college level there is an organizational trend toward the proliferation of satellite universities and junior colleges to provide for increased enrollments.

Educational program

The primary, middle, and secondary schools will provide a coordinated learning experience personalized to meet the needs of each individual student. Promotional policies and grade designations will disappear as children move ahead at their own pace.

Educational hardware such as audiovisual aids, teaching machines, and computers will be utilized more and more in the teaching process.

Electronic retrieval machinery and faster dissemination techniques will enable educators and students to keep abreast of new knowledge and new developments in education as well as in a variety of subject-matter fields.

Curriculum materials will be developed not only by educators but also by business and other specialists who possess expertise in certain areas of the curriculum. Business will also help educators in tackling pollution problems, teaching certain specialized skills in other subject-matter areas, and providing training for dropouts.

The preparation of teachers and the educational programs for students will reflect a greater stress on the behavioral sciences and on the cognitive, psychomotor, and affective domains. More study will be given to biochemical therapy as a means of improving personality, memory, and other characteristics of students.

Educational programs will be conducted on a 12-month basis in both schools and colleges. A greater number of offerings and more students, plus the waste associated with letting school buildings remain idle during the summer months, will dictate this change. There will be staggered vacations for both students and teachers. The year-round school idea will help to relieve the overcrowded conditions that exist for recreational facilities in light of the growing population and greater interest in and additional time available for recreation.

Automation, new techniques, and frontier-type ideas will be continually introduced into education. The fear of newness and change that is characteristic of many teachers will gradually be overcome as it is realized that many innovations will result in better learning for more children. Consequently, teaching machines, programmed instruction, language laboratories, educational television, tape recorders, four-speaker sound systems, super-8 cassettes, and an extensive electronics system will become part and parcel of education.

FORECAST FOR THE 70's— PHYSICAL EDUCATION

There will be many changes in physical education during the 1970's. By 1980 most of the programs that will exist will be very different from those that prevailed in the schools and colleges during the 1960's. Changes will take place in respect to the teachers, physical education programs, athletic programs, education for leisure, and facilities.

Teachers

The teacher of physical education in the future will have a specialized role to play. All teachers will not perform the same duties. For the elementary and secondary school levels, two types of teachers will be trained. First, there will be the teacher who is primarily interested in teaching physical skills. This teacher will be a specialist in this area and utilize an analytical method, breaking down the various skills into their most minute subdivisions, and then teaching from a kinesiological approach so that the student learns the basic scientific principles underlying good movement.

The other type of physical education teacher will be an expert in research techniques and will understand thoroughly the scientific basis underlying physical activity as it relates to human development. Furthermore, through his knowledge of teaching techniques, he will be able to apply this information to program development as well as communicate this knowledge to the student in an interesting, clear, and accurate manner.

These two types of teachers of physical education will make up one part of a team that handles the program in the gymnasium, playground, and swimming pool, as well as in the classroom. Other members of the team will include clerical help, student teachers, and consultants from the disciplines of biology, psychology, and sociology.

At the college and university level, both types of teachers will also be present in the basic instruction and in the professional preparation programs. As in the case of the precollege level, many members of the faculty will have released time to do research. In some cases, teachers and professors will have joint appointments in the biology, psychology, sociology, or special education departments.

In addition to these basic types of roles that physical educators will play, there will also be specialists in such areas as coaching, audiovisual media, movement education, and working with the handicapped.

Program

The physical education program for students in our schools and colleges will experience many changes in the years to come.

Students will play an increasingly active role in determining the type of physical education program that will best meet their needs and interests. This will be reflected in such innovations as more elective programs, where students select from groups of activities those in which they want to specialize. In addition, there will be independent study, where a student may spend an entire semester on some particular sport project or activity, and also provisions for students to take tests, which, if passed, will provide exemption from the physical education requirement.

The physical education program will become more instructional and sequential in nature as it proceeds through the primary, middle, secondary, and college levels of education. Some national standards will be established whereby individual schools, students, and administrators may compare themselves at any particular age or educational level with national norms. In many schools, programs will be placed on a voluntary basis rather than being required. This change will be brought about as the demand increases on the part of many subject-matter areas for more valuable space, time, and budget dollars for their programs.

Physical education will emphasize environment and ecology in their programs with involvement in total school, community, and home programs to improve such things as our polluted air and streams and protect other resources. Furthermore, there will be more community involvement on the part of physical educators in contributing to solution of the problems of the inner city.

The 70's will see a greater emphasis on research, with physical education programs reflecting new knowledge in respect to such areas as motor learning, sociology of sport, working with the handicapped, and programs that are best for the ghetto.

Physical education will grow in importance at the elementary and middle school levels as there is increased recognition among educators regarding the contribution that perceptual-motor training and movement education can make to children, such as improving their self-concept and contributing to reading and speech skills.

Evaluation will play a much more important role in determining the world of physical education programs in the future. In many cases, outside specialists will be called in to evaluate objectively the contribution of physical education programs to students in light of the time spent, space utilized, and budget costs. In some cases, physical education programs will be dropped and personnel dismissed because the value of physical education cannot be justified by objective data.

The 70's will see the extensive utilization of computers and measurement instruments to accurately group students into physical education teaching units according to abilities, traits, skills, physical fitness, and previous experiences in physical education.

A vast system of records will be kept for each student from the time he is in kindergarten until he graduates from college. These records will ensure a better organized program related to each individual's needs and a more progressive program through the grades and college. These records will follow the pupil everywhere he goes in school or college and will contain such information as physical fitness ratings, skills mastered, and knowledge accumulated. At the college level these records will have particular value in determining those students who will pursue the voluntary program in physical education and those who will have to take the required program because they have entered college with below-standard development in physical skills, knowledge, or some other aspect of fitness. Physical education will not be required of every student, only those who fall below acceptable university standards.

The program of physical education will be aimed at developing physically educated students, with a trend away from teacher-induced learnings toward student-motivated learnings. The conceptualized approach will be utilized as a result of the identification of the most important concepts to be transmitted to the student. These concepts will define the domain of physical education and the most important contributions the field makes to human beings. They will be developed in a sequential, developmental, progressive pattern from kindergarten through college, with the elimination of the overlapping, the repetition, and the trial-and-error methods of teaching that characterize some physical education programs of today.

Textbooks will be used in physical education classes and homework assigned as in other subject-matter fields. The aim will be to get at the *why* of the activity as well as the activity itself, with physical education meeting in the classroom as well as in the gymnasium. Although physical education will remain activity oriented, the goal will be to physically educate students so that they understand and identify closely with the importance of physical activity in their lives and its relationship to their physical, psychological, and sociological development. Such a goal, it has been determined, cannot be effectively accomplished without imparting a body of knowledge in the classroom that is closely related to the activity they engage in on the playground. Scientific knowledge that has been researched by our scholars will be articulately communicated to the students during the classroom sessions. Specialists in physical education will be in charge of programs starting early in the elementary school years and continuing through college. At the primary grade level, the classroom teacher will work very closely with the specialist in the conduct of the physical education program.

The movement emphasis will permeate the program throughout the school and college life of the student, showing him how to use his body most efficiently under all conditions. Physical movement will be analyzed in relation to the basic motion factors of weight, space, time, and flow. Many activities will be provided that give rise to the exploration and analysis of free and spontaneous movements of the whole body. Students will learn how a movement feels and become aware of the relationships of the different parts of their body. Furthermore,

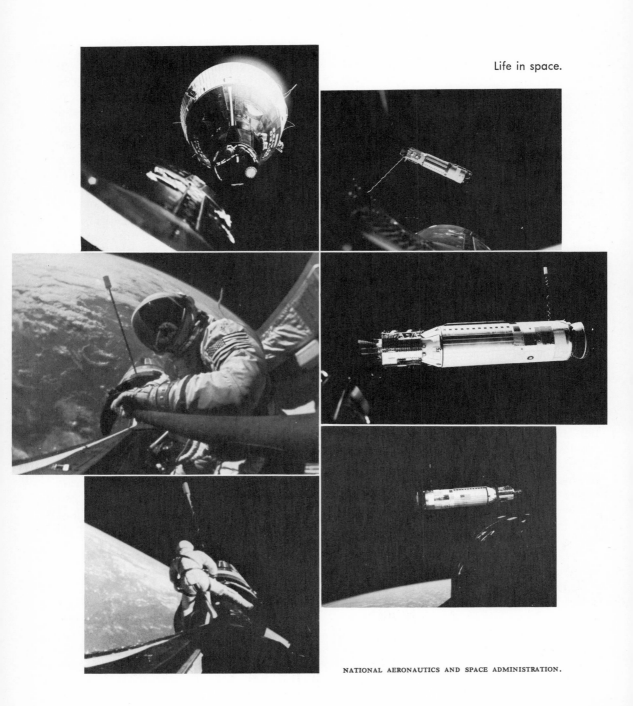

Life in space.

NATIONAL AERONAUTICS AND SPACE ADMINISTRATION.

through broad training opportunities they will enrich their movement possibilities and learn to think in terms of movement.

There will be many other program developments in physical education to provide for the mentally retarded, the orthopedically handicapped, the blind, the culturally disadvantaged, the emotionally disturbed, the poorly coordinated, all types of atypical students. Students who fall into these classifications will be identified early in their school years and educational programs will be adapted throughout their school life to meet their needs in the best way possible. Specialized programs and teachers trained for working with the handicapped will find prominent places in programs of physical education at both precollege and college levels.

The "club" movement will grow as a means of providing students and persons with special activity interests and opportunities to engage in their favorite activities. There will be all sorts of clubs including bicycling, surfing, skydiving, hiking, and skish. Faculty, school, and college sponsorship will give support to this development. The only criterion for membership will be interest in the activity. The only eligibility rule will be that the participant be a bona fide student.

Research will grow and result in the frontiers of knowledge being pushed back and new discoveries made in the relation of physical activity to mental, physical, and social development.

Effective public relations programs will continue to be emphasized so that parents and the public in general may more fully appreciate the importance and significance of physical education.

Elementary school physical education will be the focus of much professional effort, in order that a firm and strong movement education foundation may be laid for future physical education experiences of students.

The simple pleasures will continue to attract most participants: swimming, bicycling, fishing, hunting, camping, ice skating, hiking, walking, and sledding. But be-

cause of increased income, more activities usually associated with people in upper income brackets will be popular: boating, horseback riding, tennis, skiing, squash, sailing, water skiing, and golfing. Furthermore, school programs will place more emphasis on the activities that can be used throughout a lifetime. The controversial sport of boxing will not be permitted in school and college programs, and, outside of the educational setting, it will be scored as in fencing, with blows to certain parts of the body each counting a set number of points and with the head outlawed as a target.

The speed and increased frequency of travel will find many sports played on an international basis. Teams will be scheduled in Europe, South America, and Asia. There will be international sports leagues at the college level: Yale and Oxford may be battling it out for the rugby title and Reed and Nihon for the tennis championship. High schools will have television meets with their counterparts in other lands— Shaker Heights High School in Cleveland may schedule King George V High School in Hong Kong for archery.

Games that are popular in other countries will find a warm reception in the United States. The game of sipa, in which a rattan ball is kicked skillfully with the foot or hit with the head or shoulders, will be imported from the Philippines and Malaya. Japanese tennis, with three players on each side, will find wide acceptance as a means of making this sport available to more people. American boys will take a lesson from their counterparts in Asia and play field hockey on the high school and college level. Also, in the international frame of reference, there will be greater travel on the part of physical educators, more interchange of teachers both here and abroad, and a greater desire to help each of the developing countries achieve a higher level of health and fitness.

Athletic programs

In the area of athletics, there will be more interschool and intercollegiate athletic competition for women. Teams and leagues in many sports will become much more popular. In addition, many schools and colleges will have varsity and intramural teams made up of both boys and girls and men and women in the noncontact sports such as golf, tennis, and swimming. As a result of this emphasis, there will be increased involvement on the part of educators in Olympic development in order that the best girl and women athletes can be used in this international festival.

Precollege athletics will be drastically reformed over the years, with sanity becoming the byword and with athletics contributing to, rather than detracting from, a sound education.

Through the untiring efforts and dedication of many educators, a great change will come about in the control of educational sports. These devoted and informed men and women have proved they are the leaders in educational sports and the persons who determine the standards and policies to be followed. And they have rigorously and aggressively interpreted the difference between educational sport and professional sport to the American public. As a result, there is a clear distinction between the two. Educational sport will be interested solely in the participant and what it can do to make

him a better man or woman—mentally, physically, emotionally, and socially. It recognizes that sport is not an end in itself but, instead, is a means to an end—the end being the development of a better educated individual. Educators will so organize sports that players will be permitted to spend more time on their studies and pressures will be removed for championship teams. Under this system such features as the following will be instituted:

1. Athletic programs will be organized on a developmental pattern.
2. Athletic sports seasons and number of games played will be restricted in length—most school administrators feel that 10 weeks is a sufficient length of time for any one sports season.
3. Athletic practices will be limited to not more than 1½ hours per day.
4. Major sports will be made the minor sports and minor sports the major sports—the lifetime sports will get special consideration.
5. Gate receipts will be eliminated, with the cost being paid out of the general fund, the same as for English, mathematics, history, and other parts of the educational program.
6. Sport contests will be conducted only on school premises—the public arena with its gamblers, foul language, and rabid spectators will be a thing of the past.
7. Coaches will be appointed on the basis of their educational qualifications, not won-lost

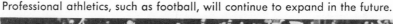
Professional athletics, such as football, will continue to expand in the future.

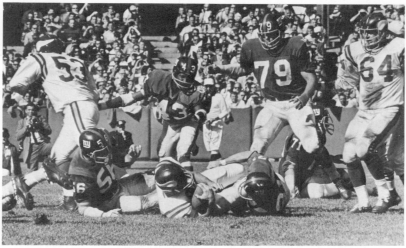

records. A knowledge of the participant physically, mentally, emotionally, and socially will be one of the most important qualifications.

8. Athletics will be an integral part of the total physical education program. The director of physical education will be assigned all the duties in regard to the athletic program.

9. All games will be played on weekday afternoons prior to days when school will not be in session—night games will be out.

At the college and university level, athletics will experience many changes. A major study of college athletics similar to the Carnegie study of the 1920's will take place. This study will expose many of the questionable practices being followed in our colleges and universities at the present time. New guidelines will be established for the future and will spell out in detail such things as: (1) the role of athletic associations to academic institutions, (2) the relationship of professional to amateur athletics, (3) the responsibility of college administrations to keep sports within a proper educational frame of reference, and (4) the role of the coach as a member of a university staff and faculty.

Intramural programs and coeducational recreational programs will increase. A further development will be the increase in the number of special club programs in many sports, including club football in many universities where there is a disinclination to be exposed to the pressures connected with "big-time" sports. Grants-in-aid for athletes will change. All monies will be deposited in a central university fund. Regardless of talent, whether in athletics, science, debating, or some other area, the student will be given financial help based on need and willingness to pay part of his own way through loans and campus work.

Athletic records

Records will fall as new training techniques are developed, more physiological research is produced, and new medical knowledge becomes known. Pills will increase energy output. Isometrics and other strength and power builders will be devel-

oped more scientifically. Practice periods will be shortened as teaching machines help football and other players to learn their plays more thoroughly. Coaches will follow more scientific procedures taught to them in college professional preparation programs specializing in such areas as psychology, sociometrics, and physiology.

The champions who break the amateur records will be teen-agers more often than not. Better training procedures, diet, and earlier maturation will produce a younger crop of record breakers. The scoreboard by the year A.D. 2000 may read as follows:

High jump	8 ft., 2 in.
Pole vault	25 ft.
Broad jump	30 ft.
100-meter dash	9 sec.
1-mile run	3 min., 30 sec.
Shot put	75 ft.
1-mile swim	14 min.
100-meter freestyle swim	49.6 sec.
100-meter breast stroke	1 min.

Participants and spectators

There will be more participants and more leagues, tournaments, and other attractive features of athletic programs. A larger, younger population will tax facilities to the hilt and consume billions of dollars worth of sports equipment. Girls will be as active as boys, with the women's liberation movement extending to physical education programs; a new hair spray will enable girls to play vigorously, take a shower, and still keep every hair in place. Even the older population will get into the act, with the flourishing Golden Age clubs directing them in active as well as passive activities.

The spectator problem will continue to be a bane on society. Automated existence, with moving sidewalks, dustless homes, snow-melting driveways, controlled grass growth, instant cooking and baking, and electrical eyes to open doors and windows in houses and offices will take its toll. Significant medical research showing the long and productive life to be associated with physical activity will go unheeded by a large number of people.

Education for leisure

Education and physical education will be vitally interested and concerned with leisure and its implications for the future. Forecasts predict that the average 38-hour work week we enjoy today will drop to 36 by 1976 and to 32 by the year 2000. In fact, there is a good possibility, according to one estimate, that only 10% of the population will be working; the rest will have to be paid to be idle. According to John Fischer, a futurist, by 1984 a man's life will be so influenced by leisure that the first 25 years will be spent getting an education, the second 25 years working, and the final 25 years enjoying the fruits of his labor. In fact, some futurists gloomily expect that the increased amount of leisure will result in a society run by a small elected elite who will preside over a multitude who have not developed their minds and who are kept happy through drugs and circuses.

The need to teach for the creative and productive use of leisure will be readily apparent. As one answer, Margaret Mead, the famous anthropologist, has suggested a new kind of vacation center where expert tutors would be provided vacationers who want to learn new languages, marine biology, food chemistry, mechanics, writing, or other pursuits.

A leisurely life in the future will not be an entire bed of roses. Problems, many of which will be created by the new technology and increased populations in the strip cities, will continually confront Americans. For example, the amount of open space available per person will tend to decrease at a faster rate than the population increases. The green spaces will be devoured by concrete and mortar, thus placing greater demands on city, county, state, and national parks. Ecological problems with polluted water, air, and other aspects of the environment will continue to plague mankind. Reservations will need to be made many months and years in advance to visit a place like the Yelowstone National Park. Cities will need to ration recreation, particularly in such an activity as golf. In the Los Angeles area at the present time, for example, it takes about four new 18-hole golf courses a year just to accommodate the growing number of golfers.

The increased amount of leisure time in the future with the shorter work week will present many mental health and other problems. People will find it difficult to know what to do. Many will become bored. Sports will offer one source of help. Education will be a major activity for all ages, since people will seek education as a way to use leisure and escape boredom.

Facilities

Increased population, rising school enrollments, city life, limited space, and skyrocketing labor and material costs will alter sports facilities. Outdoor swimming pools will be used year round, with plastic bubbles covering them when the snow comes. Playgrounds and athletic fields will also be used continuously and, in addition, will have convertible features; baseball fields and football gridirons will become hockey areas and basketball courts within an hour's time. Neighborhood playing fields on the roofs of apartment houses and civic buildings will serve inhabitants of housing developments in congested areas. Golf courses will be laid out in skyscrapers, three or four holes on each floor.

New ideas and new materials will be used in all construction. Artificial turf will make indoor facilities similar to the out-of-doors. New methods of supporting roof structures will be evidenced everywhere. This will produce large areas where activities can be engaged in free from poles, columns, and other obstructions. The "floating roof" will become common in all amphitheaters. The size of rooms and play areas will be flexible with increasing use of electrically powered equipment to change partitions, fold bleachers, and remove apparatus from play areas.

Weather will not prove a deterrent to the holding of athletic contests. Seasonal activities will operate year round, if desired. Huge arenas with roofs that roll back and form an outdoor amphitheater or, when

The simple pleasures will continue to attract most participants.

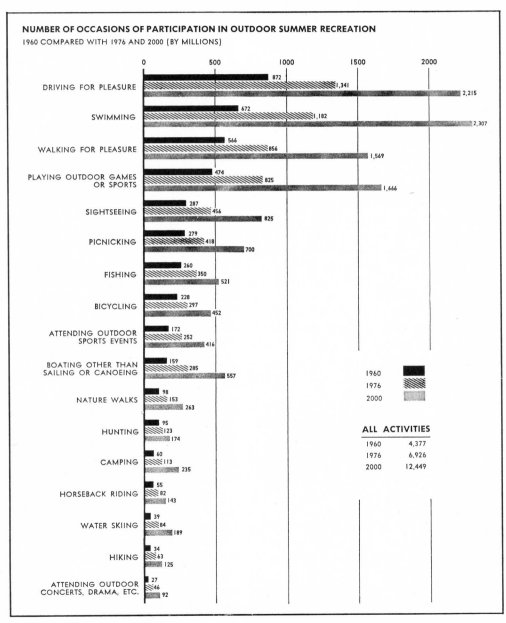

NUMBER OF OCCASIONS OF PARTICIPATION IN OUTDOOR SUMMER RECREATION
1960 COMPARED WITH 1976 AND 2000 (BY MILLIONS)

DRIVING FOR PLEASURE: 872, 1,341, 2,215

SWIMMING: 672, 1,182, 2,307

WALKING FOR PLEASURE: 566, 856, 1,569

PLAYING OUTDOOR GAMES OR SPORTS: 474, 825, 1,666

SIGHTSEEING: 287, 456, 825

PICNICKING: 279, 418, 700

FISHING: 260, 350, 521

BICYCLING: 228, 297, 452

ATTENDING OUTDOOR SPORTS EVENTS: 172, 252, 416

BOATING OTHER THAN SAILING OR CANOEING: 159, 285, 557

NATURE WALKS: 98, 153, 263

HUNTING: 95, 123, 174

CAMPING: 60, 113, 235

HORSEBACK RIDING: 55, 82, 143

WATER SKIING: 39, 84, 189

HIKING: 34, 63, 125

ATTENDING OUTDOOR CONCERTS, DRAMA, ETC.: 27, 46, 92

1960
1976
2000

ALL ACTIVITIES

1960	4,377
1976	6,926
2000	12,449

FROM REPORT TO THE PRESIDENT AND CONGRESS
BY THE OUTDOOR RECREATION RESOURCES
REVIEW COMMISSION: OUTDOOR RECREATION
IN AMERICA, WASHINGTON, D. C., JANUARY, 1962.

closed, protect against rain, wind, or snow will exist in every section of the country.

Nighttime will not prove a handicap to participation, since golf courses, tennis courses, and playfields will be illuminated so as to give daylight effect and serve the greater number of people who desire to participate.

Gymnasiums will become larger, more adaptable, more all-purpose, and more mechanical. Teachers will operate a control board, and at the push of the right buttons, the necessary equipment for each class will, in the span of a few seconds, either come out of the wall, lower from the ceiling, or come up out of special floor compartments. There will be plastic gym flooring, requiring little maintenance, guaranteed not to warp, and with all the necessary marking and lines impregnated and wear-proof. There will be wall and ceiling panels sensitive to electrical impulse instead of light bulbs.

Audiovisual centers will be readily available for individual student study on various sport skills or other aspects of physical education. Centers will contain television, movies, super-8 cassettes, tapes, and teaching machines. Materials such as rules, strategies, facts of anatomy, and first aid

will be programmed, so more time will be free for skill development.

At the college level, athletic and recreation facilities, such as tennis and handball courts, and swimming facilities will be strategically located throughout the entire campus, using the open green space around dormitories and other campus structures. Furthermore, in order to cut costs, there will be interinstitutional cooperation among colleges and universities close to one another. Colleges will share gymnasiums, libraries, cafeterias, and other facilities.

Manufacturers will continue to discover new ways to improve equipment. New and better materials for shoes and clothing will make them lighter and provide for easier movement. Uniforms for physical education classes will be made of throwaway material and will be disposed of after wearing. It will be cheaper to do this than laundering them even once.

• • •

These startling developments mean that there must be much planning and building for the years ahead. Physical educators must not be complacent. Instead, they must

Exterior of Sherwood Elementary School, Greeley, Colorado.

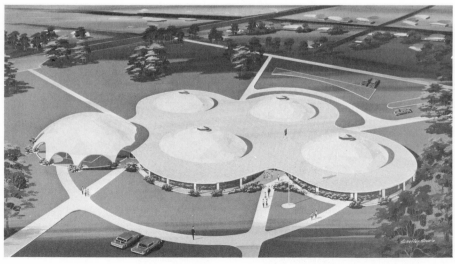

exercise vision and imagination in progressing toward this new way of life. Perhaps most important, physical educators must be ready to change.

THE INGREDIENTS ESSENTIAL TO CHANGE IN PHYSICAL EDUCATION

". . . then you had better start swimming
or sink like a stone,
For the times they are a-changing . . ."
BOB DYLAN

The implications of this verse are very clear for physical education. The world, education, and our society are in the midst of change. Unless we adapt our programs to meet the changing conditions, physical education will "sink like a stone." We must incorporate into our programs new ideas that meet the needs of our students and human beings in general.

Change is a process that takes time. The steps through which change usually occurs are: *First,* the physical educators become aware of a needed innovation, for example, movement education in the elementary school. *Second,* as more and more people become interested in the innovation, an interest stage develops. Interest in movement education has been generated through experimental programs, workshops, writings, and other means of communicating the idea to educators. *Third,* there is the evaluation stage, where physical educators determine the values that the change has for their programs—values that relate directly to the student and the goals of physical education. *Fourth* comes more extensive experimenting with the idea, and, finally, the *last step* is adoption. Movement education has gone through these steps in many school systems with the change being adopted. However, many of the elementary schools in the United States have not changed their program to incorporate movement education into their elementary schools. Therefore, more change needs to take place not only in respect to movement education but also in many other areas.

Miller,* in her article entitled "A Man to Fill the Gap: The Change Agent," points out that each profession needs to bring about change to lessen the gap between what they know and what they practice. Since there is a big gap between what we know and what we practice in physical education, change is needed and change agents are necessary to bring about the needed change. Miller defines the change agent as "a professional who has as his major function the advocacy and introduction of innovations into practice" or a professional person who tries to influence decisions that will bring about the adoption of new ideas. In bringing about change, the change agent, according to Miller, should be aware of seven principles. They are presented here in adapted form and related to physical education.

1. *The change agent must be well informed as to the needs and characteristics of the client system.* The students and other human beings, such as the physical education staff in a school or college where it is desired to effect the change, are the client system. It is important for the change agent to base his plans on their needs.

2. *The change agent must develop a close relationship between himself and the client system.* There must be a confidence in the change agent. A mutual trust and respect must exist between the client system and himself, for unless the client system has confidence in him, change cannot effectively be brought about.

3. *The change agent must realize that change is not a unilateral undertaking but, instead, is a mutually cooperative affair.* The autocratic director of physical education who orders the innovation will never succeed. Change is a cooperative procedure between the change agent and the staff of his school system. As a result, there may be compromise and modifications, but the changes that are made will be more permanent and better accepted by the staff.

---

*Miller, Peggy L.: A man to fill the gap: the change agent, Journal of Health, Physical Education, and Recreation **40**:34, 1969.

4. *The change agent should enlist the support of key leaders in the client system.* Key leaders among the students in the school system and the physical education staff, as well as other persons, can help to ensure that the change is accepted by the client system and is adopted. Their involvement is essential in getting the entire student body and staff to accept the new development.

5. *The change agent needs a well-developed plan and strategy for introducing change.* The plan for bringing about change in an organization cannot be a hit-or-miss affair. Foresight and planning must decide the timetable for moving from one step to the next in innovating change, for identifying the key leaders who in turn will influence others, and for formally approving the change. Also, the techniques to be used, the communication media to be solicited, the persons to be seen, the meetings to be held, and the information to be imparted must all be carefully planned out so that nothing is left to chance.

6. *The change agent must be willing to change himself and to keep up with the times.* In order to be effective in bringing about change in others, the change agent must be a model of change himself. He must reflect an image of self-renewal and self-improvement. Such a person is needed in order to emphathize with others and to be sensitive to the change process.

7. *The change agent needs to help others to become change agents.* The change agent's success will be determined in large measure in how well he gets other members of a staff or organization to become change agents themselves. In so doing they will be abreast of the latest research findings in their field, have a recognition of the need for innovation, possess the ability to make wise choices as to what innovations will best help the client system, and be willing to try new ideas and practices.

A TEN-POINT PROGRAM FOR THE FUTURE OF PHYSICAL EDUCATION

All the disciplines and subject-matter fields of modern education must keep abreast of new developments in order to meet the needs of their constituency. In today's educational world, to remain impervious to change and to become stagnant as a profession is to invite disaster and oblivion.

The new developments that are occurring and that have already altered the programs of other subject-matter areas also have implications for physical education. Consequently, we need to study our present programs and practices and determine whether we are meeting the needs of our students and keeping up with the times.

Although there is a risk in trying to forecast and write prescriptions for the future and in discussing such recommendations very briefly, I would like to set forth what I personally consider to be some needed changes in physical education. It is hoped that members of the profession will receive them in the spirit in which they are presented, for the purpose of discussion and consideration. As we consider these and other suggestions it will be possible to develop a dynamic program of action.

The following ten-point program is proposed for the physical education of the future:

1. *Strengthen our leadership.* Today's scholarly high school senior is as vigorously recruited by business, government, and education as the star football player is by the National Football League. A college or university gains academic prestige in proportion to the number of scholarship winners it can attract to its campus, and business and the professions thrive as they interest learned men and women in their fields of endeavor.

This is the age of the scholar. Therefore, physical education must attract scholarly students to its ranks. Physical education cannot move ahead without dynamic, erudite leadership. If we subscribe to the premise that physical education is intellectually oriented (a requirement for professional status), requiring lengthy training and preparation in such areas as foundational sciences, skills, methods, and measurement, we must be sure that each practitioner who enters the ranks is qualified and equipped mentally, as well as in other ways, to perform the required service.

The profession of physical education should be so attractive that the high school student clearly recognizes that it is a privilege to belong and that he needs strong qualifications, rather than discovering there is an "open-door" policy that admits any boy or girl who has the inclination to enter.

Although no arbitrary cut-off point is recommended on college entrance examination board tests (or similar instruments), most of our students in the future, it seems, should fall in the upper levels on both verbal and mathematical components of the test, be in the upper quarter of their high school graduating classes, possess personal characteristics that indicate they have promise for our field of endeavor, and have their application backed by strong recommendations.

The student who is interested in the physiological, psychological, and sociological aspects of physical activity and human development, has potential in the area of science, and possesses a yearning to do research should be recruited as vigorously as a student who is strong in motor skills.

Another characteristic of a profession is that it must have the machinery and ability to police and control itself. Therefore, there must be some effective means to ensure that professional preparation institutions select and train, and administrators employ, students who have met the high standards essential to quality leadership.

2. *Conduct a national inventory of our human resources.* This is an age in which many specialized human skills and talents are needed to successfully investigate, teach, and interpret the many-faceted aspects of modern-day physical education.

The profession of physical education needs to know the nature and extent of its human resources—those members who have special skills, abilities, and talents—at all educational levels and in all types of agencies. Our human resources need to be assessed in an objective, analytical manner. We need to know who has ability to do

different types of research and who are the experts in fund raising and public relations, to personally know government officials and legislators, to have skill in group dynamics and public speaking, and to have knowledge about movement analysis and adapted physical education.

After physical education's human resources are inventoried, the information should be carefully analyzed and organized in a meaningful manner. Then this information should be stored in computers so that when special talents or skills are needed anywhere in the nation or world, they can be mobilized within a very short period of time and put to good professional use.

Each physical education professional is an expert in something, but we do not have this information readily available. Such an inventory will not only provide valuable information but will also ensure a greater feeling of belonging for each of our members. How many times has a dedicated but not well-known professional and talented person said it himself or herself: "I wish I could help." But because of failure to know about this special talent and lack of proper communication, the profession has been the loser.

3. *Develop and reinforce a professional code of ethics.* To be rightfully labeled a profession in today's world means that a field of endeavor has members who adhere to desirable codes of behavior. Such a code for physical education would embody relationships with students, colleagues, employers, and the public in general. It would also point out the primary obligations of the physical educator and stress his role of service and public trust.

As a profession we have developed codes of ethics, but they have not always been known or used to guide the behavior of our colleagues. Therefore, in addition to establishing such a code of ethics, the necessary machinery would be developed to see that it is adequately publicized. Furthermore, where there is an infraction of the code, the case would be reviewed before a professional board, council, or committee. Here, the facts and circumstances would be heard and proper action taken. Although the implementation of this recommendation involves many problems, strong professional action would eventually serve to enhance desirable codes of behavior among all members.

4. *Create a center for reflective and advanced thinking.* To move ahead in the future the profession needs to exploit the wisdom and experience of the past.

My personal relationship with the late Jay B. Nash is one of my most cherished memories. I studied under Dr. Nash, assisted him in his classes, shared his confidence, and was a colleague of his for many years. I knew him particularly well for his ability to do reflective and creative thinking in physical education until the time he passed away.

Dr. Nash retired from New York University in 1953. Until the time of his death he was an energetic, dynamic individual. On the morning he died he was working on a speech to be given to the Boys Clubs that afternoon.

It often occurred to me that our national association should have tapped Dr. Nash's experience and wisdom much more that it did during the period that followed his retirement from New York University. Dr. Nash had much to offer that would have helped his profession to grow and prosper.

There are many Dr. Nash's in this country and many more to come. We still have an Ainsworth, Cassidy, Langton, Rogers, Scott, Staley, and Esslinger, to name a few. Let's utilize their invaluable ideas, suggestions, and criticisms to help us grow in the years ahead. Let's profit from their many years of experience.

A center for reflective and advanced thinking in physical education should be established where these great leaders would periodically congregate, exchange views, mull over problems facing the profession, impart their wisdom, and give those of us who are still on the action from the benefit of their thinking. Our profession will be much better for having created such an institution.

5. *Develop a "new" physical education.* Education has a "new" math, a "new" English, and a "new" physics. We should also have a "new" physical education. The first step in achieving this goal might be a major curriculum study to identify, through scientific means, the basic concepts of physical education and then assign responsibilities for each grade and education level—kindergarten through college—for fulfilling and teaching these concepts. The final blueprint would be a sequential and progressive developmental pattern for teaching skills, knowledges, appreciations, and other aspects of our professional programs. The "new" physical education would give direction to all physical educators as to *what skills* are to be taught and *when; what knowledges* are to be imparted and *when; what fitness standards* are to be achieved and *when;* and *what social outcomes* are to be expected and *when.* The progression to be followed, the sequential development to be adhered to, and the desirable standards to be met would be clearly delineated. The total of all experiences would result in graduating from our schools and colleges *physically educated* students.

6. *Expound only supported claims regarding the worth of physical education.* "Exercise will prevent disease," "Sports are a 'cure-all' for juvenile delinquency," and "Physical fitness will improve a student's IQ" are examples of claims that have been made by some physical educators in the past. They are unsupported and have misled the public and contributed to loss of respect among our academic colleagues. One reason for making such false claims may be that the facts have not been known or that they have not been adequately interpreted to the profession.

The physical education of the future should only expound claims substantiated by sound research findings. To help in implementing this recommendation, conducting more significant research, financing needed studies, and disseminating research findings to practitioners in the field, a *National Institute* should be established where research studies would be encouraged and records on all studies would be stored. Research findings would be filed away in computers on a regional basis throughout the United States and thus enable members of our profession, by a mere push of a button, to mobilize all the significant research on any particular subject with which he is concerned. For example, if a teacher in Nebraska wants the latest information on how to teach skish, a teacher in California desires to know about the role of exercise in weight control, or a doctoral student in Florida seeks the studies that have been conducted on the relation of motor skills to scholastic achievement, it would be possible to obtain answers within a few hours' time.

As the frontiers of knowledge are pushed back in regard to the worth of physical education and as the facts are made more readily available to our membership, the problem of expounding unsupported claims will diminish.

7. *Take strong professional stands on controversial issues where we provide the expertise.* The American Medical Association did not take a back seat in regard to Compulsory National Health Insurance; similarly, the AAHPER, if it wishes to be an outstanding force for the profession in the future, should speak out loud and clear on matters where it is knowledgeable and is an authoritative source of information.

As a profession we should be recognized as being the experts in certain areas of sport, physical fitness, skill teaching, the relation of physical activity to human growth and development, and other areas directly related to our training and experience. Ironically, the advice of the professional boxer, ballplayer, physical culturist, or faddist is sometimes sought before the public looks to us for help. We are still smarting from the time President Eisenhower invited several professional athletes to the White House to help him in deciding how to eliminate the physical softness of the youth of America. This situation was later corrected, thanks to some of our leaders.

One reason for this dilemma may be that we have not spoken out authoritatively and unilaterally as a profession on some of the major issues of the day. We have not agressively called attention to the fact that *we are the experts in these areas*. Too often we may have either remained silent or taken a middle-of-the-road position. Perhaps we may have been afraid of hurting someone else's feelings. Or we felt greater security by tying ourselves to the apron strings of some other educational or athletic organization. In such cases, the profession, educators, and the public in general did not benefit from a sound analysis of the problem by our profession and our leaders.

The profession needs to be heard on the major issues of the day, where we provide the expertise. After an examination of all the facts, a discussion of each of the alternatives, and a careful weighing of the evidence, we as a profession should take strong positions on such matters as whether girls should play on varsity athletic teams with boys, coaching ethics, weight-reducing gimmicks, who should teach elementary school physical education, the place of physical fitness in a well-rounded school physical education program, poorly qualified physical educators being assigned to teach health education courses, qualifications and training for coaches, swimming pools as a facility in a school, credit for physical education, small-fry sports competition, athletic standards, and other controversial issues of the day.

After the profession has arrived at a sound position, we should then use all types of communication media to gain the headlines so that we will be heard clearly in the offices of school and college administrators as well as in the homes of America. We are the experts in physical education and all that the term implies. We have a national association of more than 50,000 members. We can speak with authority and be heard.

Educators and the public in general look to us for leadership and direction on many of the controversial issues of the day where our training and experience make us the authorities. They should not be found wanting. If we are the experts in these areas, let us provide the leadership that goes with such a label.

8. *Develop a comprehensive public relations program.* The area of public relations needs considerable attention in the years ahead. There are many misunderstandings about physical education that need to be corrected. We need the help and support of general educators and the public in general. This goal cannot be achieved, however, unless they know what we are doing and the service we render to society. It is our responsibility to provide the service but we also should get credit for it—the reason for a program of public relations.

9. *Place more emphasis upon the basic instruction or service physical education program at both high school and college levels.* The basic instruction program for all students represents the "gold mine" of physical education now and in the future. This is where most students are exposed to physical education, the subpar students (poorly skilled, physically soft, physically handicapped, emotionally disturbed, culturally disadvantaged) can get attention, the future leaders of America can participate, and life-long impressions can be formed by young people as to the worth of our program.

Service programs deserve our best full-time teachers, facilities, hours for scheduling activities, and budget priorities. We should objectively determine each student's physical status and plan a program that fits his needs. Individual counseling should play an important role.

After participating in the basic instruction program, students should know that we firmly believe that the service program has top priority and does not rate second to the professional preparation courses, variety athletics, intramurals, or other aspects of our total program. It ranks first.

10. *Advocate a program of educational athletics.* Sports represent one of the most popular aspects of the American culture. Snce they are conducted in all types of settings and for many reasons that have little or no relation to education, there needs to be a clear definition of the type of program we endorse for our schools and colleges.

A program of educational athletics is needed that clearly distinguishes between athletics offered in schools and colleges and those offered in community leagues, agencies, and clubs outside the educational institution.

The platform that has been described for the future of physical education may be thought of by some members of the profession as being too ambitious an undertaking. To those members I would like to say that it is the essence of leadership that our reach must exceed our grasp. As Carl Schurz, an immigrant to this country, pointed out long ago: "Ideals are like the stars. You will not succeed in touching them with your hands. But like the seafaring man on the desert of waters, you choose them as your guides, and following them you will reach your destiny."

QUESTIONS AND EXERCISES

1. Discuss three reasons why educators should have faith in the promise of the 70's.
2. Select one of the projected changes for general education in the 70's and gather information to support the change that will take place during the next decade.
3. What challenge does the inner city have for physical education? What innovations would you propose in order that physical education may make a greater contribution to solution of the problems of the inner city?
4. Describe in detail three changes that you feel will take place in physical education programs during the 70's.
5. What implications does the women's liberation movement have for physical education and athletics?
6. How can physical educators contribute to the ecological problems that face society?
7. What are some of the requirements of a change agent? What are some of the procedures he should follow in bringing about change in physical education?
8. How will the use of textbooks help to better physically educate the youth of the future? What kinds of material should these textbooks contain?
9. Write an essay of approximately 250 words describing the contributions of physical education to modern-day living and its potential for the future.

10. What are ten inventions that have tended to make man more inactive? More active?

11. What are some of the needs of youth? How can physical education meet some of these needs?

Reading assignment

Bucher, Charles A., and Goldman, Myra: Dimensions of physical education, St. Louis, 1969, The C. V. Mosby Co., Reading selections, 7, 17, and 21.

SELECTED REFERENCES

Blake, O. William: Innovations in preparing the elementary school physical education teacher, Journal of Health, Physical Education, and Recreation **36**:60, 1965.

Bucher, Charles A.: Administrative dimensions of health and physical education programs, including athletics, St. Louis, 1971, The C. V. Mosby Co.

Bucher, Charles A., and Goldman, Myra: Dimensions of physical education, St. Louis, 1969, The C. V. Mosby Co.

Cooper, John M.: Preparation for and adjustment to change, Journal of Health, Physical Education, and Recreation **40**:36, 1969.

Douglass, Harl R.: Trends and issues in secondary education, New York, 1962, Library of Education, The Center for Applied Research in Education, Inc.

Miller, Peggy L.: A man to fill the gap: the change agent, Journal of Health, Physical Education, and Recreation **40**:34, 1969.

Report to the President and Congress by the Outdoor Recreation Resources Review Commission: Outdoor recreation in America, Washington, D. C., 1962, U. S. Government Printing Office.

Shane, Harold G., and Shane, June Grant: Forecast for the 70's, Today's Education **58**:29, 1969.

Trekell, Marianna: Speaking to the future, Journal of Health, Physical Education, and Recreation **37**:29, 1966.

Van Dalen, D. B.: Dynamics of change in physical education, Journal of Health, Physical Education, and Recreation **36**:39-41, 1965.

PART TWO

Philosophy of physical education as part of general education

5/Philosophy of education
6/Objectives of physical education
7/Role of physical education in general education

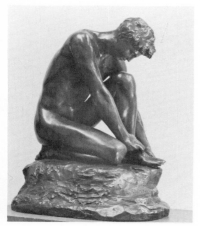

WORK OF R. TAIT
MCKENZIE. COURTESY
JOSEPH BROWN, SCHOOL OF
ARCHITECTURE, PRINCETON
UNIVERSITY.

5/Philosophy of education

I would have his outward manners, and his social behaviors and the carriage of his person formed at the same time with his mind. It is not a mind, it is not a body that we are training; it is a man, and he ought not be divided into two parts.

MONTAIGNE

It is a lamentable mistake, to imagine that bodily activity hinders the working of the mind, as if these two kinds of activity might not advance hand in hand, and as if the one were not intended to act as a guide to the other.

ROUSSEAU

The union of mind and body has to be acknowledged as being for us primary and ultimate. All voluntary movements, all sensations and passions rest on the union, neither mind by itself nor body by itself can suffice to account for their occurrence. The movements as being willed, are foreign to the body, the sensations and passions are foreign to mind as well as body.

DESCARTES

Yet some relaxation is to be allowed by all . . . there is nothing that can bear perpetual labor. . . . Boys, accordingly, when reinvigorated and refreshed, bring more sprightliness to their learning. . . . Nor will play in boys displease me; it is a sign of vivacity. . . .

QUINTILIAN

. . . what a disgrace it is for a man to grow old without ever seeing the beauty of which his body is capable.

XENOPHON

That form of exercise is best which not only exercises the body but also is a source of joy to the participant. . . . Therefore that form of exercise is recommended which contributes to the health of the body and to the harmonious functioning of the parts and to the strength of the soul.

GALEN

To learn to think we must therefore exercise our limbs, our senses, and our body organs which are tools of the intellect; and to get the best use out of these tools the body which supplies us with them must be strong and healthy.

ROUSSEAU

On July 20, 1969, over 600 million people watched on their television sets as Neil Armstrong took man's first steps on the moon. The words: "That's one small step for man, one giant leap for mankind," were heard all over the world. According to the crew of Apollo 11, it was truly the beginning of a "new age."

The peace and tranquility that Apollo 11 discovered on the moon is lacking here on earth, for we are living in an era of discontentment and dissent. The "new age" that we are facing is an age of strife and student rebellion. It is an age that needs direction. The questions that must now be asked are: How will education respond to this "new age?" What will its role be?

In the United States, education has been subject to criticism for many years. The early launchings of the Russian Sputnik gave impetus to a controversy regarding what type of training our boys and girls should have. Education in the space age is often confronted with the task of producing the answers needed to achieve the goals of our society.

Critics of education sometimes look at a subject like physical education and consider it to be a "frill." They sometimes consider physical education to be a subject that we can ill afford during the space age. They have bombarded progressive and life-adjustment education as unwarranted, unwanted, and needless educational piffle placed in the schools by the educationists to further their own destiny.

Physical education as well as other subjects in the curriculum are being attacked by students. Today's student wants an education that is relevant, and many young people cannot see the school program as relevant to what they want out of life.

Students do not want their schools to perpetuate the inequities that exist. They do not want a curriculum that makes them lose their identities as persons. In physical education, for example, they do not want meaningless drills. They do not want to become dehumanized.

Students today want to be turned on. They want to be made aware of the issues that directly affect them. Apathy and ignorance of the outside world must come to an end. Strong emphasis must be placed on activities that strengthen the relationships between people.

Educators must reexamine their roles in society. Physical educators must be aware of the needs of their students in today's complex society. All educators must be cognizant of student demands and must work in harmony with them. To achieve this goal, educators must have an understanding of philosophy, for only then will they be able to see the beginning of a truly "new age" in this country.

Philosophical thought represents the highest level of thinking. As such, it is a discipline that all educators should understand. This chapter has been written to present some considerations necessary to building an educational philosophy. It defines philosophy and discusses its component parts. It describes the importance of a philosophy of education and discusses the "good life" as a goal for educational programs. It considers the reasons why there is a need for a philosophy of physical education, then it presents some of the more popular philosophies that have prevailed through the years. Finally, a discussion is presented concerning philosophical implications for education in our current society.

WHAT IS PHILOSOPHY?

Philosophy is a field of inquiry that attempts to help man evaluate, in a satisfying and meaningful manner, his relationships to the universe. Philosophy seeks to help man evaluate himself and his world by giving him a basis with which to deal with the problems of life and death, good and evil, freedom and restraint, beauty and ugliness.

Aristotle said that philosophy is the grouping of the knowledge of the universals. A dictionary definition reports that it is the love of wisdom, the science that investigates the facts and principles of reality and of human nature and conduct. Copleston* writes: "Philosophy . . . is rooted in the desire to understand the world, in the desire to find an intelligible pattern in events and to answer problems which occur to the mind in connection with the world." In defining the word *philosophy* Webster† says: "Love of wisdom means the desire to search for the real facts and values in life and in the universe, and to evaluate and interpret these with an unbiased and unprejudiced mind." As can be seen from these definitions, philosophy offers an explanation of life and the principles that guide human lives.

In order to comprehend more clearly the meaning of philosophy, one should briefly examine the major components of which philosophy is composed.

Metaphysics

Metaphysics is associated with the principles of being. This component attempts to answer a series of related questions: What is the meaning of existence? What is

---

*Copleston, Frederick, S. J.: Contemporary philosophy, Westminster, Maryland, 1966, The Newman Press.
†Webster, Randolph W.: Philosophy of physical education, Dubuque, Iowa, 1965, Wm. C. Brown Co.

real? How are man's actions governed? How and why did the universe evolve? What is the nature of God? The question: What experiences in the physical education program will better enable students to meet the challenges of the real world? is metaphysical in nature. Will Durant, a contemporary philosopher, says that metaphysics investigates the reality of everything concerned with man and his universe.

Epistemology

Epistemology is concerned with methods of obtaining knowledge and the kinds of knowledge that can be gained. It is a comprehensive study of knowledge that attempts to define the sources, authority, principles, limitations, and validity of knowledge. In physical education we are concerned with knowledge regarding the role of physical activity and its impact on the physical, mental, emotional, and social development of human beings. We are seeking the truth about physical education, and epistemology seeks to answer the question: What is true?

Axiology

Axiology helps to determine to what use truth is to be put. It asks: How do we determine what has value, and on what criteria do we base this judgment? Axiology is concerned with the aims and values of society and is extremely important in physical education because the aims and values set by society become the basis of the curriculum used in schools and colleges. In physical education we must answer the question: How can the values that society holds so dearly be embraced in the physical education program? In our society we hold very dearly the value of "equality for all." We can see this value exemplified by having students from all walks of life playing together and developing tolerance for one another. Students who learn to respect one another on the playing fields, it is hoped, will be more likely to carry those feelings off the field.

Ethics

Ethics is a more individualized and personalized subdivision of axiology. It helps to define moral character and serves as a basis for an individual code of conduct. Ethics attempts to answer the question: What is the highest standard of behavior each person should strive to attain? The strengthening of moral conduct is an important function of physical education. In physical education the following questions must be answered: How can games and sports be utilized to help the individual learn right conduct? Is character education through physical education possible? Physical education places individuals in situations that reveal their true nature and character. One who plays on a team may soon realize that using "four-letter words" is not acceptable. The student who plays by the "rules" and acts like a "sportsman" at all times will win the respect of his fellow teammates. The relationships formed in physical education and the character that is developed, it is hoped, will carry over to behavioral situations occurring out of school.

Logic

Logic seeks to provide us with a sound and intelligent method of living. Logic describes the steps that should be taken in thinking and puts ideas into an orderly, structured sequence that leads to accurate thinking. It helps to set up standards by which the accuracy of ideas may be measured. Logic concerns itself with the orderly connection of one fact or idea with another. It asks the question: What method of reasoning will lead to the truth? Physical educators must use logical thought processes in arriving at the truth. When students ask questions such as: "Why should I play football?" the physical education teacher must not answer by saying: "Because it's in the program." The teacher should explain in clear reasoning the benefits that can be derived from playing football, for only then will the student really understand its true value.

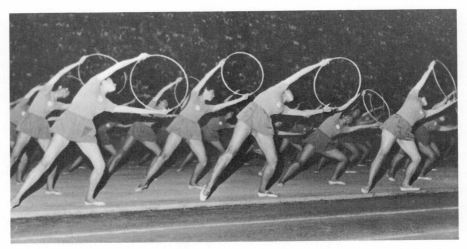

Greek physical education was developed on classical philosophical grounds, which embraced it as an essential to the education of youth.

Esthetics

Esthetics is the study and determination of criteria for beauty in nature and the arts, including dance, drama, sculpture, painting, music, and writing. Esthetics, which is a less scientific branch of axiology, is concerned not only with art but also with the artist and the appreciation of what he has created. In an attempt to determine the close relationship of art to nature, esthetics asks the question: What is beauty? There is esthetic appreciation involved in watching a gymnast perform on the trampoline, a football player leap high to catch a pass, or a baseball player dive to catch a line drive, just as there is an esthetic appreciation gained from viewing great works of art or listening to a symphony orchestra. The physical movements that one can view in athletics are often a source of great pleasure.

The components known as metaphysics, epistemology, axiology, ethics, logic, and esthetics represent aspects of philosophy. In developing a philosophy for any particular field, one would turn for information to each of these areas. These components would be applied in formulating a philosophy for any particular field within the educational endeavor, such as in health, physical education, or recreation. Philosophy yields a comprehensive understanding of reality, which, when applied to education or any other field of interest, gives direction that would very likely be lacking otherwise.

PHILOSOPHY AND LEVELS OF DISCUSSION

Broudy* lists four levels of discussion applicable to a progressive step-by-step exploration of education problems. These levels of discussion help to clarify the implications of philosophy for the physical educator.

Emotional or uncritical level

On the emotional level a person discusses the pros or cons of an issue mainly in terms of his own limited experience. The arguments presented are not based on reflective thinking but, instead, on impulse and emotional feeling. A statement by a high school basketball coach that: "All boys who play high school basketball perform better in the classroom than those who do not play" may be an emotional or uncritical statement. The coach may only have had experience with his own team and cannot

*Broudy, Harry S.: Building a philosophy of education, New York, 1954, Prentice-Hall, Inc., pp. 20-24.

know for sure whether all boys who play high school basketball perform better in the classroom than those who do not play. There is general agreement that the emotional level of thinking is the most unreliable. Few differences of opinion can be settled by using the emotional level of thought and action.

Factual or informational level

The factual level of discussion involves the gathering of evidence to support one's arguments. By mobilizing statistics and other types of factual evidence, tangible support is often given to a particular argument. However, this level of discussion can be unreliable and misleading since it depends on the facts used: whether or not they are valid and applicable, how significant they are, and other conditions that exist in the particular situation in question. A statement by a physical educaiton teacher that: "In an experiment, students who participated in the physical education program showed greater improvement in strength than those who did not participate" is a factual statement. The teacher can introduce all sorts of impressive statistics to prove his point. However, one cannot be sure whether the experiment was properly conducted. Nevertheless, the mobilizing of accurate facts in a discussion can frequently result in the solution of a problem and the satisfactory finalizing of a discussion on an argumentative topic.

Explanatory or theoretical level

Facts offer solid support, but they are most effective as they are associated with theories that make them dynamic and applicable. A statement by the physical educator that: "The jump shot in basketball should be taught as a whole and not broken down into its component parts," is theoretically valid. The teacher's statement can be supported by reference to the "Gestalt theory" and such thinkers as Kurt Koffka and Wolfgang Kohler, whose theories stress the idea that learning takes place as a whole because of the essential unity that exists in

nature. At this level of discussion the introduction of a reliable scientific explanation provides strong evidence for rational men.

Philosophical level

The highest level of discussion involves asking questions relative to what is really true, valuable, right, or real. The application of such values is universal and eternal. This is the ultimate to which any discussion can go. A statement by the physical education teacher asking: "Do students participating in team sports develop strong human relationships?" is characteristic of the philosophical level. At this level there is self-criticism of programs, and physical educators try to decide what they want to have happen to their students in the gymnasium. This level of discussion finds the greatest use when problems fail to yield a clear solution and when facts and science are limited and inconclusive. (There are many such problems in education and in physical education that merit a philosophical discussion.)

PHILOSOPHY OF EDUCATION AND THE GOOD LIFE

John Dewey* has stated: "The problem of restoring integration and cooperation between man's beliefs about the world in which he lives and his beliefs about the values and purposes that should direct his conduct is the deepest problem of modern life." Dewey has further stated that it is through one's philosophy that this problem can be solved. A philosophy is extremely valuable because of the fact that it determines one's thinking and leads one to his ultimate goals.

Philosophy has both a "synthetic" and "analytical" function. The synthetic function of philosophy is mainly concerned with formulating hypotheses. The hypotheses serve as the tools for interpreting questions

---

*Dewey, John: The quest for certainty, London, 1930, George Allen Junior, Ltd., p. 243.

concerned with the nature and experiences of man. The analytical function of philosophy attempts to determine what the key concepts are in any field. The analytical function of philosophy, as its name suggests, studies the methods of inquiry used in the various fields.

In education, as in any other field, important questions will be answered by one's philosophy. A philosophy of education is extremely important to all those who intend entering the teaching profession. One cannot be an effective teacher in today's changing society if he does not have a well-thought-through philosophy. A philosophy of education attempts to determine what kind of life one should lead. Viewing man in a systematic fashion, a philosophy of education is instrumental in giving purpose and direction to one's actions.

Before one can even begin to formulate a philosophy of education, he must have a clear concept of the person he wants to produce. Therefore, it becomes necessary to define that type of life that reflects the most satisfying and worthwhile type of ex-

istence. This is the type of life on which educational aims, methods, facilities, staff, and other essentials should be focused. For purposes of discussion this may be called the "good life."

Philosophers have used the term *good life* to indicate the happiest and most successful type of existence. For example, Bertrand Russell, in his book *Education and the Good Life,* lists vitality, sensitiveness, courage, intelligence, and love as his characteristics of the "good life." Others have said that it is characterized by pleasure. These thinkers differ, however, as to the meaning of the word *pleasure.* John Stuart Mill and Epicurus were two such philosophers. Still others have varied in saying the "good life" is the simple life, or the one characterized by vast possessions and great power, or the one devoted to worthy causes and religious fervor. Broudy, in his book *Building a Philosophy of Education,* points out that, although philosophers have not agreed entirely in their thinking, most have said that the "good life" consists of the following character-

A national survey of teachers to determine where they thought the emphasis is placed in modern-day education.

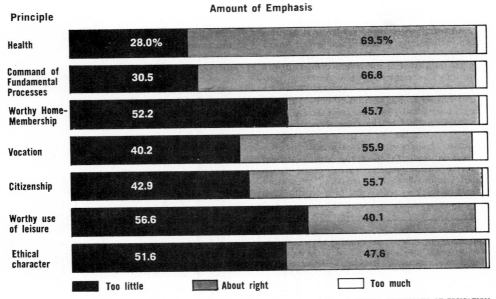

Amount of Emphasis

Principle	Too little	About right	Too much
Health	28.0%	69.5%	
Command of Fundamental Processes	30.5	66.8	
Worthy Home-Membership	52.2	45.7	
Vocation	40.2	55.9	
Citizenship	42.9	55.7	
Worthy use of leisure	56.6	40.1	
Ethical character	51.6	47.6	

FROM TEACHER-OPINION POLL: A NEW LOOK AT THE SEVEN CARDINAL PRINCIPLES OF EDUCATION, NEA JOURNAL 56:54, 1967.

istics. First, it is a life that is pleasurable with excessive pain eliminated and in which disease, poverty, and hardship are kept to a minimum. Second, the "good life" emphasizes love, emotional security, and understanding. There is freedom from fears, anxiety, frustration, despair, and loneliness. Third, the "good life" means that the individual accomplishes, achieves, renders a service, is respected, and is allowed to exercise his potentialities. There is respect for the dignity and worth of the human being. Finally, the "good life" is interesting and exciting. If the interest and excitement are permanent and of the highest type, they are tied in closely with other people and future events. They are not solely self-centered and concerned with what is going on at present.

Any analysis or definition of the "good life" must include the viewpoints of both the individual and society. Both play an important part in determining the true ingredients. Alger Hiss, for example, may have thought he was living a good life during his communist years; however, most of society felt otherwise.

In order to understand more completely the components of the "good life," it is important to discuss each aspect more fully.

A pleasurable life

A pleasurable existence is the first characteristic of the "good life." A definition of pleasure, however, is the subject of much discussion. Certainly, if a person is to enjoy life it must be a pleasant experience. A person should be happy and satisfied. The philosophers say that the greatest pleasure and happiness come from doing good and helping others. As Emerson said: "He who does a good deed is instantly ennobled." Pleasures that are temporary, sensuous, and degrading are not the kind that contribute to the "good life." True pleasure is gained through a life characterized by high ideals. Aristotle thought happiness was achieved by leading a virtuous life. John Stuart Mill felt that the things that brought happiness to the greatest number were the

ingredients that characterized this essential in the "good life." A pleasurable life also is one that is free from excessive pain and in which hardships and poverty have not been present in excessive amounts.

Education can help individuals achieve the "good life." It can help establish a philosophy of life that guides toward desired goals. It can provide the fundamental skills, knowledges, and understandings that will enable one to provide sustenance, shelter, and the essentials for maintaining life without needless pain. It can provide the ability to appreciate and enjoy the things of beauty in nature and art. It can help avoid unnecessary hardship and pain. Diseases caused by ignorance and physical suffering caused by carelessness can be eliminated through proper health knowledge and health care. Also, much pain and suffering can be eliminated by developing a strong, healthy body.

Emotional security

A "good life" is characterized by emotional security. Inner peace is a necessity. Love and a feeling of belonging are very important. Good mental health is a must. No one wants to live a life of frustration, despair, and loneliness.

Education can help to establish a sound standard of values, develop skills for a worthy use of leisure time, instill good human relations, and develop an appreciation for service to others. It can demonstrate the importance of loving and being loved; it can clarify the place of the family, church, and school in a well-ordered community. It can stress through precept and example the importance of sound moral and spiritual values. It can provide experiences that develop emotional security.

Worth and achievement

A sense of worth and achievement is an aspect of the "good life." However, it must exist not only in the individual's eyes but also in the eyes of society. A person must feel that he is recognized, is needed, and is contributing something to the group. He must feel that he has accomplished important things such as achieving prominent position or title. He must be satisfied in his own heart that he is getting ahead in the world and is developing the talents with which he has been endowed. Society, also, must feel this way about his accomplishments.

Education can help direct a person's life toward worthwhile goals, provide training for a job, develop skills to achieve, enable a person to utilize his abilities to the fullest, help him to develop physically, and give him knowledge and habits that will contribute to good health. In this case health is a means to an end and not an end in itself. It is a means of achieving greater things for mankind.

An interesting life

The last aspect of the "good life" is that it must be interesting. A person cannot be bored. A person who enjoys a "good life" looks forward to each day for new and exciting things. His future concerns not only himself but also others. He has a stake in future happenings and looks to the future and to the part he will be playing in these events. His interest in life exists because of worthwhile goals for which he is striving. Accomplishing these goals helps not only him but also other people.

Through a study of history and literature, those persons who have lived interesting and rewarding lives become known. Education can help to direct an individual to seek worthwhile, satisfying, and interesting goals. It can equip each one with skills, knowledge, and understanding that represent the basic equipment and foundation for living an interesting life.

These characteristics of the "good life," according to the great thinkers of history, represent those goals toward which all people should strive. Once we are aware of these ultimate goals in education, it becomes the role of philosophy to give purpose and direction to our actions. Educators must constantly be aware of the soundness of their philosophy. They must con-

stantly check the validity of the beliefs and values that they hold. When educators begin to ask questions such as: What is true? and What has value? we will see a more meaningful educational experience provided for mankind.

PHILOSOPHY AND PHYSICAL EDUCATION

In today's changing society, there must be a sound philosophy of physical education in order for our profession to survive in the present educational system. We must ask ourselves such important questions as: What has value in today's society? and What is relevant to the needs of today's students? We must discover the answer to these questions and a philosophy will be the means to that end. A philosophy of physical education will serve the following functions.

A PHILOSOPHY OF PHYSICAL EDUCATION GUIDES ONE'S ACTIONS. In order for man to function as an intelligent being, he needs a philosophy of life that will guide his actions. One needs knowledge about what is right before he can create any program. A philosophy will help the teacher to decide what he wants to have happen to his students in the gymnasium.

A PHILOSOPHY OF PHYSICAL EDUCATION PROVIDES THE DIRECTION FOR THE PROFESSION. Today in physical education we find that many of our curriculums lack order and direction. A philosophy of physical education will help to give direction to our programs. When assumptions are made by the physical education teacher, for example, that physical education strengthens human relationships because children play together, they should be based on a system of reflective educational thinking that embraces logic and other philosophical components. A philosophy of physical education will help to provide this system.

A PHILOSOPHY OF PHYSICAL EDUCATION MAKES SOCIETY AWARE THAT PHYSICAL EDUCATION CONTRIBUTES TO ITS VALUES. Physical education in the coming decades is going to have to face the fact that people are not going to be satisfied with only such statements as: "Students who participate in physical education show improvement in endurance." This is important, but it doesn't go far enough. In today's changing society people want to know how physical education can contribute to the solution of such problems as student unrest and how physical education programs can help stem the tide of racial discrimination. A well-thought-through philosophy of physical education will assist in interpreting those values important in society so that programs can be established to help solve the problems plaguing this nation.

A PHILOSOPHY OF PHYSICAL EDUCATION AIDS IN BRINGING THE MEMBERS OF THE PROFESSION CLOSER TOGETHER. Many members of the physical education profession are dissatisfied with what they see happening in their field today. A philosophy of physical education will enable the physical educator to better determine how he can best contribute to mankind and to society and thus provide members of the profession the opportunity to work together in making such a contribution.

A PHILOSOPHY OF PHYSICAL EDUCATION EXPLAINS THE RELATIONSHIP BETWEEN PHYSICAL EDUCATION AND GENERAL EDUCATION. A philosophy of physical education will help in the development of a rationale showing that our field has objectives that are closely related to the objectives of general education. In our definition of physical education, we stress the importance of education "of and through the physical." Our goal, as in general education, is to develop the "whole" student. A philosophy of physical education that enunciates our basic goals will give evidence that we have objectives that are related to the objectives of general education.

Physical educators must strive to develop their educational philosophies in a rational, logical, and systematic manner and to represent the best interests of all men. This means that scientific facts must be assembled and workable theories applied that support the worth of physical education as an important and necessary service to humanity.

SOME GENERAL PHILOSOPHIES

Five philosophies have prevailed down through the years and have influenced educational thinking. They are idealism, realism, pragmatism, naturalism, and existentialism.

Idealism

The philosophy of idealism has come down to us through the ages as a heritage from the earliest Greek philosophers and thinkers. The key concepts of idealism follow.

1. *A man's mind is the focus of his being.* The idealist believes that the mind of man is more real than anything else that exists. Anything that is real is essentially a product of the mind and is equated by thoughts and ideas.

2. *In the scheme of the universe, man is more important than nature.* Because to the idealist the mind and spirit are the keys to life, the physical world plays a subordinate role to man. Man interprets nature in terms of his mind, his spirit, and his being.

3. *Values exist independently of man and are permanent.* Man is capable of exercising free will. Through the use of this power, man recognizes the existence in the world of good and evil, beauty and ugliness, freedom and restraint and interprets them in relation to himself. The idealist acknowledges that man may interpret values, but he says that these values are permanent and do not change in the light of varying interpretations.

4. *Reasoning and intuition help man to arrive at the truth.* Man's mind is considered to be the basic, creative force that helps him learn more about his world. But the idealist also believes that scientific methods of investigation and research are valuable aids in seeking the truth.

The Greek philosopher Plato is often referred to as the father of idealism. He believed that ideas had an enduring quality

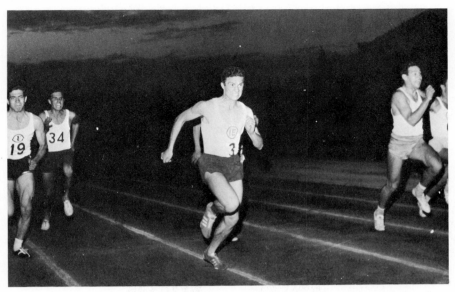

Greek physical education subscribes to the man of wisdom and the man of action.

and that physical objects were ideas expressed in a less-than-perfect fashion. Plato said that there were, in fact, two classes of ideas: those that exist in the mind of men, and those that exist outside of man's mind. Aristotle expanded on Plato's philosophy and was responsible for the earliest origins of the scientific method. Aristotle stressed arriving at the truth through reasoning and observation. René Descartes is one of the most famous of the idealist philosophers. His often-cited quotation: "I think, therefore I am" is the essential element in the philosophy of the idealist. Both Baruch Spinoza and Gottfried W. Leibniz expressed the view that something enduring and unchanging exists beyond man's universe. While Spinoza referred to this phenomenon as a "substance," Leibniz termed it a "God." George Berkeley, Immanuel Kant, and George Hegel all espoused the belief that the mind of man is the key to all things. Some of the more modern idealists, whose views encompassed many of the same elements as the men who preceded them, were Louis Agassiz, Henry Barnard, Carl Follen, Francis Lieber, Henry Wadsworth Longfellow, and Horace Mann.

IDEALISM AND EDUCATION

1. *Education develops the personality of the individual.* Idealists show great concern for the moral and spiritual values in society. In order for idealists to fulfill their moral and spiritual destiny, it becomes necessary for education to help in the development of the individual personality of each student. Education must provide opportunities for the individual to develop to his full worth.

2. *Knowledge and the development of the mind are important.* Idealism emphasizes the importance of man's rationality and the need for the cultivation of reason. Man's mind must strive to realize itself. Education is seen by the idealists as the means to this end.

3. *Education is a process that originates within the self.* Idealists view students as creative beings. The individual self contains within it the properties for its own growth. The idealistic student must initiate the learning process within himself. The idealistic educator stresses the importance of self-activity because it gives students the impetus for learning and development.

4. *The curriculum is centered around*

ideals. The idealists, because of their emphasis on the development of the personality, place great stress on programs that provide students with the opportunity to develop the essential qualities of self-reliance, self-responsibility, and self-direction. The idealistic curriculum stresses those areas of study that help the student build an ideal intellectual, spiritual, and moral character. Art, literature, and history in their classic forms are the foundation of the curriculum in the idealist school.

5. *The student is a creative being who is guided by the teacher.* The student in the idealistic school formulates ideas and learns in an environment set by the teacher. The idealistic teacher conceives the objectives and organizes the subject matter. The learning environment of the idealistic teacher would include the formulation of ideas through the project method, the lecture method, and/or the question and answer method. The idealistic teacher might tell his students what the "possible" answers are and then the students must discover their own conclusions. In this manner the idealistic teacher guides his students through a thought process that will lead to the truth.

IDEALISM AND PHYSICAL EDUCATION

1. *Physical education involves more than the "physical."* Idealists believe that the body should be developed simultaneously with the mind. Physical education should contribute to the development of the individual's intellect. For example, the physical education teacher, after describing a difficult skill such as the "kip" on the low bar, can ask students questions such as: "What angle should the hands be in when they are grasping the bar?" According to idealists, physical education activities can and must help students think for themselves.

2. *Strength and fitness activities contribute to the development of one's personality.* The idealistic physical educator must make sure that the activities that he selects are related to important aspects of life. The idealist will accept vigorous exercise activities that emphasize development of strength

and fitness because of the self-discipline and effort required. The idealistic physical educator will select such activities because they contribute to the development of one's personality; however, he will not select them if their sole aim is developing strength or fitness.

3. *Physical education is centered around ideals.* Idealists believe that activities must be offered that aid the student in developing the qualities of honesty, courage, creativity, and sportsmanship. The idealistic physical educator aims for perfection. He envisions the students becoming aware of what is true and genuine. He wants his students to develop strong moral character. The idealist will encourage student-created gymnastic routines because of the emphasis on creativity. The idealist will want "team sports" dominated by students. He will reject a basketball game dominated by the coach because the students will not get the opportunity to think for themselves. Idealistic physical educators stress the fact that students can only develop when they are playing an important part in the activity.

4. *The teacher must be a model for his students.* The idealistic physical education teacher must set a good example for his students. He will be the type of person whom students want to imitate. Through his personal example of vigorous health and personality, the idealistic physical educator will lead his students toward greater accomplishments.

5. *The teacher is responsible for the effectiveness of the program.* Idealism believes that the firm and rather paternalistic guidance of the teacher is more important in carrying out the program than are equipment and facilities available. The idealistic physical educator, believing he is responsible for the effectiveness of the program, does not confine himself to one way of teaching. The idealistic physical education teacher uses the question and answer, the lecture, the project, and other methods of teaching.

6. *Education is for life.* The idealistic physical education teacher believes that equally important to developing physical

skills or having knowledge of a sport is thinking reflectively. The idealistic physical educator believes that the ability to analyze problems is as important as knowing the rules of a game. Idealism emphasizes a well-organized, well-guided program that contributes to the full mental and physical development of the individual.

Realism

Realism asserted itself as a distinct and separate philosophy during the late nineteenth and early twentieth centuries. For many centuries preceding that time, realism was greatly overshadowed by idealism. The roots of realism date back as far as the origins of idealism, and it was, in fact, a philosophical revolt against idealism. The growth of scientific methods and the philosophy of modern realism emerged at about the same time. Realism has many subdivisions. Its adherents do not always agree on particular interpretations, but the key concepts of realism may be defined in general terms.

1. *The physical world is a real world.* The realist accepts the physical world, or world of nature, as it is. He does not contend that the world is manmade but says that it is made up of matter. The physical world is in no way dependent on man's mind. The realist says that man comes to an understanding of his physical world through his senses and through experience.

2. *All of the physical events that occur in the universe are the result of the laws of nature.* The realist contends that forces within the universe, which are physical laws, control man's physical world. This belief has given rise to the physical sciences. The realist says that man's environment is a result of cause and effect and that good, morality, and beauty conform to the laws of nature. Those things that do not conform to the laws of nature are wrong, immoral, and ugly. Man perceives the physical world through observation.

3. *The truth may be best determined through the scientific method.* The realist does not hope for or anticipate full control or complete comprehension of everything in the physical world. He does expect to modify and understand it as well as he can through the tools of science. The realist feels that science and philosophy form the best method of arriving at the truth.

4. *The mind and the body have a close and harmonious relationship.* The realists have two views on the origin of human behavior. One school of thought says that that man's behavior may be a result of natural laws. A second opinion is that all of man's behavior may be a result of learning. Both sides agree, however, that the mind and the body are inseparable and that neither takes precedence over the other.

5. *Religion and philosophy can coexist.* The realist can hold religious beliefs without compromising either religion or his philosophy. He may be a staunch atheist or a pantheist or hold beliefs anywhere between the two extremes. The philosophy of realism does not insist on any one position as being the correct one. The individual realist is free to coordinate his religious beliefs with his philosophical viewpoint.

Philosophers often lend their thinking to the shaping of more than one philosophy. Thus many of the men who helped to define idealism also adhered to elements of realistic thinking. The early realists were men who ascribed much to a belief in the powers of a supreme being, or God. Aristotle said that truth and reality were one and the same and that man's powers of reasoning made him unique. Because of this viewpoint, Aristotle is often referred to as the father of realism. St. Thomas Aquinas and René Descartes both said that matter was real and created by a God. Descartes' writing is believed to be the basis for the field of mathematical physics. Comenius, Spinoza, Kant, John Locke, and William James all helped to put forth clarifications of this philosophy.

REALISM AND EDUCATION

1. *Education develops man's reasoning power.* To the realist, education is a process

of learning how to acquire knowledge, acquiring knowledge, and putting that knowledge to practical use. The realistic educator stresses the fact that man must become the rational master of himself, for only then will he be able to control his environment.

2. *Education is for life.* The realistic educator believes that education is basic to life and that all education should have a useful purpose. The realistic educator attempts to develop his students in such a manner that they can understand and make adjustments to the "real world." The realistic educator wants his students to view the "real world." The realistic educator wants his students to view the world in an orderly and systematic fashion. Learning experiences are presented in an orderly fashion and relate to the problems of the outside world. The realistic educator believes that such experiences will aid the students in their adjustment to the "real world," the world that will enfold them when they leave the school environment.

3. *Education is objective.* The realistic educator attempts to be objective, like the scientist. He employs objective methods of teaching, testing, and evaluation. Because the realist wants his students to be exact, he presents clear facts in an objective and logical sequence. The realistic educator urges his students to master the facts that he has presented to them. Because the realist wants to bring the "real world" into the school environment, he may employ such techniques as audiovisual aids.

4. *The educational process proceeds in an orderly fashion.* The realistic educator wants his teaching to be dependable. He presents as facts only those things that have been proved by objective means. The realistic educator proceeds in a step-by-step fashion, always following scientific rules, believing this to be the only way that teaching can be dependable. The realistic teacher guides students through a process of inductive reasoning eventually leading to a unified concept of the physical world.

5. *The curriculum is scientifically oriented.* The realistic curriculum stresses the

sciences. Although mastery of fundamental facts is accomplished through drill and memorization, mastery of a body of knowledge is implemented by experimentation, demonstration, and observation. The realistic educator places great emphasis upon research and the scientific method and stresses the importance of learning as large a number of scientific facts and principles as possible.

6. *There should be standardization of measurement techniques in education.* The realist educator favors the devising of standards of performance for students in various activities. The progress of students is evaluated by objective standardized tests. The realist gathers all the possible reliable data and measures his students according to standards created. Realism has often been credited with being a major influence on the development and use of standardized tests.

REALISM AND PHYSICAL EDUCATION

1. *Education is for life.* The realist views physical education as a valuable part of the school curriculum. It is considered to be a unit of study that helps prepare the student to adjust to the world in which he lives. Participation in physical activities is viewed as a means of learning to adjust, and the emphasis is placed on the outcome of the activity in terms of adjustment. For example, the emphasis in teaching basketball is to develop such qualities as fair play and sportsmanship as well as in teaching a student how to shoot a basket.

2. *Physical fitness results in greater productivity.* The realist physical educator emphasizes the values related to man's body. He places emphasis upon "physical fitness" because of its intrinsic value. The realist physical educator stresses the point that one who possesses a physically fit body is one who may be most productive in society.

3. *Programs are based on scientific knowledge.* The realist physical education teacher accomplishes his objectives through use of a scientifically formulated curriculum. He selects activities on the basis of scientific evidence of their worth from a study

of anatomy, physiology, or kinesiology. For example, in training a young man to be a "lineman" in football, it is necessary to be aware of the proper form, which provides optimum stability. Anatomical knowledge dealing with the question of "base of support" will yield this information. A physical educator cannot be an effective teacher unless he possesses knowledge of scientific movement principles.

4. *Drills play an important part in the learning process.* The realist physical educator uses drills extensively and breaks units of work down into orderly progressions. The teaching emphasis is placed on fundamentals of games and activities, with each skill broken down into its component parts. In this manner the realist hopes to develop habits in student responses. The realist believes that breaking down the elements of a sport like soccer into all its component parts will lead to correct responses in game situations.

5. *Interscholastic athletic programs lead to desirable social behaviors.* The realist approves of interscholastic athletic programs insofar as they teach desirable social behavior. The realist approves of a team sport like baseball particularly as it develops such qualities as sportsmanship, fair play, and tolerance. The realist physical educator will not be interested in having a baseball program that only emphasizes "winning."

6. *Play and recreation aid in life adjustment.* The physical educator who is a realist believes that students who participate in play and recreational activities are better able to function in society. Through such activities students are brought into contact with aspects of the "real world" of which they will become a part when they leave the school setting.

Pragmatism

Pragmatism emphasizes experience as a key to life. Rather than being concerned with reality, this philosophy is concerned with knowledge. Because of this view, pragmatism was, in its early stages, often called *experimentalism*. The term *prag-*

matism was not coined until the late 1800's. In its modern concept, this philosophy is considered to be an American one.

1. *The experience of man causes changes in the concept of reality.* The pragmatist believes in change. He does not hold that ideas, values, or realities are inflexible. He contends, instead, that the experiences of man cause ideas, values, and realities to be dynamic. The pragmatist says that experience is the only possible way to seek the truth and that that which is not experienced cannot be known or proved.

2. *Success is the only criterion of the value and truth of a theory.* Knowledge and experience help man to discover what is true. But truth is considered to be flexible, and today's truth may be tomorrow's falsehood. The pragmatist strongly believes in the scientific method of problem solving. He considers it the best way to gain knowledge. Knowledge itself is thought to be only a steppingstone on the path to further knowledge and experimentation. The pragmatist believes that a workable theory is a true theory and that the unworkable theory has been proved false.

3. *Man is an integral part of a larger society, and his actions reflect on that society.* The pragmatist contends that man and society must live harmoniously and that the actions of one directly affect the other. He believes in democracy, that is, the needs of a group must always incorporate the needs of each individual in the group. To the pragmatist, values are an individual matter. What is right or wrong depends on the judgment of the individual, his environment, and the circumstances. However, the result of any action by an individual is to be measured in terms of its worth to society as a whole.

Heraclitus was an early Greek exponent of pragmatism. He stated the belief, still held today, that the world and its values and ideas are in a constant state of flux. Quintilian said that learning was a product of experience. Francis Bacon, an Englishman, put forth the theory that society and science must work together in order to

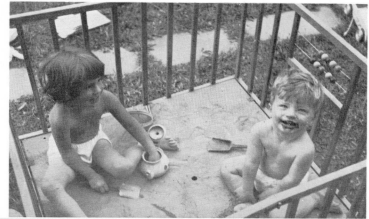

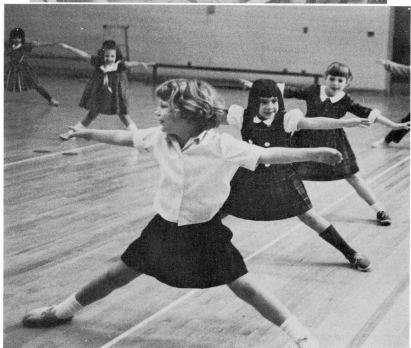

Attention in education should be focused on the child.

achieve knowledge and that one cannot function effectively without the other. The first outstanding American pragmatist was Charles S. Pierce. He wrote that the practicality of a truth was the only criterion on which that truth could be measured. William James said that a theory was good if it worked and wrong if it was not practical. The most famous of the American pragmatists was John Dewey. At times, pragmatism is referred to as "Deweyism" because of the influence of Dewey's thinking on the philosophy. Dewey brought forth the theory that everything we know is subject to change and can in no way be considered static. Dewey viewed life as a continuing, never-ending experiment. He felt that learning how to think was one of the most important goals in life. Dewey's philosophy had a most profound influence on the field of education.

PRAGMATISM AND EDUCATION

1. *The individual learns through experience.* Experience is the key word in the educational process of the pragmatist. The individual learns through experience: by inquiring, observing, and participating in various activities. Experience is viewed as the key to all learning, and the application of intelligence to new experiences is that which makes the educational process effective. Pragmatists feel that the child learns what he lives, and consequently they place great importance on student interests, devoting much time and energy in motivating those things that interest students.

2. *Education is for social efficiency.* The pragmatist believes that the major aim of the educational process is to teach the student the knowledge and skills that will enable him to take his place in society. Education provides the students with the necessary tools to enable them to adjust to their environment and solve the many problems that may arise. Pragmatists maintain that schools must provide the experiences that aid the student in becoming an active member of society. The school must be involved in community affairs and give students the opportunity to participate in discussions. Students are given the opportunity to work together as members of social groups so that they can get the valuable experience that will prove to be beneficial when they become functioning members of society.

3. *Education is child centered.* The pragmatist emphasizes the study of the child. Pragmatists recognize the importance of individual differences; therefore, each child is treated differently, thus permitting the student to progress at his own speed. The pragmatic teacher serves as an inspiration, guide, and leader. The child is viewed as the most important thing in the school and as a whole being, rather than an intellect without a body. The needs, interests, and prior experiences of the child guide the teacher toward better helping each child adjust to society.

4. *Problem solving is necessary in a world of change.* Since the pragmatist emphasizes the fact that there is constant change, education must prepare students to face situations that are still unknown. Pragmatic educators stress the point that when they leave school, students face a world that is considerably different from the one that they face when they first begin their educational career. For this reason, pragmatists emphasize the importance of having the knowledge to solve problems that may arise in an ever-changing world. Students are taught to define problems. They learn how to collect data, formulate and test hypotheses, and arrive at conclusions that will enable them to find the solution to those problems. This is the "problem-solving" method made famous by John Dewey. Pragmatic educators do not believe that it is necessary for their students to learn great numbers of facts; rather, it is more important that they learn those concepts that may be useful in solving a particular problem on which they are working.

PRAGMATISM AND PHYSICAL EDUCATION

1. *More meaningful experiences are presented when there is a variety of activity.* The pragmatic physical educator likes a varied program of physical education. He provides students with intriguing problems to solve and challenges to face in preparation for effective functioning in society. Creative activities such as dance and experiences in boating, camping, and outdoor living, as well as all types of sports, are highly valued. Through these activities the student not only learns by doing but also gains a measure of self-control and discipline and learns to cooperate with others.

2. *Activities are socializing in nature.* The pragmatic approach to physical education is one of integrating the child and society. Any activity that has social value is acceptable. Team sports and group recreational activities are found to be satisfying to the pragmatist. Calisthenic drills

and exercises are largely discarded from the pragmatic physical education program. The pragmatist sees education as life. Sports, by providing emotional involvement, competition, and interaction, contribute to the socialization of the individual.

3. *The curriculum is determined by the needs and interests of the learner.* Learning is accomplished in the pragmatic curriculum by experiencing those things that have proved to be beneficial to the learner and that result from the learner's own interests. Activities that are challenging and creative are the major ones selected by the students. Thus such activities as team sports, dance, and recreational activities are included in the pragmatist curriculum because they satisfy the needs and interests of the students.

4. *Learning is accomplished through the problem-solving method.* The pragmatic physical education teacher believes that problem solving helps to make learning more purposeful. The ability of students to recognize and solve problems encourages thinking. Dance activities prove to be very satisfying to the pragmatic physical educator because of the elements of creativity involved. Movement education, which emphasizes the problem-solving method, also is extremely valuable to the pragmatist because of the emphasis on self-discovery.

5. *The teacher is a motivator.* The pragmatic physical educator is a leader and motivator of his students. He encourages students to participate in activities that he feels are most beneficial to them. The pragmatic teacher guides his students in making the correct choices but does not direct them or tell them that they must do things his way. The pragmatic teacher employs the use of student leaders and tries to give as many students as possible a leadership experience.

6. *Standardization is not a part of the program.* The pragmatic physical education teacher dislikes standardization because he feels that such a practice makes all programs alike. Pragmatists place a higher value on evaluation than measurement. They are not as interested in measuring muscle

strength as in determining whether or not students will be able to face the challenges that life will present to them. To the pragmatist, evaluating whether a student who participates in a baseball game learns the elements of fair play is equally as important as learning to hit a ball.

Naturalism

Naturalism, pragmatism, and realism share many key concepts, although naturalism as a philosophy is the oldest one known to the Western world. Naturalism is often referred to as a materialistic philosophy, since it says that those things that actually and physically exist are the only things that have value.

1. *Any reality that exists exists only within the physical realm of nature.* To the naturalist, the physical world is the key to life. It contains all we see, observe, and think about, including the beauty or ugliness of a tree and the complexities of nuclear physics. The physical world is viewed as being in a constant state of growth and change, but it is considered to be a predictable and reliable force. Since the physical world is the key to life, the naturalist does not accept the existence of a God or any other supreme being. The philosophy of naturalism says that scientific methods are the best ways to gain knowledge about the world of nature.

2. *Nature is the source of value.* Because nature is omnipotent, anything that is of value exists only within nature and is predicated by nature. No values can exist separately from nature in any form. Like pragmatism, a thing is of value if it is workable.

3. *The individual is more important than society.* Naturalism does agree, however, that democracy comes from a group process, but it contends that each individual is more important than the group as a whole. Society reaps the benefits of the interaction of man and nature. Conversely, it is the individual who advances nature.

The men who first defined the philosophy of naturalism were in strong agreement that all things are derived from nature, including learning. This view was especially put forth by Democritus, Leucippus, Epicurus, and Comenius. In the eighteenth century, Rousseau, Basedow, and Pestalozzi set the foundations for the naturalistic process in education. Rousseau is more of a prime source for these educational objectives, but Basedow put them into actual use. Herbert Spencer further defined education under naturalism and is mainly responsible for modern educational thought among the naturalists.

NATURALISM AND EDUCATION

1. *Education must satisfy the inborn needs of the individual.* Naturalists declare that when the child is born, he already possesses certain capacities and inborn powers that determine his needs. There are fundamental forces within the individual that seek satisfaction, such as the need for social affiliation and achievement. Naturalists state that it is the role of education to satisfy these basic needs.

2. *Education is geared to the individual growth rate of each child.* Education is focused on the student. Naturalist educators believe that each child follows a logical pattern of growth and development and that education must be attuned to these natural patterns. Activities are selected according to the developing maturity level of the individual. Furthermore, according to the naturalists, the laws of growth and development are investigated when programs are developed.

3. *Education is not simply mental in nature.* Naturalists emphasize the point that education is not only mental; it is also physical and moral. Naturalists advocate the education of both mind and body, with neither taking precedence. Education encourages the development of moral character, self-discipline, and physical well-being.

4. *The student educates himself.* Naturalists emphasize the point that education involves self-activity. Students take an active part in their own educational develop-

ment. When students learn with their whole body, they establish relationships and thus educate themselves to a certain degree. According to the naturalist educators, activities are offered for exploratory purposes and for the development of natural abilities and self-expression.

5. *The teacher has an understanding of the laws of nature.* It is the role of the teacher to learn how each student learns and to guide him through the educational process. The teacher has knowledge of the laws of nature and helps the child develop according to these laws. The teacher is aware that nature has made all people different, and therefore each child has distinct learning needs that require individual types of learning activities.

6. *The teacher is a guide in the educational process.* The teacher, through example and demonstration, guides the child through an investigative procedure that helps him to draw his own conclusions. The method of instruction used is mainly inductive. The method of teaching is informal and permits students to develop naturally at their own speed and according to their own needs and interests.

NATURALISM AND PHYSICAL EDUCATION

1. *Physical activities are more than just "physical" in nature.* Naturalists agree that physical activities do more than just develop strength and fitness. The naturalist believes that activity is the main source of development of the individual. Through physical activity, the naturalist believes the child learns to become a contributing member of a group, develops high moral standards, learns to express himself in an acceptable manner, and becomes an individual who has more nearly reached his full potential.

2. *Learning is accomplished through self-activity.* Naturalists state that activity is the main source of the development of certain capabilities that have been imbedded in the individual by heredity. The need for security and recognition are such capabilities that are developed through self-activity. The

naturalist offers a wide variety of activities to the child so that he will be able to adjust to his environment. The naturalist approves of all physical activity including team and individual sports and outdoor education. He introduces new activities only when students are ready for them and have a need for and interest in them. Naturalists stress the point that students can only learn when they are "ready" physiologically, psychologically, and sociologically.

3. *Play is an important part of the educational process.* Naturalist physical educators believe that play, resulting directly from the interests of the child, provides the starting point for teaching desirable social behaviors. Through play the child becomes aware of the world of which he is a part, permitting the teacher to introduce to him many of the essential features of social relationships. In the naturalist physical educator's program, students interact with one another in playful activities and develop social habits that will prove beneficial to them when they leave the school environment.

4. *Highly competitive performance between individuals is discouraged.* Self-improvement is encouraged in the naturalist physical education program, and evaluation goes on continuously. The emphasis in evaluation is placed upon the individual's own performance. The naturalist does not approve of intense competition between groups. The child must be in competition against himself to better his performance and to improve in light of what he himself has done in past performances.

5. *Physical education is concerned with the "whole man."* According to naturalist physical educators, physical education has a mental aspect. In every physical activity one's volitional processes are at work. In a complex sport such as football, to be successful one constantly thinks and develops the correct responses. However, naturalists do not believe in making a student mentally fit and disregarding his physical fitness. Education is for the body as well as the mind. Physical education activities result in phys-

ical and mental development that prepares students to function well in society.

Existentialism

The chief concern of existentialism is the individuality of man. The existentialist fears that man is being forced to conform to society and is thus forfeiting his individuality. Existentialism, which received its impetus immediately after World War II, is entirely a modern philosophy in that it did not arise from any of the ancient philosophies. Existentialism as a way of philosophical thought had its earliest beginnings in the mid–nineteenth century.

1. *Man's existence is the only true reality.* A man is what he causes himself to become, and no more and no less. He has the ultimate responsibility for his past, present, and future. He has the choice of accepting those things that exist outside his own experience, but if he does accept them, he forfeits a part of himself. The existentialist does not contend that God does or does not exist, but only that each man must decide the answer to this question himself in the light of an objective analysis of his own being.

2. *Each man must determine his own system of values.* Any value that a man has not fully decided upon for himself cannot be a real value for him. Any value that is dictated is a meaningless value. To accept a value that is not self-determined leads away from individuality. A man can respect himself only if his ideals and values are of his own choosing and, once decided upon, he is willing to accept the responsibility for them.

3. *The individual is more important than society.* The existentialist believes that society as a whole is indifferent to the individuals who compose it. The individual can make his mark and keep contact with reality only if he continually searches for his own place as an individual. Once a man subjugates his values, personality, and ideals to those of society, he ceases to function as a man.

Sören Kierkegaard, a nineteenth century

theologian and philosopher, is considered to be the father of existentialist thought. He was concerned with seeking the meaning of each man's individuality. Most of the modern existentialist philosophers do not necessarily follow the guides set down by Kierkegaard, although they all place the major emphasis on the individual and his behavior. Jean-Paul Sartre is the outstanding atheistic existentialist. He denies that man will make any progress, and he sees the ultimate failure of both man and society. Karl Jaspers, Paul Tillich, and Reinhold Niebuhr are theistic existentialists and offer viewpoints that are far more optimistic than Sartre's. They say that man, to reach the ultimate reality, must participate in life rather than be a mere spectator. Martin Heidegger has remained fairly clear of the atheist-theist controversy and instead writes that man cannot stop searching for the meaning in life, no matter what he may find that meaning to be.

EXISTENTIALISM AND EDUCATION

1. *The individual discovers his "inner self."* Existentialist educators believe the individual discovers his inner self. The individual has an understanding of himself. The existentialist student decides those values and goals that are important and discovers his own truths. The school supplies the environment, the tools, and the opportunity for this discovery.

2. *Education is an individual process.* General education is viewed by the existentialist as an individual rather than a group process. The purpose of the school is to set an environment that allows the student to learn what he is interested in learning at the time that he is interested in learning it. The existentialist educational system permits great variety in its methods. Because of the fact that students are different, they are not educated at the same rate or in the same way.

3. *The curriculum is centered on the individual.* The existentialist student rather than the teacher selects the subject matter and the learning method. The student bases these decisions on his view of himself in the present and projected into the future. The subject matter aids the individual in discovering his inner self. Since the meaning of existence is imbedded in man himself, the curriculum is based on the individual so he can discover the true meaning of his existence. The Socratic method of learning is used because it forces the individual student to probe into his own mind. The existentialist curriculum offers many courses in the arts, humanities, and social sciences because these subjects reveal the nature of man.

4. *The teacher acts as a stimulator.* The existentialist teacher serves as a stimulus for his students. He encourages the students to discover their own truths by prodding their moral and intellectual curiosity. Existentialists encourage their students to be creative, critical, and original thinkers. The existentialist teacher enters into relationships with his students that will result in the development of their curiosity. This is essential if the student is to discover the truth. The existentialist teacher, in stimulating his students, assists them in their goal toward self-realization.

5. *Education is to teach responsibility.* The existentialist educator aids the individual in responsible decision making. The individual is presented with experiences in the school environment that enable him to be a more responsible citizen. The individual is made aware of the fact that he must take full responsibility for his decisions. Education develops the inner self of the student, according to the existentialist, for only when the individual discovers his inner self is he able to accept the responsibility for the consequences of his actions.

EXISTENTIALISM AND PHYSICAL EDUCATION

1. *There is freedom of choice.* Physical education programs should provide some freedom of choice on the part of the student. This, however, presents some difficulties when exposed to the problem of implementation. For example, if the teacher practices complete freedom in determining

the program, how can the student exercise the freedom of choice that is so vital to existentialism? And if the student is totally free to choose his own activities, does he have the ability to do so? Given absolute freedom of choice and decision making, it is conceivable that among a class of thirty students up to thirty different activities are selected for pursuit during a single class period. However, when a wide variety of individual and dual activities is offered, the existentialist aim can be carried out at least in part.

2. *There should be a variety of activity.* The existentialist physical educator provides a balanced and varied program that satisfies individual needs and interests. Within the activity selected, the student is expected to evaluate himself and, on this judgment, make a selection of the skills and activities he will pursue. It is the role of the teacher to provide the activities and to create an atmosphere in which the student learns to take the responsibility for himself, but only after he shows that he has the maturity to earn this privilege.

3. *Play results in the development of creativity.* Existentialist physical educators emphasize that when an individual is playing, he is involved in creativity. Existentialists emphasize individual and team sports; however, team sports whose only goal is winning are viewed as having little value. Dance and gymnastics fit into the existentialist curriculum because of the element of creativity involved.

4. *Students "know themselves."* The existentialist physical educator's student has a knowledge of himself, since it is necessary to have such an understanding in order to make choices that better himself and the rest of society. Through participation in individual and dual activities, the student gains knowledge about himself. Competition is acceptable; however, it is the effect of competition on the individual that is important. Existentialist physical educators also place emphasis on activities such as self-testing activities because they aid in the development of the individual's self-responsibility

and require the student to "know himself."

5. *The teacher is a counselor.* The existentialist physical educator is personally concerned about his students. Students are made to feel more responsible in the existentialist physical education program than in other programs discussed. The teacher believes that it is most important to give students the opportunity to try out their judgments in activities presented to them. In such a manner, the existentialist physical educator's students develop the quality of self-responsibility. In the learning process the teacher acts in the role of a counselor and guide, explaining the various alternatives and giving direction so that the student does not flounder.

PHILOSOPHIES OF GENERAL EDUCATION

Five general philosophies have been discussed. These have left their mark on educational thinking and practice. There are some philosophies concerned specifically with general education that also should be discussed. These represent some of the current thinking among educators as to how learning should be guided in our schools. As will be seen, some reflect traces of the general philosophies already discussed.

Instrumentalism

The first of the philosophies of general education to be discussed is labeled *instrumentalism*. Instrumentalism, identified by some thinkers as progressivism and experimentalism, comes mainly from pragmatism. Instrumentalists believe that education of the child should involve natural growth and provide physical, mental, moral, social, and spiritual experiences adapted to the age, health, interests, and abilities of each pupil. As explained by Harold Taylor, former president of Sarah Lawrence College, this philosophy looks at general education in this way.

In education, the instrumentalist holds that in order to reach the mind of the pupil the teacher must pay attention to the quality of the pupil's total experience, his desires, interests, and needs, and must take account of the social influences which produce certain attitudes of mind in the individual pupil. In other words, once the mind is conceived to be a part of nature which interacts with every other part, the development of intelligence in the human being becomes a matter of the total experience through which the human being goes. It is up to the educator to arrange things so that the pupil's experience with ideas and values is one which engages his deep attention and concern. . . . The instrumentalist insists that education must be built, not upon the materials of knowledge per se, but upon the capacities and needs of the individual student or of groups of individual students. Those materials of knowledge which are useful, important, or aesthetically exciting are then brought to the curriculum, not as a priori decisions as to what all human beings should learn, but as materials and experiences through which these human beings at this stage in their development are able to learn, to think, to enjoy, to perceive, and to know.*

In physical education the instrumentalist stresses that the development of the body is just as important as the development of the mind. The instrumentalist physical educator starts at the skill level of the child and builds upon that level. He selects his activities according to the group they are to serve. The instrumentalist physical education program also has special classes for the handicapped.

Neo-humanism

Neo-humanism or humanism has parts of several general philosophies embodied in its makeup. In the sense that it means that the answers to life and education are found within the realm of the human or natural, as opposed to supernatural experience, it can be linked to naturalism and some forms of realism. Then, too, one can discern elements of pragmatism within its explanation as the neo-humanists purport to strive for change in the light of what is considered at the moment to be something better. There is also an element of the idealistic philosophy in its emphasis upon the cultural heri-

tage and in its search for the absolutes of Good and Beautiful.

Robert C. Pooley of the University of Wisconsin interprets the neo-humanism philosophy.

Humanism as an educational philosophy means the transmission from generation to generation of what man has learned and discovered in his business of surviving, of adapting himself to his surroundings, and in striving to change these surroundings in light of what at the moment he considers better. . . . The humanist finds no goals other than what lie within the cultural heritage itself. These are relative rather than positive. Education for the humanist, then, is transmission of experience together with certain eternal questions: What is True? What is Good? What is Beautiful? And, on the contrary, what is False, Evil, Ugly? No system or scheme supplies all the answers. Man will always seek them. The cultural past supplies both the raw material toward the answers and the long history of striving; of answers partially satisfactory for a longer time. The quest continues, and this quest is the rationale of humanism.*

The neo-humanist physical education program has as its prime emphasis the stressing of knowledge of the body and its functions. The neo-humanist physical educator teaches those activities that have been embedded in the cultural tradition, according to the customs of the particular society that they are to serve.

Rationalism

Rationalism is identified in a sense with all five general philosophies, although probably drawing its main avenue of thought from the idealists and the realists. Rationalism stresses that the purpose of the educative process is to develop the mind—to develop the rational powers of the learner. All of the general philosophies would subscribe to the importance of developing the mind. The differences would arise in the method to be used in achieving this objective. The rationalist theory has been out-

---

*Association for Higher Education of the National Education Association: College and University Bulletin No. 7, November 1, 1954.

*Association for Higher Education of the National Education Association: College and University Bulletin No. 7, November 1, 1954.

Comparison of school programs guided by traditional and modern educational philosophies

Modern	Traditional
Child centered	Teacher centered
Permissive classroom atmosphere	Rigid classroom atmosphere
Based on pupil's interests and needs and relating to needs of society	Based on fact, knowledge, and subject matter, irrespective of societal changes or needs
Teacher a guide—plans along with child	Teacher a taskmaster
Focus on total development of child—physical, emotional, and social complement and supplement the mental	Focus on intellectual development
Self-directed study; opportunities for creative expression, socialization, problem solving, and experimentation	Formal drills, memorization, lectures, questions-answers, and examinations
Close school-community relationship and parental cooperation	School isolated from home and community
Self-discipline	Discipline by external authority
Broad curriculum	Limited curriculum
Healthful school environment	Austere environment
Geared to individual student	Geared to mass of students
Classroom a laboratory for testing new ideas	Classroom impervious to change

---

lined in part by Charles Wegener of Long Beach State College in California:

(1) the primary responsibility of the educational institution engaged in general education is the intellectual development of the student;

(2) the primary aim of this intellectual training is the development of a capacity for intelligent judgment in the student—a "critical" capacity appropriate to the generally or liberally educated man or woman;

(3) this critical capacity is to be "general" in the sense of being developed by a curriculum the core of which provides a systematic and comprehensive range of experience of materials in the humanities, the social sciences, and the natural sciences employed for the purpose of reflective analysis.*

The rationalist physical educator, because of his desire to develop the reasoning power of his students, stresses such things as the history of activities and the knowledge of rules and strategies of particular games.

There is lack of uniform thinking as to what philosophy should guide American education. This disagreement sometimes causes the public to comment that the educator does not know where he is going.

*Association for Higher Education of the National Education Association: College and University Bulletin No. 7, November 1, 1954.

Looking at it in another way, however, it probably is a healthy sign. Conflicting philosophies mean discussions, examinations, and perusals of what is being done. This makes it possible for all to promote and encourage that type of education that will best meet the needs of the individual and of society.

MODERN PHILOSOPHY OF EDUCATION

John Dewey's philosophy of education has resulted in much scientific research into the nature of learning, the makeup of the child, teaching methodology, and the complexity of culture. This has placed education on a much sounder footing than ever before. To link the best educational theory and practice of today with any chaos and confusion in the schools reflects a total misunderstanding of what Dewey advocated. Some of the critics need to read a little more of this great philosopher's works before they make such damaging accusations.

The purposes of education in American life are focused on all children and youth to provide them with the opportunities to become all they are capable of becoming. This is a part and parcel of our heritage as the greatest example of democratic living on this earth. We in education are commissioned to prepare the young for life. To accomplish this job our duties include such things as teaching the basic skills of learning, science, mathematics, and the arts and passing along the cultural heritage. It also means offering young people the opportunity to develop their physical, intellectual, and social selves and providing them with opportunities for self-discipline and self-direction.

What is peculiar to our education is that, in keeping with the democratic spirit, we provide for the needs of each individual in our society. For example, we offer a variety of courses to help each boy and girl capitalize on his own particular abilities and interests. This nation has been an example to the world in showing that each individual has worth. Therefore, we in education are as much concerned with the boy who has an intelligence quotient of 80 as the girl with the IQ of 140 and are as interested in the youngster who wants to be an automobile mechanic as the young person who wants to be a scientist.

The United States opens its doors to a far greater proportion of children and educates them for a longer period of time than any other nation. This is in keeping with the American way of providing opportunities for all, and for this reason it is unfair to compare the performance of *all* of our children with that of the intellectual elite who go to the selective European schools— a favorite reference for the critics. The average academic performance in America will of course be lower. If one takes the top 10% to 20% of our youth, however, and makes a comparison with the youth in Europe, the results will be much more favorable.

In leaving the latchkey out for all youth, it has been necessary to provide vocational education in our schools. And certainly there can be little disagreement that this has made a great contribution to America, whose industrial output is greater than most nations of the world. America does not be-

lieve in the "class" system. Those who earn their living by the sweat of their brows are as important to our society as those who achieve their livelihood through more academic pursuits. We are not interested only in "eggheads" and "longhairs."

We have continually increased the offering in the public schools with all types of courses, from typewriting to science, from homemaking to French. The inclusion of many of the vocational courses, incidentally, has been requested by public groups rather than by the educationists.

The schools are trying to educate the "whole" child. To listen to some of our critics you would think that children are composed of minds that are separate from their bodies. Certainly, we would agree we want to develop the intellect and the ability to reason and think clearly. And John Dewey's philosophy does not advocate doing without thinking or a life adjustment devoid of learning. However, there are other considerations.

A man is as strong as his weakest link. We are interested in developing well-integrated persons wherein the mental, emotional, social, and physical are in proper balance and complement each other in the total makeup of the human being. In this way man will be most productive and provide the type of leadership and followership America desperately needs in the space age.

Our better schools have done a masterful job. They are a paragon for the world to follow. They have shown that modern education is based on valid research and does not slight intellectual training. More of their students are taking foreign languages, science, and mathematics today than ever before. Their programs for the gifted are in operation. Discipline comes from within their students, not through some external force applied by the teachers. Their instructors are not steeped in methodology at the expense of subject-matter content. Their students who go on to college perform just as well as or better than those who come from private schools.

In some communities educational standards are not as high as we would like. Why? Because education reflects what the public wants and has the ability to pay for and what the enrollment will allow. Our schools must continue to make sure that all students are given an equal opportunity to equip themselves for the role that they are destined to play in life. It will not be an easy goal for education to accomplish. At the present time it is quite apparent that the future of American education is going to be quite turbulent. With rising costs and increased enrollments, our schools are going to have far greater demands placed upon them than ever before. Educators are going to be asked to answer the following questions: Are programs meeting the needs of the students? Is the subject matter taught in the schools "relevant" to the needs of our changing society? Every subject in the school curriculum will have to reevaluate its programs in order to determine whether they are relevant to the needs of the student and to society.

Educators must reexamine their roles in society. They must be cognizant of student demands and they must have an understanding of what "turns students on." The challenge facing American education is to make the schools responsive to the needs of its students. Education must not be apathetic to the needs of our society.

Education can accomplish its goals. We have made great progress in the last two centuries. Today, our schools are becoming more and more responsive to the needs of students. Today, many children are getting the opportunity to equip themselves for the role they are destined to play in life. The education that our children are getting today rests upon a sound scientific basis, developed by such men as John Dewey, who devoted a lifetime to thinking about the problems that are plaguing our society.

QUESTIONS AND EXERCISES

1. Why is there a need for philosophical thinking in regard to educational problems today?
2. Define philosophy. Describe its component parts.
3. Describe each of the following philosophies: (a) naturalism, (b) idealism, (c) realism, (d) pragmatism, (e) instrumentalism, (f) neo-humanism, (g) rationalism, and (h) existentialism.
4. Discuss your concept of the "good life." What implications does the good life have for the professional fields of health, physical education, and recreation?
5. Why is there a need for philosophical thinking in physical education?
6. List as many philosophical implications as you can for education in a twentieth-century world.
7. Write an essay of approximately 200 words on the title "My Philosophy of Education."

Reading assignment

Bucher, Charles A., and Goldman, Myra: Dimensions of physical education, St. Louis, 1969, The C. V. Mosby Co., Reading selections 10 to 17.

SELECTED REFERENCES

Adler, Felix: An ethical philosophy of life, New York, 1918, D. Appleton & Co.

Albert, Ethel, Denise, Theodore, and Peterfreund, Herbert: Great traditions in ethics, New York, 1953, American Book Co.

Brameld, Theodore: Philosophies of education in cultural perspective, New York, 1955, The Dryden Press.

Broudy, Harry S.: Building a philosophy of education, New York, 1954, Prentice-Hall, Inc.

Brubacher, John S.: Eclectic philosophy of education, New York, 1951, Prentice-Hall, Inc.

Butler, Donald J.: Four philosophies and their practice in education and religion, New York, 1951, Harper & Bros.

Cowell, Charles C., and France, Wellman L.: Philosophy and principles of physical education, Englewood Cliffs, New Jersey, 1969, Prentice-Hall, Inc.

Davis, Elwood Craig: The philosophic process in physical education, Philadelphia, 1967, Lea & Febiger.

Davis, Elwood Craig: Philosophies fashion physical education, Dubuque, Iowa, 1963, Wm. C. Brown Co.

Demiashkevich, Michael: An introduction to the philosophy of education, New York, 1935, American Book Co.

Dewey, John: The quest for certainty, London, 1930, George Allen Junior, Ltd.

Durant, Will: The story of philosophy, New York, 1953, Simon & Schuster.

Frankel, Charles: A review for the teacher—philosophy, National Education Association Journal **51:**50, 1962.

Friedrich, John A., and McBride, Frank A.: What is your physical education philosophy? The Physical Educator **20:**3, 1963.

Gulick, Luther Halsey: A philosophy of play, New York, Charles Scribner's Sons.

Horne, Herman Harrell: The philosophy of education, New York, 1908, The Macmillan Co.

Horne, Herman Harrell: The democratic philosophy of education, New York, 1938, The Macmillan Co.

McCloy, Charles Harold: Philosophical bases for physical education, New York, 1940, F. S. Crofts & Co.

Morris, Van Cleve: Physical education and the philosophy of education, Journal of Health, Physical Education, and Recreation 27:21, 1956.

Perry, Ralph Barton: Philosophy of the recent past, New York, 1925, Longmans, Green & Co.

Runes, Dagobert D.: Dictionary of philosophy, New York, 1942, Philosophical Library.

Russell, Bertrand: Education and the good life, New York, 1962, Liveright Publishing Corp.

Russell, Bertrand: Philosophy, New York, 1927, W. W. Norton Co.

Slusher, Howard S.: Existentialism and physical education, The Physical Educator 20:4, 1963.

VanDalen, D. B.: Philosophical profiles for physical educators, The Physical Educator 21:3, 1964.

Webster, Randolph W.: Philosophy of physical education, Dubuque, Iowa, 1965, Wm. C. Brown Co.

Ziegler, Earle F.: Philosophical foundations for physical, health, and recreation education, Englewood Cliffs, New Jersey, 1964, Prentice-Hall, Inc.

6/Objectives of physical education

A field of endeavor is characterized by the purposes or objectives for which it exists. These objectives help the members of a specialized group to know where they are going, what they are striving for, and what they hope to accomplish. Physical education has clearly stated the objectives toward which it is working. The student preparing for a career in physical education or a leader working in the field should understand the objectives and be guided by them.

WHAT DO WE MEAN BY THE TERM "OBJECTIVES"?

The word *aim* usually defines a general purpose or direction. It is a goal that is more remote, more encompassing, and less concrete. If I were to state an aim for physical education, I would use the definition of physical education on p. 7. Educators sometimes organize objectives into remote, intermediate, and immediate objectives. These usually reflect the purposes that will hopefully be realized in the distant future, near future, and the present.

In this chapter the term *objectives* is used in a general sense to include aims, purposes, and outcomes derived from participating in the physical education program. In other words, participation in physical activities under skilled leadership should result in certain constructive outcomes for the participant. These outcomes are the objectives of physical education.

Children, youth, and adults are involved with *movement*—getting their bodies into action. Movement is the medium through which physical education achieves its objectives. Boys and girls and men and women during various stages of life engage in running, jumping, hanging, walking, climbing, skipping, throwing, and leaping. Their bodies are activated in rhythms, games, stunts, exercises, and sports. Movement offers human beings an avenue for fun, recreation, physical fitness, sociability, emotional release, communication, exploration, and healthful growth. Movement is a medium for educating people in regard to their physical, mental, emotional, and social development.

There is worth in using the body as a vehicle to learn about one's self and others, games and activities, and other cultures and countries. Movement is basic to physical education as it takes place in our schools and colleges, recreation centers, hospitals, camps, and youth and adult programs.

Essentially, when discussing the objectives toward which physical educators strive, the profession is concerned with physical movement and the potentials this movement has as an educational medium. Movement is essential to human welfare and an important part of the education of people. This chapter is concerned with the objectives that can be achieved through movement.

WHY DO WE NEED OBJECTIVES IN PHYSICAL EDUCATION?

Physical educators must have clearly stated objectives. Some of the reasons for objectives are as follows:

1. *Objectives will help physical educators to understand better what they are trying to achieve.* There is purpose in

physical education. This purpose must be clearly imprinted upon the teacher's mind when he is instructing students in physical skills and upon the leader's thinking when he is instructing an activity class in a YMCA. If the objectives are clearly understood, this will have an impact on what activities are taught and how they are taught. The objectives will serve as guidelines for the physical educator in steering a course that is meaningful, worthwhile, and in the interest of human beings.

2. *Objectives will help physical educators to understand better the worth of their field in education.* Physical educators are concerned with *physical education,* not *physical training* or *physical culture.* Physical education objectives must therefore be compatible with general education objectives. The objectives of physical education that are identified and delineated represent goals compatible with and essential to the total educational effort in our society.

3. *Objectives will help physical educators to make more meaningful decisions when issues and problems arise.* Physical educators will face problems daily as they carry out their responsibilities and administer their various programs. Parents, civic clubs, booster clubs, general administrators, professional sports promoters, big league players, and others who do not understand the objectives of physical education may try to influence programs in the direction they feel important. An understanding of the objectives of physical education will help leaders in the field to make wise decisions when such pressures and issues arise.

4. *Objectives will help physical educators to interpret better their field of endeavor to general educators and lay persons.* Physical education is often misunderstood. One reason for this misunderstanding is that professional objectives are not known. Therefore, if physical educators know the objectives of their field and are imbued with their worth, they will be better able to correct the misunderstandings that exist and interpret their programs accurately.

WHAT ARE THE OBJECTIVES OF PHYSICAL EDUCATION?

The objectives of physical education have been stated many times by current and past leaders in the field. It is interesting to look first at what was conceived as the objectives of physical education in the past.

Historical analysis of the objectives of physical education

The physical education of primitive man was informal and unstructured, with the main purpose being survival. Early man needed physical strength and prowess to fight his enemies, build shelters, obtain food, and resist some of the forces of nature.

The Greeks probably represented the first people to give some structure to physical education. Some of the thinking about physical education during this time was reflected in the writings of Plato, the Greek philosopher. Plato stressed that there were objectives to physical education other than organic development when he pointed out the relation of mental development to physical development.

> They are not intended, one to train body, the other mind, except incidentally, but to insure a proper harmony between energy and initiative on the one hand and reason on the other, by tuning each to the right pitch. And so we may venture to assert that anyone who can produce the best blend of the physical and intellectual sides of education and apply them to the training of character, is producing harmony in a far more important sense than any musician.

Much of Plato's thinking has influenced philosophers and physical educators down through history to accept the premise that close mind-body relationships do exist. Although this thinking did not have much impact on the early settlers in Colonial America because of the doctrine of Puritanism, the concept of the *unity of man* became increasingly recognized.

The early history of America saw systems of gymnastics, philosophies, and objectives imported from Europe. The programs to a great extent were formal in nature and gave precedence to the development *of* the physical rather than outcomes that could be accomplished *through* the physical.

At the turn of the century, however, we saw a "new physical education" developing, which resulted in a broadening of objectives and a recognition of the contributions that physical education could make to the "whole" individual. For example, in the 1880's, Dudley A. Sargent, the Director of Physical Education of the Hemenway Gymnasium at Harvard University, cited such objectives in his program as hygienic, educative, recreative, and remedial. During this same period, Thomas D. Wood, of Stanford University and later of Columbia University, another leading physical educator of the time, stressed that physical education should contribute to the complete education of the individual. Clark Hetherington, a colleague of Dr. Wood's and one of the greatest thinkers ever produced by the field of physical education, also stressed along with Dr. Wood that physical education was concerned with mental, moral, and social contributions to the student. Jesse Feiring Williams of Columbia, also during the early 1900's, stressed the need for a physical education program that was concerned with education *through* the physical as well as an education *of* the physical.

The thinking of these early leaders constitutes the objectives of the "new physical education" that are largely embraced by physical educators today.

Objectives of physical education as indicated by research studies and professional associations

Several studies aimed at determining the objectives toward which physical educators are striving have been conducted. In 1934, the Committee on Objectives of the American Physical Education Association listed five objectives of physical education. These were: (1) physical fitness, (2) mental health and efficiency, (3) social-moral character, (4) emotional expression and control, and (5) appreciations. The committee listed knowledge, skills, and attitudes for each of these key objectives.

The Committee on Curriculum Research of the College Physical Education Association, under the direction of LaPorte, published in 1936 a review of objectives after a perusal of the literature. The committee indicated that they found 174 objectives in the literature that could be classified into ten categories.

Hartley Price, in a doctoral dissertation at New York University in 1946, analyzed the literature and ranked the professional objectives for three separate periods of American history: prior to 1900, 1900 to 1920, and 1920 to 1936. Price found that the relative importance of the various objectives differed for the historical periods studied.

In a doctoral dissertation at Stanford University in 1947, Agnes Stoodley analyzed physical education objectives as they were stated by twenty-two different authors in the professional literature. These objectives were classified under five headings: (1) health, physical, or organic development, (2) mental-emotional development, (3) neuromuscular development, (4) social development, and (5) intellectual development.

A joint committee of the American Association for Health, Physical Education, and Recreation and the Society of State Directors of Health, Physical Education, and Recreation developed a platform for physical education in 1950 that included a statement of the objectives of physical education: (1) develop and maintain maximum physical efficiency, (2) develop useful skills, (3) conduct oneself in socially useful ways, and (4) enjoy wholesome recreation.

The American Association for Health, Physical Education, and Recreation publication entitled *This Is Physical Education* incorporates a statement prepared by professional leaders of the physical education division of the AAHPER. This publication lists five major educational purposes for physical education:

1. To help children move in a skillful and effective manner in all the selected activities

in which they engage in the physical education program, and also in those situations which they will experience during their lifetime.

2. To develop an understanding and appreciation of movement in children and youth so that their lives will become more meaningful, purposive, and productive.
3. To develop an understanding and appreciation of certain scientific principles concerned with movement that relate to such factors as time, space, force, and mass-energy relationships.
4. To develop through the medium of games and sports better interpersonal relationships.
5. To develop the various organic systems of the body so they will respond in a healthful way to the increased demands placed upon them.

Rosentswieg, of Texas Woman's University, identified in 1967-1968 ten objectives of physical education from a study of the literature: (1) organic vigor, (2) democratic values, (3) social competency, (4) cultural appreciation, (5) leisure-time activities, (6) self-realization, (7) mental development, (8) emotional stability, (9) neuromuscular skills, and (10) spiritual and moral strength.

Objectives of physical education in Great Britain

Members of a study group composed of representatives of the Research Advisory Council of The Physical Education Association of Great Britain prepared a statement entitled "The Concept of Physical Education,"* which discussed the objectives of physical education as viewed by the British. There are four objectives of physical education. The first objective is a movement objective of a general nature, which includes the cultivation of good movement behavior in the total life situation. It involves such things as postural sensitivity and control and space awareness. This objective also refers to the development of a movement sense based upon both a kinetic experience and the observation of movement of other people. The second objective

is the learning of valuable skills and skilled activities that have cultural and educational value. The third objective is a concern for the right use of physical activity in the promotion of health and fitness. The fourth objective is intellectual, emotional, and social development through physical activities.

Foundations from which today's objectives of physical education are derived

In a strict sense of the term, physical education is not a discipline in itself but derives its objectives and scientific foundations from the disciplines of philosophy, biology, psychology, and sociology. Each of these areas is treated in detail in this text. The scientific foundations derived from the discipline of philosophy are discussed in Chapter 6. The scientific foundations derived from the discipline of biology are discussed in Chapters 15 and 16. The scientific foundations derived from the discipline of psychology are discussed in Chapter 17. The scientific foundations derived from the discipline of sociology are discussed in Chapter 18. As these chapters are studied, it will be possible for the reader to understand better the scientific foundations underlying his field of endeavor and the supporting evidence underlying the objective's worth in general education.

OBJECTIVES OF LEADERS OF PHYSICAL EDUCATION*

The objectives of physical education in the United States have been stated in the professional literature by many leaders in this field. These objectives are the goals toward which this profession is striving in a twentieth-century world. Space permits the listing of the objectives of only a few of the leaders of physical education.

Hetherington

Hetherington lists five classifications of objectives: the immediate objectives, the

---

*Physical Education Association of Great Britian: The concept of physical education, British Journal of Physical Education **1:**81, 1970.

*See references at the end of this chapter for publications of leaders of physical education and their objectives.

remote objectives, the objectives in development, the objectives in social standards, and the objectives in the control of health conditions.

Under the immediate objectives, Hetherington discusses the necessity of adult leadership in giving organization to the play life of children. He points out that with effective adult leadership, children's interest is increased, progress is much more rapid, the satisfaction derived from play is greater, there is more democratic organization, and play life is much more efficient.

Under the remote objectives, Hetherington stresses the role of physical education in developing abilities that make it easier for children to adapt themselves to adult group living. In the various physical education activities, growth needs are met that lay a foundation for effective group living.

In the third classification, objectives are divided into the development of instinct, intellectual, neuromuscular, and organic mechanisms.

The development of instinct mechanisms has implications for the development of character traits. As a result of participation in physical education activities, certain inherent instinct tendencies and emotions are expressed. The way a person reacts to participation in these activities depends upon the satisfactions or annoyances that result. Furthermore, whether or not character traits such as initiative, honesty, cooperation, self-subordination to the leader, and loyalty to the group are developed will depend upon the quality of the leadership provided.

The development of the intellectual mechanisms takes place through participation in a planned physical education program. Through activity, motor coordinations are learned and thus the intellectual mechanism is brought into play; strategic judgments are made in the various game situations; and, finally, a greater insight into human nature is gained through the various social experiences that take place in play activities.

The development of neuromuscular

mechanisms and nervous power, as another objective in development, emphasizes the fact that the nervous system is developed only as the muscular system is developed. Nervous connections are strengthened when muscles are exercised. Furthermore, nervous development occurs over a long period of time and after much repetition. You learn to consistently hit a golf ball straight down the fairway only after doing it hundreds of times. This nervous development must take place during the growth years. It is not developed as easily and effectively when maturity has been reached. The skill and strength gained by youth in physical activity will help to guarantee physical efficiency in the adult.

Finally, the development of organic power is, with the exception of heredity, brought about through physical activity. Organic power means vitality, vigor, capacity to assimilate food, stamina, and resistance to fatigue. The development of the circulatory, respiratory, digestive, heat regulatory, and other organic systems depends upon vigorous activity, and this development, together with sleep and proper nutrition, determines physical condition. To fulfill this objective, elementary school children should have from 4 to 5 hours and secondary school children from 2 to 3 hours of vigorous physical activity each day.

Social standards is Hetherington's fourth classification of objectives. By social standards, he refers to the criteria used in the guiding and in the judging of activities that result in adjustment to society. Children are not concerned with adult standards, and they utilize standards only as established through leadership. Physical education is concerned with objectives in respect to various social standards, including those concerned with items such as posture on the one hand and those concerned with morals, manners, and health on the other.

Hetherington's fifth classification of objectives is concerned with the control of health conditions. This refers to the steps taken to make the school a healthful place to live by eliminating all handicapping influences and encouraging and promoting healthful school practices.

Wood and Cassidy

Wood and Cassidy list two general objectives and certain specific objectives. The first general objective is the harmonious development during childhood of such qualities of the individual as interests, capacities, and abilities through the medium of natural physical education activities. The second general objective, which evolves naturally from the first, is the harmonious development of those interests, ideals, and habits that will make for a happy, healthful, and useful adult life.

The specific objectives listed by Wood and Cassidy help in the achievement of the general objectives. Such specific biological objectives are listed as muscular growth, organic vigor, nervous vitality, good health habits, correction of defects, good health service, and supervision of mental hygiene. Specific social and ethical objectives are listed that have to do with the development of the individual along social and ethical lines with a view to good citizenship. Specific intellectual objectives are listed that have to do with the development of intelligent leadership.

Nash

Nash lists four developmental objectives of physical education: organic, neuromuscular, interpretive, and emotional development. By organic development Nash means the end results of the training process that achieves physical power for the individual. This physical power is developed through big-muscle activity after freeing the body from physical defects and strains that are a drain on the human mechanism. The building of this physical power assures the individual of the ability to produce peak performance in activities requiring endurance, skill, speed, agility, and strength.

By neuromuscular development Nash means cortical control over the motor mechanism of the human body, the ability to cut down on waste motion so that ac-

tions are performed gracefully with little energy expended, and a longer period of rest between heartbeats or a longer glide in relation to the stroke of the heart. Such development implies a training period that begins early in youth and the opportunity to practice continually worthwhile and useful skills.

By interpretive development Nash means the training that helps an individual make judgments and interpret situations correctly. It implies that a person thinks through his previous experiences. The more experiences an individual has had and the better their quality, the better able he will be to interpret new experiences.

By emotional development Nash means the drives within the human being that result in action. The drives of desires, ideals, interests, and hungers impel individuals to act either in constructive or in destructive ways. If proper emotional development has taken place and has been brought under control, it can be directed toward great social advances rather than into antisocial behavior. Within physical education activities there are many inherent values that will grow and bear fruit under proper guidance. A child must have confidence, must experience success, and must have a feeling of "belonging" if he is to direct his emotions to the advantage of group living.

Williams

Williams first sets forth a broad aim of physical education as one that would provide qualified leadership, adequate facilities, and experiences having physical, mental, and social implications. Then he goes on to list general concrete objectives of physical education. These include preventive and corrective objectives of individual gymnastics as concerned with the adjustment of the various body parts to each other; objectives in games and sports that will guarantee further participation in these activities; objectives of dance involving the development of the whole individual; objectives in hiking, camping, fishing, and hunting concerned with military and social preparedness; objectives in self-testing, stunt, and combat activities, including the development of confidence, courage, and the ability to control the body effectively; objectives in fundamental skills such as walking, running, jumping, leaping, throwing, hanging, climbing, lifting, and carrying, which are important for their utilitarian value in day-to-day living; and the objectives in equipment and staff, based upon the needs of children and the social needs of society, making imperative an adequate school plant and well-qualified teachers.

Bookwalter*

Bookwalter has outlined the purposes of physical education in an interesting manner as shown in the accompanying chart. As outlined in the hierarchical arrangement, Bookwalter lists at the philosophical level the ultimate aim of physical education. At the sociological level, he lists remote adjustment objectives of health, worthy use of leisure, and ethical character. Evolving from these three objectives is the biological level and the intermediate objectives of development, namely, organic development, neuromuscular development, interpretative cortical development, and emotional-impulsive development. Finally, to give meaning and understanding to these objectives, Bookwalter lists certain controls at the next or pedagogical level. The immediate control objectives (outcomes) at the pedagogical level listed by Bookwalter are: condition controls—physical changes (physical fitness), fixed controls—habits and skills (sports habits and skills), adaptive controls—knowledge, judgments, insights, and understanding (sports understanding), and pattern controls—appreciation, attitudes, and ideals (sportsmanship). The total chart indicates that the process of education is founded on the belief that specific outcomes will occur and will lead to the attainment of the remote objectives and ultimate aim.

---

*Bookwalter, Karl W.: Physical education in the secondary schools, Washington, D. C., 1964, The Center for Applied Research in Education, Inc.

Oberteuffer and Ulrich

Oberteuffer and Ulrich list several immediate and long-range objectives or outcomes toward which physical educators should direct their efforts. The first group of these outcomes includes those that are immediate, easily recognized, and gained by the individual through participation. They are skill in an activity, organic values, and fun and amusement. The second group consists of those outcomes that, although frequently seen, are more difficult to achieve. These are psychological characteristics and social controls. The third and last group is composed of those outcomes that have outstanding value but are very difficult to achieve. However, their achievement is possible, and any physical education program designed to make the greatest contribution to the individual and to society will reach these goals. They are a deeper understanding of human nature and human relations, an understanding of the democratic way of life, and practice in reflective thinking.

OBJECTIVES OF STUDENTS IN PHYSICAL EDUCATION PROGRAMS

A survey of approximately 2,500 students at various educational levels was conducted in my classes in order to determine what students' objectives were in taking physical education. Students were surveyed who represented various kinds of individual differences and constituted the following categories: normal, academically gifted, culturally disadvantaged, poorly coordinated, emotionally disturbed, mentally retarded, and physically handicapped. Each student was asked the following two questions: What do you want to get out of your physical education class? and What should the physical education program do for you as a student? The following represents a summary of the findings of this survey.

1. *At the primary grade level* (kindergarten to third grade) the students viewed the physical education program as a place to have fun and learn games. These young-

sters also desired exercise in order that they could grow to be big and strong. Some students at this early age indicated that they wanted to learn how to become an athlete and wanted to play on a team. The poorly coordinated child hoped that he could improve his fitness in order that he could rejoin his regular class. The mentally retarded youngster indicated that he hoped physical education would make him "smarter."

2. *At the intermediate grade level* (fourth to sixth grades) students indicated that the physical education program should be a place to have fun and to learn skills and various sports. They also indicated the need for exercise in order to improve their fitness. At this age level it was almost unanimous that physical education was viewed as a place where new friendships could be made. Students also emphasized the point

that the physical education program gave them the opportunity to "show off," and that they were also able to relieve their tensions.

3. *At the junior high level* (seventh to ninth grades) students again stated that physical education should be concerned with improving one's fitness and health. Students indicated that they wanted to learn new skills and many sports. Students at this age level also indicated that physical education should do more than just develop the body; it should also develop the mind and prepare one for his future work. At the junior high level, students viewed physical education as a place to learn fair play and good sportsmanship. They also emphasized the point that they wanted to learn activities that would prove useful in their leisure hours. The majority of students at

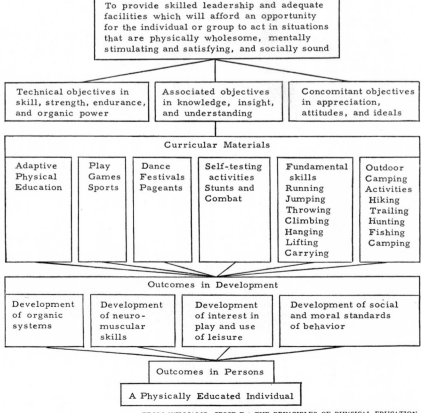

THE AIM OF PHYSICAL EDUCATION

To provide skilled leadership and adequate facilities which will afford an opportunity for the individual or group to act in situations that are physically wholesome, mentally stimulating and satisfying, and socially sound

| Technical objectives in skill, strength, endurance, and organic power | Associated objectives in knowledge, insight, and understanding | Concomitant objectives in appreciation, attitudes, and ideals |

Curricular Materials

| Adaptive Physical Education | Play Games Sports | Dance Festivals Pageants | Self-testing activities Stunts and Combat | Fundamental skills Running Jumping Throwing Climbing Hanging Lifting Carrying | Outdoor Camping Activities Hiking Trailing Hunting Fishing Camping |

Outcomes in Development

| Development of organic systems | Development of neuro-muscular skills | Development of interest in play and use of leisure | Development of social and moral standards of behavior |

Outcomes in Persons

A Physically Educated Individual

FROM WILLIAMS, JESSE F.: THE PRINCIPLES OF PHYSICAL EDUCATION, PHILADELPHIA, 1946, W. B. SAUNDERS CO.

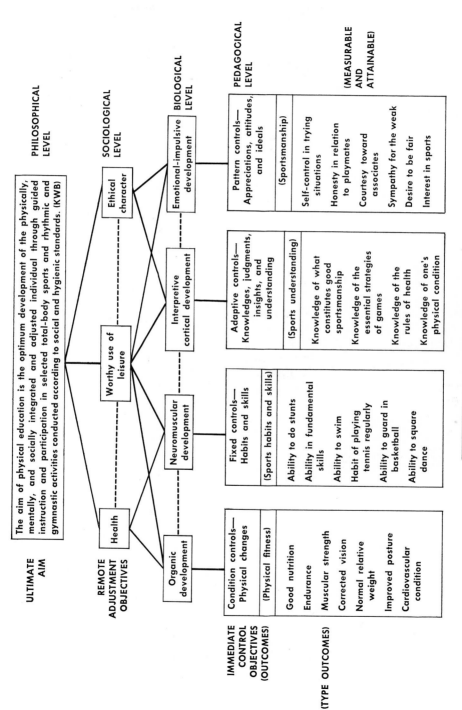

THE PURPOSES OF PHYSICAL EDUCATION

FROM BOOKWALTER, KARL W.: PHYSICAL EDUCATION IN THE SECONDARY SCHOOLS, WASHINGTON, D. C., 1964, THE CENTER FOR APPLIED RESEARCH IN EDUCATION, INC.

this age also indicated the desire to play on a team.

4. *At the high school level* (tenth to twelfth grades) students stressed the point that exercise was important because it improved one's health and fitness. Students indicated that they wanted to learn many skills and sports. They also wanted to participate in activities that will benefit them in their leisure time. At this level, students desired to play harmoniously with others and to participate in team play. Students at the high school level viewed physical education as a place where they could learn to respect their fellow students. Students also indicated that the physical education program provided them with a change of pace from their academic subjects.

5. *At the college level* students emphasized the importance that physical education plays in neuromuscular development and cardiovascular efficiency. Students indicated that physical education provided them with mental stimulation and gave them the opportunity to socialize with others. College students also indicated that physical education provided them with mental relaxation from their academic studies and introduced them to activities that would prove useful in their leisure time. College students viewed physical education as a contribution to one's mental, physical, psychological, and social development.

Most of the students surveyed, regardless of how they differed from the other students, had similar ideas as to the contribution physical education could make to their lives.

OBJECTIVES IN TERMS OF SCIENTIFIC PRINCIPLES

The professional literature has several books that discuss the principles of physical education. According to Williams,* principles are concepts that have a scientific foundation and that are based upon

facts or upon philosophical inquiry. The source of principles, therefore, can come from philosophy through insight, experience, or understanding, such as the principle that the democratic concept helps to assure the dignity of man. In the field of physical education a principle of this type might be that the welfare of the participant rather than the welfare of the school should dominate athletic programs.

Principles also are derived from scientific facts from such sources as anatomy, physiology, psychology, and other sciences. Darwin, for example, found that the principle of natural selection was valid from his study of animal life, and Cannon found that the principle of homeostasis was valid from his studies. In the field of physical education, the sciences of anatomy, physiology, and psychology, for example, provide principles regarding the developmental stages of the vital organs and the laws of learning.

Principles that give support and a scientific foundation to objectives have been set forth by Adams based on his research into the writings of many of the outstanding leaders in the field.*

1. *Education involves the whole organism.* Oneness of mind and body or the unity of man is a recognized basic tenet of education.

2. *Physical education is a phase of general education.* The objectives toward which physical education is striving are compatible and contribute to the objectives of general education.

3. *Physical education activity is conducive to growth and development.* The optimum development of the organic systems of the human body is dependent upon physical activity.

4. *Physical education contributes to the constructive use of leisure time.* Many skills and activities learned in physical education have implications for free hours during all of a person's life.

---

*Williams, Jesse Feiring: The principles of physical education, Philadelphia 1964, W. B. Saunders Co., Chapter 1.

*Adams, Miller K.: Principles for determining high school grading procedures in physical education for boys, Doctoral thesis, New York University, 1959.

5. *Physical education provides for leadership training.* There is great potential and opportunity within physical education to involve students in the planning and operation of the program.

6. *Physical education provides opportunity for expression and creativity.* There are many opportunities in physical education to utilize the body as a means of expressing one's feelings and creating new patterns of movement and ideas.

7. *Physical education provides for cultural development.* Sports and physical activities play an important role in the cultures of all peoples. These activities are a positive source of both esthetic appreciations and artistic production for the participant.

8. *Physical education provides for training emotions—sportsmanship.* The give and take of games and sports offers opportunities for both emotional release and the training of the emotions.

9. *Physical education provides for personality and character development.* Group effort, loyalty to the team, and strong ties are much in evidence on play and sports fields. As such, they provide a valuable contribution to the development of character and personality. The daily adjustments to teammates and opponents become a laboratory in personal social adjustment.

10. *Physical education provides for organic development—physical fitness.* Exercise and knowledge about one's body and its requirements contribute immeasurably to physical fitness.

11. *Physical education develops neuromuscular skills.* Skills in a variety of sports and activities present many opportunities for instructing pupils in this phase of their development.

12. *Physical education develops habits of health and safety.* The teacher of physical education instructs the pupils in habits of health and safety, and games and contests are played under conditions conducive to learning safety and health practices.

13. *Physical education provides for mental development.* The learning of game rules, techniques, and strategies, as well as the judgments necessary to good play in competitive games, requires interpretive development. Other avenues for mental development are inculcating understanding in regard to one's body and how it functions, the history of sports, the place of athletic activities in the cultures of the world, and other knowledge closely allied to physical education.

14. *Physical education contributes to democratic processes.* The physical education class is conducted in a manner that provides pupils with the opportunity to participate in planning and carrying out class activities.

15. *Physical education has biological, psychological, and sociological foundations.* Physical education has its bases in the sciences of biology, psychology, and sociology. The program is planned by teachers and administrators who draw upon these sciences for realistic and effective programs.

16. *Physical education is based on human needs.* Movement is recognized as an important human need. The need for physical activity is essential to life itself. Modern living with its sedentary aspects presents a challenge to physical education.

17. *Play is an instinctive drive that has educational potential.* The dynamic quality of play can be utilized to instill in participants proper forms of conduct and behavior.

FULLER DISCUSSION OF OBJECTIVES OF PHYSICAL EDUCATION

A study of the objectives as stated by leaders in physical education reveals a great deal of similarity. This is as it should be in that the physical education profession should be united and directing itself toward common goals. Only through a uniformity of purpose will it be possible for the thousands of professional leaders in this field to be continually conscious of what they are trying to accomplish when they meet their class, organize a game, supervise a

DEVELOPMENTAL OBJECTIVES OF PHYSICAL EDUCATION

ORGANIC

Proper functioning of the body systems so that the individual may adequately meet the demands placed upon him by his environment. A foundation for skill development.

Muscle Strength
The maximum amount of force exerted by a muscle or muscle group.

Muscle Endurance
The ability of a muscle or muscle group to sustain effort for a prolonged period of time.

Cardiovascular Endurance
The capacity of an individual to persist in strenuous activity for periods of some duration. This is dependent upon the combined efficiency of the blood vessels, heart, and lungs.

Flexibility
The range of motion in joints needed to produce efficient movement and minimize injury.

NEUROMUSCULAR

A harmonious functioning of the nervous and muscular systems to produce desired movements.

Locomotor Skills
Walking   Skipping   Sliding   Leaping   Pushing
Running   Galloping   Hopping   Rolling   Pulling

Nonlocomotor Skills
Swaying   Twisting   Shaking   Stretching
Bending   Handing   Stooping

Game Type Fundamental Skills
Striking   Catching   Kicking   Stopping
Throwing   Batting   Starting   Changing direction

Motor Factors
Accuracy   Rhythm   Kinesthetic awareness
Power   Balance   Reaction time   Agility

Sport Skills
Soccer   Softball   Volleyball   Wrestling
Track & Field   Football   Baseball
Basketball   Archery   Speedball   Hockey
Fencing   Golf   Bowling   Tennis

Recreational Skills
Shuffleboard   Croquet   Deck tennis   Hiking
Table tennis   Swimming   Horseshoes   Boating

INTERPRETIVE

The ability to explore, to discover, to understand, to acquire knowledge, and to make value judgments.

A knowledge of game rules, safety measures, and etiquette.

The use of strategies and techniques involved in organized activities.

A knowledge of how the body functions and its relationship to physical activity.

A development of appreciation for personal performance. The use of judgment related to distance, time, space, force, speed, and direction in the use of activity implements, balls, and self.

An understanding of growth and developmental factors affected by movement.

The ability to solve developmental problems through movement.

SOCIAL

An adjustment to both self and others by an integration of the individual to society and his environment.

The ability to make judgments in a group situation.

Learning to communicate with others.

The ability to exchange and evaluate ideas within a group.

The development of the social phases of personality, attitudes, and values in order to become a functioning member of society.

The development of a sense of belonging and acceptance by society.

The development of positive personality traits.

Learnings for constructive use of leisure time.

A development of attitude that reflects good moral character.

EMOTIONAL

A healthy response to physical activity through a fulfillment of basic needs.

The development of positive reactions in spectatorship and participation through either success or failure.

The release of tension through suitable physical activities.

An outlet for self-expression and creativity.

An appreciation of the aesthetic experiences derived from correlated activities.

The ability to have fun.

FROM ANNARINO, ANTHONY A.: THE FIVE TRADITIONAL OBJECTIVES OF PHYSICAL EDUCATION, JOURNAL OF HEALTH, PHYSICAL EDUCATION, AND RECREATION **41**:25, 1970.

program of activities, and evaluate their work. In unity there is strength.

The aim of all education is to enable one to live an enriched and abundant life. This is the ultimate goal on which all who are concerned with education have trained their sights. The objectives of physical education are more definite and specific than this aim, and through these objectives the ultimate goal is brought nearer to realization.

A study of the child reveals four general directions or phases in which growth and development take place: physical development, motor development, mental development, and social development. Each of these phases contributes to the well-rounded individual who will become a worthy member of society. Physical education can play a very important part in contributing to each of these phases of child growth and development. The objectives listed by present-day leaders of physical education in the majority of cases may be incorporated under these groupings. Therefore I have used these four phases as objectives for the field. It is believed that physical education will justify its existence in the educational process if it can accomplish the objectives that are set forth under these four headings.

Any discussion of objectives must be interpreted in light of the phenomenon that the individual needs to be *well-integrated,* possessing optimum development in each phase of his total development.

The AAHPER publication *This Is Physical Education* points out the importance of movement experiences in transforming the child into a fully integrated person. Thinking, learning, and body behavior are all tied closely together and function as a whole. What is very important to understand is that many ideas are translated into perceivable forms by body movement; the better a person understands movement, the better he will perform. Children are concerned with concepts, symbols, and skills of movement, and physical education can render a valuable contribution in a subject "in which children learn to move as they move to learn."

Physical development objective*

The objective of physical development deals with the program of activities that builds physical power in an individual through the development of the various organic systems of the body. It results in the ability to sustain adaptive effort, the ability to recover, and the ability to resist fatigue. The value of this objective is based on the fact that an individual will be more active, have better performance, and be healthier if the organic systems of the body are adequately developed and functioning properly.

Muscular activity plays a major role in the development of the organic systems of the body. The term *organic* refers to the digestive, circulatory, excretory, heat regulatory, respiratory, and other systems of the human body. These systems are stimulated and trained through such activities as hanging, climbing, running, throwing, leaping, carrying, and jumping. Health is also related to muscular activity; therefore, activities that bring into play all of the fundamental "big-muscle" groups in the body should be engaged in regularly. Furthermore, the activity should be of a vigorous nature so that the various organic systems are sufficiently stimulated.

Through vigorous muscular activity, several beneficial results take place. The trained heart provides better nourishment to the entire body. The trained heart beats slower than the untrained heart and pumps more blood per stroke, with the result that more food is delivered to the cells and there is better removal of waste products. During exercise the trained heart's speed increases less and has a longer rest period between beats, and after exercise it returns to normal much more rapidly. The end result of this state is that the trained individual is able to perform work for a longer period of time, with less expenditure of energy, and much more efficiently than the untrained individual. This trained condition is necessary to a vigorous and abundant life. From the time an individual rises

---

*See also Chapters 15 and 16.

in the morning until the time he goes to bed at night, he is continually in need of vitality, strength, endurance, and stamina to perform routine tasks; he must be prepared for emergencies; and he must lead a vigorous life. Therefore, physical education should aid in the development of the trained individual so that he will be better able to perform his routine tasks and live a healthful and happy existence.

Hetherington* points out that physical activity is the only source of development of the latent powers of the organism that are inherited. Although sleep, nutrition, and rest, for example, contribute to the proper functioning of the organism, they have no power to develop latent resources, which physical activity does accomplish. Hetherington also points out that a healthy nervous system depends upon vigorous physical activity during the early years of childhood and youth. He explains that the only way that nerve centers can be reached and developed is through physical activity involving exercising the muscles that the nervous system controls.

---

*Hetherington, Clark W.: School program in physical education, New York, 1922, Harcourt, Brace & World, Inc.

Hein and Ryan* did an extensive research study collecting and analyzing clinical observations and scientific findings on the contributions of physical activity to physical health. They feel the following conclusions can be justified as a result of their work:

1. Regular exercise can assist in the prevention of obesity with the result that the shortened life span and degenerative conditions caused by such a condition can be influenced.
2. Regular physical activity throughout life appears to inhibit coronary heart disease.
3. Regular physical activity assists in delaying the aging process and probably favorably influences longevity.
4. Regular physical activity contributes to a body condition that enables the individual to better meet emergencies and thus, in turn, enhance health and avoid disability.

Motor and movement development objective

The motor and movement development objective is concerned with making physical movement useful, with as little expenditure of energy as possible, and with being proficient, graceful, and esthetic in this movement. This has implications for one's work,

---

*Hein, Fred V., and Ryan, Allan J.: Research Quarterly **31:**263, 1960.

Judo contributes to physical development objective.

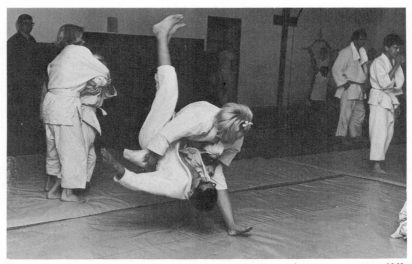

FROM MICHAELSON, MIKE: JUDO: NOW IT'S A SAFE FAMILY SPORT, TODAY'S HEALTH, FEBRUARY, 1969.

play, and anything else that requires physical movement. The name *motor* is derived from the relationship to a nerve or nerve fiber that connects the central nervous system or a ganglion with a muscle. As a consequence of the impulse it transmits, movement results. The impulse it delivers is known as the motor impulse.

Effective movement and motor behavior results in esthetic qualities of movement and in the development of a movement sense, which in essence is the development of motor skill together with appropriate knowledge about the skill and an appropriate attitude toward its development and use. In other words, proper control of skill in movement during all of life's patterns and routines takes place in the movement-educated person.

Effective motor movement is dependent upon a harmonious working together of the muscular and nervous systems. It results in greater distance between fatigue and peak performance; it is found in activities that involve such things as running, hanging, jumping, dodging, leaping, kicking, bending, twisting, carrying, and throwing; and it will enable a person to perform his daily work much more efficiently and without reaching the point of being "worn out" so quickly.

In physical education activities the function of efficient body movement or neuromuscular skill, as it is often called, is to provide the individual with the ability to perform with a degree of perfection. This will result in his enjoyment of participation. Most individuals enjoy doing those particular things in which they have acquired some degree of mastery or skill. For example, if a child has mastered the ability to throw a ball consistently at a designated spot and has developed batting and fielding power, he will like to play baseball or softball. If he can kick and throw a ball with some degree of accuracy, he will like soccer or football. If an adult can consistently serve tennis "aces," he will like tennis; if he can consistently drive a ball 250 yards straight down the fairway, he will

like golf; and if he can consistently throw ringers, he will like horseshoes. A person enjoys doing those things in which he excels. Few individuals enjoy participating in activities in which they have little skill. Therefore, it is the objective of physical education to develop in each individual as many skills as possible so that his interests will be wide and varied. This will not only result in more enjoyment for the participant, but at the same time it will allow for a better adjustment to the group situation.

Other values of skill are that it cuts down on expenditure of energy, contributes to confidence, brings recognition, enhances physical and mental health, makes participation safer, and contributes to the esthetic sense.

Physical skills are not developed in one lesson. It takes years to acquire coordinations, and the most important period for development is during the formative years of a child's growth. The building of coordinations starts in childhood, when an individual attempts to synchronize his muscular and nervous systems for such things as creeping, walking, running, and jumping. A study of kinesiology shows that many muscles of the body are used in the most simple of coordinated movements. Therefore, in order to obtain efficient motor movement or skill in many activities, it is necessary that an individual's training start early in life and continue into adulthood. Furthermore, a child does not object to the continual trial-and-error process of achieving success in the performance of physical acts. He does not object to being observed as an awkward, uncoordinated beginner during the learning period. However, most adults are self-conscious when going through a period of learning a physical skill. They do not like to perform if they cannot perform in a creditable manner. The skills they do not acquire in their youth are many times never acquired. Therefore, the physical education profession should try to see that this skill learning takes place at a time when a person is young and willing and is laying the foundation for his adult years.

The motor objective also has important implications for the health and recreational phases of the program. The skills that children acquire will determine to a great extent how their leisure time will be spent. A person enjoys participating in those activities in which he excels. Therefore, if a child excels in swimming, much of his leisure time is going to be spent in a pool, lake, or other body of water. If he excels in tennis, he will be found on the courts on Saturdays, Sundays, and after dinner at night. There is a correlation between juvenile delinquency and lack of constructive leisure-time activity. If a parent would have a child spend some of his leisure moments in a physically wholesome way, he should see that the child gains skill in some physical education activity.

While considering the value to an individual of having in his possession fundamental skills that will afford him much satisfaction and happiness throughout life, it is important to consider the balance that should exist in any physical education program between team sports and dual and individual sports. Team sports such as football, basketball, and baseball perform a great service in providing an opportunity for students to develop physical power and enjoy exhilarating competition. However, in many school programs of physical education they dominate the curriculum at the expense of various individual and dual sports, such as tennis, swimming, badminton, handball, and golf. In such cases the student is being deprived of the opportunity for developing skills in activities that he can play until the time he dies. It has been estimated that only one out of every 1,000 students who play football, for example,

Skill in bowling.

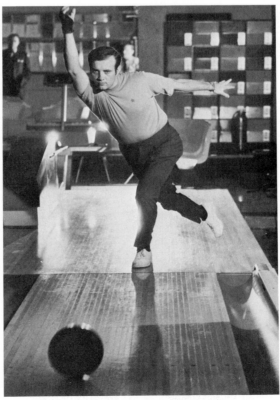

ever play the game again after they leave school. On the other hand, if they have the skill, many students will swim or play tennis, badminton, handball, or golf. Comparatively few students engage in many team sports after formal schooling ends. Team sports such as football, basketball, and baseball have much to offer and if possible should be included in every physical education program. However, it would seem wise to have an adequate program of individual and dual sports also. Only through a well-balanced program will it be possible to develop the well-rounded individual.

Ever since man first learned to coordinate his muscular and nervous systems for physical action, there has been popular interest in acts of human skill. David casting the deadly stone accurately with his slingshot, William Tell splitting the apple on his son's head with his bow and arrow, Pheidippides racing to announce the Greek victory at Marathon, and Ben Hur driving his chariot at breakneck speed down the stretch to victory—all are a part of the world's literature that inspire young and old alike.

Physical skill plays an important role in the culture of all peoples. It packs stadiums, crowds palaestras, and usurps television screens. It emblazons the names of champions on printed programs, newspaper scareheads, and advertising billboards. It captivates men's thoughts, holds them spellbound, and receives their plaudits.

Physical educators should be proud to be the teachers and the nurturers of skill. They help to shape men's lives, build a strong people, and further international peace. Their services are sought by schools, colleges, boy's clubs, Girl Scouts, hospitals, Peace Corps, churches, country clubs, and other organizations. Yes, theirs is an important business in this world.

The role physical educators play in the skill education of boys and girls is one of their most important responsibilities. Here they have an opportunity to apply their art in a manner that will influence a young person's life for the better. Just as the sculptor takes clay and with his hands molds a lifelike image of a person, so physical educators, through expert skill instruction, mold human bodies that possess esthetically beautiful qualities. To show young people how to hit a backhand shot effectively, execute a flying camel spin, and send the arrow accurately into the gold circle are contributions to human betterment well worth the time, efforts, and energies of physical educators.

Physical skill has values for many persons. The spectator thrills to the chase, struggle, competition, and challenge. The sportswriter prospers as his copy spells out the exciting action. The keeper of the coffers smiles as the coins tinkle into the treasury. Mothers and fathers brag as they bask in the glory of their children's achievements. And coaches are imbued with a sense of pride as their charges gain fame. *But,* great as these values may be for the people who vicariously profit from human skill, *none can compare to the worth it has for the participant.*

Physical educators can and should be proud of the contribution they make to humanity. It is within their power to give boys and girls physical skills and thus help them to lead healthier, happier, and more worthwhile and productive lives. The world is a better place in which to live as a result of their work, because *physical skill has worth.*

Cognitive development objective

The cognitive development objective deals with the accumulation of a body of knowledge and the ability to think and to interpret this knowledge.

Physical education has a subject matter concerned with movement. There is a body of knowledge that comes from the sciences, humanities, and other sources that interprets the nature of human movement and the impact of movement upon the growth and development of the individual and upon his culture. Scientific principles regarding movement, including those that relate to such factors as time, space, and flow, should be considered. This subject matter should be part of the education of each person who comes in contact with a physical education program.

Physical activities must be learned; hence, there is a need for thinking on the part of the intellectual mechanism, with a resulting acquisition of knowledge. The coordinations involved in various movements must be mastered and adapted to the environment in which the individual lives, whether it be in walking, running, or wielding a tennis racquet. In all these movements the child must think and coordinate his muscular and nervous systems. Furthermore, this type of knowledge is acquired through trial and error, and then as a result of this experience there is a changed meaning in the situation. Coordinations are learned, with the result that an act that once was difficult and awkward to perform becomes easy to execute.

The individual should not only learn coordinations but should also acquire a knowledge of such things as rules, techniques, and strategies involved in physical activities. Basketball can be used as an example. In this sport a person should know such things as the rules, the strategy in offense and defense, the various types of passes, the difference between screening and blocking, and, finally, the values that are derived from playing this sport. Techniques learned through experience result in knowledge that should also be acquired. For example, a ball travels faster and more accurately if one steps with a pass, and time is saved when the pass is made from the same position in which it is received. Furthermore, a knowledge of followership, leadership, courage, self-reliance, assistance to others, safety, and adaptation to group patterns is very important.

Knowledge concerning health should play an important part in the program. All individuals should know about their bodies, the importance of sanitation, factors in disease prevention, importance of exercise, need for a well-balanced diet, values of good health attitudes and habits, and the community and school agencies that provide health services. Through the accumulation of a knowledge of these facts, activities will take on a new meaning and health practices will be associated with definite purposes. This will help each individual live a healthier and more purposeful life.

Physical educators can intellectualize their activities more. Physical activities are not performed in a vacuum. Physical educators should continually provide appropriate knowledge and information for their students and encourage them to ask the question, "Why?" *Why* is it important to play this activity? *Why* should an hour a day be devoted to physical education? *Why* is exercise important? *Why* is it important to play according to the rules? Physical educators should also give their students more opportunities to think—allow them to make choices, plan strategies, and call plays and not usurp all of this responsibility themselves. *The more thinking that takes place on the part of the student, the more educational the activity becomes.*

A store of knowledge will give each individual the proper background for interpreting new situations that confront him from day to day. Unless there is knowledge to draw from, he will become helpless when called upon to make important decisions. As a result of participation in physical education activities, an individual will be better able to make discriminatory judgments, by which knowledge of values is mentally arrived at. This means that he has greater power for arriving at a wise decision and that he can better discern right from wrong and the logical from the illogical. Through his experience in various games and sports he will develop a sense of values, an alertness, the ability to diagnose a tense situation, the ability to make a decision quickly under highly emotionalized conditions, and the ability to interpret human actions.

In physical education activities a person also gains insight into human nature. Physical education, as expressed in the various forms of activity, consists of social experiences that enable a participant to learn about human nature. For all children, this is one of the main sources of such knowledge. Here they discover the individual's responsibility to the group, the need for followership and leadership, the need to experience success, and the feeling of "belonging." Here they learn how human beings react to satisfactions and annoyances. Such knowledge contributes to social efficiency and good human relations.

Social development objective

The social development objective is concerned with helping an individual in making personal adjustments, group adjustments, and adjustments as a member of society. Activities in the physical education program offer one of the best opportunities for making these adjustments, provided there is proper leadership.

Physical educators should find as many ways as possible to influence human behavior for the good. The rules of the game are the rules of the democratic way of life. Through games one sees democracy in action and appreciates an individual on the basis of his ability and performance. Economic status, background, race, or other discriminatory characteristics do not play a role. Performance is the sole criterion of success.

> I give no thought to my neighbor's birth
> Or the way he makes his prayer
> I grant him a free man's room on earth
> If his game is only square.
>
> BADGER CLARK, JR.

Another aspect of the social objective of physical education that is being recognized is the need for each boy and girl to develop an appropriate self-concept. Students need to develop wholesome attitudes toward themselves as maturing persons. During the various stages of physical growth through which young people go, they are often accepted or rejected by their classmates because of their physical characteristics. It is therefore important for each person to develop himself physically, not only for reasons of his own self-awareness but also because of the implications that his physique and physical skills have for his social image.

Another aspect of the social objective that should be kept in mind is the emergence of many social trends and forces in the American society. The demand on the part of youth to be involved, the problems of the inner city, the question of race relations, drugs, student unrest, and other social problems represent a challenge to today's physical educator.

Each individual has certain basic social needs that must be met. These include a feeling of belonging, recognition, self-respect, and love. When these needs are met, the individual becomes well adjusted socially. When they are not met, antisocial characteristics develop. For example, the aggressive bully may be seeking recognition, and the member of the gang may be seeking a feeling of belonging. The "needs" theory has tremendous implications for the manner in which we conduct our physical education programs. The desire to win, for example, should be subordinated to meeting the needs of the participants. This may mean that the fellow who is out in right field should be brought in to pitch a couple of innings or that the girl who has a great loyalty to the team but little skill should be allowed to become a member of the squad.

Social action is a result of certain hereditary and derivative tendencies. There are interests, hungers, desires, ideals, attitudes, and emotional drives responsible for everything we do. A child wants to play because of his drive for physical activity. A man will steal food because of the hunger drive. Americans are opposed to totalitarian governments because of the desire for personal freedom. The response to all these desires, drives, hungers, and the like may be either social or antisocial in nature. They are social or antisocial depending on whether the experience is pleasing or displeasing. The value of physical education reveals itself when we realize that play activities are one of the oldest and most fundamental drives in human nature. Therefore, by providing the child with a satisfying experience in activities in which he has a natural desire to engage, the opportunity is presented to develop desirable social traits. The key is qualified leadership.

All human beings should experience success. This factor can be realized through play. Through successful experience in play activities, a child develops self-confidence and finds happiness in his achievements. Physical education can provide for this successful experience by offering a variety of activities and developing the necessary skills for success in these activities.

If children are happy, they will make the necessary adjustments. An individual who is happy is much more likely to make the right adjustment than the individual who is morbid, sullen, and unhappy. Happiness reflects friendliness, cheerfulness, and a spirit of cooperation, all of which help a person to be contented and to conform to the necessary standards that have been established. Therefore, physical education should instill happiness by guiding children into the activities in which this quality will be realized.

In the democratic society in which we live, it is necessary to have all individuals develop a sense of group consciousness and cooperative living. This should be one of the most important objectives of the program. Whether or not a child will grow up to be a good citizen and contribute to the welfare of all will depend to a great extent upon the training he receives during his youth. Therefore, in various play activities, the following factors should be stressed: aid for the less skilled and weaker players, respect for the rights of others, subordination of one's desires to the will of the group, and realization of cooperative living as an essential to the success of society. The individual should be made to feel that he belongs to the group and has the responsibility of directing his actions in its behalf. The rules of sportsmanship should be developed and practiced in all activities offered in the program. Such things as courtesy, sympathy, truthfulness, fairness, honesty, respect for authority, and abiding by the rules will help considerably in the promotion of social efficiency. The necessity of good leadership and followership should also be stressed as important to the interests of society.

The needs and desires that form the basis for people's actions can be controlled through proper training. This training can result in effective citizenship, which is the basis of sound democratic living. This effective citizenship is not something that can be developed through the setting up of artificial stimuli. It is something that is achieved only through activities in which individuals engage in their normal day-to-day routine. Since play activities have such a great attraction for youth and since it is possible to develop desirable social traits under proper guidance, physical education should realize its responsibility and do its part in contributing to good citizenship, the basis of our democratic society. In this chaotic world with its cold wars, hot wars, hydrogen bombs, racial strife, imperialistic aims, human ambitions, and class struggles, human relations are more and more important to personal, group, and world peace. Only through a better understanding of one's fellow man will it be possible to build a peaceful and a democratic world.

"Plus factor"

There is another factor that should not be overlooked. This is the "plus factor." This is something above and beyond the call of duty—going the second mile, something we will have to stretch a little to accomplish. But, as Browning says: "Ah! but a man's reach should exceed his grasp or what's a heaven for?"

Physical educators cannot be content once they have developed the physical body, laid down the skills in the nervous system, and developed the amenities of social behavior. There is still something else, and this represents one of the greatest challenges to the field in which so many young people have a drive to engage. Boys and girls look to members of the profession for guidance and want to emulate them. The weight of such responsibility lies heavily upon their shoulders.

Physical educators have to make sure that all this strength, skill, and knowledge are used toward desirable ends. Hitler and Stalin used theirs to hurt people. On the other hand, Samson's strength found its highest value when he used it to deliver Israel from pagan tyranny. David's skill with the sling and Jonathan's use of the bow and arrow also served to help promote the finer things in life.

Members of the physical education profession must be concerned with ethics, making value judgments, and promoting the finer things in life. If they achieve these things their profession will grow and prosper because it has been built upon strong foundations—it will be used in the interest of helping human beings to live a more abundant life and to achieve excellence in their endeavors.

> One ship drives east and another drives west,
> With the selfsame winds that blow.
> 'Tis the set of the sails and not the gales
> That determines the way they go.
> ELLA WHEELER WILCOX

IS THERE A PRIORITY FOR OBJECTIVES OF PHYSICAL EDUCATION?

Leaders of physical education are beginning to ask such questions as: Is one objective of physical education more important than the others? Where should the emphasis in physical education programs be placed? Physical educators cannot do everything—what comes first? Does physical education have a master purpose? Is there a hierarchy of objectives?

Historically, we have seen where physical education in its early days was primarily concerned with organic development. However, at the turn of the century with the introduction of the "new physical education," other objectives more closely identified with general education, such as social development, were included. Today, there are varying viewpoints in regard to the question of priority of objectives.

A survey of selected leaders in the field of physical education, asking for their views as to a priority of objectives, resulted in some interesting information. Most professionals contacted felt that organic development and neuromuscular development are the objectives that should get highest priority. They listed such reasons as: they are uniquely tied in with physical education, they are essential for fitness throughout life, they provide the impetus for the program, and they represent the objectives that can more readily be achieved. After organic and neuromuscular development, the leaders surveyed indicated that the most widely accepted objective in terms of importance is mental or interpretive development. The reasons listed for the importance of this objective included the fact that it is important to develop a favorable attitude toward physical education if any objective is to be achieved at all. Also included was the fact that education is primarily involved with developing a thinking, rational human being in respect to all matters, whether it be concerned with his physical development or other aspects of living. Social development ranked lowest in the survey. Reasons given to support this place on the priority listing were that all areas of education are interested in the social objective and that it was not the unique responsibility of one field, such as physical education. Therefore, the other objectives should receive a higher priority rating.

The survey of national leaders in physical education brought out another important consideration. Many professional leaders stressed the point that, with the national curriculum reform movement taking place today and with increased emphasis on educational priorities, physical educators should rethink their positions in regard to their place in the educational system. They should reexamine how they can contribute their greatest effort and make their greatest contribution in today's changing world.

Rosentswieg* conducted a study in which he had 100 college physical educators in the State of Texas rank ten objec-

*Rosentswieg, Joel: A ranking of the objectives of physical education, Research Quarterly **40**:783, 1969.

Table 6-1. Comparison ranking of objectives of physical education*

Objective	Ranking
Organic vigor	1
Neuromuscular skills	2
Leisure-time activities	3
Self-realization	4
Emotional stability	5
Democratic values	6
Mental development	7
Social competency	8
Spiritual and moral strength	9
Cultural appreciation	10

*From Rosentswieg, Joel: A ranking of the objectives of physical education, Research Quarterly **40**:783, 1969.

Table 6-2. Ranking of objectives by sex*

Objective	Ranking Males	Females
Organic vigor	1	2
Neuromuscular skills	2	1
Leisure-time activities	3	3
Self-realization	4	4
Emotional stability	5	5
Social competency	6	8
Democratic values	7	7
Mental development	8	6
Spiritual and moral strength	9	9
Cultural appreciation	10	10

*From Rosentswieg, Joel: A ranking of the objectives of physical education, Research Quarterly **40**:783, 1969.

tives of physical education. Rosentswieg's findings showed that these 100 physical educators ranked the organic and neuromuscular objectives higher than all the rest. When the men physical educators were compared with the women physical educators, there was disagreement upon the primary objective of physical education. The statistical results of the study are illustrated in Tables 6-1 and 6-2.

Perhaps it will help the reader to clarify his own priority system by answering the following questions.

1. *Does the nature of education give us a clue to a priority arrangement of physical education objectives?* According to many educational leaders today, the business of education is concerned primarily with the development of the intellect, the power of good reasoning, and the application of logic. The "life adjustment" type of education is being sidetracked, and more and more emphasis is being given to the development of mental skills, the acquisition of knowledge, and cognitive development. Does this mean that physical education, since it is a part of education and since we use the term *physical education,* should also give more emphasis in this direction? The emphasis in this direction would not be for the purpose of being labeled *academic* but instead to help human beings to become more fully aware of the values of physical activity in their physical, social, and mental development.

2. *Does history give us a clue?* A historical analysis of objectives of physical education indicates that in addition to organic development and the teaching of physical skills, it is also important to consider the interpretive-mental and social development objectives. History seems to have recorded that physical educators should not limit themselves merely to muscular grace but should also be concerned with these objectives, which can be accomplished through the physical. The emphasis upon human relations—for example, the fact that this nation is a democracy and the belief that the individual has worth—should permeate programs of physical education.

3. *Do the outcomes we more readily achieve give us a clue?* Physical educators proudly demonstrate through measurement and evaluation instruments the amount of strength and other qualities of physical fitness they develop in their students. The headlines of newspapers and other communication media proclaim the success that is theirs in developing skills. However, data are not readily available to show the degree to which physical educators develop mental skills and such qualities as sportsmanship, respect for opponents, and courage. It is not difficult for physical education to show its accomplishments in the physical and

skill objectives, but the evidence is not as readily available for the other objectives. Part of the reason for this lies in the lack of objective instruments for measurement purposes, such as being able to measure qualities of sportsmanship. However, at the same time it may also mean the lack of interest on the part of many physical educators to gear their programs in these directions, their failure to recognize the importance of these objectives, the difficulties encountered in trying to achieve these goals, or a feeling that such responsibilities should be accomplished by the academic subjects or the home.

4. *Do the nature and needs of society and the individual give us a clue?* Will the study of society's social problems, including poverty, juvenile delinquency, crime, and health, give us a clue as to what we should be concerned with in physical education? If so, does this mean that objectives become more important in some segments of our society than in others? Also, what about the needs of the individual? What represents the needs of human beings for the "good life"? Are they physical, mental, neuromuscular, social? What needs are the most important for physical education to consider? What needs should be met by the home, church, and school? Which ones should be met by academic subjects—by physical education—by agencies outside the school? If a boy or girl is subpar physically, does this mean that the organic development objective should get priority? If he or she is a delinquent, should the social objective get priority? What does it mean?

5. *Does the desire for professional status give us a clue?* Chapter 1, Physial Education—Its Meaning and Professional Status, listed the criteria for a profession and then raised questions as to whether physical education meets these criteria. Does a review of Chapter 1 indicate a priority of objectives for physical education? What are the implications for physical education objectives of such professional criteria as intellectual orientation, service, code of ethics, and training?

6. *Does the term "physical education" give us a clue?* If physical education is concerned with education of and through the physical, does this indicate a priority? All the objectives of physical education are implied in the term as defined. We are concerned with the *physical* and also with *education*. This means that all objectives should be involved. But does it give us a priority rating?

7. *Does the "fitness" movement give us a clue?* As a result of the concern of the government for the physical fitness of the nation's children and youth, and as a result of the establishment of the President's Council for Physical Fitness and Sports, with its wide exposure through communication media, there has been much emphasis upon physical fitness—one objective of physical education. In some institutions of learning and in other agencies, priority has been given to the organic development or the physical fitness development objective. Has this been good or harmful?

Should all objectives get equal emphasis? Is this the answer? How do physical educators resolve this important problem? Professional associations should give considerable time and effort to resolving this answer. Leadership must be given because many practitioners are seeking the answer.

Regardless of what the outcome is, in the last analysis the individual physical educator will be the person to make the decision. What he emphasizes within his own program from day to day will be the answer. This will depend upon his philosophy, his understanding of the worth of physical education, and what physical education can and should be trying to contribute to human beings and to society. This text is designed to help the reader think profoundly about such questions and help him in arriving at an intelligent answer.

SHOULD PHYSICAL EDUCATION STATE ITS OBJECTIVES IN THE FORM OF CONCEPTS?

Jerome Bruner, in his book *The Process of Education,* discusses the structure of subject matter and states: "The more fundamental or basic the idea learned, the greater will be its breadth of applicability." A concept is an idea and is derived from the Latin word meaning "to conceive." Webster defines a concept as "a mental image of a thing formed by generalizations from particulars." In other words, it means abstracting and generalizing. Concepts are derived from facts and are expressed in understandable form. They evolve gradually. Concept formation results as the individual is exposed to material little by little. He then associates the concept with past experiences and perceives it as a familiar object.

According to Bruner, any educational discipline includes basic concepts, principles, generalizations, and insights. The curriculum should have a structure that contains subdivisions of knowledge pertinent to the field of specialization. The problem is then one of developing a structure that embraces the basic concepts around which basic principles, theories, and knowledge can be organized and discussed in meaningful terms. The real purpose of education is to teach concepts. If a student knows a concept, it will free him from remembering many isolated facts.

Physical education should consider the use of established concepts as a means of structuring its field so that physical education can be taught to students in a much more meaningful manner. The basic concepts of physical education are to be found within the stated objectives of the field.

The goal of education is to help boys and girls to become mature adults, possess ability to make wise decisions, and be capable of intelligent self-direction. The school experiences the student has in first through twelfth grades should prepare him for these responsibilities.

Physical education, as a part of education, should provide each boy and girl with carefully planned experiences that result in knowledge about the value of physical ac-

Cognitive cycle in behavior and learning.

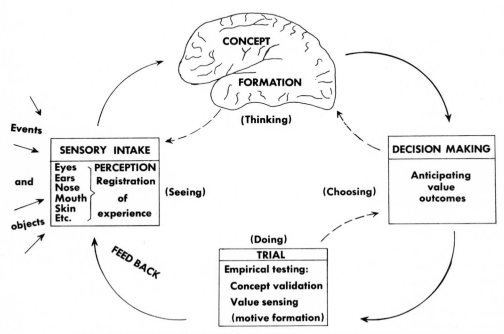

FROM WOODRUFF, ASAHAEL D.: COGNITIVE MODELS OF LEARNING AND TEACHING. IN SIEGEL, L., EDITOR: CONTEMPORARY THEORIES OF INSTRUCTION, SAN FRANCISCO, CHANDLER PUBLISHING CO.

tivity, essential motor skills, strength, stamina, and other essential physical characteristics, and the social qualities that make for effective citizenship.

Over the years, physical educators in many of our schools have attempted to achieve these goals in a dedicated and conscientious manner. However, most physical educators will agree there is still much room for improvement. Those persons who advocate change cite educational systems where there is lack of progression, sequential treatment of subject matter, and an orderly developmental pattern for teaching motor skills. Furthermore, they say, physical education curriculums vary from school to school and state to state without any degree of uniformity. As a result of these conditions, they lament, students are not becoming as physically educated as they could be, and, also, physical education is not gaining the respectability in the educational process it justly deserves.

Each subject-matter field has objectives toward which it teaches and that represent the worth of the field for the students. Physical education has traditionally advocated the four objectives of organic development, neuromuscular development, mental development, and social development. These goals have proved valuable as targets toward which both the teacher and student strive. At the same time, they are rather general in nature and do not provide the best basis for the most effective structural organization of physical education.

The student should be aware of the general objectives of physical education; in addition, as a result of his school experiences, he should be sensitive to, understand, and know the framework that constitutes the field of physical education. He should be aware of the unity, the wholeness, and the interrelatedness of the many activities in which he engages from kindergarten through grade twelve. He should even think at times as a physical educator might think, particularly from the standpoint of recognizing the importance and value of such course experiences to human beings. He should

understand what constitutes the master plan of education and the structure of physical education as it fits into this master plan.

In creating this structure of physical education, we might draw an analogy between our field and the construction of a house. Just as there are key pillars and beams that give the house form and support, so are there key unifying elements within physical education that give it a strong foundational framework and hold it together as a valuable educational experience for every boy and girl. These key elements would be identified and would tie together the various parts of the discipline into a meaningful and cohesive learning package. These elements would be the *concepts* of physical education and, as such, would represent the basic structure of physical education in the school program. They would be the key ideas, principles, skills, values, or attitudes that represent points upon which we as physical educators should focus the child's efforts throughout his school life. They would be part of both the teacher's and the student's thinking and would range from very simple ideas to high-level abstractions. They would start with simple, elementary, fundamental experiences and in a sequential, progressive, and developmental pattern gain depth and comprehensiveness over the years as schooling progresses and the student matures. These concepts would thus define the domain of physical education.

Concepts in physical education would not be memorized by the students. Rather, they would be ideas, analytical generalizations that would emerge and be understood by the student as a result of his school experiences in physical education. They would also provide him with a reservoir of information, skills, and understandings that would help him to meet new problems and situations.

The concepts, of course, would need to be carefully selected according to acceptable criteria and be scientifically sound. Furthermore, after the concepts have been identified, there would be need for extensive testing of their validity by many experts, including teachers in the field and specialists in curriculum development.

To implement the concepts within the physical education structure, there would be a need to delineate the identified concepts into meaningful units and topics that would be progressive in nature and reinforce the concepts that had been identified. The subdivisions of concepts in the structure would represent basic elements needed to develop a meaningful course of study and bring about desirable behavior. Furthermore, they would emanate and flow from the key concepts and would help to give greater meaning and understanding to them. As the conceptual unifying threads were developed at each ascending grade and educational level, the student would be provided with new challenges, where the information, skills, and understanding he has acquired could be applied. The result would be that finally the student would reach a point where he could arrive on his own at valid answers and make wise decisions in the area of physical education.

As a result of the conceptual approach, students would have a greater mastery of the field of physical education, increased understanding and power in dealing with new and unfamiliar problems related to their physical selves, and be better motivated to want to become physically educated in the true sense of the term. The approach would provide a stable system of knowledge and provide guideposts for thinking intelligently about physical education.

The conceptual approach would have particular value to physical education because of the great breadth of skills, knowledge, and values that make up this field of endeavor. It would provide a logical and systematic means for identifying among the many elements those that give form and structure to the type of physical education program professionals want taught in schools. The identified concepts would have permanence, and as the explosion of knowledge takes place in the years ahead through the efforts of our scholarly researchers, this new information can become part of the structure wherever applicable. Finally, the conceptual approach would be readily adaptable to individual differences that exist among students, as well as be sufficiently flexible to provide for the many geographical types of facilities and other factors that differentiate one community or school from another.

Some physical educators might say that the subject matter, skills, and other aspects of physical education are the same under the conceptual approach as under the traditional approach. It may be that the facts will be the same in some cases, but the approach will be different. For example, in the "new" mathematics, as developed by one professional group in grade nine, there is still concentration upon algebra, but the complete emphasis is not on the solving of algebraic equations; instead, it is on the behavior of numbers, a verbalization of concepts.

Under the traditional approach, the organization of courses involved topics and activities but without sufficient regard to the relationship of the topic and activity to what had gone on previously for the student and what lies ahead. This new method would still discuss topics and conduct activities, but topics and activities would be related to key concepts that the topic and activity are designed to elaborate upon, contribute more understanding, and make the area of learning more meaningful in the life of the student.

Health educators have developed a conceptual approach for health education.* They have identified three key concepts, ten conceptual statements, and thirty-one substantive elements that form the structure and framework for health education. Such a framework will upgrade the teaching of health and give order, form, uniformity, and meaning to the teaching of health in our schools.

A conceptual framework for social studies

---

*Health education: a conceptual approach, School Health Education Study, Washington, D. C., 1965.

has been developed for the State of Wisconsin Public Schools.* The state finds it difficult to keep up with the demand for this publication, which lists a framework of concepts for the social studies including: history, anthropology, sociology, political science, economics, and geography. In many other subject-matter areas, a conceptual approach has also been developed.

Physical education needs a national curriculum study, with careful consideration being given to the conceptual approach. At a time when the curriculum reform movement is sweeping the nation and when there already is a "new" mathematics, a "new" physics, a "new" English, and a "new" social studies, physical education can no longer be apathetic about what it teaches and how it teaches. The 85,000 public elementary schools and 25,000 public secondary schools, as well as the private institutions, need a "new" physical education. The conceptual approach is one that should be very carefully weighed for this *new physical education.*

PHYSICALLY EDUCATED BOYS AND GIRLS: AN IMPORTANT PROFESSIONAL OBJECTIVE

When a boy or girl becomes mathematically educated, we know that he or she has taken fundamental courses in arithmetic, algebra, geometry, trigonometry, and calculus. When he or she becomes science educated, we know that experiences have been provided in general science, biology, physics, chemistry, and the other sciences.

What does it mean to be *physically educated?* An important challenge facing the profession of physical education is to establish standards in regard to skills, knowledge, attitudes, and social attributes for the various educational levels, the mastery of which will result in a student being physically educated. When this job has been accomplished, we as a profession will

have taken a forward step in establishing ourselves as a more important part of the educational program.

In one of the subcommittees of the National Conference for Fitness of Secondary School Youth on which I served, the material on p. 171 was prepared as an attempt on the part of this committee to formulate some standards for the physically educated boy and girl. It represents an effort to establish standards for the profession of physical education.

Dr. Thomas Cureton, formerly of the University of Illinois, has illustrated what he believes is meant by being physically educated. His chart is reproduced on p. 170 to show one person's thinking of what it means to be *physically educated.*

Wireman* lists the qualities he feels constitute a physically educated person. They are presented here in adapted form.

1. *The physically educated person understands the history of physical education.* No person can become physically educated unless he understands and has historical perspective concerning the events that have affected the historical growth of man's feelings about physical education and what is possible in the years to come.

2. *The physically educated person is proficient in leisure-time skill and utilizes this skill for relaxation and recreation.* Some skill is necessary for enjoyment of the physical activity. Furthermore, leisure hours are utilized to some degree in putting the skill to use.

3. *The physically educated person is cognizant of the relationship of exercise, diet, and weight control.* An understanding of what constitutes a desirable weight control program and the role of exercise and diet in such a program is desirable.

4. *The physically educated person is knowledgeable about the role of sports in the nation's culture.* Sports play a significant role in the American culture, and

---

*The State Department of Public Instruction in Madison: A conceptual framework for the social studies in Wisconsin schools, Madison, Wisconsin, 1964, The Department.

---

*Wireman, Billy O.: What are the underlying values in physical education? The Physical Educator **22**:53, 1965.

Chart interpretation of what it means to be physically educated.

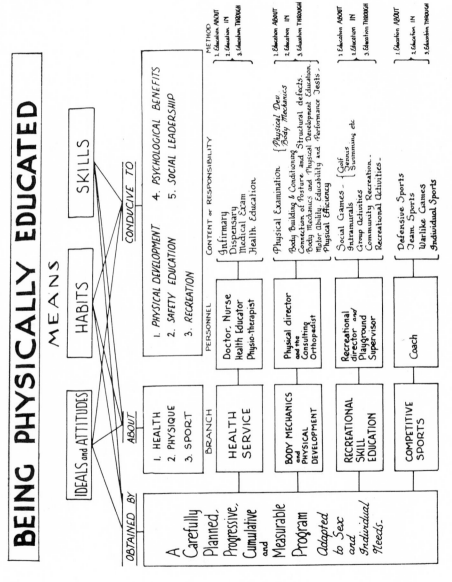

Preamble*

1. Physical education activities should be progressively administered from simple to complex levels throughout the period of the secondary school.
2. Appropriate records on all students should be maintained.
3. Appropriate provisions should be made for the handicapped and low-fitness students.
4. Comprehensive and effective intramural and interschool programs supplement the instructional program.
5. Participation in musical organizations, driver education, or military training should not be permitted to serve as a substitute for instruction in physical education since the specific objectives and the means of attaining the objectives of each differ widely.

The Physically Educated Boy and Girl

Attitudes
1. Interest in health and being healthy
2. Desire to participate in physical education activities and enjoy play with group
3. Desire to become physically educated

Knowledge and appreciations
1. Understanding and appreciation of his or her body and a feeling of responsibility for personal maintenance
2. Basic understanding of physical movement and relaxation
3. Knowledge of interrelationship of physical, mental, emotional and social aspects of the human being
4. An understanding of the rules, strategies, techniques, and history of games, sports, and other physical activities important in our culture
5. An understanding of the importance of exercise to health
6. An insight into individual capacities and limitations in regard to physical activity
7. An understanding of the signs and symptoms of fitness and unfitness

Skills
1. The body in proper balance while standing, sitting, and walking
2. Ability to relax
3. Proper rhythmic response to music including basic skills in square, folk, social and modern dance
4. Application of fundamental skills such as running, jumping, skipping, and throwing to actual game situations
5. Swim one-quarter mile and be secure in deep water
6. Skill and proficiency in a minimum of one different team sport each season of the year
7. Skill and proficiency in a minimum of one different individual sport each year
8. An annual experience during the secondary school period in self-testing activities such as apparatus, tumbling, track and field, marching, calisthenics, etc.

Social attributes
1. Secure in social situations, i.e., acts with confidence, is courteous, etc.
2. Respects his opponent
3. Respects and cooperates with authority
4. Plays within the letter as well as the spirit of the rules
5. Uses acceptable language in all situations
6. Maintains self-control at all times

*National Conference on Fitness for Secondary School Youth, Washington, D. C., Dec. 1958 (mimeographed).

therefore it is important to be informed as to the influence of sports on culture. Also within reasonable limits, a person should be an intelligent spectator as well as a skilled participant.

5. *The physically educated person has a body capable of meeting the demands of day-to-day living.* It is important to have an understanding of such factors as physical fitness, the ingredients that make it up, and how it is maintained.

6. *The physically educated person understands the concept of total health.* An understanding and appreciation of what constitutes total fitness, including the mental, physical, and psychological aspects and the interrelationship of each, are important.

QUESTIONS AND EXERCISES

1. State and discuss the objectives of physical education as listed by AAHPER, Bookwalter, Hetherington, Nash, Oberteuffer and Ulrich, Williams, and Wood and Cassidy.
2. Why are objectives essential to any profession?
3. Discuss the physical development objective and tell to what degree it is being fulfilled in the physical education program of the public schools with which you are familiar.
4. What are the implications of the motor development objective for any well-organized physical education program?
5. Discuss how physical education can help in developing the mental resources of the individual.
6. What is the human relations objective, and what implications does it have for modern-day physical education?
7. How do the objectives of present-day physical education compare with the objectives of physical education in ancient Greece?
8. To what degree do you feel the objectives, as stated in this chapter, are being achieved by present-day physical education programs in the United States?
9. Justify physical education in this twentieth-century world in the light of the objectives of the profession.
10. How do the objectives of physical education, as outlined in this chapter, meet the needs of the consumer?
11. What do you feel should be the priority arrangement for objectives of physical education?

Reading assignment

Bucher, Charles A., and Goldman, Myra: Dimensions of physical education, St. Louis, 1969, The C. V. Mosby Co., Reading selections 12, 13, and 16.

SELECTED REFERENCES

American Association for Health, Physical Education, and Recreation: This is physical education, Washington, D. C., 1965, The Association.

Annarino, Anthony A.: The five traditional objectives of physical education, Journal of Health, Physical Education, and Recreation **41:**24, 1970.

Bloom, Benjamin S., editor: Taxonomy of educational objectives, Handbook I: Cognitive domain, New York, 1956, David McKay, Inc.

Bookwalter, Karl W.: Physical education in the secondary schools, Washington, D. C., 1964, Library of Education, The Center for Applied Research in Education, Inc.

Bucher, Charles A.: Administration of health and physical education programs including athletics, St. Louis, 1971, The C. V. Mosby Co.

Bucher, Charles A.: Administrative dimensions of health and physical education programs, including athletics, St. Louis, 1971, The C. V. Mosby Co.

Bucher, Charles A.: Objectives of physical education, health education and recreation, Connecticut Teacher Education Quarterly **5:**73, 1948.

Bucher, Charles A., Koenig, Constance, and Barnhard, Milton: Methods and materials for secondary school physical education, St. Louis, 1970, The C. V. Mosby Co.

Bucher, Charles A., and Reade, Evelyn M.: Physical education and health in the elementary school, New York, 1971, The Macmillan Co.

Hess, Ford A.: American objectives of physical education from 1900-1957 assessed in the light of certain historical events, Doctoral dissertation, New York University, 1959. (microcarded)

Hetherington, Clark W.: School program in physical education, New York, 1922, World Book Co.

Krathwohl, David R., and others: Taxonomy of educational objectives, Handbook II: Affective domain, New York, 1956, David McKay, Inc.

LaPorte, William R.: Eighth annual report of the Committee on Curriculum Research, Research Quarterly **7:**99, 1936.

Lauritsen, William H.: Some techniques for measuring achievement of objectives of physical education, Doctoral dissertation, New York University, 1946. (microcarded)

Nash, Jay B.: Physical education: interpretations and objectives, New York, 1948, A. S. Barnes & Co., chapters 6 to 12.

Oberteuffer, Delbert, and Ulrich, Celeste: Physical education, New York, 1962, Harper & Row, Publishers.

Physical Education Association of Great Britain: The concept of physical education, British Journal of Physical Education 1:81, 1970.

Price, Hartley D.: The establishment of the principles which are essential for the realization of the objectives of physical education, Doctoral dissertation, New York University, 1946. (microcarded)

Rosentswieg, Joel: A ranking of the objectives of physical education, Research Quarterly 40:783, 1969.

Stoodley, Agnes L.: The stated objectives of physical education for college women, Doctoral dissertation, Stanford University, 1947. (microcarded)

Weiss, Raymond A.: Is physical fitness our most important objective? Journal of Health, Physical Education, and Recreation 35:17, 1964.

Weston, Arthur: The making of American physical education, New York, 1962, Appleton-Century-Crofts.

Williams, Jesse F.: The principles of physical education, Philadelphia, 1964, W. B. Saunders Co.

Wireman, Billy O.: What are the underlying values in physical education? Physical Educator 22: 53, 1965.

Wood, Thomas Denison, and Cassidy, Rosalind Frances: The new physical education, New York, 1931, The Macmillan Co.

7/Role of physical education in general education

What we must reach for is a conception of perpetual self-discovery, perpetual reshaping to realize one's best self, to be the person one could be.

JOHN GARDNER

The world . . . is only beginning to see that the wealth of a nation consists more than anything else in the number of superior men that it harbours.

WILLIAM JAMES

Since the time of the ancient Greeks, we have felt that there was a close relationship between a strong vital mind and physical fitness.

JOHN F. KENNEDY

But excellence implies more than competence. It implies a striving for the highest standards in every phase of life. We need individual excellence in all its forms—in every kind of creative endeavor, in political life, in education, in industry—in short, universally.

JOHN GARDNER

Experience has shown that when children have a chance at physical activities which will bring their natural impulses into play, going to school is a joy, management is less of a burden, and learning is easier.

JOHN DEWEY

Education contributes to the development, advancement, and perpetuation of the nation's culture. Educational institutions play a primary role in the development of the human resources of society. Schools, colleges, and universities are clearly the most powerful and effective institutions our society has for the achievement of intellectual skill, knowledge, understanding, and appreciation necessary to make wise de-

cisions, good judgments, and logical analysis of problems. Directly or indirectly, these educational institutions are the chief agents of society's progress, whether it is progress concerned with knowledge, arts, technology, social conscience, or other areas essential to a nation's growth. Education must meet the challenges presented in society. In the present decade this means that our nation's schools and colleges should be concerned with the well-being of the individual student in his preparation for a productive and happy life in which his potentialities as an individual are enlarged and fulfilled and where his freedom will be assured. Education must focus its attention on such areas as social equality, industrial and commercial power, economic integrity, and political wisdom. In the 1970's our nation's schools and colleges must be concerned with such problems as drug addiction, ecology, the population explosion, the racial struggle, and an accelerating crime rate. Educational institutions must also show concern for the values by which people live and by which their judgments are made and their purposes defined.

Physical education, as a phase of the total educational process, helps in realizing these purposes. It is one link in a chain of many influences that help to realize the country's ideals and contribute to the proper functioning of American society. It is continually striving for excellence so that it can become an increasingly dynamic force in general education.

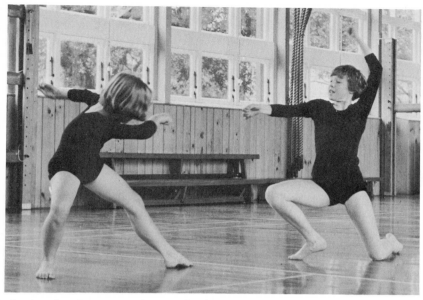

Physical education is a part of general education of students. This is creative dance at secondary girls' level in New Zealand.

EDUCATION AND SCHOOLS AND COLLEGES

The United States, in answer to the question: Who should be educated? has responded: "All our citizens!" Every child in the United States has the opportunity to receive a free elementary and secondary education. More than 50% of our high school graduates pursue some type of postsecondary education. However, education is not confined to the limits of the schools and colleges. It is much broader than this. Education is present in all the experiences an individual may go through in the home, church, clubhouse, and alley, as well as the school. However, schools and colleges represent settings where the highest organized form of education takes place in the United States. The schools and colleges exist for the purpose of orienting the youth in the spirit of democratic living and of improving on the existing social order wherever possible. The schools and colleges represent places where young people spend a great portion of their time between the ages of 4 or 5 years and up to 16 or 20 years. The schools and colleges

are locales where an attempt is made to mold children into law-abiding citizens who contribute to the welfare of society.

The schools and colleges represent a setting where growth and development take place during formative years. As such, the schools and colleges receive the main consideration in a discussion of the role of physical education in the educative process. Physical education has much to contribute during these school and college years when an individual can develop his body into a strong and beautiful machine or allow it to become weak and flabby, when an individual can learn the secret of skillful movement and coordinated action or remain awkward and lack a sense of rhythm, when an individual can develop his intellectual mechanism or allow it to become rusty, and when an individual can learn to live as a contributing member of society or be an antisocial being.

RESPONSIBILITY FOR EDUCATION

The responsibility for education falls to each of the states in the nation. The Tenth Amendment to the Constitution of the

United States reads: "The powers not delegated to the United States by the Constitution, nor prohibited by it to the States, are reserved to the States respectively, or to the people." Education comes within the interpretation of this Amendment. The states, however, do not retain complete autonomy over the educational system. Instead, in most cases they delegate the educational responsibility to a local unit of organization within their boundaries, such as the school district, village, or city. The states, however, do contribute in many ways toward helping the local communities discharge this responsibility. In many instances they give financial aid and guidance as well as supply instructional assistance and other services. The federal government also contributes in many ways toward the betterment of the educational system of the country. Although the states guard the rights endowed by the Tenth Amendment with jealous fervor, the national government has, nevertheless, contributed help in building schools, providing land, furthering health services, and in many other ways. With increased costs and expenditures, state and local governments are looking to Washington for help. The future of American education holds promise that federal aid to education on a much larger scale will become a part and parcel of our culture in the not too distant future.

MEANING OF THE TERM "EDUCATION"

The term *education* means different things to different individuals. One individual will define it as a training process that comes about through study and instruction; another person will say it is a series of experiences that enables a person to better understand new experiences; and to others it means growth and adjustment. John Dewey, an educator who has most profoundly influenced present-day education, defines education as the reconstruction of events that compose the lives of individuals so that new happenings and new events become more purposeful and more meaningful. Furthermore, through education, individuals will be better able to regulate the direction of ensuing experience. Dewey's interpretation, it seems, sums up in a few words what is meant by education. It means that a person thinks in terms of his previous experiences. It further means that the individual's education consists of everything he does from birth until death. Edu-

There is purpose in physical education.

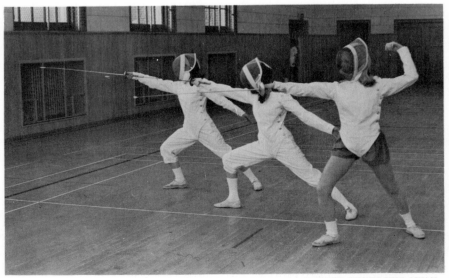

cation is a "doing" phenomenon. You learn through doing. Education takes place in the classroom, in the library, on the playground, in the gymnasium, on trips, and at home. It is not confined to a school or a church but takes place wherever individuals congregate.

The problem now arises as to what experiences will best result in a happy and rich life. The solution seems to be in the provision of experiences that will have a practical value in the lives of individuals as they live from day to day. Worthwhile experiences will enable a person to live a more purposeful, a more interesting, and a more vigorous life. The aim or goals of education, therefore, should receive consideration if a person is to know in what direction educational experiences are to be guided. The Educational Policies Commission, in discussing policies for education in American democracy, stated the following as the purpose of education:

. . . The primary business of education in effecting the promises of American democracy, is to guard, cherish, advance, and make available in the life of coming generations the funded and growing wisdom, knowledge, and aspirations of the race. This involves the dissemination of knowledge, the liberation of minds, the development of skills, the promotion of free inquiries, the encouragement of the creative or inventive spirit, and the establishment of wholesome attitudes toward order and change—all useful in the good life for each person, in the practical arts, and in the maintenance and improvement of American society, as our society, in the world of nations. So conceived, education seems to transcend our poor powers of accomplishment. It does in fact, if perfection be expected; but such is the primary business of public education in the United States; theory supports it; practice inadequately illustrates and confirms it.*

It is of interest to note, while reflecting on this statement of the purpose of education, that knowledge in itself is not enough. In addition, such a thing as ethics is also indispensable. As this report points out: "The nature of the knowledge to be disseminated is qualified by the condition, 'useful in the good life and in the maintenance and improvement of American society.' Both ethics and the nature of American civilization are drawn into immediate and inescapable consideration."*

The Commission further pointed out that education is as much concerned with the training of the body and spirit as with the transmission of knowledge.

It is not merely with the transmission of knowledge that education is deeply concerned. The functions of the schools are not fully described by a summary of programs, curriculum, and methods. No written or spoken words do, or can, completely convey the meaning of education as the day-to-day living force that it is in fact and may be—in the transactions of the classroom, in the relations of teacher and pupil, in the associations of pupil and pupil, and in the experiences of the library and athletic field. Here are exchanges, bearings, and influences too subtle for logical expression and exact measurement. Yet we cannot doubt their existence, at least those of us who recall our own educational experiences and see teachers at work. Here, in the classroom, the auditorium, laboratory, and gymnasium, are in constant operation moral and cultural forces just as indispensable to civilization as knowledge or any material elements—indeed primordial in nature and the pre-conditions for the civilized uses of material things.†

Physical education plays an important role in the educational process. The mind and body represent a unity in man. One gives strength to the other, one supports the other, and both function harmoniously in the educated person. When physical education is applied to education, it can readily be seen that it plays an instrumental role in the educational process.

---

*Educational Policies Commission: Policies for education in American democracy, Washington, D. C., 1946, National Education Association and American Association of School Administrators, p. 60.

*Educational Policies Commission: Policies for education in American democracy, Washington, D. C., 1946, National Education Association and American Association of School Administrators, p. 62.

†Educational Policies Commission: Policies for education in American democracy, Washington, D. C., 1946, National Education Association and American Association of School Administrators, p. 64.

Physical education as applied to education

The term *physical education* takes on a new meaning after a consideration of the word *education*. The word *physical* refers to the body. It is often used in reference to various bodily characteristics such as physical strength, physical development, physical prowess, physical health, and physical appearance. It refers to the body as contrasted to the mind. Therefore, when you add the word *education* to the word *physical* and use the words *physical education,* you are referring to the process of education that concerns activities that develop and maintain the human body. When an individual is playing a game, swimming, marching, working out on the parallel bars, skating, or performing in any one of the gamut of physical education activities that aid in the development and maintenance of his body, education is taking place at the same time. This education may be conducive to the enrichment of the indi-

vidual's life or it may be detrimental. It may be a satisfying experience or it may be an unhappy one. It may help in the building of a strong and cohesive society or it may have antisocial outcomes for the participant. Whether or not physical education helps or inhibits the attainment of educational objectives will depend to a great extent upon the leadership responsible for its direction.

Physical education is a very important part of the educational process. It is not a "frill" or an "ornament" tacked on to the school program as a means of keeping children busy. It is, instead, a vital part of education. Through a well-directed physical education program, children develop skills for the worthy use of leisure time, engage in activities conducive to healthful living, develop socially, and contribute to their physical and mental health.

A study of history reveals that other civilizations have recognized the important place of physical education in the training

In physical education a person gains an insight into human nature.

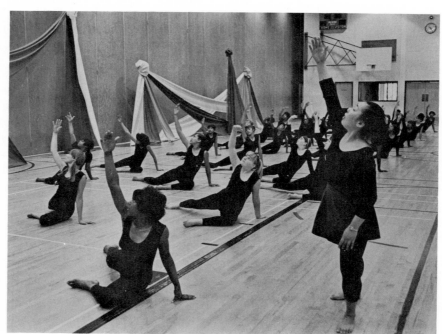

of their youth. In ancient Athens, for example, three main studies were followed by every Athenian: gymnastics, grammar, and music. Here in America the contributions of physical education in the educational program have been recognized for many years. In 1918 the National Educational Association set forth its well-known *Cardinal Principles of Secondary Education,* which listed seven objectives of education: health, command of fundamental processes, worthy home membership, vocation, citizenship, worthy use of leisure time, and ethical character. Physical education is playing a very important part in achieving these objectives. Through such contributions as the benefits of exercise to physical health, the fundamental physical skills that make for a more interesting, efficient, and vigorous life, and the social education that contributes to the development of character and good human relations, these cardinal principles are brought nearer to realization.

MEANING OF THE TERM "GENERAL EDUCATION"

The term *general education* is often confused with the term *liberal education,* and it is necessary to differentiate between the two in order to fully understand the meaning of the term *general education.* Morse* has stated that liberal education is subject centered, with content material that is logically organized. Its goal is the stimulation of reflective thinking, with little emphasis on behavior, and is primarily concerned with the intellectual person. General education, on the other hand, is more concerned with the learner than content, which may be organized with little regard for traditional fields of knowledge. Its goals are individual development, with emphasis upon behavior and social usefulness together with intellectual development as an outcome of learning.

---

*Morse, Horace T.: Liberal and general education: a problem of differentiation. Quoted by Rice, James G., editor: General education, Washington, D. C., 1964, National Education Association.

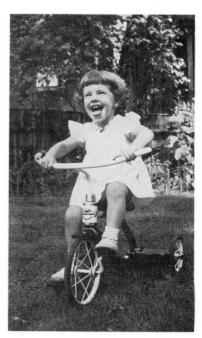

If children are happy, they are more likely to make the necessary adjustments.

General education is concerned with developing a good life for all people. It seeks to prepare students for full and meaningful lives as members of families and organizations and as future citizens. Viewing socialization as an important educational goal, general education emphasizes the point that all citizens are members of one system, be it economic or political, and unless they can function cooperatively with one another, there is going to be chaos. Wynne* has stated that one of the functions of general education is to widen the area of our common interests and concerns. Civic responsibility is looked upon as an important educational goal, and students are encouraged to communicate with one another. The learning of respect, tolerance, and self-responsibility are viewed in general education as being extremely valuable to future citizens. General education emphasizes the point that students must be given the op-

---

*Wynne, J. P.: General education in theory and practice, New York, 1952, Bookman Associates, p. 37.

portunity to participate in experiences that develop intelligence and effective thinking. The Harvard Committee,* in their report entitled *General Education in a Free Society,* emphasized this need for effective thinking. Intellectual development is not the only goal of general education. Knowledge of the body is also viewed as an important objective. Seeking to make possible the maximum development of the individual, general education enunciates the importance of health and well-being.

The Educational Policies Commission has pointed out that the function of education cannot be confined to facts but also includes training of the body and spirit. Knowledge in itself is not sufficient in the achievement of excellence.

Today, general education is looked upon as preparing the individual for a meaningful, self-directed existence. For a student to be prepared to accomplish this goal means that he must have an understanding of (1) the nature of self and others and growth in capacity for continuing self-development and for relating to others, (2) the contemporary social scene and the values and skills necessary for effective participation, (3) his cultural heritage and the ability to evaluate it, (4) the role of communication and skill in communicating, (5) the world of nature and the ability to adapt to it, and (6) the role of esthetic forms in human living and the capacity for self-expression through them. These are not new purposes of education. In 1938 the Educational Policies Commission set forth certain purposes of education that they felt included a summarization and enlargement of statements published previously by various committees and individuals representing the National Education Association. These purposes are as relevant today as they were in 1938.

These purposes are (1) the objectives of self-realization, which are concerned with developing the individual to his fullest

*General education in a free society, report of the Harvard Committee, Harvard University Press, Cambridge, Massachusetts, 1945.

capacity in respect to health, recreation, and philosophy of life, (2) the objectives of human relationship, which refer to relationships among people on the family, group, and society levels, (3) the objectives of economic efficiency, which are concerned with the individual as a producer and a consumer, and (4) the objectives of civic responsibility, which stress the individual's relationship to his local, state, national, and international forms of government.

Physical education as applied to general education

Physical education, with its emphasis on building a physically, emotionally, mentally, and socially fit society, plays an important role in general education. A heavy responsibility rests upon the shoulders of those who spend a large share of their time with the youth of today. If experiences are provided that are satisfying, successful, and directed toward enriching an individual's life, these purposes of education will be accomplished. Physical education teachers have within their power the ability to aid in the fulfillment of the objectives of self-realization, human relationship, economic efficiency, and civic responsibility in each individual. Physical education, when applied to general education, plays an important role in the development of the student. The education that takes place on the playground, in the swimming pool, and in the gymnasium can help considerably in accomplishing these purposes.

A fuller description of the role of physical education in the educational process is needed at this point. For purposes of organization such a discussion may be grouped under four headings, which have been adapted from the Educational Policies Commission's list of objectives toward which education is striving.

OBJECTIVE—TO HELP MAN ACHIEVE EXCELLENCE AS AN INTELLECTUAL BEING

The objectives of intellectual self-realization are aimed at developing the individual so that he realizes his potentialities. This development means much more than the accumulation of knowledge. It means that the individual in the process of constant interaction with his environment has achieved his rightful place, that a proper relationship has been established, and that he recognizes and associates with what is best in his culture. It means that education is interested not only in shaping the individual for his future role as a member of society but is interested also in his development and growth as he progresses toward adult life. Physical education should contribute to the objectives of intellectual self-realization in the following ways.

1. *Physical education should contribute to academic achievement.* Research findings indicate that physical education programs can contribute to academic achievement by providing daily movement experiences and instruction in selected basic motor activities, consistent with the developmental level of the students; by promoting physical fitness; by providing knowledge and modifying behavior in regard to good health practices; and by aiding in the process of social and emotional development, which leads to a more positive self-concept. Research findings also indicate that the intellectual, physical, and emotional developments are closely associated. Endocrinology has shown that mentality changes as body chemistry changes. Biology has linked the cell to the learning experience. Psychology points to the fact that the child's earliest learnings are factual and kinesthetic. Just as it is important to teach English so that students can communicate effectively with one another, history so that they have an understanding of their cultural heritage, and mathematics so they can understand the technology of our society, it is also important to educate students regarding their physical selves so they can function most efficiently as human beings. For further explanation of the evidence to support the relationship between physical education and academic achievement, see Chapter 17, Psychological Interpretations of Physical Education.

2. *Physical education should contribute to an inquiring mind.* An inquiring mind is essential to the educated person. Only through curiosity is it possible to probe into the makeup of one's environment.

The motor mechanism of the child enables him to explore, to cruise, and to see his environment. It stimulates his curiosity. He wants to see what is on the other side of the fence, how hot the stove is, what happens when he pulls the light cord, what is in the box with the cover, how people react to certain situations, and the like. Motor activity helps develop the inquiring mind and aids in the solving of problems that at times thwart the individual. In fact, psychologist Newell C. Kephart, former Executive Director of the Achievement Center for Children at Purdue University, points out that motor activity is related to higher thought processes. He also indicates that a child's behavior cannot function better than the motor abilities upon which it is based.

Today, in education, the independent study movement is becoming more popular in our schools and colleges. Alexander and Hines,* in their book entitled *Independent Study in Secondary Schools,* describe the independent learner as one who makes optimum use of his intellectual and other powers. He is one who undertakes on his own initiative learning tasks important to him. The student in the independent study movement desires the opportunity to participate in activities that will provide him with answers to questions that are perplexing him. Physical education provides the opportunity for students to participate in such activities. One may visit a school at 7 A.M. and observe a youngster running around a track with an interested coach holding a stopwatch for him. Physical education activities open up new fields of curiosity. The student seeks to discover the answers to such questions as why a vigorous workout

---

*Alexander, William M., and Hines, Vynce A.: Independent study in secondary schools, New York, 1967, Holt, Rinehart and Winston, Inc., p. 4.

and a shower are exhilarating and why exercise improves his appetite, circulation, respiration, stamina, and endurance; why Jim can lift his own weight in the air and Dick cannot; why Henry can wield a tennis racquet with great skill; and why Sally can swim so gracefully. A new and interesting phase of living is opened to the individual through activity. His inquiring mind is active, and he seeks the answers to his health and physical problems. Many opportunities should be provided the student to do independent study in various physical education activities that interest him.

3. *Physical education should contribute to the ability to speak, read, and write effectively.* Physical education, through the various activities that it sponsors, can indirectly help an individual to speak, read, and write with more effectiveness and clarity.

Through the development of a healthy and physically fit body one may possibly have better poise to command the attention of one's listeners. Francois Delsarte, a French teacher of voice and dramatics, pointed this out when he developed a special system of physical exercises that were aimed at more effective dramatics and singing. This system spread to America, where it was received with a great deal of interest. Many teachers of oratorical public speaking were in accord with Delsarte's methods, combined them with their own ideas, and developed a system of exercises that contributed to health, poise, grace, and beauty of face and figure.

The ability to read efficiently is important to an individual's development. It has been pointed out that there are three types of illiterates. First, there are those who cannot read; second, those who have mastered the mechanics of reading but do not use this acquired art; and, third, those who read material of insignificant value. Physical education can contribute to discrimination in reading by pointing out scientific materials available in regard to the maintenance and promotion of one's health and physical fitness. It can discount the litera-

ture of health and physical culture "faddists," quacks, quick-cure artists, and medicine men who are exploiting the public. It can refer students to sources of information where scientific information may be obtained. It can develop in the student a critical attitude toward quick health cures and other misleading advertising that is chronicled daily in newspapers and magazines and broadcast over radio and television. Through this medium of discriminatory reading, physical education can contribute to self-realization.

Physical education should aid an individual to write effectively. The ability to express one's views in a clear, concise manner is a medium that contributes immensely to the solving of problems. In the presentation of physical education reports on activities, in health lessons, and in the writing of examinations, there should be a constant alertness on the part of the physical education teacher to see that acceptable standards of written work are followed. This work should not be the sole prerogative of the English profession. Instead, it is the duty of all educators to utilize every "teachable moment" in the improvement of the writing ability of their students.

4. *Physical education should contribute to knowledge of exercise, health, and disease.* The educated person has an understanding of the facts pertinent to exercise, health, and disease. To a great degree, a person's success is dependent upon his health. His state of health and physical fitness will determine to a great extent whether or not he succeeds in realizing his potentialities. An individual cannot expect to be a top executive in the business world if he is sick and stays away from work 2 or 3 days a week. He cannot expect to achieve stardom in professional athletics without a physically strong and healthy body. He cannot expect to be accepted by members of his community if his life is controlled by drugs such as heroin and LSD. He cannot aspire to a high-salaried position in radio, engineering, the ministry, education, advertising, law, medicine, or

dentistry unless his body can stand the rigors of long hours of study and work. He cannot expect to achieve happiness in living unless he is in good health. Therefore, a knowledge of exercise, health, and disease is a contributing factor to self-realization so that health obstacles, handicaps, and strains may be guarded against.

Physical education contributes to this knowledge by instructing the individual in regard to the importance of nutrition, physical activity, rest, and sleep; by informing him of the dangers of drugs; by exploring with him the preventive and control measures that exist to guard against disease; by providing opportunities for vigorous out-of-doors activity; by motivating the formation of wholesome health attitudes and habits; by following up the correction of defects; by stressing safety factors for the prevention of accidents; and by establishing various health services. Through the experiences and knowledge provided by a physical education program, the objectives of self-realization are brought much closer to attainment.

5. *Physical education should contribute to family and community health.* The educated person protects his own health, his dependents' health, and the health of the individuals within the community where he resides. The educated person has a knowledge of health and disease and applies these facts to himself, to his family, and to his community. He sees that his body is cared for in the manner prescribed by the authorities on health and disease and has periodic health examinations. He gets adequate amounts of exercise, rest, and sleep; eats the right kind of food; engages in activity conducive to mental as well as physical health; and sees that others also have the same opportunities to maintain and improve their health in accordance with his standards. He realizes that health is a product that increases in proportion as it is shared with other individuals, and he knows that health is everybody's business. In many ghetto areas where the horror of drug abuse has taken countless lives, the edu-

cated person who has knowledge of such horrors is the one who can inform members of the community of the dangers to them if they use drugs.

Physical education provides a program of activity to improve the physical and mental health of the individual, his family, and the entire community. In the schools a planned program of physical activity is offered as an essential to the optimum body functioning of young people during this developmental period of their lives. It enables them to experience many pleasurable emotions and to develop organic power essential to a healthy, happy, and interesting existence, so that they will not have to turn to antisocial pursuits as an outlet for their frustrations. The groundwork for adult years is laid during this formative period. Recreational programs provide facilities and opportunities for the adult to continue, after leaving school, physical activity adapted to his needs. They offer adults the opportunity to lose themselves in wholesome activity and thus be relieved of some of the tension experienced in modern-day living. Such a program is essential to the health of all.

6. *Physical education should contribute to skill as a participant and spectator in sports.* Recognizing that the body and mind represent a unity in man, the educated person recognizes the value of physical activity. Sports and physical education activities are an important part of our culture. Furthermore, the stress of modern-day living, with its quest for material possessions, its machine type labor, its sedentary pursuits, and its competitive nature, has implications for all who would enjoy some of the simple, natural, and wholesome forms of activity. Modern-day man has been bitten by a bug that has destroyed to some extent his sense of values in regard to entertainment. Many persons no longer wish to find entertainment through their own resources but, instead, desire to have professionals satisfy these needs. Too frequently they turn to night clubs, horse races, or games of chance for amusement. The edu-

cated person selects the manner in which he will spend his leisure time with discretion and with regard for enriched living.

Participating in a game of softball, tennis, or badminton or going for a swim not only provides an interesting and happy experience during leisure hours but at the same time contributes to mental and physical health. The development of physical skills in all persons rather than in just a few select individuals is an educationally sound objective and should be encouraged more and more by educators. The so-called recreational sports should receive greater emphasis so that activities may be better adapted to the older segment of the population. Swimming, golf, tennis, camping, and similar activities should occupy a prominent place in all physical education programs.

Physical education not only develops skill in the participant but at the same time develops an interest and knowledge of other activities that at times may be engaged in by individuals from the standpoint of a spectator. Although it seems the benefits from participation would outweigh the benefits of being a spectator in regard to physical activity, nevertheless many leisure hours may be spent in a wholesome manner observing a ball game or some other sports activity. The wise person, however, discovers the proper balance between the amount of time he will utilize as a participant and as a spectator. The balance is destroyed if a person fails to realize that being a spectator cannot result in the same values for an individual as being a participant. Physical education can help by supplying a knowledge of various sports so that the role of the spectator may be more meaningful and interesting.

7. *Physical education should contribute to resources for utilizing leisure hours in mental pursuits.* The educated person has mental resources for the utilization of leisure hours. Recreation is not confined to sports and exercise. Instead, there is a whole gamut of activities that are more inactive in their nature but that offer entertainment and relaxation after working hours for a great many people. Such activities as reading, photography, music, and painting may be included in this group. Physical education contributes here by providing the material for interesting stories of great athletes, such as Babe Ruth, Jackie Robinson, Glenn Cunningham, Ben Hogan, and Kareem Jabbar. These individuals, through the stories that have been written about them, allow others to live vicariously their struggles in attaining fame and fortune amidst obstacles that seemed almost insurmountable. Physical education offers photography and painting enthusiasts subjects for their pictures. Everyone has seen works of art that were inspired through some sports event. Physical education also offers many hobbies. A sport such as fishing motivates a hobby such as tieing flies. Many other examples could be listed.

8. *Physical education should contribute to an appreciation of beauty.* The educated person has developed an appreciation of the beautiful. From the time of early childhood the foundation of an appreciation of beautiful things can be developed. Architecture, landscapes, paintings, music, furnishings, trees, rivers, and animals should ring a note of beauty in the mind of the growing child and in the adult.

Physical education has much to offer in the way of beauty. The human body is a thing of beauty if it has been properly developed. The Greeks stressed the "body beautiful" and performed their exercises and athletic events in the nude so as to display the fine contours of their bodies. Nothing is more beautiful than a perfectly proportioned and developed human body. Physical activity is one of the keys to a beautiful body. Also, there is a beauty of movement that is developed through physical activity. When a person picks up an object from the floor, it can be done with great skill and grace, or it can be done crudely and awkwardly. When a football pass is caught, a basketball goal made, a high jump executed, a two and one-half somersault dive performed, or a difficult dance displayed, there can be included in the performance of these acts rhythm, grace, poise, and ease of movement that is beauty in action. Anyone who has seen Jim Ryun run, Jack Nicklaus drive a golf ball, Rod Laver stroke a tennis ball, Wilt Chamberlain hook a shot through the net, or Johnny Bench hit a home run knows what beauty of performance means. Such beauty comes only with practice and perfection.

9. *Physical education should contribute to directing one's life toward worthwhile goals.* The educated person conscientiously attempts to guide his life in the proper direction. Upon the shoulders of each individual rests the responsibility of determining how he will live, what religion he will choose, the moral code he will accept, the standard of values he will follow, and the code of ethics in which he will believe. This is characteristic of the democratic way of life. In a democracy man can in reality "half control his doom."

Man must develop his own philosophy of life. The way he treats his fellow men, the manner in which he assumes responsibility, the objectives he sets to attain on earth, and the type of government in which he believes will all be affected by this philosophy. Through the philosophy that he has established, man forms his own destiny.

Physical education can help in the formulation of an individual's philosophy of life. Through the medium of physical education activities, guidance can be given as to what is right and proper, goals that are worth competing for, intrinsic and extrinsic values, autocratic and democratic procedures, and standards of conduct. Children and youths are great imitators, and the beliefs, actions, and conduct of the coach and the teacher are many times reflected in the beliefs, actions, and conduct of the student. In education, leadership is the key that unlocks the door to self-realization for many of our youth.

OBJECTIVE—TO HELP MAN ACHIEVE
EXCELLENCE AS A SOCIAL BEING

Human relationships may be defined as the relationships that exist between individuals. Good human relations may be summed up in the Golden Rule: "Do unto others as you would have others do unto you." Good human relations imply that people live together, work together, and play together harmoniously. Each individual appreciates the other person's viewpoint and attempts to understand his actions. Good human relations are found in families where brother and sister, mother and father, father and son, and mother and daughter live cooperatively and happily together. They are found among friends who are willing to help each other in time of need, among classmates who share responsibilities, among neighbors who thrill to the accomplishments of others, and among workers who help solve each other's problems. Poor human relations also exist. These occur when a business competitor seeks an unfair advantage, when a football player drives a cleated shoe into an opponent's face, when a boy shows disrespect for his parents, and when a fellow worker condemns a colleague.

The question of human relations is one of the most pressing problems of this day and age. Good human relations is the key to a happy and successful life and a peaceful world. Therefore it is important that education play its role to the fullest extent in accomplishing the objectives of human relationships.

Physical education can make a worthwhile contribution in this area of human relations. This can be done through placing human relations first; enabling each individual to enjoy a rich social experience through play; helping individuals play cooperatively with others; teaching courtesy, fair play, and good sportsmanship; and contributing to home and family living.

1. *The physical education program aimed at excellence places human relations first.* The human being is the most valuable and the most important consideration in this life. One human life is worth more than a handful of diamonds or any other abundance of material possessions that could be accumulated. Therefore, human welfare should receive careful consideration in all walks of life. When a new law is passed

by Congress, there should be due consideration for its effect on human welfare; when a machine is invented, we should take into consideration whether it will affect human beings beneficially or adversely; and when an accusation is made, the effect on human welfare should be considered. The more human welfare is considered, the happier are all.

The ideal physical education program places human welfare first on its list. When an activity is planned, it takes into consideration the needs and welfare of the participants; when a rule or regulation is made, the player's welfare is considered; when a student is reprimanded, his welfare and that of others are considered. The desire or convenience of the teacher is not the first consideration. The physical education program takes into consideration the weak and the less skilled and makes sure that adequate arrangements have been made for such individuals. It is a student-centered program, with the attention focused on the individuals for whom the program exists. Throughout the entire procedure there is prevalent among students, teachers, and administrators the thought that the human aspects are the most important consideration. Through the media of precept and example, consideration of others is the keynote of the program. When the student plays, he considers the welfare of others; when the teacher plans, he considers the welfare of all. By placing human relations first, a spirit of good will, fellowship, and joyous cooperation exists.

2. *The physical education program aimed at excellence enables each individual to enjoy a rich social experience through play.* Play experiences offer an opportunity for a rich social experience. This experience can help greatly in rounding out a child's or youth's personality, in helping him to adapt to the group situation, in developing proper standards of conduct, in creating a feeling of "belonging," and in developing a sound code of ethics.

Children and youths need the social experience that can be gained through as-sociation with other persons in a play atmosphere. Many children and youths live in cities, in slum areas, and in communities where delinquency runs rampant, where their parents do not know the next door neighbor, and where the environment is not conducive to a rich social experience. In such neighborhoods the school is one place where children and youths have an opportunity to mingle, and physical education offers a place where they have opportunity to play together. The potentialities are limitless in planning social experiences through "tag" and "it" games, rhythms, games of low organization, and the more highly organized games. Here the child or youth learns behavior traits characteristic of a democratic society. Because of his drive for play, he will be more willing to abide by the rules, accept responsibility, contribute to the welfare of the group, and respect the rights of others.

Today, the dropout rate is becoming a greater problem in education, and students are looking to sources other than the schools to provide them with the experiences that they feel are necessary to equip them for their roles in society. Physical education, through its various activities, can prove instrumental in limiting the dropout rate. In Cleveland, Ohio, one inner city high school reported that of the students who participated in the athletic program during a 3-year period, only two became dropouts, within a setting where 60% of the general student body drops out.* Play experience in physical education can prove to be beneficial in keeping students in school and off the streets.

3. *The physical education program aimed at excellence helps individuals to play cooperatively with others.* The physical education program should stress cooperation as the basis for achieving the goals an individual or group desires. Each member of the group must work as though he were

---

*Briggs, Paul W.: The opportunity to be relevant, Journal of Health, Physical Education and Recreation **41:**43, 1970.

a part of a machine. The machine must run smoothly, and this is possible only if every part does its share of the work. Pulling together and working together bring results that never are obtained if everyone goes his separate way. In a speech delivered at Madison, Wisconsin, former President Truman stressed the effectiveness of cooperation in our day-to-day living, citing such examples as farm cooperatives, cooperative stores, and the bringing of electricity to rural areas through cooperative means. He then went on to stress that world peace is possible only through cooperation among the nations of the world and that the problems confronting the nations of the world today will be solved only through working together.

Cooperation must be an important objective in physical education. A physical education program that would teach individuals to play cooperatively should stress leadership and followership traits. The success of any venture depends on good leadership and good workers or followers. Everyone cannot be a captain on a basketball, relay, or soccer team. Everyone does not have leadership ability. Those who are good leaders should also be good followers. A leader in one activity might possibly make a better follower in another activity. These are a few of the points that should be brought out. The important thing to stress is that both leaders and followers are needed for the accomplishment of any enterprise. All contribute to the undertaking.

A physical education program that would teach individuals to play cooperatively should stress cooperation as the first consideration, rather than competition. Students in our schools compete for grades, to make the honor roll, to receive a bid to certain societies, to be a member of the squad, and to be an officer of their class. This may be good if conducted according to proper procedures, but in many of our schools it breeds discontent, cheating, and cliques and results in personality maladjustments. The person who takes home the honors, accumulates the prizes, and makes the headlines is too often the hero in the eyes of the public, whereas the diligent, hard-working, quiet individual who cooperates to his utmost for the success of a group enterprise receives nothing for his efforts. The success of the democratic way of life depends on cooperation among members of society and not on the exploits of a few who seek honor, prestige, and glory. The "all for one and one for all" motto will accomplish much more than the "all for me" motto. In adult life people follow many of the objectives formulated in their youth. If competition rather than cooperation receives the main consideration in school, it will aggravate the competitive "survival of the fittest" existence so characteristic of modern-day living. Cooperation is the secret of successful living.

4. *The physical education program aimed at excellence teaches courtesy, fair play, and good sportsmanship.* The amenities of social behavior are a part of the repertoire of every educated person. They have developed as part of our culture just as the playing of baseball, eating hot dogs, and democratic living have. Some individuals in our societies are referred to as "ladies" and "gentlemen," whereas others are called "hussies" and "rowdies." Many times such courtesies as saying "please" or "thank you," tipping one's hat, offering a lady your arm, and acting in a polite, quiet manner have made the difference in these labels being attached to certain individuals.

Courtesy and politeness are characteristic of good family training, just as fair play and sportsmanship are characteristic of good training in physical education activities. On the one hand, it reflects the character of the parent or guardian and, on the other, the teacher or coach. When a player kicks his opponent in the groin, trips him up, or does not play according to the rules, he often reflects the spirit of his leader. Some coaches and teachers will use any means to win a game or achieve a goal. Others feel that winning is not the prime objective. Instead, their main objective is to provide an experience that will help the members of a group realize values that will help them live an enriched life.

Courtesy, fair play, and sportsmanship contribute to good human relations. The player who is a gentleman on the field is usually a gentleman off the field as well. Such an individual makes friends easily, builds good will, and inspires trust among those with whom he comes in contact. Others know that he believes in playing according to the rules, that he will not take unfair advantage, that he assumes responsibility, and that he is considerate of others. These characteristics should be developed in every child who visits a physical education class or tries out for any athletic team.

5. *The physical education program aimed at excellence contributes to family and home living.* Physical education has a contribution to make to family and home living. The makeup of a child depends to a great extent on the type of family and home environment in which he lives. Many times such an environment determines whether an individual is kind or mean, quiet or boisterous, or polite or rude. In view of the imprint of the home and family upon the child, the school has the educational responsibility to improve and nurture the child, to interpret society to him in its correct light, and to strengthen family ties. Physical education can assume part of this responsibility.

The coach and the physical education teacher are many times the ones in whom a child puts his trust and confidence and whom he desires to emulate. The nature of physical education work and its appeal to youth probably are the causal factors of such practice. Consequently, physical education personnel should utilize their advantageous position to become better acquainted with the youth and his home and family life. Many times divorce and separation have affected children's lives. A change from rural to urban life with the difficulties of adjustment might be an experience through which a child is passing. There may be a lack of "belonging" or a pro-

tected existence, which causes anxiety and worry. By having a knowledge of the whole problem, the teacher or coach will be able to help in the adjustment process and in making for better home and family living. This could be done through proper counseling and guidance, helping youth to experience success in play activities, talks with parents, and home visitations. The ghetto youth who participates in the physical education program is often given experiences that are different from his everyday life. The youth who has been brought up in the slums of the city who makes the team is admired by his friends and family for this accomplishment.

The increased complications of family living, because of such factors as the prevalence of divorce, the desire for careers on the part of women, the turmoil of urban existence, and juvenile delinquency, place more and more responsibility upon education to help children make proper life adjustments. Physical educators, because of their program in which children have a natural desire to engage and because children look to them for guidance and help, can contribute considerably in these adjustments.

Objective—to help man achieve excellence as an economic being

A third objective of education deals with the production and consumption of goods and services. Education has the opportunity of informing the young in respect to both the vocational aspects of living and the consumer aspects. Both are important and are necessary for a happy and successful life. Most people select and follow various vocations in the matter of earning a living, placing them in the role of a producer. At the same time they buy goods and services, which places them in the role of a consumer. Schools and colleges should prepare youth to be both good producers and good consumers. Physical education can aid in more efficient production of goods and services and also can aid in the establishment of certain standards that will guide the public in the wise consumption of certain goods.

1. *Physical education should contribute to good workmanship.* Excellence in workmanship is tied in with intellectual, physical, social, and emotional qualities. The total individual must be developed if good workmanship is to be achieved. A man will be as strong as his weakest link. Work is an essential for all individuals. Through work one contributes goods and services to the wider community of which he is a part. Everyone, by reason of his ability, skill, and knowledge, can contribute to the needs of a great population. The man who screws a bolt on an assembly line at an automobile plant, the woman who types a letter, the boy who washes a car, and the girl who sweeps the living room all contribute goods or services. It is characteristic of the democratic way of life for everyone to contribute according to his capacity and ability. Only through work is democratic living achieved.

Children and youths should have opportunities for work. As part of their educational training children and youths should be assigned tasks around the house and around the school or college. In physical education, children could help in developing playfields, taking care of equipment, and instructing those with less skill. Through regular duties, a young person can discover that he is contributing to the welfare of the group and is providing goods or services that will help others to live a little more comfortably, happily, and successfully. A young person also takes pride in achievement. He feels a sense of satisfaction in accomplishment. Such an educational experience has implications for successful living in a democracy.

2. *Physical education should contribute to vocational placement.* The happiness and success of an individual is dependent to a great extent upon his selecting the right position or field of work. There are thousands of positions to which one may turn for work. The individual is anxious to select the one that is best suited to his personal ability, skills, and makeup. This process of selection can prove very disheartening without some type of professional guidance. Schools should assume part of the responsibility of seeing that students are guided into those positions where they will be the happiest and where they will be able to serve society best. Physical educators should be constantly alert for individuals who can become desired members of their profession.

The physical educator in the secondary school is in a most advantageous position to guide youth either into or away from the physical education profession. Many students who are not suited for this profession turn to him for vocational guidance. Others, because of their skills, good human relations, scholastic achievements, personality, and health, are wanted in this expanding profession. The undesirable candidates can be guided into work where their qualifications are needed, and to the desirable candidates can be explained the advantages of being in physical education work. The physical educator should be a virtual talent scout on the lookout for good material. The physical educator performs a service for the students by guiding them into a profession where they will be happy in their work, and he also performs a service for the profession of physical education and ultimately for the public at large that receives the benefits of the services of properly guided individuals. Such students should be taken into the confidence of the physical educator and opportunities provided for continuous development of their interest in physical education. Opportunities for working in various phases of the physical education program could be provided, deficiency in skills could be made up, and desirable personality traits emphasized.

3. *Physical education should contribute to successful work.* The success of any job depends to a great degree upon the health and physical fitness of the worker. If one is in the best of health and is physically fit, it is expressed in many ways. His human relations are such that he greets his col-

leagues with a cheery "good morning," his personality reflects enthusiasm and an abundance of energy, his capacity for work is great, he is not absent from work because of illness, his poise and leadership qualities are enhanced, and he reflects a satisfaction in his work that instills confidence in his employers.

The benefits of participation in various forms of physical education activities have proved of financial value. Thisted, in studying various groups of graduates of the University of Iowa, found that individuals who had participated in varsity basketball and football earned higher income than nonathletes in similar groups. This study is not sufficient to provide conclusive evidence in this respect. However, it seems that experience in physical education activities should contribute to physical health, mental health, human relations, and other social assets that could not help but contribute to better work.

4. *Physical education should encourage professional growth.* A person's training is not complete when he graduates from college or trade school, finishes a training course, or works in a particular vocation for a certain number of years. There is always some additional knowledge or skill that can be further developed that will make the work a little more productive. One individual has stated that the more a person learns, the more he realizes how little he knows. Conversely, many individuals with little knowledge about a particular subject sometimes gives the impression that they know everything there is to learn about the field. There is so much to know in this world that it is a physical and mental impossibility to do anything but scratch the surface. In order to compromise in this situation, we specialize; but even as we specialize there are multitudinous skills and items to master. Therefore, if a person wishes to make a success of his chosen vocation, it is necessary to continually learn new things. It is necessary to keep abreast of current developments in the field and to be constantly vigilant so that services and goods to the public may be improved.

The profession of physical education should continually provide for in-service training. Such items as new skills should be mastered. The implications of new ideas pertinent to child growth and development should be considered in the light of physical activity. Standards should be established in regard to the types of programs that should be administered at various school and college levels. New coaching techniques should be discussed, and an attempt should be made to solve the problems that arise from the tension of modern-day living. Physical education is a growing profession, and new facts in the areas of biology, psychology, and sociology that have implications for this profession are continually evolving. Only if physical educators are constantly studying new developments will they serve human welfare in the most favorable light.

5. *Physical education should contribute to the wise consumption of goods and services.* The educated person buys his goods and services with wisdom. He is well informed as to the worth and utility of various goods and services. He utilizes standards for guiding his expenditures, and he follows appropriate procedures to safeguard his interests.

Physical education can help to inform children and adults as to the relative values of goods and services that influence their health and physical fitness. The field of health is an area in which goods and services of doubtful value find a ready public market. If a person selects many of the more popular magazines and reads the advertisements with care, it would seem that he would need to eat certain types of cereal to be an outstanding athlete, drink certain whiskeys to be a man of distinction, take certain pills for proper elimination, smoke certain cigarettes to keep the throat healthy, visit certain salons and slenderizing parlors to have a well-developed body, use special types of toothpaste to keep teeth shiny, and use specially prepared tonics to keep hair from falling out. Literature that offers advice on health matters occupies prominent places on newsstands, drugstore counters, and various shops throughout the country. Advice is also seen and heard through billboards, posters, press, radio, and films. Much of the material is specially prepared and disseminated as a money-making scheme to exploit the public. Human welfare has no consideration in much of the advice being given.

By nature of their position and background in health matters, physical educators have the opportunity to help the student and the adult to take a critical view of such literature and pronouncements. Physical educators should instill in all persons the necessity for disregarding every remedy or cure until it has been successfully proved worthwhile through research and experimentation. The need for consulting the family physician should be impressed on all persons. The practice of self-medication should be discouraged. Many times harm rather than help results if such practice is followed. The individual should be a shrewd and intelligent buyer when it concerns his health and physical well-being. He has only one body, and this has to go with him throughout life. The physical educator should also be careful not to trespass on medical domain in giving advice. He should never attempt to diagnose or treat. These are the physician's prerogatives.

OBJECTIVE—TO HELP MAN ACHIEVE
EXCELLENCE AS A CIVIC BEING

Civic responsibility falls upon each member of a democracy. Only as each individual assumes his civic responsibility and contributes to group welfare will democratic ties be strengthened. Education can do much in teaching the wide disparities that exist among men and the action that is necessary to correct these conditions.

1. *Physical education should contribute to humanitarianism.* Youth should be well informed as to the needs of mankind everywhere. There should be established in each individual the desire to contribute to human welfare. This desire should not be passive but should be translated into action.

Physical education can, within reason,

emotionalize democratic play experiences to the point where youth sees the importance and the value of cooperative living and contributing to the welfare of all. Here is an ideal setting for developing humanitarian values. Children and youth from all walks of life, all creeds, colors, and races are brought together for a social experience. Interest and a natural drive for activity provide a laboratory for actual practice in developing these values.

2. *Physical education should contribute to tolerance of other people's views.* It is the prerogative of every person to think out solutions to various problems, form his own opinions, and attempt to bring others around to his point of view. At the same time, he should realize that it is everyone else's prerogative to do the same thing.

Physical educators can help in developing tolerance of other people's opinions in the various activities they conduct. Students can be trained to participate intelligently in the discussion of common problems that develop in a game situation. All can be encouraged to contribute their thinking. Thoughts and ideas are respected by all, and the final settlement of the problem can be made by group opinion. When the time occurs for the election of captains for the basketball team, there usually is a difference of opinion; when Johnny, Jim, Dick, and Harry all want to pitch in the softball game, there is a difference of opinion; when Mary, Ruth, and Nancy feel the umpire has made a bad call and Dorothy, Diana, and Lee think it is a good call, there is a difference of opinion; and when there are twenty-five in a class and there are twenty-two positions on teams to be filled, there is a difference of opinion as to who should play. All of these situations present opportunities for the physical educator to allow the democratic process of respecting the opinions of others to operate. Physical educators should be alert to take advantage of such "teachable moments."

3. *Physical education should contribute to conservation of natural resources.* Part of the great wealth that is America's is represented in terms of wildlife, fish, forests,

water, soil, and scenic beauty. These resources of the nation contribute to the living standard, appreciation of beauty, recreation, and pride that characterize this country. Every resident should feel it his personal responsibility to maintain and improve these resources whenever possible.

Physical education must be concerned with ecology, and physical educators should be especially concerned with preserving such national resources as wildlife, fish, water, and forests. These represent the media through which many enjoyable moments are spent by sportsmen, campers, and seekers of recreation and relaxation. If these resources are destroyed or allowed to deteriorate, many of the nation's chief sources of beauty and happiness will have been lost. Therefore, physical educators should inform the youth and the public of the value of such resources to the health and physical fitness of the country. It is important to impress upon all persons the value of knowing the right method and procedure of making a camp fire, the laws concerned with the taking of wildlife and fish, the importance of preventing forest fires, the contribution of forests in preventing floods and soil erosion, and the harmful results of recklessly destroying the nation's resources. Through an educational program that points out that natural resources are directly related to the welfare of each resident of this country, much good can be done in conserving this form of the nation's wealth.

4. *Physical education should contribute to conformance with the law.* In a democracy laws are made by the people and for their benefit. Therefore, these laws should be adhered to by everyone. Obedience is essential to a well-ordered society. Laws should be obeyed even though a person is not in agreement with them. Such statutes are on the books because the people directly or through their representatives voted for them. They are designed to protect the people's interest and welfare. If a person feels that they are not in accordance with public welfare, then every attempt, through democratic means, should be made to erase them. The solution to the problem is not to break laws. They should either be followed or be discarded through legislative action.

The prevalence of crime in this country is evidence of the fact that many people in the nation do not live within the law. The growing crime rate represents a grave concern for the democratic way of life. People should realize that laws are for their benefit and that any failure to live up to the law infringes upon the rights of others. When a law is passed stating that a person should not drive more than 50 miles per hour, it is to protect not only the driver but other people who may be driving or walking along the road. Everyone should appreciate this fact and stay within the laws that have been created for their benefit.

Schools and colleges can do much toward developing law-abiding citizens. There are certain rules and regulations that are established in school and college for the protection and benefit of all. The library should be kept quiet so that students may study. No one should swim alone because of the danger involved, and all should attend classes regularly, since this is deemed necessary in order to get the right kind of education. These rules and regulations are similar to the laws outside of school and college. They are for the protection and welfare of all concerned.

Physical education can contribute to developing a law-abiding attitude in youth. The rules of safety that have been established for the playground, gymnasium, and other places where physical education activities are held should be made clear to each student. Furthermore, the purpose behind such rules should be explained.

Physical educators can set a good example for students by being law-abiding citizens. They should abide by the rules and laws that have been established. They should teach through example as well as precept. Organizations, leagues, and athletic conferences have rules governing them. The National Collegiate Athletic Association

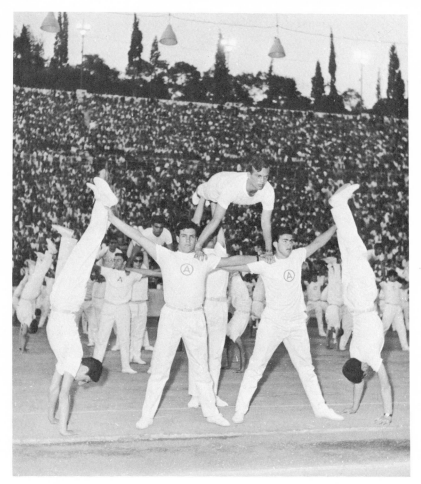

Greek physical education. The Greeks have a rich tradition in physical education as a part of general education.

(NCAA) sets up certain eligibility rules for intercollegiate participation. When these rules are broken by certain members, it is not in keeping with the democratic way of life. The NCAA is a representative athletic body. Each member has a vote. When a rule is passed by the majority, it should be accepted by all and strictly adhered to. If some are in disagreement, they can work for its repeal, but in the meantime the letter and spirit of the rule should be kept. This is setting the right example for that great mass of youths and adults who attend or follow the field of sport. Representatives of every athletic league and conference should draw up rules and regulations to govern competition in accordance with the general welfare of the participants, the educational institutions concerned, and society in general. Through such a procedure, athletics may be conducted in a much more meaningful and purposeful manner.

5. *Physical education should contribute to civic responsibility.* It is the responsibility of every citizen to have a clear understanding of his civic duties and to see that they are carried out in an intelligent manner. The principal duties that involve action on the part of the citizen are voting intelligently, developing an appreciation of the various governmental services, and knowing the law.

Every citizen should cast his vote in an intelligent manner. In order to vote intelligently a citizen must know the issues involved and the arguments pro and con. He should make a thorough study of the whole problem in the light of what it means for the general welfare. This means that a citizen should know about local, state, national, and international affairs. He should be well informed. He should not be influenced by all the propaganda cast in his direction. He should think through the issues in a calm, intelligent manner. The physical educator, when faced with important decisions, should follow a similar plan in determining what course he will follow. Many times the decision arrived at will not be popular with one's colleagues. However, a person must have a skin that is tough rather than sensitive to the interests of those who are often more concerned with their own welfare than with the welfare of the participants or of the students. This seems especially true of many coaches who have public, alumni, and student pressure on them to produce winning teams.

6. *Physical education should contribute to democratic living.* The educated citizen believes in the democratic way of life, and his every action is symbolic of his loyalty to its ideals. He is aware of the freedom of worship, speech, and assembly; of the worth of the individual; of equality for all; and of the right to be a part of and to participate in government. At the same time, he realizes that in order to participate in these benefits he must contribute to the group, must work for the happiness of all, and must live up to the ideals that are characteristic of democratic living. The educated citizen is the chief contributor to the preservation of America's freedom.

The word *freedom* is an unusual word. Each young person should know what it means and how it is protected and preserved for himself and for future generations.

All young persons should know that freedom is not an end but a means to an end, *that freedom is a catalyst that releases their energies.* It is the key that unlocks doors to opportunities and makes it possible for them to become all they are capable of becoming. It is an instrument for their self-realization—mentally, physically, socially, and spiritually. It is their avenue for achieving excellence. Without this freedom they would be like the boy in East Berlin who is brainwashed with communist thinking and must crash through "the wall" in order to breathe free air.

All young persons should know that freedom is never a "fait accompli." Freedom was not won with the surrender of Cornwallis at Yorktown. It was not a permanent possession of the United States with the signing of the Declaration of Independence by Benjamin Franklin and his colleagues in Philadelphia. Woodrow Wilson stated that freedom cannot be laid away in a document—"Democratic institutions," he stressed, "are never done, they are like the living tissue, always amaking." Young people must clearly see that freedom is never complete as a result of a successful political campaign, the election of a famous man to public office, or the winning of a war. Americans must never lower their guard, be complacent, or drop their vigilance. Freedom is an elusive thing and can vanish into the air like a soap bubble when those persons who share its benefits fail to put forth daily efforts to guarantee its preservation. The Czechoslovakians, Poles, and Hungarians will attest to this fact.

Young people should know that, in the long run, whether or not our freedom is preserved for them and future generations will not be determined by bombs but by wisdom; not by having been the first on the moon but being the first to help in the elimination of poverty and suffering wherever it exists in the world; not by seeking some magic political formula but by seeking the truth; and not by possessing great wealth but by possessing knowledge and dynamic ideas. Young people must not be deceived into thinking that freedom can be won through military power and dollars rather than through sound thinking and wise decisions. Freedom lies in their minds, guided by truths that each of them has the opportunity to possess.

Education should help young people to see themselves as contributors and builders of democratic ideals. It should help them to be worthy examples to the world that they are free to make choices on their own, formulate their own standard of values, and fulfill their destinies. Then it should guide them in the use of their freedom so that they act wisely, direct their lives meaningfully, search for the truth, achieve excellence within their abilities, and continually seek opportunities for self-realization and self-fulfillment.

Despite all the advantages and opportunities offered for democratic living in America, there are many shadows that fall across its path. America is being challenged as to whether this shining star of democracy will continue to shine as a hope and a goal for all civilizations to attain or whether it will dim and fade with time. Such factors as unbridled science, failure of government to meet the needs of human welfare, lack of interest in religion and moral codes, racial inequality, the war effort, and settlement of controversial issues by force help to darken the road to democracy. There must be a change toward the principles and way of life that are truly democratic. All individuals, organizations, and professions must contribute in this movement. Education, by reason of its close association with youth who are at a formative period in life when the values of democratic living can become a part of them, should carry its share of responsibility. Physical education, with its activities in which children have the natural desire to engage, can help to provide one of the most natural laboratories for the right social experiences. Nowhere is democracy better served, for the lessons that are learned on the playing fields and in the gymnasium have aided in keeping America free. A Brown, Cohen, Murphy, and Rizzo, all members of one team, working together, cooperating, and doing their best to achieve common goals, will show those people struggling for freedom in the far corners of the earth that our way of life, "American style," is worth waiting for, fighting for, sacrificing for, and dying for. The cry will reverberate throughout the world that the future lies with democracy and freedom and not with those nations that proclaim freedom through their mouthings but in actual practice make a mockery of the ideal. We know what freedom is because our every thought and action express it clearly.

QUESTIONS AND EXERCISES

1. In approximately 300 words discuss the role of physical education in the educational process.
2. Comment on the statement: "All education takes place within the walls of the public schools."
3. What level of government has responsibility for public education? Comment on the advisability of leaving this responsibiilty at this level.
4. In what ways does the federal government contribute to education?
5. What is meant by the term *education?*
6. What are the objectives of education as outlined by the Educational Policies Commission?
7. What is meant by the term *general education?*
8. Discuss the objective of self-realization. How does physical education contribute to its achievement?
9. Discuss the objective of human relationship? How does physical education contribute to its achievement?
10. Discuss the objective of economic efficiency. How does physical education contribute to its achievement?
11. Discuss the objective of civic responsibility. How does physical education contribute to its achievement?
12. To what extent is the physical education profession, through the programs that exist today, contributing to the objectives as set forth by the Educational Policies Commission?
13. In the light of the discussion in this chapter, why should the public feel that physical education is an essential to the educational program in the schools?

Reading assignment

Bucher, Charles A., and Goldman, Myra: Dimensions of physical education, St. Louis, 1969, The C. V. Mosby Co., Reading selections 11 to 14 and 16.

SELECTED REFERENCES

Brameld, Theodore: Philosophies of education in cultural perspective, New York, 1955, The Dryden Press.

Briggs, Paul W.: The opportunity to be relevant, Journal of Health, Physical Education, and Recreation **41:**43, 1970.

Bucher, Charles A.: Administration of health and physical education programs including athletics, St. Louis, 1971, The C. V. Mosby Co.

Bucher, Charles A.: Administrative dimensions of health and physical education programs, including athletics, St. Louis, 1971, The C. V. Mosby Co.

Bucher, Charles A.: Health, physical education, and academic achievement, NEA Journal **54:** 38, 1965.

Bucher, Charles A., Koenig, Constance, and Barnhard, Milton: Methods and materials for secondary school physical education, St. Louis, 1970, The C. V. Mosby Co.

Bucher, Charles A., Olsen, Einar A., and Willgoose, Carl E.: The foundations of health, New York, 1967, Appleton-Century-Crofts.

Educational Policies Commission, National Education Association and American Association of School Administrators, Washington, D. C:
Education for all American children, 1948.
Education for all American youth, 1944.
Education and the defense of American democracy, 1940.
Education of free men in American democracy, 1941.
Policies for education in American democracy, 1946.
The purpose of education in American democracy, 1938.
The unique function of education in American democracy, 1937.

Fraleigh, Warren P.: Should physical education be required? Physical Educator **22:**25, 1965.

Gardner, John W.: Excellence, New York, 1961, Harper and Row, Publishers.

General Education in a Free Society: Report of the Harvard Committee, Cambridge, Massachusetts, 1945, Harvard University Press.

Morse, Horace T.: Liberal and general education: a problem of differentiation. Quoted by Rice, James G., editor: General education, Washington, D. C., 1964, National Education Association.

Oberteuffer, D.: Some contributions of physical education to an educated life, Journal of Health, Recreation, and Physical Education **16:** 3, 1945.

Radler, D. H., and Kephart, Newell C.: Success through play, New York, 1960, Harper and Row, Publishers.

Whitehead, Alfred North: The aims of education, New York, 1929, The Macmillan Co.

Wynne, J.: General education in theory and practice, New York, 1952, Bookman Associates.

PART THREE

Relationship of physical education to health, recreation, camping, and outdoor education

8/School health program

9/Recreation

10/Camping and outdoor education

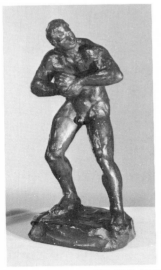

WORK OF R. TAIT
MCKENZIE. COURTESY
JOSEPH BROWN, SCHOOL OF
ARCHITECTURE, PRINCETON
UNIVERSITY.

Introduction

The next three chapters are devoted to areas of endeavor with which physical educators are frequently associated. Health, recreation, camping, and outdoor education are specialties that have grown rapidly during the last decade. With this growth many questions have been raised as to their relationship with physical education. Should they be associated with physical education? Should each of them go it alone? Are health, physical education, and recreation closely related? Should each of these fields of endeavor be a part of the same professional organization? How should these specialties be administered—separately or collectively?

The student of physical education needs to know the relationship of physical education to health, recreation, camping, and outdoor education. He needs to understand how the various fields evolved and the pros and cons of furthering a close relationship among the special areas or encouraging the separateness of each.

The next three chapters outline each of these fields of endeavor so that the reader may have a better understanding of the nature and scope of each and the relation of physical education to each. First, however, this introduction identifies several statements of fact about the relationship that exists among physical education, health, recreation, camping, and outdoor education.

1. *History indicates that physical education is the parent.* Physical education is as old as primitive man. Historically, physical education has reached many heights, including the great emphasis placed upon this area during the early Greek civilization. Physical education was also emphasized later on in history in the Scandinavian countries and in Germany. Various gymnastic systems from these countries were introduced into America. In 1885, physical education's largest professional organization was established under the title of the American Association for the Advancement of Physical Education. In 1903, the name was changed to the American Physical Education Association.

The areas of recreation, camping, outdoor education, and health education as organized fields of endeavor came into being later in history. The birth of recreation is frequently marked with the construction of the sand gardens in Boston. Health, in its early history, was concerned as much with facilities as with the health of the child. Early health instruction took place primarily at the college level. In the later nineteenth century a majority of the colleges had courses in hygiene. The association of camping and outdoor education with schools and colleges is the most recent entrant into educational circles.

Common interests and goals prompted the Department of School Health of the National Education Association in 1937 to join the national association to form the American Association of Health and Physical Education. In 1938, recreation was also added to the title of the national association. Camping and outdoor education have never been included in the title of the national organization, but sections have been established within the association.

Each of the special fields of health, physical education, recreation, camping, and outdoor education has grown considerably since it joined together professionally with the allied special areas. The purpose of the national association is to bring about a closer relationship among the various members, upgrade the standards of each area stimulate an interest in and understanding of the work being accomplished, distribute informative materials, and take other necessary actions to make for a greater contribution to our society by each of the special areas.

2. *Health, physical education, recreation, camping, and outdoor education are viewed today as distinct and separate fields of endeavor.* Today, each of these professional fields of specialization has its own distinct program, teachers and leaders who have special training, and its own subject matter and underlying philosophy. The emphasis upon specialization has helped to clarify the uniqueness of each area. It is difficult for a person to be trained in more than one of these fields. Each field has become a specialty that requires many years of preparation in order to acquire the knowledge and skills peculiar to the area.

3. *Professional organizations frequently incorporate all areas.* Such organizations as the American Association for Health, Physical Education, and Recreation; the Society of State Directors of Health, Physical Education, and Recreation; and the Canadian Association for Health, Physical Education, and Recreation are examples of organizations that incorporate all of these subject areas. In addition, other organizations such as the American Academy of Physical Education, Delta Psi Kappa, and Phi Epsilon Kappa include members in these areas and are involved in activities peculiar to each of the fields.

4. *Administrative units in colleges, universities, and schools frequently incorporate all areas.* Institutions of higher learning engaged in the preparation of leaders for these special fields and some agency programs have administrative units that carry such titles as: School or College of Health, Phys-

ical Education, and Recreation; Division of Health, Physical Education, and Recreation; and Departments of Health, Physical Education, and Recreation. Many of these administrative units also include camping and outdoor education. Similarly, many school districts incorporate these areas into their administrative structure.

5. *Publications and course offerings in colleges and universities frequently incorporate all these areas.* A check of professional libraries, magazines, articles, and courses offered in colleges and universities will result in the realization that all areas are frequently referred to in the same publication or course.

6. *Physical education is related to health.* Physical education is designed to further the health of those who participate in its programs. Opportunities abound for the development of physical, mental, emotional, and social health in human beings. Physical education helps in the correction of remediable physical defects, alleviates tension, develops vitality, and offers a chance for emotional expression. The physical educator needs to be familiar with sound health practices and should have experiences in the field of health. He will be a better physical educator if he has some preparation in health. Physical educators are involved with such things as injuries, medical examinations, physical fitness, and facility management, all of which have implications for the health of the participant.

Health education recognizes that physical activity contributes to health and sees games and sports as a means of making contributions to mental as well as other aspects of health.

Desirable health practices are objectives of both the fields of health education and physical education.

7. *Physical education is related to recreation, camping, and outdoor education.* Physical education develops many skills in such activities as dancing and sports, which can be utilized in recreation, camping, and outdoor education settings. Physical education develops wholesome attitudes that em-

phasize the need and motivation for constructive recreational, camping, and outdoor education pursuits. Physical education facilities are frequently a part of recreation and camping programs. The basic instructional physical education program helps to develop proper attitudes for recreation. One of the strongest reasons for physical education programs to exist is the teaching of recreational skills.

8. *Health, recreation, camping, and outdoor education are related.* A widely accepted belief by professionals is that wholesome play and recreation are important to the total health of the individual. Practitioners of health, recreation, camping, and outdoor education are interested in the well-being of the people they serve. They are interested in relieving fatigue and tensions and in rehabilitating the sick, injured, and infirm. They are interested in helping people to live a healthy, vigorous, happy, and productive life.

9. *A rationale exists for a close relationship among health, physical education, recreation, camping, and outdoor education.* Leaders in all the special fields have pointed out why they feel the fields are related and why they should work together to achieve their objectives. All fields have some objectives that are similar. A strong unity among the fields can add strength to each area's place in education and society and its success in achieving educational goals. A strong professional association combining all areas can help in furthering each separate area and the unique contributions each makes to the good of mankind. Personnel who are knowledgeable in two or three areas can help in furthering administrative efficiency and in contributing to the growth and prestige of these areas. Duplication of efforts can be avoided and less expense incurred as a result of a close coordination of all areas.

10. *A rationale exists for separating the areas of health, physical education, recreation, camping, and outdoor education.* Leaders in each of the special areas have also indicated reasons why the fields should

be separated. Each has its own subject matter and trained specialists. An area like recreation is primarily voluntary in nature, whereas health and physical education are more formal in nature and primarily serve a captive audience. Recreation is more directly related to park executives, municipal recreation, and social agency personnel than it is to educators in the schools. Physical education is primarily concerned with such physical activities as games and sports, whereas recreation is concerned with the whole gamut of activities in which people engage, including drama, music, and arts and crafts. Health education is concerned with instruction in scientific health matters. The science and skills associated with health are different from those associated with physical education. Health education is as much related to medicine and public health as it is to physical education. Camping and outdoor education are not related to physical education in some school, college, and agency programs.

11. *The relationship of health, physical education, recreation, camping, and outdoor education needs considerable study.* The very nature of the problem and the complexities involved defy a ready answer. Perhaps it would help to point out what Wegener* sets forth as functions of education.

The functions of education are: (1) to contribute to the systematic development of each individual toward his full potentialities in the intelligent pursuit of the good life, (2) to coordinate the progressive and conservative functions of an enduring society, (3) to serve the individual and society, and (4) to give man systematic assistance in the development of his whole self: intellectually, morally, spiritually, socially, economically, politically, *physically,* domestically, esthetically, and *recreationally.*

Health, physical education, recreation,

---

*Wegener, Frank C.: The organic philosophy of education, Dubuque, Iowa, 1957, Wm. C. Brown Co.

camping, and outdoor education contribute to the systematic development of man. Each of these fields has a unique and important contribution to make. Each of these fields is related in many ways to the other. The question to be decided is how each can make its contribution most effectively. In making the decision, personal considerations, petty annoyances, and selfish motives must be cast aside. The answer must rest with what is best for mankind and an enduring democratic society. In addition to considering the relationships of the special areas under discussion, it would also be wise to explore relationships with other disciplines, such as history, social work, medicine, social science, philosophy, and psychology. All professional disciplines might be viewed as potential members of a team. Such exploration may result in an arrangement where our special programs can make even greater contributions to the attainment of broad educational objectives and the development of man.

8/School health program

Health as a curricular offering in the nation's schools and colleges is taking on an added dimension of importance during the 70's. The increased drug addiction on the part of young people, the public awareness regarding pollution of the environment, the changed thinking of society in regard to sexual mores, and the research showing the dangers inherent in smoking are a few of the concerns receiving the attention of educators and the public alike. These concerns are resulting in such developments as the mandating of health courses in our schools and government appropriations for purposes of training teachers, conducting research, and providing programs to cope with these problems. In addition, many new health books are being published on such topics as drugs, ecology, and sex education, as well as about health in general.

Health education is emerging as one of the important subjects in the curriculum. If health problems are to be solved, an informed public is essential. Furthermore, young people must be aware of the effects on their health of such things as drugs, tobacco, venereal disease, and accidents. Only if young people are provided with the scientific facts will they be able to make informed choices regarding matters that relate to their health. It is felt that schools and colleges have a responsibility to do something to alleviate health problems— that health education can play a very important role in eliminating many of the problems that adversely affect young people, adults, and society.

Public health officials, medical doctors, dentists, and other representatives of professional services are taking more interest in health. Research in the health area is providing new and better direction to help schools and colleges in changing the health behavior of young people.

The future of America depends to a large degree upon what is done to improve the health of the students in the nation's schools and colleges and to provide an environment that represents a healthy and safe place to live. Although parents, industry, and the public in general must help, institutions of learning must assume a major responsibility for health education.

Unfortunately, research shows that health is not being taught properly in many schools at the present time. In some educational systems the curriculum is not planned, the teacher is not qualified, classes are too large and do not meet regularly, and the information imparted is not scientifically accurate. Consequently, there is much work to be done to improve the school health curriculum.

DEFINITION OF HEALTH

Health has been defined in many ways. Jesse F. Williams,* nearly 50 years ago, proposed the definition that health is "the quality of life that renders the individual fit to live most and to serve best." Oberteuffer,† more recently, defined health as "the

---

*Williams, Jesse F.: Personal hygiene applied, Philadelphia, 1925, W. B. Saunders Co.

†Oberteuffer, Delbert: School health education, New York, 1960, Harper and Row, Publishers.

A shocking 15% of all children studied so far in the National Nutrition Survey show evidence of growth retardation.

FROM TODAY'S HEALTH **47**:33, 1969.

condition of the organism which measures the degree to which its aggregate powers are able to function."

Other authorities in the field of health have stressed such concepts as the three-dimensional makeup of health—physical, mental, and social—and not merely the absence of disease or infirmity; the homeostatic balance that enables human beings to function harmoniously; the adaptability of the individual to various environmental factors affecting his well-being; and the readiness of the individual to meet the needs of the present and future.

All of these concepts reflect what is meant by health. Each of the concepts reflects a state of being essential to a full and productive life. Furthermore, in order to have this state of being, certain health practices are essential, otherwise the homeostatic balance or the steady state may be disrupted and ill health result. Consequently, health education is essential in order to better assure that proper health habits are established early in life.

Nolte,* after citing several definitions of health, some of which are listed previously, has graphically portrayed what she feels constitutes the discipline of health. This

*Nolte, Ann E.: Variations on a theme, Journal of School Health **38:**425, 1968.

diagram gives greater meaning to the nature and definition of health by showing how it is affected by the interaction of the organism with the environment and how the discipline of health must be concerned with the cognitive, affective, and action domains.

HISTORY OF THE SCHOOL HEALTH PROGRAM

The health program in the schools is a phase of the educational process that attempts to build in the student a sound foundation of scientific health knowledge, health attitudes, and health habits.

Health science, a comparatively new subject in the school program, derives its foundations from the biological, behavioral, and health sciences. It is an academic field and subject. It helps human beings to apply scientific health discoveries to their daily lives. It is best conducted in institutions of learning by professionally trained health educators.

The earliest forms of health programs in the schools were evidenced in the latter part of the nineteenth century and were concerned primarily with the temperance movement. A large amount of time was devoted to discussing the ill effects of alcohol on the human body. A state program of health instruction was introduced in

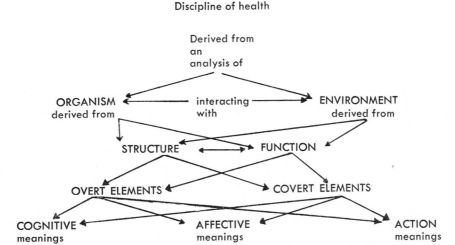

FROM NOLTE, ANN E.: VARIATIONS ON A THEME, JOURNAL OF SCHOOL HEALTH **38:**425, 1968.

Ohio in 1872 as a result of pressure on the part of the Women's Christian Temperance Union. Early instruction in health, other than that of temperance, emphasized a knowledge of the structure and function of the human body.

During the early part of the twentieth century a movement started that emphasized the formation of healthful attitudes and habits. Instead of stressing the names of the various anatomical parts of the human body or the harmful effects of alcohol, the emphasis was along the lines of better living.

On June 28, 1937, the Department of School Health and Physical Education of the National Education Association and the American Physical Education Association were combined to form the American Association for Health and Physical Education. This was in keeping with the rise of health to a place of importance in the educational system.

The results of the medical examinations reported to Selective Service officials during World War II, which pointed out the incidence of dental caries, postural abnormalities, and other defects, gave impetus to an increased emphasis on health in our schools. These statistics also did much to stimulate thinking toward better preparation of health teachers. Teacher-training institutions were called upon to make provision in their programs for such preparation.

Today, health programs in schools and colleges are gaining increasing stature as educators recognize the importance of instilling in young and old alike a body of health knowledge based on scientific fact, wholesome health attitudes, and desirable health practices. Health education is not unique to the United States. It is included in many educative programs throughout the world.

School health programs have made progress over the years. Six ways in which they have improved are as follows:

1. *Health education has changed from a hygiene class to one that is dynamically involved in the total health of the child.*

Whereas old programs were concerned with anatomy and physiology, today's health education programs include topics involving the basic needs and interests of students. Teaching methods and textbooks have been changed to meet the challenge by presenting health material in an interesting, attractive, challenging, and thought-provoking manner designed to develop desirable health attitudes and practices in students.

2. *There is greater emphasis on saftey and mental health.* The health problems of school children have changed in the last few decades. Communicable diseases are being brought under control, but in their place accidents have evolved as one of the important causes of death among school children. Also, emotional disturbances are widespread, making imperative the need for health instruction and health services aimed at furthering good mental health.

3. *Curriculum studies have become an important part of the health picture.* The School Health Education Study, a national project, and many state and local curriculum studies have taken place in recent years. As a result, there has been a continuous flow of curriculum materials and courses of study for our schools and colleges. Particular emphasis in many of these studies has been placed on the conceptual approach to teaching health. Furthermore, topics that represent health problems for the American society such as sex education, environment, drugs, alcohol and tobacco, and mental health have been highlighted in these curriculum studies. The result of these projects has provided a more meaningful, systematic, and scientific approach to the teaching of health.

4. *Professional organizations contribute leadership.* Such organizations as the American Association for Health, Physical Education, and Recreation, American School Health Association, National Education Association, and American Medical Association have sponsored in-service programs, workshops, and research and provided other forms of help and leadership for school health programs in the United States.

5. *Teacher preparation has been upgraded.* Numerous professional conferences have been held that have tended to raise the standards of preparation for classroom teachers, health educators, physical educators, and other personnel associated with school health programs.

6. *Books have been published that have resulted in a broader understanding of health education in the schools.* Such publications as *Health Education, Healthful School Living,* and *School Health Services,* sponsored by the Joint Committee on Health Problems of the National Education Association and the American Medical Association, as well as those publications authored or sponsored by many leaders and organizations in the field of health, have served to assist in communicating articulately the important place that health plays in modern educational programs.

CONCEPT APPROACH TO HEALTH EDUCATION

The last decade has witnessed considerable progress in the utilization of the concept approach to the teaching of health. The concepts and conceptual frameworks that have been identified represent the key or central ideals that should be emphasized in health education curriculums at various educational levels. These concepts, which are essential to good health practices, are designed to make the student aware of the many health choices he must make, the responsibility he has for making wise choices, and the results of the decisions that he does make. The concepts that are utilized are identified by such methods as research regarding the health needs and characteristics of children and youth and an analysis of critical health problems. Then these concepts are translated into instructional units.

School Health Education Study

A significant study in the area of health education that utilized the conceptual approach is the School Health Education Study. The Study conducted a nationwide status study of health education in the public schools, including the testing of students at all grade levels. It produced information on the kind of instruction students receive, what health misconceptions they have, who does the teaching, the content areas that are emphasized, how the subject is organized and scheduled, and many other factors of importance to educators and persons interested in the health of children and youth.

The Study was initiated in September, 1961, and involved such procedures as surveys of 135 public school systems and of the health practices of approximately 6 million students in more than 1,000 elementary schools and 359 secondary schools. It also included the development of experimental curriculum materials and an experimental curriculum demonstration project in four school system tryout centers: Alhambra, California; Evanston, Illinois; Great Neck–Garden City, New York; and Tacoma, Washington.

The Study had the services of an interdisciplinary advisory committee of individuals, with representatives from national health education–related organizations serving as ex-officio members of the committee. Dr. Elena M. Sliepcevich served as Director of the School Health Education Study.

Since the concept approach had been used in teaching other subject-matter fields and had won much acclaim in educational circles, the School Health Education Study felt that this was the approach they should use. They reasoned that the decisions that people make as well as their behavior patterns are determined largely by their knowledge of and attitudes toward certain basic health concepts.

Concepts that evolve from their research, the School Health Education Study concluded, can have an impact on the cognitive (knowledge, intellectual abilities, and skills) and affective (values, attitudes, and appreciations) domains. Recognizing the value of the concept approach, the School Health Education Study developed, on an experimental basis, an outline, *A Conceptual Approach to Health Education.*

The concept approach outlined by the School Health Education Study recognized the three closely interwoven dimensions of health: mental, physical, and social. Furthermore, it stressed the triad of health education—the unity of man in respect to his physical, mental, and social aspects; the knowledges, attitudes, and practices important to influencing health behavior; and the focus of health education upon the individual, family, and community. All of these components of the triad are interdependent and constantly interacting.

The Study identified three key concepts, ten conceptual statements, and thirty-one substantive elements that represent the con-

ceptual framework for health. The three key concepts for health education identified by the Study are growing and developing, interacting, and decision making, all of which are closely interrelated. Ten additional concepts were identified as a framework around which health education could take place.* These ten concepts are:

1. Growth and development influences and is influenced by the structure and functioning of the individual.
2. Growing and developing follows a predict-

*Payne, Arlene (reviewer): Health education: a conceptual approach to curriculum, The National Elementary Principal **48:**70, 1968. Copyright 1968, National Association of Elementary School Principals, NEA. All rights reserved.

HEALTH CONCEPTS
guides for health instruction

Concepts and supporting data pertaining to major health problems facing youth today

American Association for Health, Physical Education, and Recreation

FROM AAHPER HEALTH EDUCATION DIVISION: HEALTH CONCEPTS—GUIDES FOR HEALTH INSTRUCTION, WASHINGTON, D. C., 1967, THE ASSOCIATION.

able sequence yet is unique for each individual.

3. Protection and promotion of health is an individual, community, and international responsibility.
4. The potential for hazards and accidents exists, whatever the environment.
5. There are reciprocal relationships involving man, disease, and environment.
6. The family serves to perpetuate man and to fulfill certain health needs.
7. Personal health practices are affected by a complexity of forces, often conflicting.
8. Utilization of health information, products, and services is guided by values and perceptions.
9. Use of substances that modify mood and behavior arises from a variety of motivations.
10. Food selection and eating patterns are determined by physical, mental, economic, and cultural factors.

The School Health Education Study has also prepared a set of instructional materials for various grade levels (lower elementary, upper elementary, junior high, high school) for each of the identified concepts. In addition, there are behavioral objectives for each of the four educational levels.

Curriculum Commission of the AAHPER

Another important health education study is the one conducted by the Curriculum Commission of the American Association for Health, Physical Education, and Recreation.*

This study included the identification of key concepts and supporting data pertaining to some of the major health problems of today and those that will exist in the next decade. This material is helpful as a reference for teachers, curriculum committees, and other persons interested in some of the main health problems facing young people today. It covers such important health areas as accident prevention, aging, alcohol, disaster preparedness, disease, economics of health care, environmental conditions, food

protection, occupational health, air pollution, radiation, family health, international health, mental health, nutrition, and smoking.

TERMINOLOGY FOR SCHOOL AND COLLEGE HEALTH PROGRAMS

The following definitions were drawn up by the Committee on Terminology that represented the American Association for Health, Physical Education, and Recreation, the Society of Public Health Educators, and the American Public Health Association. They are presented here for the reader's information.*

Dental examination. The appraisal, performed by a dentist, of the condition of the oral structures to determine the dental health status of the individual.

Dental inspection. The limited appraisal, performed by anyone with or without special dental preparation, of the oral structures to determine the presence or absence of obvious defects.

Health appraisal. The evaluation of the health status of the individual through the utilization of varied organized and systematic procedures such as medical and dental examinations, laboratory test, health history, teacher observation, etc.

Health observation. The estimation of an individual's well-being by noting the nature of his appearance and behavior.

Medical examination. The determination, by a physician, of an individual's health status.

Screening test. A medically and educationally acceptable procedure for identifying individuals who need to be referred for further study or diagnostic examination.

Cumulative school health record. A form used to note pertinent consecutive information about a student's health.

School health program. The composite of procedures used in school health services, healthful school living, and health science instruction to promote health among students and school personnel.

Healthful school living. The utilization of a safe and wholesome environment, consideration of individual health, organizing the school day, and planning classroom procedures to favorably influence emotional, social, and physical health.

Health school environment. The physical, social, and emotional factors of the school setting

---

*American Association for Health, Physical Education, and Recreation: Health concepts—guides for health instruction, Washington, D. C., 1967, The Association.

*Report of the Joint Committee on Health Education Terminology, Journal of Health, Physical Education, and Recreation **33**:27, 1962.

which affect the health, comfort, and performance of an individual or a group.

Health science instruction. The organized teaching procedures directed toward developing understandings, attitudes, and practices relating to health and factors affecting health.

School health services. The procedures used by physicians, dentists, nurses, teachers, etc., designed to appraise, protect, and promote optimum health of students and school personnel. (Activities frequently included in school health services are those used to [1] appraise the health status of students and school personnel; [2] counsel students, teachers, parents, and others for the purpose of helping school-age children get treatment or for arranging education programs in keeping with their abilities; [3] help prevent or control the spread of disease; and [4] provide emergency care for injury or sudden sickness.)

School health education. The process of providing or utilizing experiences for favorably influencing understandings, attitudes, and practices relating to individual, family, and community health.

Safety education. The process of providing or utilizing experiences for favorably influencing understandings, attitudes, and practices relating to safe living.

Health counseling. A method of interpreting to students or their parents the findings of health appraisals and encouraging and assisting them to take such action as needed to realize their fullest potential.

School health coordination. A process designed to bring about harmonious working relationship among the various personnel and groups in the school and community that have interest, concern, and responsibility for development and conduct of the school health program.

RELATIONSHIP OF
PHYSICAL EDUCATION TO THE
SCHOOL HEALTH PROGRAM

For many years the relationship of physical education to health has been a confused issue. Among professional persons working in these specialized programs this confusion has abated to some degree since the end of World War II, but among educators and lay people in general there is still considerable misunderstanding. Many school administrators feel that a program of physical activity satisfies the health needs of children. Some persons feel that training in physical education qualifies a person for full-time work in health. Still others

feel that health and physical education are allied but not the same and that each requires trained specialists. The continued emphasis on having qualified teachers of health has resulted in better programs being established in professional preparation institutions.

From the foregoing discussion it can be seen that health and physical education are not synonymous and that their activities are different. At the same time, they have common goals and are closely related, and physical education personnel can play an important part in school health programs. Although concentrated or direct health instruction is needed, health education should take place not only in the classroom but on the athletic field, playground, swimming pool, and gymnasium and in every other room and part of the school plant. The health program utilizes the services of the doctor, nurse, dentist, physical educator, home economics teacher, and other specialized personnel in furthering its program of health instruction, health services, and healthful school living.

Many schools find it economically impossible to have both a health educator and a physical educator on the staff. In such cases the physical educator who has adequate training in health can do much in the way of organizing and coordinating a working health program. In larger communities where sufficient funds make it possible to have personnel with broader training and experience in the health education area, the physical educator can still play a prominent part in helping in various health activities. Through the program of physical activities, he can play a major role in contributing to the health of every child with whom he works.

Physical educators interested in contributing most to the health of the child should, in addition to having a working knowledge of many health areas, know the health aspects of physical activity and the outcomes of sports and activity programs that have implications for the individual's physical, emotional, and social welfare. There is also

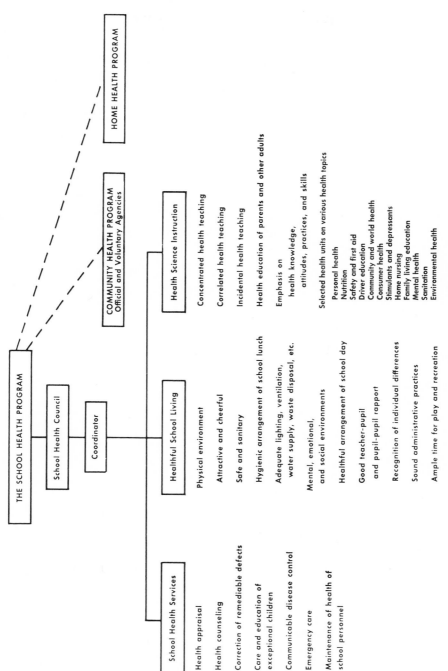

Suggested health education for the schools of the United States.

a need for physical educators to know what constitutes desirable activities, the special problems of physical education relating to girls and women, and the need for a knowledge of such things as first aid, body mechanics, and adapted physical education.

The Third National Conference on Physicians and Schools sponsored by the American Medical Association recommended that coaches should be adequately prepared in: "(1) principles of growth and development; (2) health needs of adolescent boys and girls; (3) desirable health practices, particularly those related to the conduct of athletics; (4) principles of first aid and accident prevention; (5) physiology of exercise; (6) conduct of interscholastic athletics so their maximum contribution may be made to the physical, emotional, mental, and social development of youth."*

In discussing the relationship of physical education to school health, it can be seen that each is closely related to the other, but at the same time, each is distinct. Each area has its own specialized subject-matter content, its specialists, and media through which it is striving to better the living standards of human beings. In the larger professional preparation institutions, each area has its own separate training program. In several states each area has its own certification requirements.

Health and physical education teachers must work closely together since, in many cases, they use the same facilities, perform duties in each other's area, work on committees together, and have professional books and magazines that cover the literature of both fields. Both are concerned with the total health of the individual. Both are concerned with the physical as well as the social, mental, emotional, and spiritual aspects of health. Both should help one another and follow practices that will provide the most benefits for the greatest number of people.

How many physical educators teach health

A survey conducted a few years ago by Sliepcevich,* which involved writing to each of the state directors of health, physical education, and recreation in the fifty states and requesting information as to what percentage of the health education offered in the junior and senior high schools was taught by physical educators, provided the following information, presented here in adapted form.

1. The health education being taught in the schools by physical educators ranges all the way from 10% to "nearly all."
2. More than 90% of the health education is being taught by physical educators in eight states.
3. Approximately 90% of the health education is being taught by physical educators in nine states.
4. From 80% to 85% of the health education is taught by physical educators in five states.
5. About 75% of the health education is being taught by physical educators in four states.
6. From 50% to 70% of the health education is being taught by physical educators in sixteen states.

These statistics showed that in approximately one-third of the states, 75% or more of the health education was being taught by physical educators, and in twenty-one states 70% or less of the health education was being taught by physical educators. The record shows clearly that at the time this survey was conducted, most of the health education classes in this country were being taught by physical educators.

A more recent study in the state of Michigan shows the undergraduate field of preparation for those persons who teach health (Table 8-1) and the area of emphasis in graduate study for those who teach health (Table 8-2).

There is a trend toward more trained health educators assuming the responsibility for teaching health classes. However, many

---

*Dukelow, Donald A., and Hein, Fred C., editors: Physicians and schools, report of the Third National Conference on Physicians and Schools, Chicago, 1952, American Medical Association, pp. 29-30.

*Sliepcevich, Elena M.: The responsibility of the physical educator for health instruction, Journal of Health, Physical Education, and Recreation **32:** 32, 1961.

Table 8-1. Undergraduate majors—teachers of health*

Major	Teachers	Major	Teachers
Physical education	775	Psychology	4
Health education and physical		Business	4
education	289	Nursing	4
Science	173	Education	3
Biology	100	Special education	3
Home economics	99	Recreation	3
Social studies	32	Physiology	2
English	24	Physics	2
History	18	Guidance	2
Social science	16	Music	2
Health education	15	Industrial arts	1
Elementary education	13	French	1
Chemistry	8	Theology	1
Mathematics	6	Speech	1
Art	5	Political science	1
Physical science	4		

*From Patterns and features of school health education in Michigan public schools, East Lansing, Michigan, 1969, Michigan Department of Education.

Table 8-2. Graduate emphasis of health teachers*

Area	Teachers	Area	Teachers
Physical education	52	Special education	2
Guidance and counseling	20	Secondary education	2
Education	18	Nursing	2
Administration	13	Traffic safety	2
Health education	11	Library science	1
Science	4	Mathematics	1
Biology	4	Public health	1
Health and physical education	3	Earth science	1
Recreation	3	Psychology	1
Chemistry	3	Ecology	1
History	2	Family living	1
		Geography	1

*From Patterns and features of school health education in Michigan public schools, East Lansing, Michigan, 1969, Michigan Department of Education.

physical educators still continue to teach health classes in the nation's schools.

Sliepcevich* listed some guides that needed to be followed if the quality of health instruction by physical educators is to be improved.

1. Physical educators need training in physical and life sciences, such as anatomy, chemistry,

bacteriology, and genetics. There is also a need for training in the behavioral sciences, such as social anthropology and psychology.

2. All physical educators should have the equivalent of at least a minor in health education because it is likely they will be required to teach health.

3. When assigning health teaching to physical educators, school administrators should recognize the great amount of time needed for the preparation and teaching of health. In addition, the variety of teaching methods required, resources available, and need for motivating pupils also require enormous amounts of time and effort on the part of the teacher.

*Sliepcevich, Elena M.: The responsibility of the physical educator for health instruction, Journal of Health, Physical Education, and Recreation **32:** 32, 1961.

Table 8-3. Health worries of secondary school students*

Health worries										

	Percent indicating worries									
	Grade level						Total	G†	B	P
Health worries	9	10	11	12	13	14	Total	G†	B	P
Cancer	50	73	53	47	49	53	54	59	50	—
What I'll be like in 15 years	34	70	43	43	40	30	44	47	40	—
Automobile accidents	27	63	43	30	30	33	38	39	37	—
Personal grooming	30	33	40	37	37	37	35	45	26	0.01
Dental problems	44	47	33	34	7	27	33	36	31	—
Lack of exercise	30	33	30	17	38	44	31	39	23	0.01
Dandruff	27	43	43	30	23	20	31	31	31	—
Acne	14	50	33	37	35	10	30	35	24	0.01
Overweight	13	30	30	24	47	33	29	45	13	0.01
Lack of sex knowledge	23	47	37	24	17	30	20	27	30	—
Leukemia	14	47	23	34	33	20	28	31	27	—
Mental illness	17	47	17	23	20	40	27	39	15	0.01
Childbirth	40	30	17	20	30	10	25	48	3	0.01
Ability to have children	40	27	20	20	14	27	25	38	11	0.01
Drowning	27	33	17	20	20	20	23	26	20	—
Underweight	44	10	13	27	13	20	22	14	29	0.01
Unpleasant breath odor	17	53	3	10	37	20	22	20	23	—
Blindness	24	37	23	10	20	17	21	21	22	—
Vitamin deficiencies	14	7	23	14	20	30	18	18	18	—
Being burned	20	33	7	17	7	10	16	21	12	—
Frequent headaches	17	24	17	7	23	10	16	17	14	—
Body odor	14	30	10	14	10	7	14	16	12	—
Losing leg or arm	14	22	7	7	22	7	13	9	13	—
Venereal diseases	14	17	10	7	15	7	11	10	11	—
Poison by gas	4	7	10	16	4	4	7	8	7	—

*From Dowell, Linus J.: A study of selected health education implications, Research Quarterly **37:**29, 1966.

†Symbols read: G = girls; B = boys; P = level of confidence found by the chi square test of significant differences between boys and girls in health worries.

Table 8-4. Health interests of secondary school students*

Health interests	Percent indicating interest by grade level						Percent of interest			
	9	10	11	12	13	14	Total	G†	B	P
Emotions	57	43	47	67	57	57	54	67	42	0.01
Fitness	53	47	73	67	47	33	53	48	59	0.01
Drugs	54	33	43	60	43	67	50	59	41	0.01
Heredity	27	37	47	46	40	60	47	51	43	—
Weight control	40	43	50	37	64	44	46	62	30	0.01
Reproduction	44	33	63	33	53	46	45	49	42	—
Posture	64	57	53	30	40	30	45	55	35	0.01
Diseases (communicable)	34	47	53	30	43	43	42	40	44	—
Alcohol	37	33	33	27	37	53	37	30	43	0.01
Medical care	33	50	37	33	30	33	36	41	31	0.01
Skin	27	30	37	37	44	34	35	55	15	0.01
Rest and sleep	43	53	23	14	27	37	33	30	36	—
Noncommunicable diseases	23	60	40	24	13	33	32	40	24	0.01
Eyes	30	37	43	20	24	30	31	40	21	0.01
Nutritional needs	27	10	40	10	30	34	24	27	21	—
Foods	17	13	33	17	33	17	21	21	22	—
Immunity	17	13	20	10	10	20	15	15	16	—
Water	14	7	7	17	17	10	13	13	13	—
Ears	4	20	20	7	13	7	12	9	14	—
Ventilation	7	10	0	7	0	13	6	7	6	—
Digestion–utilization	4	0	10	0	7	7	5	5	5	—

*From Dowell, Linus J.: A study of selected health education implications, Research Quarterly **37**:28, 1966.

†Symbols read: G = girls; B = boys; P = level of confidence found by the chi square test of significant differences between boys and girls in health interests.

4. Physical educators need to be impressed with the responsibility they have for making a contribution to the improvement of health instruction. This requires adequate preservice and in-service preparation, which in addition to subject-matter content in health also requires a familiarity with curriculum development and the basic principles involved in the integrating and correlating of health content with other subjects in the school program.

5. Physical educators who are interested in and have the necessary competencies for good health teaching should strive to become certified in this special field.

AREAS OF SCHOOL HEALTH PROGRAM

The school health program is divided into three parts: teaching for health, living healthfully at school, and services for health improvement.

Teaching for health*

The school has a major responsibility in the area of health instruction. It should instruct children and youths in such subjects as the structure and functioning of their bodies, the causes and methods of preventing certain diseases, the factors contributing to and maintaining good health, and the role of the community in the health program. Such an instructional program, if planned wisely and taught intelligently, will contribute to sound health habits and attitudes on the part of the student.

Health instruction should avoid too much stress on the field of disease and medicine. This is pointed out by Dr. Bauer, health

*See also discussion of development of health knowledge, p. 228.

authority, in an article entitled "Teach Health, Not Disease." He says that teachers should primarily teach health, how to live correctly, and how to protect one's body against infection, rather than teaching disease and medicine. Proper health instruction should impress upon each individual his responsibility for his own health and, as a member of a community, for the health of others.

Teaching for health should take place in many ways in the school. There should be provision for concentrated health teaching in courses specifically set up for this purpose. Health teaching should also take place in other subjects in which aspects of health pertinent to these subjects are covered. An example would be the subject of nutrition in a home economics course. In addition, such instruction should take place incidentally when a "teachable moment" occurs. An example would be when some young person has become hooked on drugs and is hospitalized. Furthermore, through many school experiences such as the school lunch and the medical examination, opportunities arise for teaching health.

The School Health Education Study indicated current practices in the health topics offered in schools throughout the United States. Content areas most frequently covered in health science courses at all grade levels included food and nutrition, exercise and relaxation, accident prevention, cleanliness and grooming, and dental health. From the fourth to twelfth grades, such topics as posture and body mechanics, rest and sleep, vision and hearing, and communicable diseases were introduced. At the seventh grade, boy-girl relationships, smoking, and structure and function of the human body were introduced in a majority of the school districts surveyed. Topics most frequently omitted by school districts include boy-girl relationships, consumer education, health careers, international health activities, sex education, venereal diseases, noncommunicable diseases, and foot care.

The Committee on Health Education for Pre-School Children of the American School Health Association* lists the following as a topical outline of content for this age group:

Cleanliness and grooming
Dental health
Eyes, ears, nose
Nutrition
Rest and sleep
Safety
Growth and development
Family living
Understanding ourselves and getting along
Prevention and control of disease

The Committee on Health Education for Elementary School Children of the American School Health Association† lists the following as a topical outline of content for this age group:

Grades 1, 2, and 3

Cleanliness and grooming
Rest and exercise
Sleep and rest
Growth
Posture
Role of physician and dentist
Individual responsibility for one's health
Responsibility for the health of others
Dental health
Vision and hearing
Babies
Nutrition
Making new friends
Being alone sometimes
Family time
Protection from infection
Food protection
Safety

Grades 4, 5, and 6

Health care
Cleanliness and grooming
Vision and care of eyes
Hearing and care of ears
Heart
Teeth
Exercise, rest, and sleep
Nutrition
Growth and development
Family living
Understanding ourselves
Getting along with others

---

*Health instruction: suggestions for teachers, Journal of School Health **39**:11, 1969.

†Health instruction: suggestions for teachers, Journal of School Health **39**:22, 34, 1969.

Making decisions
Environmental health
Prevention and control of diseases
Safety and first aid

The Committee on Health Education for Junior High School of the American School Health Association* lists the following as a topical outline of content for this age group:

Junior high school

Health status
Cleanliness and grooming
Rest, sleep, and relaxation
Exercise
Posture
Recreation and leisure-time activities
Sensory perception
Nutrition
Growth and development
Understanding ourselves
Personality
Getting along with others
Family living
Alcohol
Drugs
Smoking and tobacco
Environment
Air and water pollutions
Consumer health
Disease

The Committee on Health Education for Senior High School of the American School Health Association† lists the following as a topical outline of content for this age group:

Senior high school

Health status
Fatigue and sleep
Exercise
Recreational activities
Sensory perception
Nutrition
Growth and development toward maturity
Family living
Alcohol
Drugs
Smoking and tobacco
Health protection
Noise pollution

Health agencies
Health careers
World health
Safety and accidents

The health education content areas and the number of schools that include each area in their health science course, as reflected in a survey conducted in the fall of 1968 in which 810 schools returned the questionnaire, are shown in Table 8-5.

The health education program in Los Angeles includes in the junior high and senior high school programs the topics listed on p. 218.

Content and basic aims of the New York State Health Education Programs are reflected in the diagram on p. 219.

In respect to the basic health science course in colleges and universities, a survey conducted a few years ago showed that better than 80% of the institutions covered by the survey offered a personal health course for their students. In some cases the course was offered on an elective basis, while in other cases it was required. Teacher preparation programs, in particular, were the setting for most of the required courses.

The college survey also showed that in most cases the basic health science course was offered by the health and physical education department. However, in other cases it was offered by departments of biology or zoology, science, general education, or home economics; college health service; College of Medicine; and College of Nursing.

The survey further showed that the basic health science course was offered on the average for 2 or 3 semester or quarter hour credits and was taught by a variety of persons including health educators, physical educators, biologists, and physicians. Some of the topics covered in the courses included mental health, family health, nutrition, reproduction, tobacco, alcohol, narcotics, preparation for marriage, personal appearance, disease control, health appraisal, and care of the body.

The personnel chiefly involved in instructing and in transmitting health knowl-

---

*Health instruction: suggestions for teachers, Journal of School Health **39**:48, 1969.

†Health instruction: suggestions for teachers, Journal of School Health **39**:71, 1969.

Table 8-5. Health education content areas*

Subject area	Schools	Subject area	Schools
Personal health	263	Hit and miss	5
Smoking, tobacco	155	Child care	4
Drugs	150	Menstruation	4
Sex education	150	Civil defense	3
Alcohol	148	Heart	3
Anatomy and physiology	113	Sanitation	3
First aid	112	Self-help	3
Communicable diseases	109	Those required by state law	3
Nutrition	81	Sight and hearing	3
Mental health	52	Genetics	2
Safety	41	Major health problems	2
Growth and development	37	School health	2
Physical fitness	30	Immunization	1
Marriage and family living	20	Psychology	1
Public and community health	19	Recreation	1
All areas	10	Young adult problems	1
Dental health	9	Regular physical examination	1
Cancer	6	Daily shower in physical	
Personality	6	education	1
Personal relations	5		

*From Patterns and features of school health education in Michigan public schools, East Lansing, Michigan, 1969, Michigan Department of Education.

	Junior high	Senior high
Unit 1	Introduction to health science	Orientation to health needs
Unit 2	Growing and maturing	Guidelines for improved nutrition
Unit 3	Achieving personal health	Transitions to maturity
Unit 4	Food for growth and health	Narcotics, alcohol, tobacco, and other harmful substances
Unit 5	Addicting, habit-forming, and other dangerous substances	Progress in public health
Unit 6	Progress in community health	Consumer health protection
Unit 7	First aid and safety	Essentials of first aid

edge to students include the health educator, elementary school teacher, physical education teacher, biology teacher, general science teacher, home economics teacher, social studies teacher, school nurse, dental hygienist, school lunch manager, and parents.

The physical educator who is teaching health should:

1. Discover the health needs and interests of pupils
2. Organize meaningful health units in terms of health needs and interests of pupils
3. Know thoroughly the subject matter that is imparted to pupils
4. Possess an understanding of what constitutes a well-rounded school health program and the teacher's part in it
5. Utilize problem solving and other recommended methods in teaching for health
6. Possess an enthusiasm for the teaching of health
7. Take time to prepare thoroughly for classes

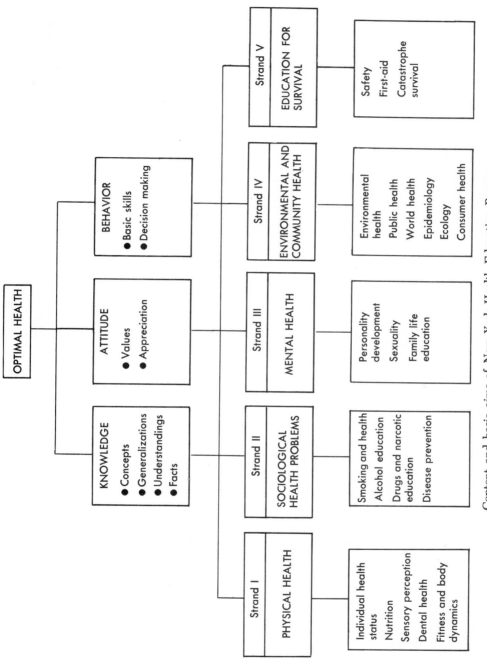

Content and basic aims of New York Health Education Program.

8. Make classes interesting and exciting experiences for the students
9. Provide students with opportunities to participate and exercise their initiative
10. Use up-to-date textbooks that have been carefully evaluated as to their worth for classes
11. Provide an attractive setting for classes
12. Tap the many resources in the school and community that are available and that will make health teaching more dynamic
13. Assist students in solving their own health problems

Critical health areas

Certain health areas are receiving increased attention from educators because of the acute problems associated with them in today's world. For this reason they have been called "critical health problems." Five of the most pressing of these problems are concerned with family life education, tobacco smoking, use of drugs, use of alcohol, and the environment. Health education should strive to ensure proper understanding and appreciation of these health areas when young people are faced with decisions concerning them. Teachers have a responsibility for developing key concepts in each of these health areas.

FAMILY LIFE EDUCATION. Family life education, which includes sex education, should play a prominent role in schools and colleges. Through adequate planning, effective community interaction, outstanding teaching, and appropriate subject matter, much good can be done. The emphasis throughout the program should be on human sexuality, or how boys and girls and men and women fulfill their roles in life. Each student should be helped to identify his own masculine or feminine role in school, at play, at home, and at work. The core of one's identity is one's sexual role.

Family life education should be designed to help young people grow and develop in a way that will be meaningful and lead to the achievement of maturity, emotional independence, and a responsible relationship with the opposite sex. In order to achieve these goals, boys and girls and young people need a knowledge of their physical, mental, social, and emotional selves and an understanding of their role in the family and the means of achieving good human relationships. Teachers should know their subject matter, be comfortable in using the language of sex, and be aware of the great social changes in progress in our society. Audiovisual aids, books, and other materials used should be up to date and appropriate for students. Resource people, such as nurses, clergymen, doctors, psychologists, and social workers, can make a valuable contribution to the program.

In general, a family life education program should concern itself in early childhood with such matters as an understanding of sex differences, developing a wholesome attitude toward sex, helping boys and girls to relate emotionally to their peers, showing them to be good family members, and providing an understanding of such physiological facts as how a baby grows in the body of his mother. In middle childhood an attempt should be made to help boys and girls develop wholesome attitudes toward themselves, respecting their right to have opinions, and helping them to experience success and to develop confidence. Furthermore, there is a need to help boys and girls to understand the growth process and the role of inheritance in this process, to develop respect for social customs, and to respect life itself. Later childhood should find the student recognizing his appropriate sex role, mastering the social graces in boy-girl relations, and developing a sound standard of values in human relations. Early and later adolescence should find boys and girls accepting masculine or feminine roles through appropriate behavior in boy-girl relations and developing an understanding of the physical change they experience as adolescents.

TOBACCO SMOKING. The smoking of tobacco is a very ancient practice. Early Anglo-Saxon, Chinese, and Roman history indicates that people long before the first century were using a potent mixture and implements for drawing smoke through the nose and mouth for the purpose of deriving pleasure. Today, the American public carries on this practice by smoking billions of cigarettes, cigars, and pipefuls of tobacco each year.

It is obvious to anyone who is willing to observe that poisons present in tobacco smoke taken into the body can cause damage to the person doing the smoking. The physiological effects of smoking are not compatible with a healthy, efficient body. Cigarette smoking is damaging to the cilia of the lungs, affects heart and respiration rate, and affects blood pressure. It is linked with cancer of the lung, chronic bronchitis, and heart disease. Cigarette smokers have a higher death rate from certain diseases than nonsmokers. Smoking sometimes interferes with physical activities. Smoking is the greatest single cause of fires.

Perhaps the most significant change in

smoking in recent years is the increase in the number of smokers at an early age. One frequently sees students in the elementary and middle schools puffing on cigarettes. Partly as a result of intensive advertising that glamorizes the habit and partly because parental influences have relaxed, young people now smoke in public and sometimes at home with little adult disapproval. Slightly less than one out of every three American teen-agers smokes, and an estimated 2 million new smokers between the ages of 12 and 17 are added each year, many of them acquiring the habit early in life. According to the U. S. Public Health Service, if present lung cancer rates continue, an estimated 1 million of today's school children will develop lung cancer during their lifetime. Nearly 10% of habitual smoking starts at the seventh-grade

SMOKING AND LIFE EXPECTANCY

PRESENT AGE	PACK-A-DAY SMOKERS can expect to live to age	2-PACK-A-DAY SMOKERS can expect to live to age	NON-SMOKERS can expect to live to age
25	68.1	65.3	73.6
30	68.4	65.8	73.9
35	68.8	66.3	74.2
40	69.3	66.9	74.5
45	70.0	68.0	75.0
50	71.0	69.3	75.6
55	72.4	71.0	76.4
60	74.1	73.2	77.6
65	76.2	75.7	79.1

DATA:
American Cancer Society

level, with youngsters experimenting at earlier ages. It is very important, therefore, to start adequate instruction in the intermediate grades concerning the use of tobacco and continue on into high school and college years.

The school period is an excellent time to provide the beginning of instruction on tobacco and smoking. It provides an opportunity to acquaint boys and girls with an understanding of such things as what tobacco is, the health hazards associated with smoking, and the economics of smoking. Through meaningful instruction, proper understanding and attitudes can be developed that can result in intelligent decisions on the part of students as to whether or not they will use tobacco.

DRUGS AND DRUG ADDICTION. Americans spend more than $5 billion each year on medical drugs. Drugs as they are used to treat disease have proved to be a very worthwhile contribution to humanity. New discoveries by scientists are constantly producing new drugs that assist in fighting disease, alleviating pain, and providing treatment for various human ailments.

In order that drugs may be used properly and constructively by human beings, there is need for an educational program to help adults and especially youths understand their use, the contributions they make, and the dangers involved when they are misused.

There is increasing concern among many health authorities and interested citizens regarding not only the indiscriminate use of drugs by adults but, even more important, drug experimentation among our youth. Narcotic, or habit-forming, drugs detach a person from reality. They make him unaware of danger. Some drugs induce a sense of well-being by postponing feelings of fatigue. Some drugs have been used by participants in sports where a high level of energy is required, but such practice is denounced by physical educators, coaches, and sports medicine associations.

Marijuana is a drug that young people sometimes experiment with, thinking it will not be harmful; however, its use can result in intoxication and reckless and even violent behavior. The immediate effect of smoking marijuana is a temporary mental disturbance. The user of marijuana loses touch with reality and is likely to act on suggestions that he would not consider in a more normal state of mind. The user of marijuana is dangerous not only for these reasons but because it may pave the way to addiction to more powerful and dangerous drugs. The user learns to depend upon a drug for pleasure. Later, in an effort to get pleasure, he may turn to stronger drugs such as morphine, heroin, and lysergic acid diethylamide (LSD). These stronger drugs are usually peddled by the same law-breaking individual who first introduced the victim to marijuana. This constant search by the "pusher" for new victims, and new markets for his illegal wares, has caused much crime and the practice of preying upon young and innocent youth. The typical drug addict needs from $10 to $40 per day to maintain his habit. Thus, as the illegal sellers push their drugs on the market, the drug user must turn to petty thefts, shoplifting, burglary, and other crimes to secure the price of a fix.

Plastic cement, model airplane glue, gasoline, and other chemical substances have been used in recent years by unsuspecting youths who sniff these materials to acquire sensations that resemble acute alcoholic intoxication. The results of such sniffing can be very harmful. Continuous inhaling can produce double vision, hallucinations, stupor, amnesia, and unconsciousness. The fumes can seriously damage the liver, the kidneys, the brain, and other parts of the body. Moreover, the use of such chemicals may also lead to using stronger drugs and ultimately to addiction with its dreaded withdrawal sickness.

The time to help youth with respect to drugs and drug addiction is before they are tempted to experiment with dangerous drugs. This, of course, means an educational program regarding drugs and drug addiction starting in the early school years.

If youngsters are well informed regarding drugs—their nature, use, and abuse—when they encounter this problem and are tempted they will have a resource of information that will enable them to make an intelligent choice as to whether they want to experiment—with all the harmful impact upon their health, success, and future that it implies. Without such information they may readily fall prey to addicts and other uninformed youth who are seeking some form of a "kick" of which they do not know the consequences.

ALCOHOL. Seven out of ten Americans use alcoholic beverages at the cost of more than $12 billion a year. Drinking enjoys a place in the social scheme that is accorded few other practices. Millions of dollars are spent on advertising by alcohol producers to promote the sale of alcoholic beverages. Tax revenues from the sale of alcoholic beverages help fill local, state, and federal treasuries in the amount of approximately $4 billion annually.

Despite the large role that alcohol and drinking play in our economy, their use presents serious personal and social consequences that cannot be ignored. Drinking may well lead to absenteeism from work, crime, and automobile accidents; an increased work load and cost are placed upon hospitals, jails, and welfare agencies; innumerable problems accrue to the alcoholics' children and families.

Although some persons drink to relax and to socialize, others use alcohol as a means to escape from their problems or for other deep-seated psychological reasons. Young people sometimes start drinking as a result of giving in to social pressures or because of a desire to go along with the group. What these people want is the approval of their friends; they fear that if they do not drink, they will not be accepted. Some young people drink because they think it is adult to do so. Others say they drink to have fun or excitement.

Persons vary in the way they behave under the influence of alcohol. The only general statement that can be made is that they will not display their normal personality, but, instead, one which has been altered by the depression of the mental processes by intoxication or the accumulation of the toxic effects of alcohol. Some persons will be happy or silly, while others become belligerent, noisy, vulgar, or morose.

One of the truly serious problems concerned with alcohol is alcoholism. One of every fifteen drinkers will fall victim to that sickness. Unfortunately, there is no way to predict who that one will be.

In making the choice whether or not to drink, the important thing for young people is to make a decision based on the facts. Most young people know the arguments in favor of social drinking in moderation. But it is also important for them to know about drinking in our society as it involves lawbreaking, automobile deaths, wrecked lives, and broken homes. If they choose to drink, young people should look at the health risks they run and, most importantly, at the responsibility the drinker must bear for his actions. If young people choose not to drink they will have decided that the liabilities of alcohol far outweigh its benefits and that good health habits suggest they abstain. Whatever their choice, it should be their own, made freely, based upon the facts as to what is best for them.

The early school years are not too early to develop concepts that will help children better to understand the role of alcohol in our culture and whether or not they should drink when they are older.

THE ENVIRONMENT. In recent years the subject of environment and its pollution has become a critical health area. The study of the environment and its relation to the living creatures in it—including their relations to one another—is called *ecology*. Understanding of ecology and research in it are becoming more and more important, because man has been placing ever larger demands on his environment and, in the process, bringing about ever more severe changes in it. The result has been serious damage to some parts of the environment to the point that scientists are wondering how much longer the environment will be able to meet the demands that man places upon it.

Ecology, among other things, studies the resources of the environment, or of a particular portion of it, together with the demands placed upon those resources by the creatures that live in it. For example, we study the ecology of a pond by determining what resources the pond has—how much oxygen in the water, how much mineral nutrients that living organisms require. It is also important to know what creatures live in the pond, how they live, how fast they reproduce, which of them eat the others, and so on. If we study a pond over many years, we will probably note certain changes in the ecology. For example, as vegetation and vegetable debris build up at the bottom of the pond, these may absorb oxygen, reducing the oxygen content of the pond's water. If there is a natural flow of water into or out of the pond, changes in this flow will change the ecology of the pond as well. And if life forms in the pond change—perhaps as a result of men fishing in it or polluting it—the pond itself will change, because different life forms produce different conditions in the environment. The ecology of a small pond is of no great concern to mankind, with one important exception: the things we learned from a limited, small environment such as the pond often have implications for a much larger environment—the nation and the world. The study of ponds, among many other things, shows us that natural forces and living creatures other than man do not change the environment rapidly or in a very large way. Man, by contrast, affects his environment in enormous ways and in very short periods of time.

In recent years it has been increasingly recognized that we are polluting the air we breathe, the waters where we swim or fish, the food we eat, and many other things. There are also such things as noise pollution, which is affecting our hearing. The car that we drive, the detergents that wash our dishes, and the DDT that is used to kill insects are affecting our way of life and, particularly important to health educators, they are affecting our health.

The schools and colleges have a responsibility to bring to the attention of our young people and the public in general the consequences of such pollution, and particularly the implications it has for our health and well-being. Since environmental pollution has become so deadly in its impact and so critical to our way of life, it is a subject that should be taught in all our health education programs.

Living healthfully at school

The second area into which the school health program may be divided is that of healthful school living. This implies that the time children spend in school should be spent in an environment and atmosphere conducive to physical, social, mental, and emotional health. The environment will be sanitary and cheerful, the teacher will have a pleasing personality, the school program will be well balanced, and educational methods will be in accordance with good health standards.

A sanitary and cheerful school environment has implications for healthful school living. Such factors as proper lighting, ventilation, facilities, play areas, and seating should be taken into consideration. The teacher, administrator, and custodian all play an important part in accomplishing this objective. The teacher must assume responsibility for the classroom. Among other things, he should see that the classroom is at an optimum temperature, is clean, has adequate lighting, and is equipped with seats that fit the children. The administrator and custodian should see that the school in general meets proper healthful living standards and that the teacher is given help and support in his attempts to accomplish this objective.

The teacher's personality has a strong bearing on the health of the child. The teacher should have a sense of humor, ready smile, sympathetic attitude, and good health. This will help the child to adjust satisfactorily to school living, to enjoy his time in school, to have a successful experience, and to feel that he belongs.

A well-balanced school program is a necessity for healthful school living. There must be adequate time for rest, relaxation, play, and study. Close work with books and writing materials should not be of such length as to cause undue fatigue. Play periods should be of adequate length to enable the child to have sufficient exercise. Lunch periods should be long enough to allow for leisurely eating.

Educational methods should be in accordance with good health practices. Class size should be such as to allow the teacher to give personal attention to each student and at the same time allow for group experiences. The teaching load should not be too demanding of the teacher's time and efforts. Promotion policies should conform to what is in the best interests of the child's health. Home-school relationships should allow for adequately knowing the child's background and permitting parents to be informed as to the child's progress in school. Homework should contribute to the development of the whole child, which takes into consideration his so-called academic needs and also his needs in respect to such essentials as recreation, leisure, and play.

Personnel involved in providing a healthful school environment are the school administrator, classroom teacher, custodian, city health department, sanitarian, school physician, school nurse, health educator, physical educator, school bus driver, and school lunch director.

The physical educator interested in students living healthfully at school should:

1. Meet with the school physician, nurse, and others in order to determine how best to contribute to a healthful environment
2. Participate in the work of the school health council; if none exists, interpret the need for one
3. Provide experiences for living healthfully at school
4. Help pupils assume an increasing responsibility for a clean and sanitary environment
5. Try in every way possible to obtain good mental health in order to be a living example for the students
6. Set an example for the child in healthful living
7. Motivate the child to be well and happy
8. Help supervise various activities that directly affect health, such as school lunch, rest periods, and the like
9. Be aware of individual differences of pupils
10. Keep emotions under control at all times
11. Provide in every way possible for the safety of pupils so that accidents may be kept to a minimum
12. Check regularly the temperature, ventilation, lighting, water supply, waste disposal, and other physical features to see that they provide for the health of students

Services for health improvement

A survey of Head Start children points up the need for an effective health services program. More than 1 million children needed measles vaccinations, 740,000 children had not received polio vaccinations, the average Head Start child had five dental cavities, more than 2,000 active cases of tuberculosis were uncovered, about 7,400 children were found to be mentally retarded, 188,000 children had disorders of eyes, bones, and joints, and from 5% to 10% of the children had psychological disorders.

Health services are an important part of any school health program. The health services of the school should include health appraisal and counseling, correction of remediable defects, emergency care of sickness and injury, communicable disease control and prevention, and education of the exceptional child.

Health appraisal and counseling are achieved in the schools as a result of medical, dental, and psychological examinations; teachers' observations; screening tests for vision and hearing; and records of growth and height statistics. The best results in these various phases of health appraisal are obtained when medical examinations are given to children before entering school and each year that the child is in school, when vision and hearing tests are given annually, and when there is continual teacher observation. As a result of the findings of the various examinations and observations, health counseling with both pupils and parents should take place as conditions warrant.

Although it is usually recognized by authorities in the field of health that it is desirable to have complete medical examinations every year, this is not regarded as being practical by many school administrators. In such cases a *minimum* program would provide for medical examinations before entering school and approximately every third year the child is in school.

Health appraisal and counseling will be of little value unless there is a "follow-through" to see that remediable health defects are corrected. This is an important health service. There should be periodical checks to see that such things as dental caries are remedied, eyeglasses are provided, and other defects attended to. School health programs can render a valuable service if they follow through to see that the remediable defects they discover are corrected.

Emergency care of sickness and injury is needed for the great number of children who are regularly injured through accidents or who become unexpectedly sick while at school. The teacher, as well as the nurse,

school physician, and administrator, has responsibilities in this emergency program. Through proper first-aid procedures, safety education, and regard for the health of children, the injured or sick child will be properly and quickly cared for and accidents reduced.

Communicable disease prevention and control should be included in school health services. In carrying out this function, schools should coordinate their program and work with the local department of health. Such measures as isolating the child suspected of having a contagious disease, educating the parents to take advantage of immunization and other preventive measures, informing the health department of suspected cases of communicable disease, encouraging sick children and teachers to stay home, and teaching the causes of the development and spread of diseases are a few of the services that may be rendered in this phase of school health.

Another health service that should be included in the school health program is the provision of an adequate educational program for the exceptional child. This includes children handicapped by physical or mental disabilities; speech, vision, hear-

A thorough medical examination should be one of the main bases for the selection of physical activities.

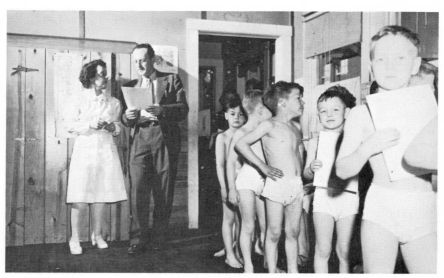

LAWRENCE CENTRAL HIGH SCHOOL, LAWRENCE, IND.

ing, and nutritional deficiencies; and those with emotional disorders needing special attention. It also refers to the gifted child who needs special attention. Special provisions for these children guarantee a better educational experience, with a greater saving of human resources. For example, sight-saving classes may be held for the children with vision defects, lip-reading instruction for some of those with hearing defects, and a restricted program for children with a history of rheumatic heart disease and those convalescing from serious illness.

The personnel involved in the school health services program include school and family physicians, school and public health nurses, school and family dentists and dental hygienists, school dietitian, health educator, physical educator, classroom teacher, school administrator, guidance counselor, psychologist, and parents.

The physical educator interested in health services for students should:

1. Meet with the school physician and nurse to determine how to contribute most to the health services program
2. Become acquainted with the parents and homes of students
3. See that children needing special care are referred to proper places for help
4. Be versed in first-aid procedures
5. Continually be on the alert for children with deviations from normal behavior and signs of communicable diseases
6. If feasible, be present at health examinations of pupils
7. Follow through in cooperation with the nurse to see that remediable health defects are corrected.
8. Prescribe a physical education program to meet the physical needs of each student
9. Utilize their position to provide wise health counseling to both students and parents
10. See that athletes are given a medical examination and provided with other health services as needed.

KEY PERSONNEL IN SCHOOL AND COLLEGE HEALTH PROGRAMS

The key personnel in school and college health programs are as follows:

Teacher of health. Is the most important person for an effective school health program.

Health coordinator. Has the job of developing effective working relationships with school, college, and community health programs and coordinating the total school or college health program with the general education program.

School administrator. Can provide leadership that ensures a sound health program, qualified personnel, adequate budget, proper facilities, and the sympathy and support of faculty and parents.

Physician. Plays key role in the conduct of medical examinations, correction of remediable defects, and support to the total school health program.

Nurse. Provides liaison with medical personnel on the one hand and with students, teachers, and parents on the other. She can stimulate support for and give direction to all phases of the school health program.

Physical educator. Can contribute much to the school health program. Is in a position to impress upon students the importance of gaining desirable health knowledge, developing desirable health attitudes, and forming desirable health practices. Many teachable moments are present in a physical education program to teach about health opportunities closely related to the health and fitness of students.

Dentist. Conducts dental examinations, gives or supervises oral prophylaxis, and advises on curriculum material in dental hygiene.

Dental hygienist. Usually assists dentists and does oral prophylaxis. Has the opportunity to relate her work to educational outcomes.

Custodian. Helps to ensure healthful school living by providing a sanitary school environment.

Nutritionist. Plans student meals and can also be of help with nutritional problems of students and as a consultant on subject matter for health education.

Guidance counselor. Concerned with area of health as it relates to student effectiveness and productivity and has the opportunity to impress upon students the role of health in scholastic and vocational success.

WHAT OUTCOMES SHOULD BE EXPECTED FROM THE SCHOOL HEALTH PROGRAM?

The long-term, overall outcome to be expected from the school health program is improved health of human beings. This refers to all aspects of health, including physical, mental, emotional, and social. It applies to all individuals, regardless of race, color, economic status, creed, or national origin. The school has the responsibility to do everything within its power to see that all students achieve and maintain optimum health. This applies not only from a legal point of view but also from the standpoint that the educational experience will be much more meaningful if optimum health exists. A child learns more easily and better when in a state of good health.

The commonly mentioned educational outcomes to be expected from the school health program are concerned with the development of health knowledge, desirable health attitudes, desirable health practices, and health skills.

Development of health knowledge

In order to develop health knowledge, health education must present and interpret scientific health data that will then be used for personal guidance. Such information will help individuals to recognize health problems and to solve them by utilizing valid and helpful information. It will also serve as a basis for the formulation of desirable health attitudes. In the complex society that exists today, many choices confront the individual in regard to factors that affect his health. For this reason a reliable store of knowledge is essential.

Knowledge of health will vary with different ages. For younger children there should be an attempt to provide experiences that will show the importance of living healthfully. Such settings as the cafeteria, lavatory, and medical examination room offer these opportunities. As the individual grows older, the scientific knowledge for following certain health practices and ways of living can be presented. Some of the areas of health knowledge that should be understood by students and adults include nutrition, the need for rest, sleep, and exercise, protection of the body against changing temperature conditions, contagious disease control, the dangers of self-medication, and community resources for health.

If students are properly health educated, for example, they should understand the germ theory of disease and also have a desire to prevent disease whenever possible through desirable health practices. Boys and girls should understand where to find the health services necessary to cope with various types of health problems. Young people should know the effects of using tobacco, narcotic drugs, alcohol, and other depressants and stimulants. In addition, they should appreciate the fact that

Health instruction lecture at Evergreen Park High School, Evergreen Park, Ill.

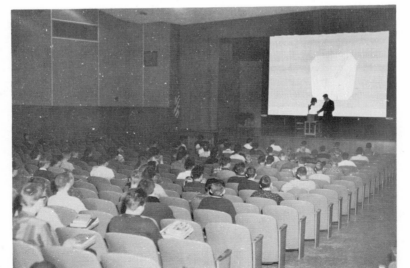

health is everybody's business—each person has a responsibility for the health of others in the family, community, nation, and world. This is especially important in today's world if environmental pollution is to be stopped. There should be a recognition of the part played by nutrition, physical activity, rest, and sleep in physical fitness; the part played by safety in accident prevention; and the importance of good mental health. If such topics are brought to the attention of persons everywhere and if the proper health attitudes and practices are developed, better health will result.

Development of desirable health attitudes

Health attitudes refer to the health interests of the individual or the motives that impel a person to act in a certain way. Health knowledge will have little worth unless the person is interested and motivated to the point that he wants to apply this knowledge to everyday living. Attitudes, motives, drives, or impulses, if properly established, will result in the person's seeking scientific knowledge and utilizing it as a guide to living. This interest, drive, or motivation must be dynamic to the point where it results in behavior changes.

The school health program must be directed at developing those attitudes that will result in optimum health. Students should have an interest in and be motivated toward possessing a state of buoyant health, feeling "fit as a fiddle," being well rested and well fed, having wholesome thoughts free from anger, jealousy, hate, and worry, being strong, and possessing enough physical power to perform life's routine tasks. They should have the right attitudes toward health knowledge, healthful school living, and health services. If such interests exist within the individual, proper health practices will follow. Health should not be an end in itself except in cases of severe illness. Health is a means to an end, a medium that aids in achieving noble purposes and contributes to enriched living.

Table 8-6. Many colleges offer a health course for students. This table gives the title of academic department offering personal health course by number of colleges reporting*

Department	Number of colleges	Percentage
Health, physical education, and recreation	161	43.63
Physical education	108	29.27
Health education	22	5.96
Biology	22	5.96
Science (natural and behavioral)	11	2.98
Life science	10	2.71
Education	8	2.17
Nursing education	7	1.90
Other	17	4.61
No response	3	.81

*From Mayshark, Cyrus, and Kirk, Robert H.: Status of the personal health course in junior colleges, School Health Review **2:**19, 1971.

Another factor that motivates people to good health is the desire to avoid the pain and disturbances that accompany ill health. They do not like toothaches, headaches, or indigestion because of the pain or distraction involved. However, developing health attitudes in a negative manner through fear of pain or other disagreeable conditions does not seem to be a sound approach.

A strong argument for developing proper attitudes or interests centers around the goals a person is trying to achieve in life and how optimum health can help to achieve such goals. This is the strongest incentive or interest that can be developed in a person. If a person wants to become a successful artist, businessman, dancer, housewife, or parent, it is very beneficial to possess good health. This is important so that the study, training, hard work, trials, and obstacles that one encounters can be met successfully. Optimum health will aid in the accomplishment of such goals. As Jennings, the biologist, has pointed out, the body can attend to only one thing at a time. If its attention is focused on a backache or an ulcer, it cannot be focused satisfactorily on essential work that must be done. Centering health attitudes or interests on life goals is dynamic because it represents an aid to accomplishment, achievement, and enjoyable living.

Development of desirable health practices

Desirable health practices represent the application of scientific health knowledge to one's living routine. The health practices that a person adopts will determine in great measure the health of that person. Practices or habits harmful to optimum health, such as failure to obtain proper rest or exercise, overeating, drug addiction, overdrinking, and oversmoking or failure to observe certain precautions against contracting diseases, will usually result in poor health.

Knowledge does not necessarily ensure good health practices. An individual may have at his command all the statistics as to the results of speeding at 70 miles an hour, yet, unless this information is applied, it is useless. The health of an individual can be affected only by applying that which is known. At the same time, knowledge will not usually be applied unless an incentive, interest, or attitude exists that impels its application. Therefore, it can be seen that in order to have a good school health program it is important to recognize the close relationship that exists among health knowledge, health attitudes, and health practices. Each contributes to the other.

Development of health and safety skills

There are certain skills that should be learned through the health and safety education program in the schools. These include neuromuscular skills in first aid, home nursing, and safety and driver education. It takes skill to put splints on a broken leg or to administer artificial respiration. It takes skill to read a thermometer or to care for a sick person. It takes skill to effectively put out a fire or help in the case of an accident. And it takes skill to drive in city traffic or to park on a steep hill. These skills

are taught in various aspects of the school health and safety program and are outcomes that are expected from students who participate in these educational experiences. It should be remembered, however, that skill requires refresher training periodically in order that a person is always ready in the event of an emergency.

INTERRELATIONSHIPS BETWEEN SCHOOL AND PUBLIC HEALTH PROGRAMS

The health of the school child is a major consideration of our educational systems. In 1918 it was placed first on the list of cardinal principles for education. In 1938 it was reemphasized by the Educational Policies Commission. Conferences have been held, legislation passed, personnel appointed, and programs planned for the express purpose of promoting the health of youth in our schools. This great emphasis focused on the health of the child and the happiness and fitness of future citizens of the United States means that every effort must be made to accomplish this objective in the most efficient and best way possible. Therefore, all the personnel and resources available in the community must be mobilized for this purpose. This is not a job for one agency. Instead, it requires the help and assistance of all organizations affecting the health of the child. Voluntary and official agencies, hospitals, boards of education, and interested individuals and organizations must pool their resources, facilities, equipment, and knowledge in order that the health of the child may receive utmost consideration.

In addition, the solving of community health problems outside the school needs the concerted effort of every agency. Public health programs are to a great degree based upon an enlightened public that understands the health problems of the community and gives its support to the solving of these problems. The school can play a major part in helping to educate the citizens of the community so that health progress may be realized. The school health program should fit into the total community health program in a well-coordinated manner so as to render utmost service to all concerned.

In discussing interrelationships between school and public health programs, it is important to consider the controversy between community health groups and the schools as to who is responsible for administering the various phases of the school health program.

There are primarily three points of view as to where the responsibility lies. One group believes that the board of education should be responsible, another group believes that public health officials should assume the responsibility, and a third group thinks that school health is a joint responsibility of both the board of education and public health officials. It is advisable to consider briefly some of the arguments in favor of each point of view.

Those individuals who advocate board of education control of the school health program set forth many pertinent arguments in their behalf. These arguments can be summed up in the following statements. They point to the fact that the Tenth Amendment to the Constitution of the United States places the authority for education in the hands of the states. The states delegate this authority to the local communities, which in turn vest the authority in a board of education. The board of education, in the absence of legislation to the contrary, is responsible for all education, and therefore health education falls logically under their jurisdiction. They point to the fact that teachers, as a result of their training in such areas as psychology and methodology, are much better prepared to instruct children in health matters than are public health officials. They are better prepared to make health services meaningful educational experiences for all pupils. As another argument, they maintain that if public health officials were responsible for the school health program, the teachers would have two bosses, thus making for inefficient administration.

Those individuals who advocate that the school health program should be controlled by public health officials also list many pertinent arguments in their favor. Public health supporters say that health is logically a province of the medical profession and should therefore be under the supervision of medical personnel such as those found in most public health departments. They point to the fact that the school is part of the total community and claim that such an important thing as health is therefore a responsibility of community health officials. Furthermore, the pupil is in school only 5 days a week, 180 days or so a year. The rest of the time he is in the larger community outside the school environment. They argue that public health nurses, as a result of their training and experience, are the best qualified to develop and administer a health services program, especially in respect to home-school-community relationships. They maintain that, according to law, the control of communicable diseases is a prerogative of public health officials and that they can do the job much more efficiently than can the board of education.

Finally, there is a group of persons who maintains that the school health program should be controlled jointly by both the board of education and public health officials. They point out that there will be bet-

Who Administers School Health Services?

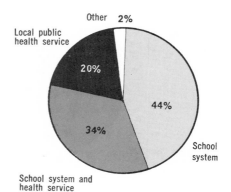

390 reporting school systems with 12,000 or more enrollment, 1965-66

FROM NEA RESEARCH BULLETIN 44:107, 1966.

ter utilization of personnel, facilities, and community resources and that, consequently, greater health progress can be made if there is joint control with both working together for the good of all.

There does not seem to be a simple solution to this controversy as to where the responsibility lies for school health. Probably the answer to this problem will vary according to the community. The solution would seem to depend upon how each community can best meet the health needs of the people who inhabit its particular geographical limits. The type of administrative setup that most fully meets the health needs and makes for greater progress should be the one that is adopted. Vested interests should not be considered; the health interests of the consumer should be the primary concern. Health is everybody's business and everyone should strive for the best health program possible in his community, state, nation, and world.

PROFESSIONAL PREPARATION OF HEALTH EDUCATORS*

Various individuals, committees, and surveys have stressed the need for more adequate preparation of those teachers who assume health education responsibilities.

Oberteuffer (1946), in a panel discussion before the College Physical Education Association, stressed the lack of adequate preparation in the field of health. He stated that the number of courses being offered in this area was insufficient and that individuals must have training to be good teachers of health.

Langton has emphasized this same point, believing that at least 20% of the specialized area, in addition to the basic sciences, should be set aside for health education work. He further has pointed out that only through such a division is it possible for the prospective teacher to obtain adequate training in health education.

The Joint Committee on Physical Fitness of the American Medical Association and of the National Committee on Physical Fitness stated the need for the same kind of organized teaching of health that has been developed for the teaching of mathematics, English composition, history, and languages.

The National Committee on School Health Policies, formed in 1945 by the National Conference for Cooperation in Health Education, listed the policies under which school health programs should operate and brought out the need for better qualified teachers in health education.

The results of one study, in which forty teachers and forty administrators participated, indicated that teachers are deficient in health education knowledge. The conclusion reached was that a teacher of health in the schools should be as well prepared as a teacher of any other subject.

In 1962 a major conference on the preparation of health, physical education, and recreation teachers and leaders was held in Washington, D. C. This conference, attended by many health leaders, stressed the need for adequate preparation of health teachers and outlined the requirements for such preparation. Furthermore, recommendations were made in the areas of student personnel, faculty, curriculum, laboratory experiences and facilities, and instructional materials.

The latest standards for the professional preparation of health educators were established by the Conference on Teacher Preparation in Health Education, sponsored by the School Health Division of the AAHPER.* Guidelines and standards were set forth in each of four areas, namely, (1) certification standards, (2) recruitment and placement, (3) appraisal of undergraduate and fifth-year programs, and (4) minimum standards for professional preparation programs.

The minimum professional preparation requirements for certification in health edu-

---

*See also Chapter 2.

*Conference on Teacher Preparation: Recommended standards and guidelines for teacher preparation in health education, Journal of Health, Physical Education, and Recreation **40:**31, 1969.

cation, according to this report, should include appropriate study in the following specific areas:

1. The school health program, including the areas of healthful school environment, health services, and health instruction
2. Mental, emotional, and social health; alcohol, drugs, and tobacco
3. Dental health, vision, hearing
4. Emergency care, including first aid
5. Safety education, including occupational, home, and recreational safety; manmade and natural disasters
6. Community health, including such aspects of environmental health as air pollution, water pollution, and radiation; fluoridation; agencies promoting community health; official, voluntary, and professional health agencies and organizations
7. Nutrition in respect to health education, including knowledge of basic food nutrients, wise selection and use of foods; obesity and weight control; food faddism, food fallacies, and controversial food topics
8. Disease prevention and control, including the communicable and the degenerative diseases and chronic health disorders
9. Family life education, including human sexuality, and the psychosocial and cultural factors promoting successful marriage and family relations
10. Consumer health, including intelligent selection of health products and health services, consumer protection agencies, health misconceptions and superstitions, health insurance plans, and health careers
11. Study in methods and materials for health instruction
12. Student teaching in health education

A health educator has the job of improving health practices, attitudes, and knowledge of children and adults. He should be interested in community as well as personal health problems and be devoted to encouraging and stimulating people to recognize the importance of good health for themselves and others. The health educator may act in the capacity of a teacher of concentrated courses in health education, a coordinator of a school or public health program, or a staff member of some voluntary health association such as the American Red Cross.

The personality of the health educator is of particular concern. This individual should be well adjusted and well integrated emotionally, mentally, and physically if he is to do a good job in developing these characteristics in others. Such a person must also be interested in human beings and possess skill and understanding in human relations so that health objectives may be realized.

It is important that the health educator have a mastery of certain specialized health knowledge and skills and have proper attitudes. Such knowledge, skills, and attitudes will help the health educator to identify the health needs and interests of individuals with whom he comes in contact, provide a health program that will meet these needs and interests, and promote the profession so that human lives may be enriched. This means that many experiences should be included in the training of persons entering this specialized field. These experiences may be divided into general education, professional education, and specialized education.

General education experiences will constitute about one-half of the total curriculum and include knowledge and skill in the communicative arts, understanding of sociological principles, and an appreciation of history of various peoples, with their various social, racial, and cultural characteristics, and the fine and practical arts that afford a medium of expression, of releasing emotions, for richer understanding of life, and for promoting mental health. The science area is very important to the health educator and should include such sciences as anatomy and kinesiology, physiology, bacteriology, biology, zoology, chemistry, physics, child and adolescent psychology, human growth and development, general psychology, and mental hygiene.

In professional education it is important for the health educator to have a mastery of the philosophies, techniques, principles, and evaluative procedures characteristic of the most advanced and best thinking in education. Professional courses in educational philosophy, methods of teaching, and practice teaching would come in this area.

The specialized health education area should include personal and community health, nutrition, family and child health, first aid and safety, methods and materials, organization and administration of school health programs, public health (including the basic principles of environmental sanitation and communicable disease control), and health counseling.

Health education minor program

Although it is hoped that sometime in the future all persons who teach health will have a major in this special subject, this is not true at the present time. Therefore, in order to be realistic in terms of the need to improve the present quality of health teaching, a minor program is suggested. This, however, should be considered the minimum, and it is believed that physical educators who desire to teach health should have this minimum preparation. The prerequisites to the minor program should include biological, physical, and social sciences.

Physical education majors, as part of their regular program, should take human anatomy, physiology, first aid and safety, body mechanics, physiology of exercise, health observation, and adapted physical education. The minor program should contain 15 to 20 semester hours or 22 to 30 quarter hours in health education courses. This should include such subjects as personal and community health, first aid, nutrition, health problems of school children, accident prevention, environmental sanitation, methods and materials, safety education, and organization and administration of the school health program.

Johns* has developed a set of guidelines for effective health teaching based on such things as research data, thinking of experienced teachers, and personal experience. They are presented here in outline and adapted form.

---

*Johns, Edward B.: Effective health teaching, Journal of School Health **34:**123, 1964.

Effective health teaching requires an outstanding teacher because:

The teacher is the key to good health teaching. Therefore, the teacher must be well prepared, interested, emotionally stable, intelligent, and resourceful.

Effective health teaching requires adequate time comparable to other important academic subjects. Adequate time is needed in the school program if the desired information is to be communicated and the lives of children and youth are to be affected.

Effective health teaching means the teacher should view health teaching as a science and an art. The teacher must keep up to date in regard to the latest information in regard to health and also teach in a manner that enables the student to identify with the material being taught.

Effective health teaching means that the resources of both the school and the community are utilized. Such school resources as health materials, library, and health office must be utilized. In addition, the resources of the community, such as provided by professional, voluntary, and official health agencies, must be mobilized.

Effective health teaching means careful planning. The health teacher must plan in a meaningful manner for the teaching experience, including conferences with such persons as the school nurse and school physician, an analysis of home and community health conditions, and meetings with students.

Effective health teaching means that the teacher knows his students. The teacher of health must know the problems and needs of his students, the health knowledge they possess, the health practices they follow, and other vital information about their health status. In addition, the teacher must be acquainted with the instruments and techniques utilized to obtain this information.

Effective health teaching means that the teacher formulates objectives in relation to outcomes desired. The teacher must know the behavioral changes desired in his students, not just the knowledge to be gained.

Effective health teaching means that the teacher organizes material and experiences so they are meaningful to the student. This means that the teacher can so organize the material to be used that key concepts are identified and have meaning and purpose for the students.

Effective health teaching means that methods, procedures, and techniques are functional. Motivation is one of the most important considerations in an effective learning situation. As such, methods, procedures, and techniques will play an important role in determining the effectiveness of health teaching.

Effective health teaching means that the ma-

terials are **scientifically accurate and up to date.** This means that textbooks must be up to date, current periodicals used, and criteria established and used for selecting authoritative materials.

Effective health teaching means that evaluation takes place. The teacher should utilize an evaluation procedure using scientific instruments and techniques to determine the degree to which objectives that have been established are met.

Effective health teaching also means provision for a healthful and wholesome environment. A proper environment takes into consideration proper lighting, heating, and ventilation standards; audiovisual instruction; and other factors conducive to learning.

CAREERS IN HEALTH EDUCATION

A physical educator with interest, training, and qualifications for health work may be interested in exploring the possibilities of a career in this field. In the years ahead there will be many positions available in the elementary and secondary schools and in colleges and universities. The expansion in school enrollments plus the increased emphasis given to health education augurs well for job opportunities in our community and educational programs throughout the country. Furthermore, some insurance companies, youth agencies, and organizations, such as the American Social Hygiene Association, National Tuberculosis Association, and Young Men's Christian Association, employ people trained in the health field. The attention being given to safety education means more positions for people with special training in this field in industry and government, as well as in the schools and other settings.

For professional as well as career purposes, the physical educator should be familiar with such health organizations as the following:

Selected educational health associations:
1. American School Health Association
2. American Public Health Association
3. American Association for Health, Physical Education, and Recreation
4. Society of State Directors of Health and Physical Education

Selected governmental health agencies:
1. United States Public Health Service
2. State department of health
3. County health department
4. Local health department

Selected professional health associations:
1. American Medical Association
2. American Nurses' Association
3. American Dental Association

Selected voluntary health agencies:
1. American Cancer Society
2. National Tuberculosis Association
3. American Red Cross
4. National Association for Mental Health
5. National Society for Crippled Children and Adults
6. American Heart Association

Selected international health organization:
1. World Health Organization

For those persons interested in specializing in safety education, several job opportunities prevail in schools, colleges, industry, transportation agencies, and other organizations and agencies. Safety educators devote their time to promoting safety considerations and reducing accidents. Jobs are available as supervisors of safety education and teachers of driver education in schools; as safety supervisors or safety directors in industry and government; as supervisors or consultants in community safety; or as teachers of safety and/or driver education in colleges and universities.

QUESTIONS AND EXERCISES

1. Trace the history of health in the schools from the latter part of the nineteenth century to the present.
2. Define each of the following: (a) school health program, (b) school health services, (c) health appraisal, (d) school health counseling, (e) school health education, and (f) healthful school living.
3. Define and discuss each of the three main areas of the school health program
4. What are the objectives of the school health program? Compare to the objectives of the physical education program.
5. What is the relationship of the school health program to the public health program?
6. What professional preparation does a health educator need? To what extent does this preparation overlap with that required in physical education?
7. What part can the physical educator play in the school health program?

Reading assignment

Bucher, Charles A., and Goldman, Myra: Dimensions of physical education, St. Louis, 1969, The C. V. Mosby Co., Reading selections 18 to 20.

SELECTED REFERENCES

American Association for Health, Physical Education, and Recreation: Health concepts—guides for health instruction, Washington, D. C., 1967, The Association.

American Association for Health, Physical Education, and Recreation: Preparing the health teacher, Washington, D. C., 1961, The Association.

Anderson, C. L.: School health practice, ed. 4, St. Louis, 1968, The C. V. Mosby Co.

Bucher, Charles A.: Administration of school health and physical education programs, including athletics, St. Louis, 1971, The C. V. Mosby Co.

Bucher, Charles A.: Administrative dimensions of health and physical education programs, including athletics, St. Louis, 1971, The C. V. Mosby Co.

Bucher, Charles A., Olsen, Einar A., and Willgoose, Carl E.: The foundations of health, New York, 1967, Appleton-Century-Crofts.

Committee on Terminology in School Health Education: Report, Journal of Health, Physical Education, and Recreation 33:27, 1962.

Grout, Ruth E.: Health teaching in schools, Philadelphia, 1963, W. B. Saunders Co.

Harris, William H.: Suggested criteria for evaluating health and safety teaching materials, Journal of Health, Physical Education, and Recreation 35:26, 1965.

Hein, Fred V.: Critical issues in health and safety education, Journal of School Health 35:70, 1965.

Hoyman, Howard S.: An ecologic view of health and health education, Journal of School Health 35:110, 1965.

Joint Committee on Health Problems in Education, National Education Association and American Medical Association, Washington, D. C., National Education Association:
Health education, 1961.
Healthful school living, 1957.
The nurse in the school, 1955.
School health services, 1961.
Suggested school health policies, 1962.

Mayshark, Cyrus, and Irwin, Leslie: Health education in secondary schools, St. Louis, 1968, The C. V. Mosby Co.

Means, Richard K.: A history of health education in the United States, Philadelphia, 1962, Lea & Febiger.

Oberteuffer, Delbert, and Beyer, Mary K.: School health education, ed. 4, New York, 1966, Harper & Row, Publishers.

Pollock, Marion B.: The significance of health education for junior college students, Journal of School Health 34:333, 1964.

Report of the Study Committee on Health Education in the Elementary and Secondary School of the American School Health Association: Health instruction—suggestions for teachers, Journal of School Health, vol. 34, December, 1964 (entire issue).

School Health Education Study: A summary report, Washington, D. C. 1964, School Health Education Study.

School Health Education Study: Health education: a conceptual approach, Washington, D. C., 1965, School Health Education Study.

Smolensky, Jack, and Bonevchio, L. Richard: Principles of school health, Boston, 1966, D. C. Heath & Co.

9/Recreation

Recreation is concerned with those activities in which a person participates during hours other than work. It implies that the individual has chosen certain activities in which to voluntarily engage because of an inner, self-motivating desire. Such participation gives him a satisfying experience and develops physical, social, mental, and/or esthetic qualities contributing to a better existence. To be more specific, the kind of recreation that education is advocating can be characterized by five descriptive terms:

1. *Leisure time.* To be recreation the activity must be engaged in during one's free time. From this point of view work cannot be one's recreation.

2. *Enjoyable.* The activity engaged in must be satisfying and enjoyable to the participant.

3. *Voluntary.* The individual must have chosen, of his own volition, to engage in this pursuit; there must have been no coercion.

4. *Constructive.* The activity is constructive. It is not harmful to the person physically, socially, or in any other way. It helps him to become a better integrated individual.

5. *Nonsurvival.* Eating and sleeping are not recreational activities in themselves. One may engage in a picnic where a dinner is involved, but other facets of the affair, such as the social games and fellowship, are important parts of the recreational activity.

OBJECTIVES OF RECREATION

There are many worthwhile objectives for the field of recreation. The American Association for Health, Physical Education, and Recreation states that this special field contributes to the satisfaction of basic human needs for creative self-expression; it helps to promote total health—physical, emotional, mental, and social; it provides an antidote to the strains and tensions of modern life; it provides an avenue to abundant personal and family living; and it develops good citizenship and vitalizes democracy.

According to George D. Butler, who spent more than a quarter of a century with the National Recreation Association, recreation contributes to human happiness, mental and physical health, character development, crime prevention, community solidarity, morale, safety, economy, and democratic living. These benefits are derived from a program that serves the entire population, including children and adults, boys and girls, men and women. Most programs are organized in respect to the needs and interests of those they serve.

One of the best statements of objectives has been discussed by The Commission on Goals for American Recreation.* The objectives are six in number:

1. *Personal fulfillment.* The need for each person to become all that he is capable of becoming and the contribution that recreation can make to this goal.

2. *Democratic human relations.* The rec-

---

*The Commission on Goals for American Recreation: Goals for American recreation, Washington, D. C., 1964, American Association for Health, Physical Education, and Recreation.

ognition by recreation that it has goals that contribute to the individual as well as to the democratic society of which he is a part.

3. *Leisure skills and interests.* Recreation has the goal of meeting the interests of people and developing skills that will provide the incentive, motivation, and medium for spending free time in a constructive and worthwhile manner.

4. *Health and fitness.* Recreation recognizes the importance of contributing to the alleviation of such conditions as mental illness, stress, and physical inactivity that prevail in many segments of the American society.

5. *Creative expression and esthetic appreciation.* Recreation attempts to provide the environment, leadership, materials, and motivation where creativity, personal expression, and esthetic appreciation on the part of the participant exist.

6. *Environment for living in a leisure society.* Recreation plays an important role in encouraging such things as preservation of natural resources, construction of playgrounds and recreation centers, and awakening the population to an appreciation of esthetic and cultural values.

Four objectives that merit discussion are the health development objective, includ-

The use of time in three generations.

AVERAGE LENGTH OF LIFE (ACTUAL YEARS)		40	70	75
DIFFERENT ERAS		1885	1950	2000
PERCENTAGE OF TOTAL LIFETIME SPENT IN ACTIVITIES SHOWN	SCHOOL	5.6	4.0	4.8
	WORK	26	15.3	7.9
	LEISURE	7.8	20.7	27.1
	EAT & SLEEP	60.5	59.9	60.2

FROM STILL, JOSEPH W.: GERIATRICS **12**:577, 1957.

ing physical fitness, human relations objective, civic development objective, and self-development objective.

Health development objective, including physical fitness

Health development is an important objective in the field of recreation. Health, to a great degree, is related to activity during leisure hours as well as during hours of work. The manner in which a person spends his free time determines in great measure the quality of his physical, mental, emotional, and spiritual health. Through recreation, adaptive physical activity conducive to organic, mental, emotional, and spiritual health is available. A wide range of activities exists that offer opportunities for every

individual to promote his organic health. These activities provide relaxation, an escape from the tensions of work, and a chance to forget about problems; thereby, they contribute to mental health. Activities are planned and conducted to provide enjoyment and pleasure and in this way contribute to emotional health. Activities are included that require the participation of many persons. This is conducive to better social relations and thus promotes spiritual health. Public recreation programs are designed to counteract the deteriorating effects of strenuous or routine work or study and thus complement the overall day-to-day tasks that a person follows. Recreation overcomes many of the shortages that exist when the man leaves the office, the child

A suggested community physical fitness organizational plan.

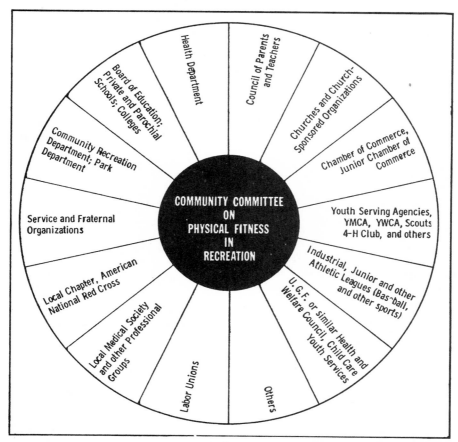

FROM PRESIDENT'S COUNCIL ON PHYSICAL FITNESS AND SPORTS: PHYSICAL FITNESS ELEMENTS IN RECREATION, WASHINGTON, D. C., 1962, U. S. GOVERNMENT PRINTING OFFICE.

leaves school, or the housewife completes her work. In this way it contributes to the integration and development of the whole person.

It can be seen from the description of the health development objective that *recreation contributes to physical fitness*. The President's Council on Physical Fitness and Sports has prepared a special publication stressing the contribution that recreation programs can make to the physical fitness of the population.* The chart on p. 239 shows a community organizational plan for accomplishing this objective. The community committee on physical fitness in recreation, which represents the hub of this chart, should undertake to accomplish the following objectives:

1. Develop and carry out a community program of physical fitness involving all organizations and agencies having recreation interests
2. Provide opportunities for and encourage daily participation in vigorous physical activities adapted to all age groups
3. Provide year-round opportunities for the development of physical fitness
4. Utilize available leadership and facilities and strive for the enactment of state-enabling legislation and local ordinances authorizing use of public property or funds for recreation

Human relations objective

The human relations objective represents a major contribution of recreation to enriched living. Recreational programs develop many individual qualities. Such attributes as courage, justice, patience, tolerance, fairness, and honesty are only a few that can be developed while people are playing and recreating together in the many activities that comprise the total recreation program. Attitudes that promote good human relations are also developed. Wholesome attitudes of social cooperation, loyalty to the group, recognition of the rights of others, and the belief that a person receives from the group in direct proportion to what he gives make for better relations

---

*President's Council on Youth Fitness: Physical fitness elements in recreation, Washington, D. C., 1962, U. S. Government Printing Office.

and enable the accomplishment of worthy goals. The growth of family recreation also helps to make for a more unified home life. This is essential, since the family group represents the foundation on which good human relations are built. Furthermore, to develop good social traits it is necessary to bring people together in a situation where there is a feeling of belonging and where each individual is recognized. There are innumerable opportunities for such interaction in the many recreational programs that exist throughout the country.

Civic development objective

The civic development objective is a noteworthy goal for recreation. Recreation contributes in many ways to the development of any community. It contributes to community solidarity by uniting people in common projects, regardless of race, creed, economic status, or other discriminatory factors. It helps to build the morale of the members of the community. It is a contributing factor in alleviating crime in that it provides settings and activities in which youth and other individuals may engage in constructive, worthwhile activities rather than in destructive, antisocial activities. It helps to make the community a safer place in which to live through adequate playgrounds and other recreational centers that keep children and youth off the streets. It helps to make the community more prosperous by contributing to the health of the individual, by cutting down on the dollar appropriation for combating crime, and by increasing the total work output of an individual. It helps the growth and development of the individual so that he becomes a more valuable citizen in the community and has more to contribute in its behalf.

Self-development objective

The self-development objective refers to the potentialities that participation in a program of recreation activities has for developing the individual to his fullest capacity. Recreation does this through a variety of means. It contributes to the balanced growth of a person. It allows for growth in ways other than through the production of material things for utilitarian purposes. In other words, it satisfies the human desire for creativity through such things as music, art, literature, and drama. It allows a person to create things not for their material value but, instead, for the joy, satisfaction, and happiness that occur when producing something through one's own efforts. It allows for the development of skills and abilities that are latent and dormant until they are aroused by leisure hours with proper settings and inspiration. These skills help to make a better integrated person. They provide an avenue for him to experience joy and happiness through an activity in which he has the desire to engage. People, when engaging in recreation, revitalize themselves through the medium of activities that provide smiles, hearty laughs, and release from the tension associated with day-to-day routine. Such activities afford a place for many to excel. Such an urge is many times not satisfied in one's regular job or profession. Recreation provides an opportunity to satisfy this desire. It provides an educational experience. The participant learns new skills, new knowledge, new techniques, and develops new abilities. He files away new and different experiences that will be helpful in facing situations that he will encounter from day to day.

HISTORY

Recreation, to some extent, has always been a part of the lives of all people, of every race, nation, and creed. In many cases man has spent his leisure hours in a constructive and worthwhile manner by participating in such activities as music, dances, games, sports, painting, and other arts. In early history the Chinese, Hindu, Persian, Egyptian, Babylonian, and Greek peoples left evidence of these pursuits.

In the United States there have been many milestones in the progress of recreation to a place of national importance. The land that is now Central Park in New York City was purchased in 1853, and the Boston sand garden for children was opened by the Massachusetts Emergency and Hygiene Association in 1885. In 1889 playgrounds were opened in New York and in 1892 at Hull House in Chicago. The "playground" idea spread to other cities, which included Brookline, Massachusetts, Louisville, Kentucky, and Los Angeles, California. The Playground Association of America was founded in 1906 with Dr. Luther H. Gulick as president. This same association became known as the National Recreation Association and today it is part of the National Recreation and Park Association. The development of Community Houses, the Works Progress Administration, and the National Youth Administration of the depression years and the large recreation program for service personnel of World War II have played an important part in the progress of recreation.

In 1938 the word *recreation* was officially made a part of the title of the American Association for Health, Physical Education, and Recreation. In 1940-1941 the Federal Highway Act authorized expenditures of monies for roadside parks. In 1948 the President's Committee on Religion and Welfare in the Armed Forces was established. In 1952 the First National Recreation Workshop was held at Jackson's Mill, West Virginia. In 1954 the Council for the Advancement of Hospital Recreation was organized. In 1956 the International Recreation Association was established. In 1958 the Federal Outdoor Recreation Resources Review Commission was created. In 1962 the Bureau of Outdoor Recreation was established in the U. S. Department of Interior. In 1965 five of the leading organizations most directly concerned with the profession of recreation merged and formed the National Recreation and Park Association.

Since the turn of the century, recreation has been considered more and more to be a fundamental human need. Such social factors as modern science and technology with their added leisure, urbanization with its need for publicly sponsored recreation, the changing impersonal and mechanized nature of work with its need for activities of a more personal nature, new attitudes toward recreation such as less religious objection with the church sponsoring programs for its membership, the growth of transportation with its implications for greater travel during leisure hours, the schools' interest in recreation and its sponsorship of programs, an affluent America with its implication for increased monies spent on recreation, and the expansion of commercial recreation with its many opportunities for leisure-time pursuits have been responsible for a great growth in recreation in recent years.

More than 3,000 communities in this country are sponsoring public recreation programs under school and/or local government auspices. In addition, such volunteer and private organizations as the Boy Scouts, American Red Cross, camps, settlement houses, YMCA and YWCA, industry, and the armed forces have recreational programs. More than $1 billion is spent each year on community recreation and from $9 to $25 billion on recreation of all kinds. By the mid-70's it is estimated that the American public will spend about $50 billion on recreation. It is estimated that on sports equipment alone Americans will spend more than $4 billion each year. Pleasure boats account for approximately $800 million, winter sports approximately $70 million, tents $70 million, golf $300 million, and firearms $500 million of the total.

One report notes that families earning at least $10,000 spend more than $500 a year on recreation, including $90 on participant sports. Those families with income of $5,000 or less spend $125, with $14 going for participant sports.

Research* shows that education is a factor in the amount of money spent on recreation. Families headed by a college graduate spend significantly more than those headed by a person who has only a high

school diploma. Also, the higher the occupational level, the greater the amount of money spent on sports.

The American people are becoming recreation conscious, with nine out of ten Americans taking part in some form of outdoor recreation; nearly one out of two participates in some form of water recreation, one out of three works around the yard and in the garden, one out of ten has special hobbies such as woodworking, one out of about twenty sings or plays a musical instrument, and approximately one out of twenty participates in the nation's camp grounds.

In the last 10 years the population of the United States has increased by 15%, and during the same period use of the national parks has increased 86%. In the future the population explosion will create an even larger market for recreation. In addition to population, income will jump skyward in the years ahead. Disposable consumer income will rise to $706 billion by 1976 and to $1,437 billion by the year 2000. The percentage of people in this country with incomes of $10,000 is estimated to reach 40% by 1976 and 60% by the year 2000. The increase in income will mean more leisure-time activities for most people.

The amount of free time available to people will increase. The standard scheduled work week will decrease from 39 hours to 36 hours by 1976 and 32 hours by the year 2000. Much of this additional leisure time will be devoted to recreational pursuits.

The future is bright for those persons who seek to guide the recreational destinies of human beings into constructive channels.

A great theologian, Peter Marshall, once said: "It is not the length of life that matters but how it is lived. That is the thing that counts. It is not how long, but how well." Constructive recreation adds to the quality of living. It contributes to a well-balanced life. It acts as a dash of fresh, cool water on the brow of the tired worker. It is refreshing and invigorating.

---

*The Reporter Dispatch, White Plains, New York, September 30, 1969, p. 20.

AMERICANS WILL SEEK MORE OUTDOOR RECREATION ...
Because They Will Have More Money and Leisure Time

ESTIMATED CHANGES IN POPULATION, INCOME, LEISURE, AND TRAVEL FOR THE YEARS 1976 AND 2000, COMPARED TO 1960

1960 = 100%

1960 FIGURES	
POPULATION (MILLIONS)	180
G.N.P. (BILLIONS)	$503
PER CAPITA DISPOSABLE INCOME	$1970
WORK WEEK (HOURS)	39
PAID VACATION (WEEKS)	2.0
PER CAPITA MILES OF INTERCITY TRAVEL	4170

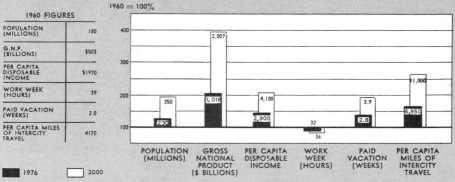

■ 1976   □ 2000

Incomes Will be Higher ...

DISPOSABLE CONSUMER INCOME IN BILLIONS
1960 AND PROJECTED, 1976 AND 2000

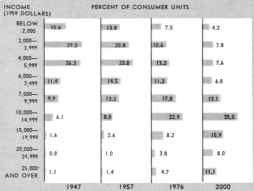

PERCENT OF CONSUMER UNITS IN EACH INCOME CLASS
1947, 1957, AND PROJECTED, 1976 AND 2000

INCOME (1959 DOLLARS)	PERCENT OF CONSUMER UNITS			
	1947	1957	1976	2000
BELOW 2,000	15.6	13.8	7.5	4.2
2,000– 3,999	27.2	20.8	10.6	7.8
4,000– 5,999	26.3	23.8	13.2	7.6
6,000– 7,499	11.4	14.5	11.3	6.8
7,500– 9,999	9.9	13.3	17.8	13.1
10,000– 14,999	6.1	8.8	22.9	25.5
15,000– 19,999	1.6	2.6	8.2	15.9
20,000– 24,999	0.8	1.0	3.8	8.0
25,000· AND OVER	1.1	1.4	4.7	11.1

People Will Have More Free Time to Spend on Recreation

AVERAGE SCHEDULED WORK WEEK FOR NONAGRICULTURAL WORKERS BY INDUSTRY
1960 AND PROJECTED, 1976 AND 2000, HOURS

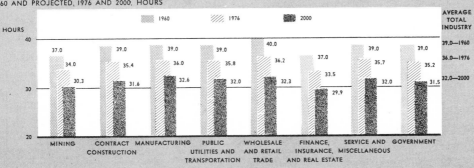

FROM U.S. DEPARTMENT OF COMMERCE:
A PROPOSED PROGRAM FOR SCENIC ROADS
AND PARKWAYS, WASHINGTON, D. C., 1966,
U.S. GOVERNMENT PRINTING OFFICE.

NEED FOR RECREATION
IN MODERN-DAY LIVING

Every individual should experience the joy that comes from engaging in recreation activities that fit his needs, interests, and desires. The Constitution of the United States sets forth a fundamental belief that the Creator endowed each individual with certain inalienable rights; among these are life, liberty, and the pursuit of happiness. Recreation can contribute to the attainment of such vital concepts.

The need for recreation in our changing society is increasing. History-shaking events have made this true. Paul F. Douglas, a leader in recreation, points out that two events that go hand in hand have happened since the turn of the century. In 1905 Albert Einstein set forth his famous formula $E = MC^2$. This represented the foundation for the atomic age. This new era of atomic energy brought increased leisure to man. A year later, in 1906, the National Recreation Association was founded. This organization was established to help man enjoy this leisure.

A shorter work week and more labor-saving gadgets have been the constant goal of many persons in our society. Man is being given less work and more leisure. But has increased leisure given man more happiness? Howard Mumford Jones says that this century has been one of increasing horror. The desire for life, liberty, and the pursuit of happiness is not being fulfilled for millions of Americans. A candid view of the public does not find an abundance of laughter, smiles, and happiness. People today are seeking many forms of escape from reality in sleeping pills, liquor, eating, cheap literature, and drugs. Some of these persons are beginning to realize that an accumulation of material things and ample leisure do not in themselves ensure happiness. Happy people need to be creative, have a feeling of belonging, and have opportunities to direct their energies into constructive activities away from the job as well as on the job.

A survey conducted at New York Uni-versity included many thousands of people, covering a wide range of occupations and including an age range of 4 to 80 years. This study pointed up the fact that the leading characteristics of happy people were (1) interest in work, (2) interest in hobbies, (3) interest in others, (4) lack of interest in material things, and (5) rendering a service to individuals and groups.

Dr. William Menninger, the famous doctor and psychologist, pointed out in a speech before the National Recreation Association that the happy and healthy person today is the one who has recreational pursuits. He participates in some recreational activity to supplement routine daily work. He further states that "good mental health is directly related to the capacity and willingness of an individual to play. Regardless of his objectives, resistances or past practice, any individual will make a wise investment if he plans time for his play and takes it seriously." However, too few persons know how to play. They lack skills, interest, and other motivating factors. They do not feel that it has an important place in their lives. Many persons think that when their mortarboards and commencement gowns are put away it is also time to cast off such things as tennis racquets, bathing suits, or paints and easels.

Play is an important part of every person's life, and as Hjelte, a leader in recreation, pointed out, nothing is recreation in the full sense unless it is practiced in the spirit of play. Pleasure must come from engaging in the activity. It matters not if one is young or old, rich or poor, strong or weak, active or bedridden, man or woman, or boy or girl, recreation can contribute to better living. One recreation leader has stated that activities should range everywhere from the informal play of the child to highly competitive athletics for youth, from the make-believe play of the novice to the expertly staged dramatic presentation of the trained individual, from shaping a crude form in a sandpile to forming a beautiful object in marble, from discordant singing to classical composition, from the superficial reading of an average novel to the complete absorption in a literary masterpiece.

A survey of student opinion regarding extracurricular activities, which has some implications for school recreation programs, was made at Calhoun High School in Port Lavaca, Texas.* The survey revealed that more than half of the students questioned indicated that their involvement in such activities was based on enjoyment of the activities themselves. Some 68% of the students considered extracurricular activities as important as their classwork. Most students engaged in one or two activities. Students were influenced most to participate in extracurricular activities by their classmates, with teachers having only a limited influence. However, one out of every three students felt the need for additional professional guidance in selecting school activities outside the classroom.

A doctoral study by Norvel Clark, which was done at New York University in 1962, investigated the needs and interests of junior high school students in the Bedford-Stuyvesant area of Brooklyn, New York. The study was done with the purpose in mind of developing a recreation activity program based on the identified needs and interests.

The study revealed the rank order of needs of children as evaluated by experts in the field of education, social group work, recreation, and community education. The needs were as follows: (1) the need to achieve, (2) the need for economic security, (3) the need to belong, (4) the need for love and affection, (5) the need for self-respect through participation, (6) the need for variety as relief from boredom and ignorance, (7) the need to feel free from intense feelings of guilt, and (8) the need to be free from fear.

The study also revealed that more than 85% of the students were interested in team and individual sports, which the panel of experts rated high as to the contribution they made to the objectives of the organization.

Recreation programs in communities from coast to coast are being challenged to provide all types of activities that cut across the needs, interests, and desires of human beings. Such activities must include arts and crafts, boating, nature study, gardening, all sorts of games and sports, literary activities, music, dramatics, nature study, camping, parties, and many others. In addition to offering a broad and varied program, it is a further essential that all the resources of a community be mobilized and coordinated so that the best possible program can be offered. Such groups as the church, YMCA, industry, business, schools, Camp Fire Girls, Boy Scouts, and labor unions must all do their share in providing for these essential human needs. Many communities across the country are providing board recreation programs. These range from trips to museums in Sacramento to camping for handicapped children of the Butte County Schools in California, from dramatics in Natchitoches to fishing in Oregon.

LEISURE

There have been several definitions and interpretations of *leisure.* The word comes from the Greek *scole,* and this means that there is a relationship between leisure and education. The English word *leisure* is more closely related to the Latin *licere,* which means "to be free."

The classical interpretation of leisure, according to Sebastian de Grazia in his book *Of Time, Work and Leisure,* was that free time cannot be identified directly with leisure since leisure implies such things as a state of being, a mental attitude involving contemplation and serenity. Thus, according to de Grazia, anyone can have free time but not every person can have leisure.

Aristotle thought of leisure as a state of existence or being where one engages in activity for its own sake. Furthermore, leisure was in contrast to work in the formal

---

*McKenzie, Ronald F.: Those extra-curricular activities, Texas Outlook **52:**35, 1968.

sense. Instead, it involved such activities as art and philosophical discussion.

Today, the most common definition and interpretation of leisure is that it represents the free time that man has after he takes care of his necessities and after his work has been performed. It represents the time when the person has a choice of that which he will do. He can travel, study, play a musical instrument, or play a sport. He makes the choice.

One important implication for the physical educator regarding leisure is that it represents a time when many individuals engage in sports or other forms of physical education activity. In a sense they utilize their leisure to play. The word *play* comes from the Anglo-Saxon word *plega,* which means a game or sport. The Latin word *plaga* refers to a blow, stroke, or thrust. Thus one plays a game by striking a ball, stroking a racquet, or thrusting as in fencing. Leisure, then, is a time when one can play and enables one to express and enjoy himself.

The amount of leisure available to most persons is increasing as a result of our automated existence and common belief that one should enjoy the fruits of his labors. At the same time, educators recognize that in order to have a strong society, leisure hours must be spent in a constructive rather than a destructive manner. It should be utilized to help individuals to develop those areas of self where shortages exist in their personal development. For example, one may wish to know more about and appreciate the fine arts, and thus leisure time represents an opportunity to achieve this goal. Another example would be the opportunity leisure provides the person who spends long hours every day at a desk doing mental work to spend time engaging in some physical activity.

Education, including physical education, can do much to provide the skills, understanding, appreciations, attitudes, and values that will motivate human beings to spend their leisure hours in a profitable manner.

Charlesworth's plan for leisure

James C. Charlesworth, Professor of Political Science, University of Pennsylvania, and President of the American Academy of Political and Social Science, proposes a comprehensive plan for the wise use of leisure.* This plan is a milestone in the professional literature, and, as such, the reader will benefit from reading a few of the highlights of the plan that have implications for physical education and recreation.

CHARLESWORTH'S CATEGORIES OF LEISURITES

The categories of persons who are in a position to make use of free time are: old people, children and teen-agers, wives, vacationers, week-enders, patients in mental and general hospitals, armed forces, prisoners, and the unemployed.

A PRACTICAL PHILOSOPHY OF LEISURE

1. *The wise use of leisure time is more creative, constructive, and wholesome than work.* The admonition that idle hands will do the devil's work applies only to empty time.

2. *Programs for the wise use of leisure are a public and government responsibility.* Social dangers, including disease, illiteracy, crime, and mental disorders, have implications for public and government responsibility for leisure.

3. *The present philosophy in this country of growth for growth's sake should be repudiated.* The desire to beat Russia and to prove the worth of capitalism is ill founded.

4. *One works in order to enjoy leisure.* The old adage that work is its own reward is outdated. People in recreation and education, however, must insist upon putting first things first.

5. *The leisure pattern in America must not be imitative.* It is interesting to read

---

*The American Academy of Political and Social Science: Leisure in America: blessing or curse? Philadelphia, 1964, The Academy, pp. 30-46.

about the Greeks and the Romans, but a pattern of leisure in America should be based on its culture, economy, and other pertinent factors.

ORGANIZATION FOR LEISURE IN
GOVERNMENT AND EDUCATION

ORGANIZATION PLAN FOR LEISURE. This plan should provide for a department in state governments responsible for leisure. This department would give its attention to promoting the constructive use of leisure by inhabitants of its state.

INSTRUCTION. Activities for leisure should be compulsory throughout schooling and available throughout life. Emphasis should be on activities that evoke such qualities as pride, human understanding, and development of the mind and spirit. Softball leagues, for example, represent the elementary level of recreational thinking. Emphasis on championship records and sustained athletic practice is a low form of leisure objective. People should be taught self-fulfillment rather than encouraged to be spectators.

LEISURE PROGRAM OBJECTIVES. Objectives should include intellectual development, esthetic appreciation, social qualities, skill in nonathletic and athletic games and in noncompetitive hobbies and sports, sightseeing, nature study and outdoor life, loafing, and resting.

ADMINISTRATIVE UNITS FOR LEISURE ACTIVITIES. Programs should be coordinated by governmental leisure agencies but administered by such nongovernmental units as universities, churches and synagogues, clubs and organizations, neighborhood circles, housing developers, housing authorities, and settlement houses.

RECREATION SETTINGS AND AGENCIES SPONSORING RECREATION PROGRAMS

Recreation activities are conducted in many settings. These settings afford many job opportunities for the person with training in recreation. A few of these settings will be discussed here.

GOVERNMENT. Recreation programs are carried on at all governmental levels: federal, state, county, township, municipal, and school district. For example, approximately fifty federal agencies and 230 state agencies play important roles in respect to recreation and park development. The National Park Service, National Forest Service, U. S. Army Corps of Engineers, the Bureau of Land Management, the Bureau of Indian Affairs, the Bureau of Reclamation, the Tennessee Valley Authority, the Fish and Wildlife Service, and the Bureau of Outdoor Recreation are a few of the federal agencies that participate or are involved in recreational services. State park departments, state conservation departments, and state education departments are involved in recreational services at the state level of government. Community recreation is provided by the local government. It is controlled, financed, and administered by the community. Community recreation departments and park departments, for example, sponsor recreation programs.

INDUSTRIES. The nation's great industrial concerns, such as Lockheed Aircraft and Eastman Kodak Company, sponsor recreation programs for their employees.

HOSPITALS. Recreation programs are provided in many veterans, municipal, county, and other hospitals for the benefit of patients. The therapeutic values have been well established for the ill and handicapped.

SCHOOLS AND COLLEGES. Elementary and secondary schools and colleges and universities in some sections of the country provide recreation programs. School recreation is frequently provided by a board of education for the students and in some cases for the adult population.

HOME. The family unit is becoming a center for much recreation.

COMMERCIAL ESTABLISHMENTS. Amusement parks, movie houses, bowling alleys, and many other forms of recreation abound from coast to coast.

SERVICE CLUBS FOR THE ARMED FORCES. The United Service Organization is an example of a recreation program provided for individuals who serve in the armed forces.

CHURCHES AND RELIGIOUS ORGANIZA-TIONS. Today, many churches and religious organizations, especially in large metropolitan areas, have extensive recreation programs for their parishioners.

VOLUNTARY YOUTH-SERVING AGENCIES. Many agencies for young people such as the Boy Scouts and the Girl Scouts are interested in how these boys and girls spend their free time, and therefore they sponsor recreation programs. Other voluntary agencies offering recreational services are museums, libraries, and granges. Also, private voluntary agencies organized around special interests of certain groups, such as music specialities and photographic specialties, offer recreation programs.

CLUBS. Boating, tennis, golf, and other clubs represent private recreation agencies that operate their own facilities for the benefit of the membership of the club.

RECREATION PROGRAM

The primary purpose of recreation is to provide program service to its constituency. This means that a wide variety of activities must be offered so that the needs and interests of the entire population are met as far as practical and possible.

Activities that comprise the offerings for recreation programs may be classified into several groups. Some of the more common activities are as follows.

Musical activities
1. Instrumental
2. Orchestral
3. Community sings
4. Choral groups
5. Barber shop quartets
Dance
1. Folk
2. Square
3. Social
4. Modern
Arts and crafts
1. Plastics
2. Leathercraft
3. Graphic arts
4. Ceramics
5. Metalcraft

6. Photography
7. Stenciling and block printing
8. Sewing
Sports and games
1. Archery
2. Badminton
3. Bowling
4. Fencing
5. Golf
6. Hopscotch
Dramatics
1. Plays
2. Festivals
3. Clubs
Outdoor activities
1. Campfires
2. Outdoor cooking
3. Woodcraft
4. Camping
5. Canoeing
6. Conservation
7. Fishing
8. Orienteering
Miscellaneous
1. Horticulture
2. Forums
3. Cards
4. Hobby clubs

SCHOOL AND RECREATION

The school has a definite relationship to recreation. It has the responsibility of utilizing such resources as pupils, facilities, personnel, and programs to help in the attainment of recreation objectives, and it also has the responsibility of providing recreational experiences within the framework of the educational program. The cardinal principle of "worthy use of leisure time" can be fulfilled to a considerable extent if school authorities accept their responsibilities in achieving recreational objectives.

School-centered recreation

Some recreation leaders have raised the question as to whether or not recreation should be school-centered. Hjelte and Shivers* list some arguments, pro and con, in respect to this issue. The reasons that they list *for* a school-centered program are as follows: The school possesses the facili-

*Hjelte, George, and Shivers, Jay: Public administration of parks and recreational services, New York, 1963, The Macmillan Co.

ties essential to a good recreation program, and duplicating these facilities results in waste and inefficiency. Schools are located within a community in much the same way as recreational centers are located—to meet the needs of the people within a particular geographical area. The school comes in contact with all the children, and therefore the consumer of recreation can best be met through this agency. The objectives of schools and the objectives of recreation are similar. The schools are a source of leadership for recreation programs.

Hjelte and Shivers' arguments listed as being *against* a school-centered recreation program are as follows: Education should restrict itself to intellectual training and should not be concerned with experiences that are only indirectly related to intellectual training. Public schools have too many responsibilities without adding any more. Teachers are poorly paid and facilities are inadequate in many localities, and so a heavier burden should not be placed upon these resources. Recreation is hampered by the formality of the school environment and becomes regimented. Consequently, recreation is able to realize its potentialities to a greater extent through the establishment of a special agency. School facilities, equipment, and supplies are damaged through a recreation program and alterations are necessary, which raises the question as to whether other facilities might not be provided more economically. Finally, in attempting to join the forces of education and recreation, difficulties are encountered in securing financial aid for both. Greater public support can be gained if recreation is not grafted onto the educational program.

Regardless of the arguments for or against school-centered recreation, the schools should play a vital part in the field of recreation. At the present time they are contributing staff and facilities. The program of studies in the schools, however, has a long way to go before it realizes its potentialities for developing resources for leisure.

According to the report of the National Conference on School Recreation the responsibilities of the school in the area of recreation are fivefold*:

1. *Schools should educate for the worthy use of leisure.* The schools must contribute their services in preparing young people for the increasing amount of leisure time they will have in an automated society. These services include the development of skills and appreciations and understandings in many educational areas, such as music and art, with which the school is concerned.

2. *Schools should achieve maximum articulation between instruction and recreation.* The articulation can be most effectively achieved by having an enlightened administration in charge of school affairs. By enlightened is meant an understanding and appreciation of the importance of constructive recreation in our society. Furthermore, this articulation can be achieved by providing leaders in the school-connected recreation program who develop effective teacher-pupil relationships and who plan and administer a dynamic educational program.

3. *Schools should develop cooperative planning of recreation programs and facilities.* School district officials should recognize and enthusiastically work toward the utilization of elementary schools, secondary schools, and community and junior colleges as centers for recreational activities. Such a goal should be implemented by cooperative planning between the school and officials representing the various agencies and organizations of the community.

4. *Schools should coordinate and mobilize total community resources for recreation.* The school should act as a hub around which recreation becomes an effective force throughout the community. School staffs, facilities, and a widely diversified program of recreation will help in achieving this goal.

5. *Schools should interpret recreation to*

---

*Danford, Howard G., editor: School recreation, National Conference report, Washington, D. C., 1959, American Association for Health, Physical Education, and Recreation.

the people. The public should become aware of the need for recreation in today's world. Only as the need and importance of recreation are communicated to them will the proper support and participation accrue. There is a special need to interpret recreation to such key people as government officials, communications media officers, school leaders, parents, and students.

The Second National Conference on School Recreation* made the following recommendations, which included setting forth a series of principles and statements regarding school-centered recreation and municipal-school recreation. These principles and statements are presented in adapted form.

School-centered recreation

1. Schools should accept, as a major responsibility, education for leisure.
2. Schools and colleges should provide their students with opportunities for participation in wholesome, creative activities.
3. The facilities and resources of a school should be made available for recreation purposes when needed.
4. Where community recreation programs are missing or inadequate, the school should take the initiative and provide recreation programs for young and old alike.
5. The school should cooperate with community organizations and agencies interested in or already sponsoring recreation programs.
6. The school should appoint a person to act as a community school director who would be responsible for the recreation-education program in the school.
7. Recreation and education are not identical, but each has its own uniqueness and distinctive features.
8. The community school director should provide in-service recreation education for his staff.
9. The federal level of government has a responsibility to stimulate recreation programs.
10. Recreation depends upon public understanding and support for its existence.

11. Recreation should be concerned with exploiting the interests of people.
12. The recreation program should consist of many varied activities.
13. Recreation should be concerned with contributing to the mental health of the individual.

Municipal-school recreation

1. The school should accept the responsibility to educate for the worthy use of leisure, contribute to recreation in the instructional program, mobilize community resources, and cooperatively plan facilities for recreation. The college and university should promote research in recreation and provide professional preparation programs in this specialized area.
2. There should be joint planning of municipal school recreation based on stated principles and brought about by state departments of education and local boards of education.
3. School facilities should be available for recreational use.

Ways in which the school program can develop resources for leisure

How people express themselves during their leisure hours will depend upon the resources they have developed for their free time. Human beings have a tendency to pursue during leisure hours those activities that are familiar to them and that are geared to their interests and abilities. Many want to spend their time doing something in which they have developed some skill and where they are recognized. A boy will go swimming in his free moments because he has learned how to swim or dive well. A girl will paint because she knows how to apply the principles of color dynamics. A man and woman will participate in dramatics because they have developed some acting ability and are recognized and accepted by the group. It is because these resources for leisure have been developed in these individuals that they engage in such activities. These activities in turn contribute to a more interesting, vigorous, and satisfying life.

Although there is controversy over who should be responsible for leisure education, the schools seem best equipped to play a major role. Such essentials as leadership,

---

*Report of the Second National Conference on School Recreation: Twentieth century recreation: reengagement of school and community, November 7-9, 1962, Washington, D. C., 1963, American Association for Health, Physical Education, and Recreation.

facilities, and equipment are readily available. In addition, it is the center of community life and represents a common meeting ground for the entire population as well as the children who attend school. Furthermore, because some students do not go on to college, the major part of this work must be done in the elementary and secondary schools. The ironical part of this whole problem of leisure-time education, however, is that, although the schools are best equipped to do the job, they are not accepting the challenge.

To a great degree school programs are still geared to preparation for college, to a mastery of the three R's, to an acquisition of subject matter content geared to some vocation or profession. Some time ago Dr. Paul Douglass, a former President of American University, conducted a survey. He discovered that only 3% of some 30,000 women graduates thought their education had been valuable for the development of resources for leisure-time pursuits. This is an indictment of our educational program in the United States. If schools are going to be practical and functional, then surely they should develop skills and other resources for leisure-time activities— especially in this age when leisure time is continually increasing.

Yet, here are some illustrations of what is happening in some schools. A music teacher in one of our supposedly "better" schools would point to those students who could not carry a tune and ask them to please refrain from singing. This was a regular practice in her classes—only those who could sing well were allowed to join in. The others remained silent and were mere spectators. If the teacher is trying to develop in the child a resource for leisure, what difference does it make whether he has a good voice, can harmonize, or can hit the high notes? Another illustration points up a similar problem. A teacher of art used to say: "You must not draw a flower that way—draw it this way." The children were required to adhere to a fixed, rigid pattern that few of them were interested in or could master. Why should the child not be allowed to express himself? *If the flower looks beautiful to him and he enjoys himself, education for leisure has taken place.*

It is important for teachers to realize that they are not developing star performers. Instead, they are working with individuals who vary in ability and skill. The important thing is to give them a satisfying experience and sufficient knowledge and skill so that they will be motivated to do more of the same thing when they get away from the classroom and the teacher. This will not take place if the schoolroom becomes a place where only the most skilled youngsters can perform and where things have to be done in a rigid, prescribed pattern.

All subjects in the educational program have a contribution to make in developing resources for leisure. The science subjects, for example, should emphasize to a greater degree than they do at present a study of birds, trees, rocks, and flowers, as an incentive to forming hobbies. The art department should be concerned with making jewelry and artificial flowers, decorating furniture, painting designs on materials, and painting as a hobby instead of turning out highly skilled work. English could do a better job with informal dramatics, storytelling, and creative writing. The social sciences could create a greater desire to participate in community activity and develop a better environment in which to live. They could also study the furniture of various periods of history as an incentive to antique collecting. Why not include more costume designing in home economics and stimulate to a greater degree the creative joy of cooking? Geography classes, while studying the various countries of the world, could obtain stamps from each as an incentive to stamp collecting.

Physical education could emphasize to a greater degree the individual activities such as fishing and tieing trout flies. When it is realized that only one out of approximately 1,000 persons ever plays football after leaving school, it can be seen that there should be at least equal stress on such activities as bait casting, swimming, bowling, and golf. Educators must realize that recreation is related not only to physical education but to all areas. Dr. Jay B. Nash, formerly of New York University, conducted a survey of 1,000 adults and found that only 2% utilized sports and games for their leisure-time activities. As one grows older there is a tendency to do other things.

The school with its wide and varied educational offering has infinite opportunities to develop resources for leisure. During this day and age of mass production, application of atomic energy to industry, and increasing amounts of leisure, the schools are being challenged to accept this responsibility.

Schools should help young people to adjust to the way of life that they will encounter after leaving school, aid them in solving the problems they will meet, and help them to become responsible citizens. Education most certainly must concern itself with leisure-time education. The day of the 30-hour work week is rapidly approaching. If one considers that 8 hours a day are spent in sleeping and 3 hours for eating, this still leaves 61 hours a week for potential leisure-time activity, twice as much as for work. These leisure hours represent a challenge facing the nation's schools.

LEADERSHIP FOR RECREATION PROGRAMS

All professionally minded major fields of endeavor strive for high standards of leadership. These standards are possible largely through the efforts of unified professional organizations. These organizations establish standards for the professional training of practitioners, promote legislation to advance the field, develop a public relations program, and are active in achieving such other goals as certification standards and accreditation.

National Recreation and Park Association

In 1965 the American Institute of Park Executives, the American Recreation So-

ciety, the American Zoological Association, the National Council of State Parks, and the National Recreation Association were merged into a unified national organization known as the National Recreation and Park Association. Laurence S. Rockefeller was elected as the first president of this association. The merger was designed to bring together a single organization supported by private citizens and professional groups and dedicated to helping all Americans devote their free time to constructive and satisfying activities. (For further discussion, see Chapter 22.)

The National Recreation and Park Association is a nonprofit organization concerned with such projects as the conservation of natural resources, wise use of leisure time, beautification of the American environment, and improvement of park and recreational facilities and programs. Financial support comes from members' dues, contributions, and publication sales.

Structurally, the NRPA has been divided into six branches:

1. Association of Recreation—Park Boards—Commissions
2. American Association of Zoological Parks and Aquariums
3. American Park and Recreation Society
4. National Conference on State Parks
5. National Therapeutic Recreation Society
6. Society of Park and Recreation Educators

The NRPA has eight district offices and representatives in the United States located in the various geographical parts of the country. The organization is under the direct supervision of a sixty-three–member Board of Trustees that meets several times each year to guide its operations.

THE PROFESSION AND RECREATION

The Recreation Division of the AAHPER has prepared a policy statement on what it feels are its contributions to the recreation program.* This statement was approved by the Board of Directors of the AAHPER. It envisions its concern with recreation at the present time in five areas of endeavor:

1. *Education for leisure.* The profession has an important role to play in developing, communicating, and implementing a national philosophy of leisure and recreation.

2. *Professional preparation and personnel standards.* The profession has a concern for the recruitment and preparation of recreators and for the improvement of personnel standards and practices.

3. *Research and evaluation.* The profession has a responsibility for proposing, formulating, and encouraging interdisciplinary and interagency exchange of information and for furthering the application of sound research concerned with recreation and leisure.

4. *Recreation services.* The profession has the responsibility of promoting the most productive relations possible between school and community recreation programs. Such relations may involve personnel, facilities, and other essentials to adequate recreational services. The profession supports the community-school concept in recreation.

5. *Planning and development.* The profession has the responsibility for encouraging greater participation by agencies at all governmental levels and other organizations in the process of coordinating, planning, developing, and financing resources and services for recreation.

Project ME (Man's Environment)

The AAHPER has launched the Project for Man's Environment to encourage school use of such areas as urban parks and recreation and wilderness areas in an attempt to sensitize children and parents to the importance of our cultural and natural world

and the need to have a quality living environment. The National Park Service of the federal Department of Interior is financing the project. Some of the specific activities with which Project ME will be involved include evaluating curriculum materials of the National Park Service, developing resource materials relating to the environment, creating a model in-service education environmental program, and conducting a national study to determine how extensive is the utilization of environmental resources by schools.

TYPES OF POSITIONS IN RECREATION

The field of recreation has developed to the point where it offers a promising area of employment for individuals trained in this specialized work. In recent years training institutions have developed curriculums to provide the necessary leadership for the field of recreation. Many positions are open for the qualified person, including the following: superintendents, general supervisors, directors, play leaders, and supervisors of special activities in recreation departments; directors' assistants and area specialists in youth-serving organizations; consultants, executive officers, research workers, and assistants in government agencies; teachers in colleges, universities, and professional schools; administrative positions in commercial recreation; directors and area specialists for hospital recreation programs; positions with such organizations as 4-H clubs; and directors of church recreation programs.

Various types of recreation positions for which the aspiring student can prepare are as follows:

1. Superintendent of recreation
2. Assistant superintendent of recreation
3. Recreation director
4. Recreation supervisor
5. Recreation center director
6. Consultant in recreation
7. Field representative
8. Executive director
9. Hospital recreation supervisor
10. Camp recreation coordinator
11. Extension specialist

---

*American Association for Health, Physical Education and Recreation: Recreation policy statement, Journal of Health, Physical Education, and Recreation 37:43, 1966.

12. Service club director
13. Girls' worker or boys' worker
14. District recreation supervisor
15. Recreation leader
16. Supervisor of special activities
17. Recreation therapist
18. Recreation educator

Positions are also available in programs for the mentally retarded, ill, and disabled. This phase of recreation service is concerned with programs for the ill, disabled, handicapped, and aged persons who, because of their condition, are not able to participate in community recreation programs for the normal, physically active person. In addition to rendering direct services to such people, there are also opportunities to supervise and administer programs in a variety of medical settings and other places that support such programs. Persons working with the ill, disabled, mentally retarded, and the like should take courses such as survey of physical defects, group dynamics and human relations, psychology of the physically handicapped, abnormal psychology, recreational crafts, social recreation, and physical rehabilitation.

QUALIFICATIONS FOR THE RECREATOR

The person who works in the field of recreation, whether full time or as a physical educator or other specialist, needs particular qualifications in order to carry out his responsibilities. Some qualifications that are of special importance are an interest in and liking for people, emotional maturity, enthusiasm and skill, desire to render a service, professional preparation, and professional mindedness.

A recreation curriculum
FRESHMAN YEAR

	Hours
English and American literature	3
English composition	4
Introduction to psychology	3
Introduction to mathematics	4
	14

English and American literature	3
Man and society	3

Educational psychology	2
Nature of matter	4
Introduction to music	3
	15

Summer camp

Aquatics and land sports	2
Organization and supervision of camping or camp crafts	2
	4

SOPHOMORE YEAR

Philosophical analysis	3
Government and politics	3
Social psychology	3
Speech 1	2
Introduction to anthropology	3
Introduction to human relations	2
	16

Man in a biological world	4
The American economy	3
Emotion and motivation	3
Group dynamics in the classroom	2
Man and society	2
Creative art experiments	2
	16

Intersession

Activities for camp programs	2

JUNIOR YEAR

Culture and personality	3
Activities for social recreation	2
Crafts in recreation	2
Physical activities in recreation	2
Rhythms	2
First aid and safety procedures	2
Games	2
	15

Child psychology	3
Leadership in recreation	2
Folk dance	2
Organization and conduct of social recreation	2
Physical activities for recreation	2
Music in recreation	2
Recreational dramatics	2
Field work	2
	17

SENIOR YEAR

Psychology of adolescence	3
Crafts in recreation	2
Field work in recreation	3
Philosophy of recreation	2
Electives	5
	15

Field work in recreation	3
Introduction to social research	2
Social agencies in the community	2
Organization and administration of recreation	2
Electives	5
	14

Interest in and liking for people

The person who works in recreation must have faith in people and recognize the worth of each individual. The recreation leader should have qualifications that permit easy access to people of all races and creeds; he should be sympathetic and understanding in the many human associations related to work in the recreation program. People participate in the recreation program on a voluntary basis. They come of their own choice, and they can also leave of their own free will. Therefore, it is important to provide all individuals with experiences that will satisfy the needs for which they attend.

Emotional maturity

The person who works in recreation must be an adult in his outlook on life. He must have good mental and physical health, the ability to accept others' opinions and personalities for what they are, and a pleasing, friendly personality.

Enthusiasm and skill

The person who works in recreation should be enthusiastic about recreation and the contribution such programs can make to human welfare. He should have skill in working with people and also in the organization and administration of particular activities or the program as a whole. The recreation leader should possess productive energy that can be channeled in the right directions.

Desire to render a service

The person who works in recreation should be interested in rendering a service to mankind. He must like work and count rewards not in terms of material things but in terms of what he does for people.

Education

The person who works in recreation must be educated in the true sense of the word. The recreation leader should have a broad background of general education and, in addition, be well prepared in the activities taught and the particular specialized tasks performed.

Interest in profession

The person who works in recreation should be interested in building the profession. He should maintain a high code of professional ethics, join professional associations and be active in them, conduct himself in a manner that will bring credit to the profession, and continually try to work toward a better profession that renders greater services to humanity.

PROFESSIONAL PREPARATION OF THE RECREATOR

The preparation of the recreation leader should be thorough and complete. The recreation curriculum on p. 254 gives the requirements for a professional student in a large university. An examination of the courses and experiences required will show the extent to which the biological sciences, general education, social sciences, arts, humanities, and professional recreation courses are required over a 4-year period. Important areas where competencies are needed include the principles involved in the organization and administration of recreation agencies, philosophy of recreation, laws and governmental organization that affect recreation programs, and skills and technical knowledge relating to such areas as music, arts and crafts, athletics, and social activities.

According to the survey reported by Anderson,* most of the undergraduate curriculums in recreation and/or park administration in colleges and universities are

---

*Anderson, Jackson M.: Professional preparation for recreational and park personnel, Journal of Health, Physical Education, and Recreation **39:** 85, 1968.

located in a department or a division of health, physical education, and recreation, and the college in which these special areas are located is usually the college of education. The types of degrees offered include the B.S., B.A., and the A.A. This survey showed that more than 100 colleges and universities now offer professional preparation programs in recreation and park administration.

PERFORMANCE OF RECREATION WORK BY PHYSICAL EDUCATORS

Physical education and recreation are not synonymous, but they are closely related, and physical education personnel can play a prominent part in recreation programs. The field of recreation utilizes not only physical education activities but also many other activities in which an individual desires to participate during his leisure hours. This means that, although games and sports play a prominent part, many other activities less physically active in nature are utilized. However, physical education activities have implications for recreation. The skills that are developed and instruction that takes place in physical education classes have a definite carry-over value. People want to engage in activities in which they have mastered some skill. People like to excel.

A person trained in physical education has a great contribution to make to recreation. Many physical educators are playing prominent roles in this field today. When recreation was in its embryo state, the physical educator was usually the logical person to assume leadership for such a program. Today, however, in many of our large municipal recreation programs and in other areas, those with specialized training in recreation are providing much of the leadership. The physical educator, however, still plays a very prominent part in this work. Because of the nature of his training, the physical educator directs many recreation programs in communities where insufficient funds make it impossible to hire a full-time recreational leader; he acts as a specialist in the area of athletics and other physical education activities in large city, industrial, and other recreational programs; and he plays an important part in communities that utilize school facilities for the community recreation program. The physical educator is also called upon to serve in many other recreational capacities such as playground director, supervisor, and camp director.

In discussing the relationship of physical education and recreation, one thing should be stressed above all others—there must be cooperation between the two. Both are primarily interested in furthering the health and happiness of people. In attempting to attain this objective, personnel must be utilized in a way that will be most advantageous in furthering the health and happiness of all. In many cases facilities must be utilized by both programs. Supplies and equipment must be shared. Programs must be planned cooperatively and the ultimate objective kept closely in mind. Each should help the other and follow practices that will result in the most benefits for the greatest number of people. Both should be well acquainted with the program in each area. Only in this way will the best interests of the people be served.

OPPORTUNITIES AND CHALLENGES IN RECREATION WORK

Many new developments in our changing society are creating new opportunities and challenges for the recreation profession. Some of these new developments are discussed here briefly.

There is a national awareness regarding the need to protect our environment

Americans are increasingly beginning to realize the degree to which healthy land, air, and water are essential to the nation's and world's well-being. The quality of the environment is one of the major considerations of our government and people. Park and recreational professionals, for example, have an opportunity to participate and play a major role in making our communities, cities, and suburbs healthy environments.

This can be done through such means as developing education programs that stress proper use and enjoyment of the environment, increasing recreation opportunities for all persons, making parks more active centers of city life, and building recreation and natural beauty into housing programs.

Inner city problems require more attention to recreational possibilities

The problems of our growing cities, with their increased crime rates, higher costs of living, growing welfare rolls, transportation difficulties, and lack of proper recreation facilities, provide fertile ground for major contributions by the recreation profession. Among other innovations being suggested and/or tried are new concepts regarding park-school development to further recreational opportunities for all city inhabitants, recreation-education parks with transportation being provided for city youth, and recreation plazas that might involve closing off streets, putting in swimming pools, and providing indoor spaces for youth activities.

States join forces to meet recreational needs of their citizens and visitors

On April 1, 1969, the states of Vermont and New Hampshire signed a Plan of Cooperation whereby the recreational services of each state work cooperatively together. This is the first such formal agreement between the recreation services in two states, and it is expected to develop into a trend throughout the country as the demand for recreation services increase. The Vermont–New Hampshire plan of cooperation calls for an interchange of publications, discussions of state Directors of Recreation, and leadership training programs in recreation.

There is federal government involvement in attempting to preserve and improve the beauty of America

The national government recognizes that our growing population is swallowing up areas of natural beauty, and therefore it is taking measures to provide for a beautiful America, such as making the capitol the nation's showcase, beautifying locations throughout the United States, planning land acquisition for conservation purposes, conducting research, preserving wildlife, retaining and improving scenic and historical sites, offering improved outdoor recreation to more people, improving water and waterways, and controlling pollution of streams and rivers.

American communities are becoming recreation minded

Many villages, cities, and communities from coast to coast are acquiring and developing their green spaces, restoring national shrines, rehabilitating depressed neighborhoods and ghettos, providing for "senior citizens," setting aside acreage for recreation, advocating "See America First," establishing neighborhood playgrounds, making provision for the physically handicapped and mentally ill and retarded to share in the benefits of recreational programs, stressing the performing arts, and developing sports programs.

There is community-school cooperation in recreation programs

Two examples will support this statement. In Flint, Michigan, as a result of the impetus provided by Charles Stewart Mott and the Mott Foundation, recreation programs exist in the schools. It brings people of all nationalities, economic status, and other types of backgrounds together on commonly owner property: the public schools. More than 12,000 visitors come each year to see the Flint program. The program includes all types of recreational activities ranging from roller skating to an international program that involves approximately 1,000 athletes and their families in Flint, Michigan, and Hamilton, Canada.

Another example of community-school connected recreation is in Los Angeles, California, where the city school district, through its Youth Services Section, sponsors a program where millions participate over the course of any one year. More than 550 recreation sites are utilized and more than 4,000 full-time and part-time personnel are involved in the leadership phase of the program. A year-round, 107-acre camp is utilized where outdoor education is carried on. A day camp is also in operation. The program utilizes the recreational experiences in the Youth Services Program as a laboratory experience for skills learned in the classroom.

Religion recognizes the value of recreation

The Puritan colonists encouraged the belief that recreation and spiritual teachings were not compatible. Today, however, religion and the church feel that it is their responsibility to help people make the most constructive and creative use of leisure. It is recognized that recreation can complement the church program and help to meet the needs of church members. As a result, many churches throughout the United States have gymnasiums and recreation centers as part of their facility complex. The Southern Baptists, for example, in one year spent approximately $150 million on facilities used primarily for recreation.

The cultural explosion has an impact on recreation

The increased national interest in music, art, concerts, exhibitions, and other cultural interests is affecting recreation. Recreation programs are expanding their offerings to include specialists in the various arts. The public is encouraged to participate more. Opportunities are being increased for new forms of participation in the arts. Additional appropriations of money are being made. As a result, recreation is being afforded the opportunity to meet the increased interest in cultural activities and thereby contribute to a better America.

The National Recreation and Park Association is giving leadership to recreation

This new association that combines the efforts of the leading recreation and park people is furthering recreation in America.

This agency is concerned with both natural and manmade beauty in America and the human environment. It is attempting to help people in this country have a better and healthier place in which to live, work, and enjoy their leisure. Its goal is to provide the populace with good parks and playgrounds and to instill the need for proper use of land and water. Better recreation programs and a better climate for recreation should evolve as a result of the formation of this new association.

OPPORTUNITIES FOR PLACEMENT

The continued and expanded interest in recreation means many job openings in the years to come. There are more than 3,000 publicly sponsored local and county agencies engaged in recreation. Many more will be needed in the future. Thirty thousand companies now have recreation programs, and this number will expand considerably in the next decade. As people get more leisure time there will be a greater need for professional people to help them spend this leisure in as constructive a way as possible.

The growth in recreation is assured because of such factors as the increase predicted in the population of this country by the year 2000, the growth in disposable income, the increase in the amount of leisure time, and, finally, the increase in auto travel.

By 1980, employment in the administration and management of public recreation facilities and tourist and private recreation services is expected to be approximately 1.4 million. This represents an increase of more than three-quarters of a million new positions since 1960.

The growth of recreational services does not stop here, however. In rural areas, it is expected there will be an estimated 350,000 full-time positions available in farm and other rural recreational enterprises by 1980.

New careers and areas of specialization are available as a result of the expansion and growth of recreational services. These include such areas of concentration as rural recreation, industrial recreation, therapeutic recreation, forest recreation, recreation

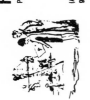

Choose a Career in RECREATION

Choosing a career in Recreation, Parks, and Conservation is choosing a life of Leadership.

Few fields of endeavor offer the variety of experience and responsibilities as does the recreation, park, and conservation field. Administration, finance, public relations, planning, community action, group leadership, and personnel direction are all part of the daily life of the recreation leader. And, when the day is done, the personal satisfaction which results from the contributions you have made to the better life of the community and the enrichment of our nation is proof of the wise selection in choosing recreation as a career.

PUBLIC

Public recreation includes administration, supervision and leadership in:
Community Sponsored Programs.
School Sponsored Programs.
County Sponsored Programs.
State Sponsored Programs.
Federal Recreation Agencies.
(All public recreation is paid for by taxes through city, county, state or national government, depending upon the position described.)

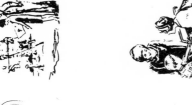

INDUSTRIAL

Industrial Recreation includes administration, supervision and leadership in:
Management Sponsored Programs.
Employee Sponsored Programs.
Cooperative Programs Financed by Management:
and (A) Operated by Employees or
(B) Operated by Both Management and Employees.
Association or Institution Type Programs.

ILL and HANDICAPPED

Recreation for the Ill and Handicapped includes administration, supervision and leadership in medically approved recreation programs for hospitalized patients and for ill and handicapped persons in special schools and institutions. Recreation activities are used as a means of stimulating healthy response in patients, enriching their lives and in helping them achieve a better social adjustment.

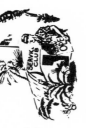

ARMED FORCES

Civilian positions with the Armed Forces include direction of clubs, libraries, hobby shops and entertainment (sports, drama and music) for active duty military personnel and their dependents.

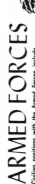

RECREATION EDUCATION

Recreation education is a basic responsibility of the home and school for preparing the individual for worthy use of leisure. Professionally it includes the continual responsibility on the part of the recreationist, as well as the teaching of recreation professional courses in a junior college, college or university.

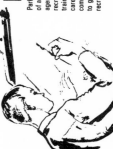

VOLUNTARY

Voluntary and youth serving programs include scouts, boy's and girl's clubs, Y's, and other agencies which derive support from public and private subscription.

COMMERCIAL

Commercial recreation includes the operation and management of privately owned enterprises offering recreation and entertainment to the public for a set individual charge.

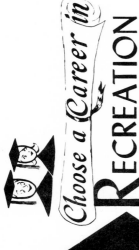

PARKS

Parks management is closely allied with recreation as a result of a growing trend in government to join park management agencies with recreation agencies to better serve the total recreational needs of the people. Because recreationists are trained to plan for the effective use of facilities, as well as their care and upkeep, the recreation professional with the proper combination of training and experience will be the logical person to guide the total development and management of park and recreation facilities and programs for the public benefit.

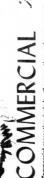

Prepared by:
The Middle-Atlantic District Advisory Committee
of the
National Recreation and Park Association

COURTESY NATIONAL RECREATION AND PARK ASSOCIATION.

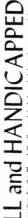

planning, recreation and/or park administration, and public or community recreation.

The rewards for those young people who go into recreation as a career will include the satisfaction of improving the social well-being of human beings, contributing to community development and a better environment, providing the resources for the worthy use of leisure time, and a financial return that compares favorably with many other professions. Salaries for recreation leaders now range from $4,000 to $7,000 to start and go to as high as $25,000 for key positions. As the cost of living increases and as teachers and other persons with comparable professional training find increased pay in their monthly envelopes, so will recreation leaders.

QUESTIONS AND EXERCISES

1. Define the term *recreation*. What is the history of the National Recreation and Park Association?
2. List and discuss each of the objectives of the recreation profession.
3. Survey your community to determine how many recreation activities are available for young people.
4. Why is there a need for good recreation programs in the space age in which we are living?
5. Select ten adults and find out how they spend their free time.
6. What part do physical education activities play in a recreation program?
7. What are the arguments for and against a school-centered recreation program?
8. How can the schools play a more important role in preparing for the student's leisure time?
9. For what jobs could a physical educator qualify in a municipal recreation program?

Reading assignment

Bucher, Charles A., and Goldman, Myra: Dimensions of physical education, St. Louis, 1969, The C. V. Mosby Co., Reading selections 21, 22, 25, and 26.

SELECTED REFERENCES

American Academy of Political and Social Science: Leisure in America: blessing or curse? Philadelphia, 1964, The Academy.

American Association for Health, Physical Education, and Recreation: Recreation policy statement, Journal of Health, Physical Education, and Recreation **37**:43, 1966.

Bucher, Charles A.: Administration of school health and physical education programs, including athletics, St. Louis, 1971, The C. V. Mosby Co.

Bucher, Charles A., Administrative dimensions of health and physical education programs, including athletics, St. Louis, 1971, The C. V. Mosby Co.

Bucher, Charles A., editor: Methods and materials in physical education and recreation, St. Louis, 1954, The C. V. Mosby Co.

de Grazia, Sebastian: Of time, work, and leisure, New York, 1962, The Twentieth Century Fund.

Dulles, Foster Rhea: A history of recreation, New York, 1965, Appleton-Century-Crofts.

Hunter, O. N., and Jensen, Clayne R.: Recreation and a changing world, Journal of Health, Physical Education, and Recreation **36**:32, 1965.

Kleindienst, Viola, and Weston, Arthur: Intramural and recreation programs for schools and colleges, New York, 1964, Appleton-Century-Crofts.

Kraus, Richard: Recreation and leisure in modern society, New York, 1971, Appleton-Century-Crofts.

Kraus, Richard: Recreation today—program planning and leadership, New York, 1966, Appleton-Century-Crofts.

Kraus, Richard: Which way—school recreation? Journal of Health, Physical Education, and Recreation **36**:25, 1965.

Lee, Robert: Religion and leisure in America, Nashville, 1964, Abingdon Press.

Meyer, Harold D., and Brightbill, Charles K.: Community recreation—a guide to its organization, Englewood Cliffs, New Jersey, 1964, Prentice-Hall, Inc.

President's Council on Youth Fitness: Physical fitness elements in recreation, suggestions for community programs, Washington, D. C., 1962, U. S. Government Printing Office.

Report to the President and Congress by the Outdoor Recreation Resources Review Commission: Outdoor recreation in America, Washington, D. C., 1962, U. S. Government Printing Office.

Saake, Alvin C.: Recreation is big in Hawaii, Journal of Health, Physical Education, and Recreation **37**:31, 1966.

10/Camping and outdoor education

The out-of-doors is nature's laboratory. It is a setting that offers excellent opportunities to learn many knowledges and skills and to develop wholesome attitudes. L. B. Sharp, one of the pioneers in the fields of camping and outdoor education, stated it this way: "That which can best be learned inside the classroom should be learned there. That which can best be learned in the out-of-doors through direct experience, dealing with native materials and life situations, should there be learned."

Over the course of the last three decades, many experiments have been conducted based on the premise set forth by Sharp. These experiments have provided the evidence to show that boys and girls who use nature's classroom will learn more readily those things that directly relate to the out-of-doors and be more interested in doing so.

What L. B. Sharp stated several years ago was demonstrated by a kindergarten teacher who took her class out of the school to study the clouds in the sky, a third-grade class that utilized a compass to measure distances and determine directions preliminary to beginning a map for social studies, a sixth-grade class that went to a park and discovered fossils, and an eighth-grade class that found a spider web and related it to what they were doing on conservation. Outdoor education is not just nature study, it represents a vital part of the educational program at all educational levels and in all subjects including art, social studies, mathematics, physical education, and industrial arts.

School camping and outdoor education are not synonymous. Outdoor education is education in the out-of-doors and also education about the out-of-doors. Outdoor education includes school camping. The camp provides a laboratory by which many facets of the out-of-doors can be studied firsthand. And the camp experience helps to develop qualities important to preparing young people for the lives they will live.

The worth of camping and outdoor education in the school program has been well established. The teacher of physical education, as well as all teachers at the elementary, secondary, and college levels, can benefit from studying the objectives, contributions, program, administration, and other aspects of these important fields. In the future, education will utilize these programs more and more, and individuals trained in these areas will find many opportunities to apply their knowledge and experience.

The public concern about the environment and ecology today accents the importance of students knowing more about the out-of-doors and how they can help in preventing it from becoming polluted.

CAMPING AND OUTDOOR EDUCATION AND TODAY'S ENVIRONMENTAL PROBLEMS

Former United States Education Commissioner James E. Allen recommended that every school should have an opportunity for environmental study, so that students would grow up with the realization that the environment represents everything that makes up the world and that all of its numberless elements are interdependent.

In a natural undisturbed situation, life of all kinds tends to assemble, to live, to reproduce, and to furnish food for each other. Basically, this ecological system (relationship between organisms and their environment) consists of the predator living off the prey. However, there are many factors that can enter into this picture of undisturbed natural situation and bring about change.

Through a rapidly increasing population and the demand for a higher and higher standard of living, man has succeeded in destroying many valuable insects, fish, and animal life by polluting the air and water, by producing excessive amounts of man-made radiation, by carelessly using insecticides, and by constantly increasing the nuisance of noise. As a consequence, man is threatening to destroy himself as well as other living things.

Since his advent upon the earth, man has been adjusting to his environment so as to improve his security and comfort. At the same time, however, urbanization—with its increased congestion and noise, the development of chemicals for a myriad of uses, the multitude of waste products cast off by industrial plants, and the intensified use of streams and lakes for purposes of refuse disposal—has contributed to the artificial contamination of the environment.

As a result of all of this, man has multiplied his traditional problem of water pollution, has initiated a new set of problems in the protection of his food supply, and has succeeded in thoroughly contaminating his most abundant natural resource, the atmosphere.

As former Commissioner Allen indicated, the schools must do something about environmental problems facing our nation and the world. A logical school experience in which some of this education can take place is the camping and outdoor education program. Of course, this in turn has implications for physical education, since the environment represents a very important setting for various sports and other physical activities. As he reads this chapter, the reader will see that through a better understanding of our natural environment, which

Camping and outdoor education program.

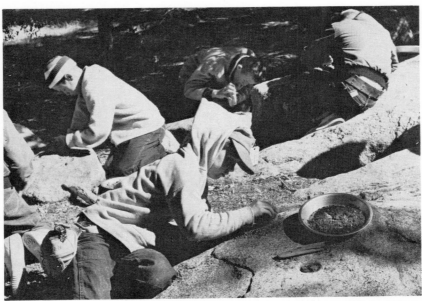

can best be gained through a direct experience, he can be helped to understand ecology and the contributions that he can make to preserve our valuable natural resources.

HISTORY

In May, 1948, representatives of such well-known organizations and agencies as the American Association for Health, Physical Education, and Recreation, United States Office of Education, National Secondary School Principals Association, American Association of School Administrators, and the American Council on Education made recommendations that camping experience should be a part of every child's educational experience, that cooperative arrangements should be worked out with conservation departments and other agencies directly related to natural resources, and that experimental camping programs, as a phase of the educational program, should be established in Michigan and in other states that were interested in trying out this educational trend.*

The state of Michigan led the way in this experiment to show the values that may be derived from making the camping experience a part of the regular school program. Twelve camps were set up in Michigan on an experimental basis. In one year alone they utilized 200 teachers and 1,000 students. There were also hundreds of educators and leaders in closely allied fields who visited these camps. The project was subsidized by the Kellogg Foundation. This was only the beginning of the school camping and outdoor education movement. Since that time it has grown rapidly. Schools all over the country are recognizing its value and importance in the educational program.

In 1962 100 leaders in education, conservation, and recreation participated in a National Conference on Outdoor Educa-

tion. This Conference reaffirmed the importance of outdoor education and came to the following conclusions*:

1. There is a greater need today than ever before for education in the out-of-doors.
2. Outdoor education needs to be stressed more in all schools and colleges and in conservation, recreation, and other agency programs.
3. All agencies and organizations concerned with outdoor education should work very closely together in order that such experiences can be provided for more boys and girls and also adults in our society.
4. The American Association for Health, Physical Education, and Recreation should provide strong leadership for the outdoor education program.

AAHPER Outdoor Education Project, 1955 to 1970

In 1955 the AAHPER initiated the Outdoor Education Project in cooperation with business and industry in order to give added impetus to school and college programs.† Some highlights and accomplishments of this project are:

Teacher and leadership preparation in the field of outdoor education was furthered by national conferences, state and regional workshops, college courses in outdoor skills (50,000 prospective physical education teachers and recreation leaders took such courses).

Interpretation of outdoor education was provided through such media as newsletters, films and filmstrips, and other materials.

Publications in the forms of books, articles, and other materials cover a variety of subjects, including casting and angling, archery, and shooting and hunting.

More than 2,000 school districts now have resident outdoor schools, as compared to 300 in 1955.

Teaching of outdoor skills in schools and colleges (archery, casting, angling, shooting) is now done in approximately 40% to 50%, of these institutions, as compared to 12% to 20%, in 1955.

Other types of outdoor education programs have been introduced, such as winter programs and farm programs.

*Professional Report from the National Conference on Outdoor Education: Journal of Health, Physical Education, and Recreation 33:29, 1962.

†Smith, Julian: AAHPER Outdoor Education Project 1955-1970, Journal of Health, Physical Education, and Recreation 41:44, 1970.

*Smith, Julian W.: Adventure in outdoor education, Journal of Health, Physical Education, and Recreation 26:8, 18, 1955.

Outdoor education programs extend to Europe and other countries

On June 16, 1970, twenty-eight teachers from all over the United States enrolled and participated in the first Foreign Outdoor Education Tour sponsored by Northern Illinois University. This tour included an in-person study of outdoor experiences of European children in such countries as Germany, Denmark, East Germany, Berlin, Austria, Switzerland, and France.

Growth of camping*

In 1970 the estimated number of camps of all types was approximately 20,000.

---

*Shivers, Jay S.: Camping, administration, counsel, programming, New York, 1971, Appleton-Century-Crofts.

These camps served about 6 million children during the summer months. There are approximately 15,000 persons hired full-time in the camping field, with an additional 200,000 employed during the summer seasons. The potential of camping is very great, and more and more of the nation's students are participating in such an experience.

Outdoor education and camping have become firmly established in the American educational system. Schools are recognizing the values that relate to education in the out-of-doors that can be correlated closely to what is going on in the classroom. Also, educators are becoming more aware of the importance of education about the out-of-doors and all the resources that are em-

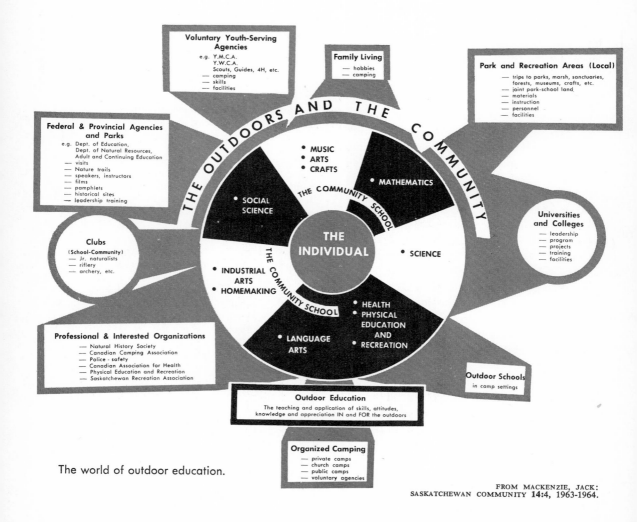

The world of outdoor education.

FROM MACKENZIE, JACK:
SASKATCHEWAN COMMUNITY **14:4,** 1963-1964.

bodied in the world of nature. The years ahead will see further progress in this direction.

OBJECTIVES OF CAMPING AND OUTDOOR EDUCATION

Many objectives have been listed for camping and outdoor education programs. Some of the more important objectives that have been enumerated over the years as being the reasons why such programs should exist in our schools are as follows:

1. Students learn to live democratically with other children and adults.
2. Students learn more about the physical environment, the importance of our vast wealth of natural resources, and how to preserve them. They also learn about the ecological aspects of the environment.
3. An appreciation for the out-of-doors and the contributions it can make to enriched living is developed.
4. Those qualities that make for good citizenship, such as responsibility, leadership, teamwork, and honesty, are developed.
5. The contribution that the out-of-doors can make to good health is more appreciated.
6. The love of adventure, which is part of the makeup of children and youth, is satisfied.
7. Students are stimulated to learn about native materials and to see their relationship to the learning that takes place in the classroom.
8. Worthwhile skills in recreation such as map reading, fishing, and how to use a gun are developed.
9. Benefits are derived from wholesome work experiences.
10. Students learn to depend on personal resources in practicing the rules of healthful living.
11. Students learn some of the basic rules of safety.

These objectives are worthy goals and tie in closely with the social, intellectual, and health aims of general education. The child develops socially by learning to live democratically. Responsibilities for maintaining a camp are assumed by all. Each child, regardless of national origin, color, or other difference, is respected as an individual who can contribute to the group enterprise. He also develops intellectually as he satisfies his lust for adventure. He

sees the wonders of nature firsthand. He learns about conservation, soil, water, and animal and bird life. A camping experience also promotes good health. The out-of-doors, together with healthful activity, interesting projects, and congenial classmates, improves the general fitness of the child. He usually leaves camp with a ruddy glow to his cheeks, sparkling eyes that reflect the new things he has seen and learned, and an extra notch in his belt. If education is "preparation for life," then surely camping and outdoor experiences are an essential and worthwhile part of it.

Freeberg and Taylor* list four objectives for the outdoor education program: democratic group living, conservation education, leisure-time education, and healthful outdoor living.

The Cleveland Heights, Ohio, public schools list as objectives for outdoor education the following:

1. To teach citizenship
2. To teach principles of natural science
3. To teach principles of conservation
4. To teach health and physical education
5. To teach other subject-matter aspects related to the camping situation

SOME SETTINGS FOR OUTDOOR EDUCATION

School and community gardens and farms. Experiences can be provided relating to such things as agriculture, bird and animal study, conservation, gardening, and milk production.

School areas in general. Experiences can be provided for studying such products of nature as plants, shrubs, birds, trees, and fish.

School forests. Where large wooded areas exist, experiences can be provided in relation to such things as reforestation, conservation, and the growth and wise use of forests.

Museums. Many different types of museums offer opportunities for experiences in

---

*Freeberg, William H., and Taylor, Loren E.: Programs in outdoor education, Minneapolis, 1963, Burgess Publishing Co.

such areas as archeological exploration, art appreciation, historical milestones, scientific accomplishments, and bird and animal life.

Zoos. Zoos provide opportunities for experiences in the study of animals.

CAMPS. Camps offer opportunities for such things as group living, work experience, and development of outdoor skills.

Opportunities for outdoor education are available everywhere in the country. In addition to the fields, woods, and lakes, many private or public sanctuaries, museums, parks, camps, and zoos can be used for such purposes.

PROGRAM

Camp Quest is the setting for the camping and outdoor education program for the LeMars Community School District of LeMars, Iowa. The program, for students enrolled in grades seven and eight, includes such recreation and physical education activities as archery, croquet, softball, volleyball, soccer, horseshoes, and basketball, and such projects as astronomy, rocks and

minerals, fossils, entomology, agronomy, forestry, aquatic life, and ornithology. Six 1-week camps are held, Monday through Friday, during the months of June and July. Recently, as a means of improving the camp, permission was secured from the board of education to have an abandoned schoolhouse moved to the camp site. This now provides a facility for carrying on instruction and project activities during inclement weather.

The Frederick County, Maryland, school system provides an outdoor teaching experience for their sixth-grade children that involves an interesting project called the "Field Notebook Technique." Each student finds an object that is unfamiliar to him, examines it closely, makes a sketch of the object, writes a description of it, and then, when he returns to the classroom, checks the library and other resources and gathers as much information as possible about the object.

Queens College in the City of New York initiated a program in outdoor education and camping in the Department of Health

The outdoor education program.

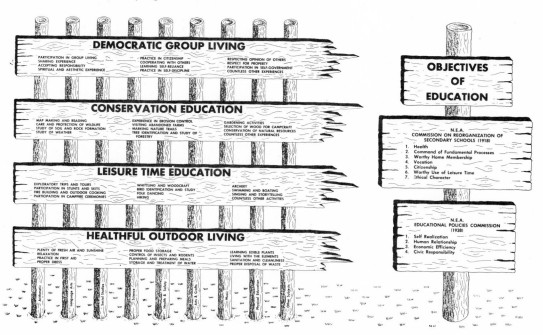

FROM FREEBERG, WILLIAM H., AND TAYLOR, LOREN E.:
PROGRAMS IN OUTDOOR EDUCATION,
MINNEAPOLIS, 1963, BURGESS PUBLISHING CO.

and Physical Education. This program is designed to familiarize students with the various natural environments, develop outdoor skill techniques, recognize the need for a cooperative interdisciplinary approach to studying natural areas, and develop positive attitudes toward the conservation of natural resources. One project included Professor John Loret taking a group of students on a 3-week course of study on the tropical island of St. John in the United States Virgin Islands. Activities included snorkeling, swimming, studying marine life, listening to geologists, botanists, and government administrators, and scuba diving to see the natural environment and become more familiar with the ecological aspects of the Virgin Islands.

The San Diego city schools utilize the school camp experience to make studies in science and conservation more interesting and meaningful. Some of the learning experiences they describe are as follows:

Astronomy. Studying about stars and planets by looking at them through telescopes; visiting the Palomar Observatory and Museum

Geology. Digging into the earth to find rocks and minerals for study; reading the story of the soil profiles; studying soil and earth features

Meteorology. Observing and identifying weather; measuring weather phenomena at camp with accurate instruments; maintaining a weather station at camp

Ecology. Hiking to see and study the relationship of living things to their environment

Conservation. Learning about the problems of the land and working to help the land through soil erosion control, beetle control, tree planting, reduction of fire hazards, and forest improvement

Botany and biology. Studying birds, insects, animals, and plants in the field and pond; collecting specimens

Forestry. Learning woodmanship and the safe use of forestry tools and equipment

Survival skills. Using map and compass on

Camping and outdoor education at Westchester County Recreation Camp, Croton, N. Y.

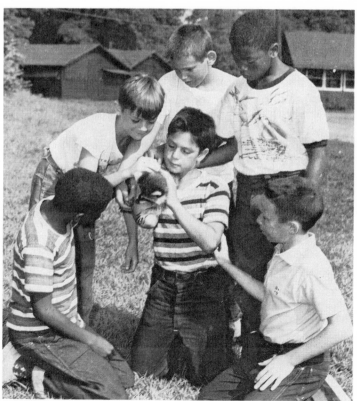

JOHN GOSS.

hikes; considering problems of food, shelter, and safety on a "survival hike"

Many other school systems throughout the country have developed outdoor education and camping programs. The University School in Carbondale, Illinois, involves their fourth-, fifth-, sixth-, and seventh-grade school children in such programs. Orange Local School District in Chagrin Falls, Ohio, has access to Hirman House Camp. Stiles School in Rockford, Illinois, has established a nature area. Snohomish County, Washington, conducted a successful pilot outdoor education program. Long Beach, California, schools provide valuable camping experiences for their school children at Camp Hi-Hill. Many other schools in other states have also had successful camping and outdoor education experiences.

Paul E. Harrison of Northern Illinois University has pointed out the contributions various departments in many schools are making in camping and outdoor education programs. These suggestions clarify the role of the total school offering in such an educational experience.

Speech department
Activities in speech and dramatics can take many forms:
1. Short plays, comedy, drama
2. Pageants
3. Folk festivals
4. Readings, recitations
5. Marionette and puppet shows

Music department
Campers can spend many happy hours with music:
1. Informal campfire sings
2. Pageants
3. Camp orchestra

Mathematics
Arithmetic is a must in many camp activities:
1. Food costs
2. Surveying and mapping
3. Camp stores and banks
4. Figuring land areas, elevation, tree heights, lumber footage, tree age

Industrial arts
Using appropriate tools and interesting natural materials where they are found:
1. Camp maintenance and repair
2. Building new camp equipment
3. Reading blueprints

4. Camp activities, dramatics, staging
5. Craft programs

Homemaking
Good food and appropriate clothing make for a happy camp:
1. Planning and preparing foods for cook-outs, camp-outs, and regular menus
2. Care of clothing and camp equipment
3. Social graces
4. Helping with camp food service

English department
The camp can provide an opportunity for the practice of effective communication and appreciation of literature:
1. Proper language usage
2. Writing letters, plays, poems
3. Storytelling
4. Reading

Social science
The history of the area—its land, its people, and its customs—is always an interesting problem for study:
1. A study of the area's industries
2. Indian lore and the lumber camps
3. Use of public property
4. Camp government

Science, physical and biological
A study of the land, water, and living things is always interesting and useful:
1. A study of forest and forest life
2. Experiences in botany
3. Activities in geology
4. Study of the skies, stars, constellations, weather stations
5. Soil
6. Sanitation
7. Rivers and lakes
8. Fish and fishing
9. Fire protection
10. Photography, aerial and other
11. Map development
12. Reforestation

Physical education department
Physical exercise is basic to camp happiness:
1. Hiking
2. Cook-outs and camp-outs
3. Swimming and boating
4. Snowshoeing
5. Archery
6. Bait casting and fishing
7. Hunting and tracking
8. Wood crafts
9. Camping out
10. Games and athletic events

Art department
The camper has a chance to study nature as it develops:
1. Creative drawing and sketching
2. Painting (dramatic-music pageants)

SAMPLE STUDY UNITS IN OUTDOOR EDUCATION

The teachers and administrators of Clear Lake Camp, operated by Battle Creek public schools, Michigan, have developed an excellent program of study for outdoor education. In this course of study are listed such items as a statement of philosophy, suggestions to teachers and counselors, and more than forty units of study covering various aspects of camping and outdoor education. Two of these units are given to show the reader how camping and outdoor education can be made a functional part of general education.

Bird hikes

    I. Time—varies with the purposes of various groups

    II. Description of destination—may be one or more of the following: swamp, marsh, lake shore, woods, fields, homes, or roadsides

    III. Equipment—binoculars or field glasses and cameras must be brought from home; bird identification books available at camp

    IV. Learning possibilities

        A. Identification of birds
        B. Habitat of birds, and reasons
        C. Economic value or lack of value
        D. Enemies of birds
        E. Living habits of birds, their nests, their food, their family life
        F. Interdependence of birds and man
        G. Balance in nature
        H. How birds are or may be protected
            1. Game laws
            2. Reasons for game laws
            3. Sanctuaries
            4. Planting of trees
            5. International migratory laws
        I. Migration
            1. Routes
            2. Distances
        J. Why people "bird watch"
            1. Enjoyment of songs and actions and colors
            2. Feeling of at-homeness with nature
        K. Adaptation of body of bird to mode of life: claws, wings, beaks
        L. Evolution in bird families

    V. Possible implications for curriculum

        A. Studies in science
        B. Studies in conservation
        C. Studies in geography
        D. Studies of grains

Boating

    I. Place—Clear Lake

    II. Safety precautions

        A. Safety is of prime importance in using the boats
        B. Children must be seated at all times while in a boat
        C. A teacher or counselor must be in the boat with the children

    III. Equipment (available at camp)—five boats with oars and anchors attached

    IV. Learning possibilities

        A. Proper way to enter a boat
        B. How to shove off from shore
        C. How to sit in a boat and keep it balanced
        D. Identifying the stern, bow, gunnel or gunwale
        E. How to row
        F. How to turn
        G. Beaching a boat properly
        H. Why a boat floats (displacement of its own weight)
        I. Awareness of and practice of safety
        J. Uses of boats for recreation
        K. Uses of boats for making a living

    V. Possible implications for curriculum

        A. Open up possibilities for thinking in terms of self-development and the place of recreation in balanced living
        B. Understanding more about water transportation
        C. Science learnings
            1. Displacement of weight causes an object to float
            2. Principle of leverage
            3. Principle of inertia
            4. Principle of momentum
            5. Principle of friction

    VI. Resource materials—Boy Scout Merit Badge Pamphlet on Rowing

WORTH OF CAMPING AND OUTDOOR EDUCATION

The values of school camping and outdoor education are very much in evidence as a result of the many experiments that have been conducted throughout the United States. For purposes of discussion, it might be said that the values of such experiences are threefold: (1) they meet the social needs of the child, (2) they meet the intellectual needs of the child, and (3) they meet the health needs of the child.

A camping and outdoor education experience is an essential part of every child's school experience because it helps to develop the child socially. In a camp setting children learn to live democratically. They mix with children of various creeds, national origins, races, economic status, and abilities. They aid in planning the program that will be followed during their camp stay; they assume part of the responsibility for the upkeep of the camp, such as making their own beds, helping in the kitchen, sweeping their cabins, and fixing the tennis courts; and they experience cooperative living. The children get away from home and from their parents. They lose their feeling of dependency upon others and learn to do things for themselves. This is especially necessary in modern-day society where divorce, separations, and the desire of the mothers to seek careers of their own are so prevalent. The child learns to rely on his own resources. The camp experience also provides an enjoyable experience for the child. A child is naturally active and seeks adventure. This experience provides the opportunity to release some of this adventure and satisfy the "wanderlust" urge.

A camping and outdoor education experience is an essential part of every child's school experience because it helps to develop the child intellectually. While living in a camp or in another outdoor education setting, the child learns about such things as soil, forests, water, and animal and bird life. He learns about the value of the nation's natural resources and how they should be conserved. He learns by doing rather than through the medium of textbooks. Instead of looking at the picture of a bird in a book, he actually sees the bird chirping on the branch of a tree. Instead of reading about soil erosion in a textbook, he sees how it really occurs. Instead of being told about the four basic groups of food, he has the opportunity to plan a diet that meets the right standards. Instead of reading about the values of democratic living, he actually experiences it. The child experiences many new things that he cannot possibly experience at home or within the four walls of a school building. Camp-

ing is also of special value to children who do not learn easily from books. In many cases the knowledge accumulated through actual experience is much more enlightening and beneficial.

A camping and outdoor education experience is an essential part of every child's school experience because it helps to meet the health needs of the child. Camps are located away from the turmoil, confusion, noise, and rush of urban life. Children have their meals at a regular time, obtain sufficient sleep, and participate in wholesome activity in the out-of-doors. They wear clothing that does not restrict movement, that permits the absorption of healthful sun rays, and that they are not afraid to get dirty. The food is good. They are doing things that are natural for them to do. It is an outlet for their dynamic personalities. It is much more healthful, both physically and mentally, than living in a "push-button" existence with its lack of recreation, relaxation, and opportunity for enjoyable experiences. It is like living in another world, and children come away refreshed from such an experience.

Another way to determine the worth of camping and outdoor education is to evaluate the comments of students, teachers, school administrators, and parents who have experienced these programs. The Long Beach Unified School District in Long Beach, California, has compiled a sampling of such statements, a few of which follow.

What the students say:

"I like being in the out-of-doors because I feel I understand wildlife better than reading a book about it or having someone tell me about it. I feel happy and carefree when I am around wildlife. Wildlife is something more to me than words on a paper. I hope you will understand how I feel about conservation."

"I like playing and working with others because it helps me to get along with my schoolmates and to be a better person. Because of this I have done much better in all my work and play."

"I felt that I could take care of myself because I didn't have to depend upon my mother, and I had a lot of fun trying to prove it to myself."

"I learned how all living things depend upon each other for something. Man depends on certain insects to carry pollen from one plant to another. Insects, in turn, depend on certain flowers to help them with their food supply, nectar. It all keeps revolving in this way to make life possible."

"Before I went to camp I didn't care about stars, plants, rocks, trees, or animals. Now I want to know more about them. Since camp I have read several books and seen several nature movies."

What the teachers say:

"The class has a much better understanding and interest in the ways and means of conserving our natural resources."

"For many, camp has opened a world which they have read about or studied but never experienced. A knowledge of and an appreciation of nature are clearly evident in the children and will provide them a richer life."

"Quietness of the evening and the campfire has excellent spiritual value."

"I went to camp in doubt. I came back completely sold."

What the parents say:

"It is the grandest thing that has ever been presented by our schools."

"I consider it a very necessary part of the curriculum, and the experience gained is a necessary part of growth."

"I sincerely hope the camp program will be continued and in my opinion [it] should be made compulsory for all children. I can't begin to express my appreciation."

"One of the finest projects the city schools have ever undertaken. A rare treat and privilege."

"They learned so much in so short a time."

What the school administrators say:

"Space does not permit saying all that might be said in praise of this fine educational experience provided for sixth graders, but I feel that it represents a very rich addition to our program."

"It was my privilege to see two groups in action and I have every confidence that we have in this phase of our educational program something that will grow in popularity and usefulness as it becomes better known by our community."

"They [the children] themselves seemed to feel that this was one of the most important and enjoyable experiences of their lives and one which really gave them some new values. They evidenced this in improved attitudes and habits, new appreciations and interests."

IMPLICATIONS FOR THE PHYSICAL EDUCATION TEACHER

If camping and outdoor education are to render their greatest service to the pupil, good leadership must be present. Regardless of how elaborate the camping facilities, the size of the budget, and the number of opportunities available for educational trips, true education will not take place unless the teachers, counselors, and leaders can interpret, discuss, guide, and educate the student. Physical education teachers can provide much of this leadership. The close alliance that exists between their field and that of camping, through a common interest in such things as the out-of-doors, sports, and other activities, makes it possible for them to take a leading role in this movement.

Physical educators are proficient in the teaching of many outdoor activities being stressed by specialists in the field of outdoor education. These include casting and fishing; shooting and hunting; boating, sailing, canoeing, and other water activities; and winter sports such as skiing and skating. Persons must be trained as camp administrators, camp counselors, and instructors. Classroom teachers must receive special instruction to orient them to the camping program. School administrators must be informed and their cooperation and support enlisted. These are only a few of the opportunities and challenges facing leaders in camping and outdoor education. Physical education personnel should play a major role in meeting these opportunities and challenges.

Those interested in becoming active in the camping and outdoor education movement should have special preparation in this area. Such courses as camp counseling, camp administration, crafts, guidance, and psychology, together with an actual camp experience, will prove helpful.

Smith has outlined three essential features of training for outdoor education: (1) an understanding of human beings, (2) the ability to interpret the outdoors, and (3) skills and techniques to teach and guide in the out-of-doors. He goes on to give his suggestions for leadership in this important area.

Colleges and universities will need to provide more actual and direct experiences in the outdoors along with methods and techniques adapted to teaching in informal situations. A multidisciplinary approach, involving all appropriate fields and departments, is needed to provide adequate training. Preparation must include realistic outdoor field experiences with children and teachers in communities.

The interested physical educator can contribute to camping and outdoor education by preparing himself through study as well as experience for leadership in these fields. Furthermore, all physical educators can do much to contribute to the objectives of these specialized areas by stressing outdoor activities. There is a need for more teaching of swimming, archery, tennis, boating, skin and scuba diving, water skiing, skating, bicycling, hiking, and many other activities conducted in the out-of-doors. These activities can be enjoyed at all ages. They are important parts of physical education programs. For those undergraduate students, as well as the physical education leaders in the field whose interests and desires tend toward camping and the out-of-doors, this is a field where participation has vast possibilities. It deserves special consideration by those who wish to pioneer in a new field of endeavor, render an outstanding contribution to children, youth, and adults, help in the achievement of educational objectives, and build a healthier and better society.

QUESTIONS AND EXERCISES

1. How do camping and outdoor education contribute to the goals of general education?
2. Compile a list of objectives for camping and outdoor education programs.
3. List ten outdoor education experiences that every child should have.
4. What contributions can each of the subject-matter departments in the school make to camping and outdoor education programs?
5. Consult several authoritative camping books and draw up what you feel would constitute a desirable camp program.
6. What is the relationship of physical education to camping and outdoor education?
7. What contributions can the physical educator make to camping and outdoor education programs?

Reading assignment
Bucher, Charles A., and Goldman, Myra:

Dimensions of physical education, St. Louis, 1969, The C. V. Mosby Co., Reading selections 23 and 24.

SELECTED REFERENCES

Bucher, Charles A.: Administration of school health and physical education programs including athletics, St. Louis, 1971, The C. V. Mosby Co.

Bucher, Charles A.: Administrative dimensions of health and physical education programs, including athletics, St. Louis, 1971, The C. V. Mosby Co.

Bucher, Charles A., and Reade, Evelyn M.: Physical education and health in the elementary school, New York, 1971, The Macmillan Co.

Bureau of Outdoor Recreation, U. S. Department of the Interior: Outdoor recreation action, published regularly by the Department of the Interior, Washington, D. C.

Donaldson, George W.: Journal of Outdoor Education, Northern Illinois University, DeKalb, Illinois (back and current issues).

Freeberg, William H.: Programs in outdoor education, Minneapolis, 1963, Burgess Publishing Co.

Gabrielsen, M. A., and Holtzer, Charles: Camping and outdoor education, New York, 1965, Library of Education, The Center for Applied Research in Education, Inc.

Knapp, H. G.: Outdoor science laboratories, Montana Education Journal **44:**19, 1967.

Leyh, Gene: Outdoor teaching, Today's Education **58:**27, 1969.

Loret, John: A happening in the out-of-doors, Journal of Health, Physical Education, and Recreation **40:**45, 1969.

Marsh, Norman F.: Outdoor education on your school grounds, State of California, The Resources Agency, Office of Conservation Education, Sacramento, 1968.

Outdoor education, Journal of Health, Physical Education, and Recreation **36:**75, 1965.

Report to the President and Congress by the Outdoor Recreation Resources Review Commission: Outdoor recreation in America, Washington, D. C., 1962, U. S. Government Printing Office.

Shivers, Jay S.: Camping, administration, counseling, programming, New York, 1971, Appleton-Century-Crofts.

Smith, Julian: AAHPER outdoor education project 1955-1970, Journal of Health, Physical Education, and Recreation **41:**44, 1970.

Smith, Julian W., and others: Outdoor education, Englewood Cliffs, New Jersey, 1963, Prentice-Hall, Inc.

Taft Campus Newsletter, published by Department of Outdoor Teacher Education, Northern Illinois University, Lorado Taft Field Campus at Oregon, Illinois (all issues).

PART FOUR

Changing concepts of physical education

11/Changing concepts from early times to modern European period
12/Changing concepts from beginning of modern European period to present
13/Movement education—a developing concept in physical education
14/International physical education in our contemporary world

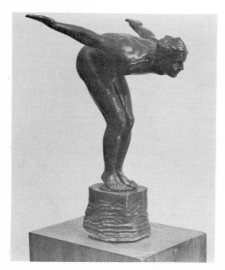

WORK OF R. TAIT
MCKENZIE. COURTESY JOSEPH
BROWN, SCHOOL OF ARCHITECTURE,
PRINCETON UNIVERSITY.

11/Changing concepts from early times to modern European period

The principal aim of gymnastics is the education of all youth and not simply that minority of people highly favored by Nature.

ARISTOTLE (350 B.C.)

Lack of activity destroys the good condition of every human being, while movement and methodical physical exercise save it and preserve it.

PLATO (380 B.C.)

Intellectual progress is conditioned at every step by bodily vigor. To attain the best results, physical exercises must accompany and condition mental training.

COMENIUS (1650)

If you would cultivate the intelligence of your pupil, cultivate the power that it is to govern. Give his body continual exercise.

ROUSSEAU (1750)

The greatest of follies is to sacrifice health for any other advantage.

SCHOPENHAUER (1850)

We do not yet sufficiently realize the truth that as, in this life of ours, the physical underlies the mental, the mental must not be developed at the expense of the physical. . . .

HERBERT SPENCER (1860)

I hope that here in America more and more the ideal of the well-trained and vigorous body will be maintained neck and neck with that of the well-trained and vigorous mind.

WILLIAM JAMES (1890)

The young child perhaps learns more and develops better through his play than through any other form of activity.

HERBERT S. JENNINGS (1917)

There is danger at the present time in the enthusiasm for the cramming of the brains of our young people with facts, scientific or otherwise, that there will be inadequate time for the establishment and perpetuation of physical fitness, which should never stop.

DR. PAUL DUDLEY WHITE (1960)*

It is interesting to note the various purposes for which physical education has existed in the lives of people of various countries and cultures. From the time of primitive man to the present, either directly or indirectly, physical activity has played a part in the lives of all people. Sometimes this activity has been motivated by such a factor as the necessity for earning a livelihood, whereas in other instances it has resulted from a desire to live a fuller life. Furthermore, it is clear that the objectives of physical education have changed over the course of history, so that at the present time they are directed at the better development of man, not only physically but also emotionally, socially, and intellectually. These changing concepts of physical education have come about as a result of many years of experience and study in regard to the values inherent in participating in physical activity under qualified leadership. This chapter proposes to briefly review the concepts of physical education in leading ancient and medieval civilizations.

---

*Quoted on a wrestling tournament program, January 29, 1963, Health and Physical Education Department, Norfolk, Virginia.

HISTORY OF PHYSICAL EDUCATION*

Let's roll back the years and let our minds wander
Back to the days of the Great Alexander,
When the Greeks' concern for strength and speed
Was geared to the objective of the nation's need.
There was reasonable pride in masculine muscle
And no person sneered at the concept of bustle,
And Demosthenes and Aristotle
Were pressing with logic the national throttle
The Grecian leaders in education
Had never heard of integration.
The Norsemen and Gauls had not yet bowed
To the power of Caesar and his Roman crowd.
Jousts and skill with the sword and bow
Were the accepted routine of the weekend show.
Came the Renaissance with its freedom new-born
Which sneered at the medieval as outmoded corn,
Jahn and Ling and old Guts Muths
Suddenly discovered the startling truths,
That the proper road to physical education
Could be trod only by regimentation.
And the Turnverein with emphasis formal
Was considered to be the training most normal.
Then Catherine Beecher and her calisthenics
Were accepted as the acme of rhythm mechanics,
Came Sargent's concept that human strength
Could be measured best by weight and length
But suddenly out of the routine and drill
The voice of free play arose with a shrill
Demand for concomitant outcome and aims
That could only be reached by a program of games.
Williams urged activities informal,
Obedience to command was considered abnormal,
Disciples were enlisted throughout the nation
Against the "whistle-blowers" and regimentation.
Williams held court in old York State

Along the Hudson with Nash, his mate.
Assisted by Brownell, Cassidy and others
They dried the sweat from their muscular brothers.
Then mental hygiene and safety and sex
Were solved at conventions so they'd no longer vex
The disciples of the new inanimation
Which some claimed was withering the legs of the nation.
Elmer Mitchell favored another variation
In the fields of intramurals and recreation.
The happy student found there was no need
To move around at the former high speed.
He could shoot his arrows and cast his flies
In a program which claimed to humanize.
But suddenly the Axis war machine
Challenged the disciples of the new routine,
The American youth who had trained in cars
And purportedly absorbed their rhythms in bars,
Were transformed o'ernight into Army sad-sacks
Trudging on foot with rifles and packs,
Thousands of miles all over the world
Wherever the Stars and Stripes were unfurled.
The scions of this soft and decadent nation
Which had taken the muscles out of education
Out-stouted, outfought, outlasted the men
Trained from the cradle in drill regimen.
Mussolini, then Hitler, then Tojo were taken,
Our boys lived on Spam and brought home the bacon.
Back from the wars to school and college
Once again in search of knowledge,
Where philosophers talk themselves into condition
And shudder at the evils of competition,
Youth continues to fight and to play,
To develop and grow in the time-honored way.
And the members of the world's greatest profession
By precept and deed in daily session,
Inspire and lead the youth of the nation
To prepare for citizenship and vocation.
The methods are varied, but the goal's within reach
So long as the teachers continue to teach.

*Gary, M. J.: Bulletin of Connecticut Association for Health, Physical Education, and Recreation, June, 1956.

PHYSICAL EDUCATION IN ANCIENT ORIENTAL NATIONS

Primitive society did not think of physical education as people do today. There was no organized physical education program in primitive society nor in the cultures of any of the ancient oriental nations. From the physical point of view, primitive man did not need to set aside a period during the day when he could participate in various forms of activity—activity was a part of his daily regimen. Well-developed bodies and sound organic systems were commonplace among primitive people. Their physical activity was obtained in the search for food, such as berries, fish, and wild game, in erecting shelters from the adverse elements, and in protecting themselves from a hostile environment.

History has shown that there are certain tendencies in man that have been responsible for his formal and informal participation in physical activity. Some of the more important of these throughout history have been the search for food to satisfy hunger, the desire for protection against enemies, innate drives for mating and propagation, the urge to manipulate brain and brawn, fear of the strange and unknown, and man's gregarious nature. Hunting, fishing, warfare, dancing, and play evolved as a result of these general tendencies exhibited by man. These explain to some extent why primitive man and all men in general have been prone to engage in motor activities whether they wanted to or not. Whether or not these activities should be characterized as "work" or as "play" depends upon the motive behind the participation in the activity. "Work" is characterized by need and necessity and is more or less compulsory. On the other hand, "play" is spontaneous, internally driven, and utilized for fun and relaxation.

Civilization has brought the need for an organized physical education program. As a result of labor-saving devices, sedentary pursuits, and security, the need has arisen for some type of planned program whereby individuals may realize the physical benefits that were once a part of early man's daily routine, as well as many emotional, sociological, psychological, and intellectual benefits. Therefore it is interesting to examine certain of these ancient countries in order to determine the part physical education played in the lives of their people. Through an understanding of the past or history of physical education, a person is better able to understand and interpret present-day physical education.

China

Ancient China followed a policy of isolation. It did not care to associate with the rest of the world but, instead, desired to live unto itself. At first, the topography of the land provided China with the necessary protection against invaders. When the Himalaya Mountains no longer served this purpose, the Great Wall was built; and when the wall became obsolete, laws were passed to keep invaders out of the country.

The fact that ancient China lived an isolated existence was detrimental in many ways to a belief in physical education. Since China did not fear aggression, it lacked the military motivating factor of being physically strong. Furthermore, the teachings of the people of ancient China were mainly concerned with memorizing the works of Confucius. Ancestor worship was also an important part of their religious life. Individuality was suppressed, and all persons were destined to live a rigid and stereotyped existence. In a country where such beliefs held sway, there was little room for organized physical education. Physical activity meant stress on the importance of the body and individual freedom of expression, which were contrary to the teachings in this ancient country. China felt secure behind its natural and manmade barriers and did not have an incentive to be physically strong, as was found in many of the ancient countries.

There were certain evidences of participation in physical education activities in China, however, despite the emphasis on intellectual excellence and the influences

Track and field training in a girls' school in Tainan, Taiwan.

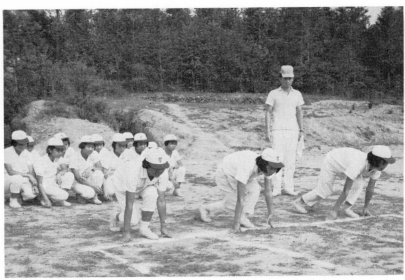

COURTESY DR. GUNSUN HOH, REPUBLIC OF CHINA.

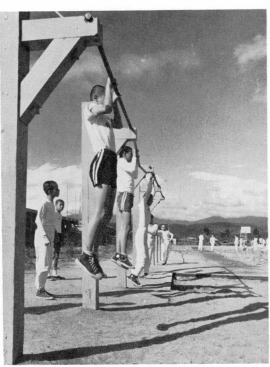

Chinese students chin themselves during physical education class.

COURTESY DR. GUNSUN HOH, REPUBLIC OF CHINA.

of Taoism, Confucianism, and Buddhism, which emphasized the studious, quiet, and contemplative life. In many Chinese classics there abound discussions of how sons of rich families engaged in music, dancing, and archery. Dancing especially was popular, with such special dances as "split-feather dance," "whole-feather dance," "regulating dance," "tail dance," "shield dance," "battle-axe dance," and the "humanity dance" being engaged in. Wrestling, jujitsu, boxing, football (ts' u chu), polo, tug-of-war, water games, ch' ui wan (in many respects similar to golf), shuttlecock, and flying kites were also popular.

It is interesting to note that the Chinese felt certain diseases were caused from inactivity. As a result, history discloses that the "Kong Fu" gymnastics were developed in 2698 B.C. These were medical gymnastics intended to keep the body in good organic condition. It was believed that illnesses were caused by internal stoppages and by malfunctioning of organs. Therefore, if certain kneeling, bending, lying, and standing exercises could be performed, together with certain types of respiratory training, the illness could be alleviated.

Although there does not seem to have been much participation in formal physical activities by the masses in early China, play was engaged in by the more favored classes.

India

Ancient India in many ways was similar to ancient China. People in this country lived an existence that was very religious in nature. Hinduism stressed the fact that man's soul passed through several reincarnations before being united with Brahma, the supreme goal. The quickest and most certain way to attain this goal was to refrain from catering to the body and enjoying worldly things. The person who desired to be holy ignored the physical needs of his body and concentrated solely on his spiritual needs. It can readily be seen that physical activity had little place in the culture of this religious people.

Buddha's prohibitions of games, amuse-ments, and exercises in ancient India did not totally prevent participation in such activities. Evidence is available as to such pastimes as dice, throwing balls, plowing contests, tumbling, chariot races, marbles, riding elephants and horses, swordsmanship, races, wrestling, boxing, and dancing. Yoga, an activity common in India and involving exercises in posture and regulated breathing, was very popular. This disciplining of mind and body required the instruction of experts, and a person fully trained in this activity followed a routine involving eighty-four different postures.

Ancient Near East

The civilizations of ancient Egypt, Assyria, Babylonia, Syria, Palestine, and Persia mark a turning point in the history of physical education. Whereas the objectives in China and India had stressed religious and intellectual matters, these countries were not restricted by a static society and religious ritual. On the contrary, they believed in living a full life. Therefore all types of physical activity contributed to this objective. It is in these countries that physical education also received an impetus from the military, who saw in it an opportunity to build stronger and more powerful armies.

Egyptian youths were reared in a manner involving much physical activity. While yet young boys, they were instructed in the use of various weapons of war, such as bow and arrow, battle-axe, mace, lance, and shield. They were required to participate in exercises and activities designed to make the body supple, strong, and capable of great endurance and stamina. These activities included marching, running, jumping, wrestling, pirouetting, and leaping. Before their military training started they had numerous opportunities to engage in many sports and gymnastic exercises. They also found great enjoyment in going on hunting and fishing expeditions.

In the countries between the Tigris and Euphrates rivers, there was also great stress placed upon physical education activities. This was especially true of the upper classes.

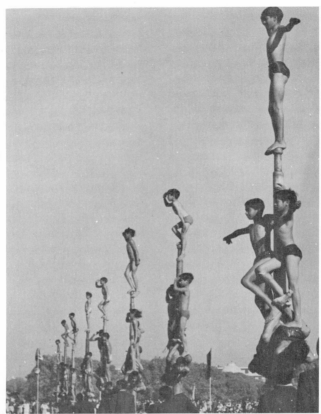

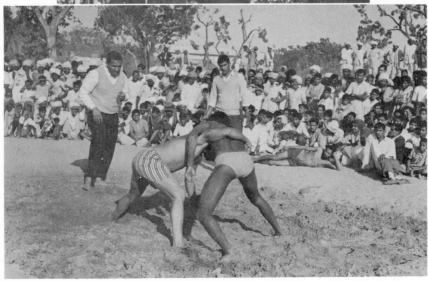

Physical education activity in India.

Whereas the lower social strata of the population found few opportunities for recreation and play, the upper classes indulged themselves in these pastimes at regular intervals. Horsemanship, use of bow and arrow, water activities, and training in physical exercises were considered on a par with instruction that was more intellectual in character.

Persia is a good example of a state that had as its main objective the building of an empire through military aggression. A strong Persian army meant a healthy and physically fit army. Under King Cyrus the Great, the imperialistic dreams of Persia were realized. At the end of his rule in 529 B.C., the Persian Empire encompassed the area that we refer to today as the Near East. The success of King Cyrus' campaigns was largely the result of the moral and physical conditioning of his soldiers. At the age of 6 years, the state took all boys away from their homes for training. This training consisted of such events as running, slinging, shooting with a bow, throwing the javelin, riding, hunting, and marching. The soldier had to be able to travel without much food and clothing and was compelled to endure all sorts of hardship.

Intellectual training was thought useless in a state that depended upon a strong army to realize its ambitions. Physical education was aimed at imperialistic ends. The program of physical activity was directed toward building strength and power in each member of the armed forces, with the major objective of destruction, conquest, and aggrandizement. Strength, endurance, stamina, agility, and other physical characteristics were not developed so that the individual could live a full, vigorous, and more interesting life but, instead, so that the state could utilize these physical attributes in achieving its own selfish aims. In directing physical education toward such ends, this profession loses one of its most vital potentialities—that of helping to build a peaceful world characterized by objectives aimed at the development of each individual's capacities to their fullest extent.

PHYSICAL EDUCATION IN GREECE

Physical education experienced a "golden age" in ancient Greece. The Greeks strove for physical perfection, and this objective affected all phases of their life. It had its influence on the political and educational systems, on sculpturing and painting, and in the thinking and writings of that day. It was a unifying force in Greek life, played a major part in the national festivals, and helped in building strong military establishments. No country in history has held physical education in such high respect as did ancient Greece.

As early as 3000 B.C. there were evidences of physical education activities being popular in Cretan culture. Archeological investigations at Mycenae and other centers of Aegean civilization have unearthed buildings, pottery, and other materals that point to the important place of physical education in this ancient culture. Literature such as Homer's *Iliad* and *Odyssey* also is a source of this information. Hunting seems to have been one of the most popular pastimes in this era. Lion hunting, deer hunting, bull grappling, boxing, wrestling, dancing, and swimming are commonly referred to by historians who have written about these ancient civilizations.

Physical education was a vital part of the education of every boy in Greece. Gymnastics and music were considered the two most important subjects. Music was for the spirit and gymnastics was for the body. "Exercise for the body and music for the soul" was a common pronouncement. Gymnastics, it was believed, contributed to courage, discipline, and physical well-being. Furthermore, gymnastics stressed a sense of fair play, development of the individual esthetic values, amateurism, and the utilitarian values inherent in the activity. Professionalism was frowned upon. An individual ran, wrestled, jumped, danced, or threw the javelin not for reward but for what it would do for his body. Beauty of physique was stressed, and everyone participated in the nude, which motivated development of the "body beautiful."

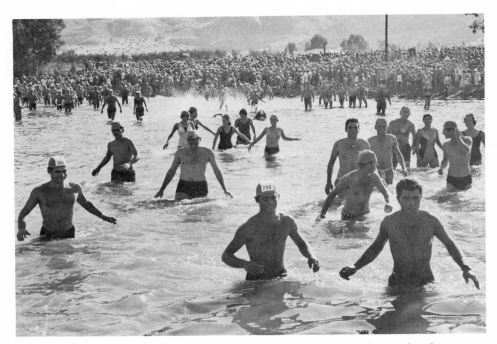

Modern-day Israel emphasizes mass recreational activities. Five thousand swimmers participate in a popular crossing of the Sea of Galilee.

Because of the topography of the land and for various political reasons, Greece was composed of several city-states, each exercising its own sovereignty and existing as a separate entity. It waged war and conducted all of its affairs separately from the other city-states. This situation had an influence not only on the political aspects of each city-state but also on the objectives of physical education within each state. Sparta and Athens exemplify two such city-states.

In Sparta, a city-state in the Peloponnesus district of Greece, the main objective of physical education was to contribute to a strong and powerful army. The individual in Sparta existed for the state. He was subservient to the state and was required to help defend it against all enemies. Women as well as men were required to be in good physical condition. It was believed that healthy and strong mothers would bear healthy and strong sons, which in turn would strengthen the state. It is believed that Spartan women may have begun their physical conditioning as early as 7 years of age and continued gymnastics in public until they were married. Newborn infants, if found to be defective or weak, were left on Mount Taygetus to die. Only strong and vigorous babies were welcome in this military state. Woody points out that mothers bathed babies in wine to test their bodies and to temper them for future ordeals. A boy was allowed to stay at home only for the first 6 years of his life. After this he was required to stay in the public barracks and entered the agoge, a system of public, compulsory training, where he underwent a very vigorous and rigid training schedule. If he failed in this ordeal, he was deprived of all future honors. A major part of this training consisted of such physical activities as wrestling, jumping, running, throwing the javelin and discus, marching, horseback riding, and hunting. This conditioning program secured for Sparta a strong army that was second to none. However, it was developed at the expense of personal freedom.

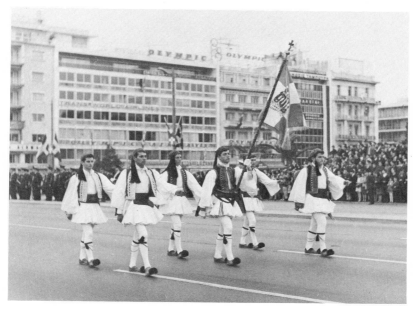

Greece.

Athens, a city-state in eastern Greece, was the antithesis of Sparta. Here the democratic way of life flourished, and consequently it had a great bearing on the objectives of physical education. Athens did not control and regulate the individual's life as rigidly as Sparta. In Athens the people enjoyed the freedom that is characteristic of a truly democratic government. Although the military emphasis was not as strong in Athens as in Sparta, the emphasis on physical education was just as great or greater. Athenians engaged in physical activity to develop their bodies, for the esthetic values, and to live a fuller and more vigorous life. An ideal of Athenian education was to achieve a proper balance in moral, mental, physical, and esthetic development. To the Hellenes, man was a whole, and he was as strong as his weakest part. One part of him could not be sound if the other parts were not also sound.

Gymnastics for the youth were practiced in the palaestra, a building that provided rooms for various physical activities, for oiling and sanding their bodies, and an open space for such activities as jumping and wrestling. The proprietor of the palaes-

tra was called a paidotribe (from the Greek word *paidotribes,* meaning demonstrator). He was responsible for demonstrating the exercises and games to the Greek youth. He demonstrated the exercises called for by the *gymnastis,* the head physical educator. The *gymnastis* was the man who planned the activity program and diet for each member. A third person in the palaestra was the *alyptis* or masseur. There were also flute players, since many activities were conducted with music.

Some of the more noted palaestras were those of Taureas, Timeas, and Siburtios. The paidotribe was similar to a present-day physical educator. He taught many activities, understood how certain exercises should be adapted to various physical conditions, knew how to develop strength and endurance, and was an individual who could be trusted with children in the important task of making youthful bodies serve their minds. As a boy approached manhood, he deserted the palaestra and attended the gymnasium.

Gymnasiums became the physical, social, and intellectual centers of Greece. Although the first use was for physical activity, such men as Plato, Aristotle, and Antisthenes were responsible for making such gymnasiums as the Academy, Lyceum, and Kynosarges outstanding intellectual centers as well. Youth usually entered the gymnasium at about 14 to 16 years of age. Here special sports and exercises received the main attention under expert instruction. Although activities that had been engaged in at the palaestra were continued, other sports such as riding, driving, racing, and hunting were added. Instruction in the gymnasium was given by a paidotribe and also a gymnast. The paidotribe had charge of the general physical training program, whereas the gymnast was a specialist responsible for training youth in gymnastic contests. The chief official at the gymnasium, in overall charge of the entire program, was called a gymnasiarch. In keeping with the close association between physical education and religion, each gymnasium recognized a particular deity. For example, the Academy recognized Athena; the Lyceum, Apollo; and Kynosarges, Hercules.

The national festivals were events that were most important in the lives of the Greeks and were also very important in laying the foundation for our modern Olympic games, which are conducted every fourth year in various parts of the world. These national festivals were in honor of some hero or divinity. They consisted of feasting, dancing, singing, and events involving physical prowess. Although there were many of these national festivals conducted in all parts of Greece, four of them are of special importance and attracted national attention. The first and most famous of the four was the Olympia festival in honor of Zeus, the supreme god, which was held in the western Peloponnesus district. Another was the Pythia festival in honor of Apollo, the god of light and truth, held at Delphi, which was located north of the Corinthian Gulf. A third was the Nemea festival held in honor of Zeus at Argolis near Cleonae. The fourth was the Isthmia festival in honor of Poseidon, the god of the sea; it was held on the isthmus of Corinth. Athletic events were the main attraction and drawing force in each. People came from all over Greece to see the games. At Olympia the stadium provided standing space for approximately 40,000 spectators.

During the time the games were held, a truce was declared by all the city-states in Greece, and it was believed that if this truce were broken the wrath of the gods would be visited upon the guilty. By the middle of the fifth century this truce probably lasted for 3 months.

A rigid set of requirements had to be met before anyone could participate as a contestant in the games. For example, the contestant had to be in training for 10 months; he had to be a free man; he had to be of perfect physique and of good character; he could not have any criminal record; and he had to compete in accordance with the rules. An oath also had to be taken that he would not use illegal tactics to win, to which fathers, brothers, and trainers also had to swear. Once enrolled for a contest, the athlete had to compete. Physical unfitness was not a good excuse. Events consisted of such feats as foot racing, throwing the javelin, throwing the discus, wrestling, high jumping, broad jumping, weight throwing, boxing, and horse racing. The victor in these events did not receive any material reward for his victory. Instead, a wreath of olive branches was presented. However, he was a hero in everyone's eyes and had many receptions given in his honor. Furthermore, he had many privileges bestowed upon him by his home city-state. To be crowned a victor in an Olympic event was to receive the highest honor that could be bestowed in Greece. The Olympic games were first held in 776 B.C. and continued every fourth year thereafter until abolished by the Romans in A.D. 394. However, they have since been resumed and today are held every fourth year in a different country.*

Physical education in ancient Greece will always be looked upon with pride by members of this profession. The high ideals that

---

*For an evaluation of Olympic games, see Bucher, Charles A.: Sports Illustrated, August 8, 1955; Reader's Digest, September, 1955.

motivated the various gymnastic events are objectives that all should try to emulate. Such great men of history as Socrates, Plato, Aristotle, Hippocrates, and Galen proclaimed their value for all. The large expanse of ruins excavated at Olympia and the relics, sculptures, and statues, especially the one of Hermes by Praxixteles, are evidence of the emphasis on physical perfection and pride in Hellenic culture that exalted Greek civilization.

Another aim of physical education held by the Greeks was that in addition to serving as a recreational pursuit and as an aid to esthetic development, physical education should also be utilized as therapy for the infirm and for the diseased. The growth of this phase of physical education was stimulated as a result of increased medical knowledge and of a social trend in later Greek history. Many individuals, because of wealth and idleness, obtained inadequate exercise and indulged in luxurious living at the expense of their health. Adapted physical exercise proved to have therapeutic value in many such cases. By paying attention to diet and exercise, health could be enhanced.

The use of physical education as an aid to medicine can be identified as early as the middle of the fifth century B.C. Its worth was also emphasized by outstanding Greeks at later dates. Galen stated that physical education is a part of hygiene and subordinate to medicine. Hippocrates proclaimed the law of use, stating that through use all parts of the body are kept in a state of good health, whereas disuse results in imperfect development and ill health. He also pointed out that some exercises are natural, whereas others are violent, and that many should be engaged in on a progressive basis. Hippocrates divided the year into the four seasons and recommended suitable diet and exercise for each. For example, in the winter one should eat lightly, and exercise should be procured by engaging in many kinds of activity. He listed running on the double, wrestling, and brisk walks as possible sources of activity.

In concluding this section on Greek phys-

ical education, the views of certain outstanding philosophers and Greek leaders to whom the world today turns for understanding and intellectual insights are recorded.

Socrates stressed the general utility of physical education and the importance of health in achieving life's purposes. He pointed out that even in thinking, where it appears the body is used very little, bad health can contribute to grave mistakes.

Plato recognized the importance of physical education for both men and women. He thought that both physical education and music were important phases of education.

Aristotle held that the body and soul are closely interrelated and that mental faculties are affected by bodily movement and conditions of body health. He thought that one should engage in lighter exercises such as dancing, running, jumping, and throwing until 14 or 15 years of age. Heavier exercises could be engaged in later. Excessive or deficient exercise, he stressed, is similar to excessive or deficient food and drink; both result in harm to the body. Physical education should help one to live a virtuous life and not one of conquest.

Xenophon, a contemporary of Plato, thought of physical education as important for the development of a strong army. He felt that soundness of body and of mind was essential to success in life. However, Xenophon's main thoughts were of war, and his thinking in regard to physical education was mainly in terms of the military.

PHYSICAL EDUCATION IN ROME

While the Hellenes were settling in the Grecian peninsula about 200 B.C., another Indo-European people was migrating to Italy and settling in the central and southern parts of this country. One of these wandering tribes, known in history as Latins, settled near the Tiber River, a settlement that later became known as Rome. The Romans were to have a decided effect not only upon the objectives of physical education in their own state but also upon that of the Greek world, which they conquered.

The Romans, through their great leaders

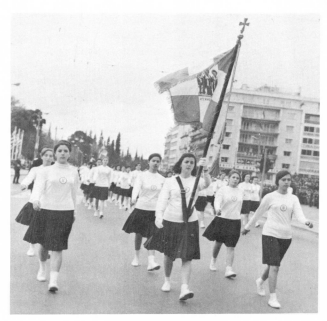

Greece.

and well-disciplined army, extended their influence throughout most of the Mediterranean area and the whole of Europe. However, this success on the battlefield brought influences into Roman life that affected Roman ideals. Many Romans became interested in material things as a result of the conquests. They were not truly interested in the cultural aspects of life, although sometimes some of the finer aspects of Hellenic culture were taken on as a means of show. Wealth became the objective of most citizens, and vulgar display became the essence of wealth. Luxury, corruption, extravagance, and vice became commonplace in the various phases of Roman living.

In respect to physical education, the average Roman believed that exercise was good only for health and military purposes. He did not see the value of play as an enjoyable pastime. During the period of conquest, when Rome was following its strong imperialistic policy and before the time of professional troops, citizens were liable for military service from 17 to 60 years of age. Consequently, during this period of

Roman history, army life was considered very important, and physical activity was considered essential in order to be in good physical shape and ready to serve the state at a moment's notice. Soldiers followed a rigid training schedule that consisted of such things as marching, running, jumping, swimming, and throwing the javelin and discus. However, during the last century of the Republic, mercenary troops were used, with the result that the objectives of physical training were not considered as important for the average Roman. As a spectator, he could enjoy life without all this waste of time building up the body.

After the conquest of Greece, Greek gymnastics were introduced to the Romans, but they were never well received. The Romans lacked the drive for clean competition. They did not believe in developing the "body beautiful." They did not like nakedness of performers. They preferred to be spectators rather than participants. They preferred cruel, gory, gruesome games to clean, wholesome events played for the benefit of the participants. They preferred professionalism to amateurism.

Roman dislike of Greek physical education was voiced in numerous ways. Cicero thought the physical exercises performed by the Greeks were absurd. Scipio was criticized for going to the palaestra. Horace felt the Greek system did not develop endurance and stamina enough for the Roman. Martial referred sarcastically to the wrestling grounds of Greece. Tacitus criticized the habit of taking off one's clothes to exercise.

Athletic sports were not conducted on the same high level as in ancient Greece. The Roman wanted something exciting, bloody, ghastly, and sensational. At the chariot races and gladiatorial combats, excitement ran high. Men were pitted against wild animals or against one another and fought to the death in order to satisfy the craving of the Roman for excitement and brutality. Frequently large groups of men fought each other in mortal battle before thousands of pleased spectators.

The rewards and incomes of some individuals who engaged in the chariot races were enormous. Diocles of Spain retired at 42 years of age, having won 1,462 of 4,257 races and rewards totaling in the neighborhood of $2 million. Other famous contestants were Thallus, Crescens, and Scorpus.*

The thermae and the Campus Martius in Rome took the place of the gymnasium in Greece. The thermae were the public baths, where provision was also made for exercise, and the Campus Martius was an exercise ground on the outskirts of the city. Most of the exercise was recreational in nature.

Many leaders in physical education have drawn parallels between Roman conditions and those that prevail in present-day United States. In making these comparisons, they raise the question as to whether the United States is following the same road that Rome followed. They point to the influence of wealth and materialism on our way of life, the political corruption that exists, the class struggle, the passing out of doles, the cry for "bread and games," the professionalism in the world of athletics, the desire of thousands of Americans to see pugilists knock each other into unconsciousness, the growing habit of being a spectator rather than a participant, and the desire to please and help the individual in the gallery rather than the participant, on the field.

PHYSICAL EDUCATION DURING THE DARK AGES

The fall of the Roman Empire in the west about 476 A.D. resulted in a period of history that is frequently referred to as the Dark Ages. This period, however, was anything but dark in respect to the physical rejuvenation brought about by the overrunning of the Roman Empire by the Teutonic barbarians.

Before considering the Dark Ages, it is interesting for the student of physical education to note a cause of the fall of Rome, which brought on this new period in history. Historians list many causes for the breakdown of the Roman Empire, but the most outstanding cause was the physical and moral decay of the Roman people. The type of life the Romans led, characterized by divorce, games, and suicide, caused a decrease in population. Extravagance, doles, slave labor, and misuse of public funds caused moral depravity and economic ruin; luxurious living, vice, and excesses caused poor health and physical deterioration. The lesson is borne out in Rome, as it has been in many civilizations

---

*At the site where once the inhabitants of Rome yelled with delight at the skill and daring of their favorite charioteers and gladiators, Romans of today are applauding the exploits of soccer players, who have replaced the chariot drivers and slaves in the public estimation.

The Circus Maximus, the oldest and greatest of the Roman circuses, was situated at the foot of the Palatine Hill and dated back to the last king of Rome, Tarquinius the Younger (534-510 B.C.). It reached its greatest splendor in imperial times and seated as many as 200,000 persons. It reached its final form under Trajan (A.D. 53-117). The Rome Municipal Council decided that this unusual site, formerly occupied by the Circus Maximus, should be transformed into a sports center.

that have fallen along the way, that in order for a nation to remain strong and endure it must be physically as well as morally fit.

As a morally and physically weak Roman Empire crumbled, morally and physically strong Teutonic barbarians overran the lands that once were the pride of the Latins. The Visigoths overran Spain, the Vandals overran North Africa, the Franks and Burgundians overran Gaul, the Angles and Saxons overran Britain, and the Ostrogoths overran Italy. These invasions brought about the lowest ebb in literature and learning known to history. The so-called cultural aspects of living were disregarded. Public works projects were neglected. Bridges and buildings were allowed to collapse. In government, centralization of authority began to be abandoned, and in its place, tribes looked to their chieftains or lords for protection.

Despite all the backwardness that accompanied the invasions in respect to learning, public works, and government, and resulted in the name "Dark Ages" being attached to this period of history, the entire world still received physical benefits. The Teutonic barbarians were a nomadic people who lived out of doors on simple fare. They were mainly concerned with a life characterized by hunting, caring for their cattle and sheep, and participating in vigorous outdoor sports and warfare. A regimen such as this built strong and physically fit bodies and well-ordered nervous systems. The Teutonic barbarians came at a time when the physical deterioration caused by the excesses in Rome needed a change. They helped to guarantee a stronger, healthier, and more robust stock of future generations of people.

Asceticism and scholasticism

Although the Teutonic invasions of the Dark Ages supported the value of physical activity, two other movements during approximately this same period in history worked to its disadvantage—asceticism and scholasticism.

Out of pagan and immoral Rome, Christianity and asceticism grew and thrived. Certain individuals in ancient Rome became incensed with the immorality and the worldliness that existed in Roman society. They believed in "rendering unto Caesar the things that are Caesar's and unto God the things that are God's." They would not worship the Roman gods, attend the baths, or visit the games. They did not believe in worldly pleasures and catered to the spirit and not to the body. They believed that this life should be used as a means of preparing for the next world. They thought that all sorts of physical activity were foolish pursuits in that they were designed to improve the body. The body was evil and should be tortured rather than improved. They preached that the mind and body were distinct and separate entities in man and that one had no bearing on the other. A Christian emperor, Theodosius, abolished the Olympic games in 394 A.D. as being pagan.

The spread of Christianity resulted in the rise of asceticism. This was the belief that evil exists in the body, and therefore it should be subordinated to the spirit, which is pure. Worldly pursuits are evil, and one should spend his time by being alone and meditating. The body is possessed of the devil and should be tortured. Individuals wore hair shirts, walked on hot coals, sat upon thorns, carried chains around their legs, and exposed themselves to the elements so that they might bring their worldly body under better control. Such practices led to poor health and shattered nervous systems on the part of many.

As Christianity spread, there also developed monasteries where Christians could isolate themselves from the world and its evils. Later, schools were attached to these monasteries, but it can be readily understood that any institution so clearly associated with early Christianity would not allow physical education to become a part of the curriculum. The medieval university also frowned upon physical education, thinking it unimportant in the lives of students.

Another influence that has had a major

impact on the history of physical education is scholasticism. This is the belief that facts are the most essential items in one's education. If one knows the facts, if one has developed his mental and intellectual powers, he will have the key to a successful life. It deemphasized the physical as being unimportant and unnecessary. This movement, developed among the scholars and universities of the Middle Ages, has been passed down from generation to generation and still plagues physical educators today. In many leading universities and among many outstanding scholars, there still is a tendency to disregard the physical as not having any relationship to the mental. A dean of a famous college in the East recently referred to the gymnasium as a "muscle factory," and from his speech one could readily discern that for him it existed only as a necessary evil. Scholasticism presents a challenge to physical education. Only through a true interpretation of the values inherent in physical education under proper guidance can a respected position for physical education be secured in the schools of this country.

PHYSICAL EDUCATION DURING THE AGE OF FEUDALISM

As a result of the decentralization of government during the period of the Dark Ages, the period of feudalism came into being. Although Charlemagne established an empire over which he ruled effectively for some time, his death in 814 marked the disintegration of his empire, and it crumbled almost immediately. For the next few centuries effective, centralized leadership was lacking. A new social order was established. The period during which this social order existed is called the period of feudalism and extended between the ninth and fourteenth centuries. The type of government, judicial system, human relations, methods of waging warfare, land ownership, industry, and social life were all affected by feudalistic practices.

The feudalistic period appeared because man needed protection, and since there was a shortage of strong monarchs and governments that could supply this protection, the people turned to noblemen and others who built castles, had large land holdings, and made themselves strong. Feudalism was a system of land tenure based upon allegiance and service to the nobleman or lord. The lord who owned the land, called a fief, let it out to a subordinate who was called his vassal. In return for the use of this land the vassal owed his allegiance and certain obligations to his lord. The large part of the population, however, was made up of serfs, who worked the land and shared little in the profits. They were attached to the land and, as it was transferred from vassal to vassal, they were also transferred.

The lord lived on a large estate or manor that was a self-sufficient community in itself. The house or castle was usually erected on an easily defensible site and was quite frequently surrounded by high walls and a moat.

There were two careers open to sons of noblemen during feudalistic times. They might enter training for the church and become members of the clergy, or they might enter chivalry and become knights. If they decided in favor of the church, they pursued an education that was religious and academic in nature, and if they decided in favor of chivalry, they pursued an education that was physical, social, and military in nature. To the average boy, chivalry had much more appeal than the church.

The training that a boy experienced in becoming a knight was long and thorough. Physical training played a major role during this period. At the age of 7 years a boy was usually sent to the castle of some nobleman for training and as preparation for knighthood. First, he was known as a page, and his instructor and teacher was usually one of the women in the lord's castle. During his tenure as a page, a boy learned court etiquette, waited on tables, ran errands, and helped with household tasks. During the rest of the time he participated in various forms of physical activity that would serve him well as a knight and that would harden and strengthen him for the arduous years ahead. He practiced for such events as boxing, running, fencing, jumping, and swimming.

At the age of 14 years the boy became a squire and was attached to some knight. His duties included keeping the knight's weapons in good condition, caring for his horses, helping him with his armor, attending to his injuries, and guarding his prisoners. During the time the boy was a squire, there was more and more emphasis placed on physical training. He was continually required to engage in vigorous sports and exercises, such as hunting, scaling walls, shooting with the bow, running, swordsmanship, horsemanship, and climbing.

If the squire proved his fitness, he became a knight at 21 years of age. The ceremony through which he passed to become a knight was very solemn and memorable. The prospective knight took a bath of purification, dressed in white, and spent an entire night in meditation and prayer. In the morning the lord placed his sword on the knight's shoulder, a ceremony known as the accolade; this marked the conferring of knighthood.

Jousts and tournaments were two special events in which all knights engaged several times during their lifetime. These special events served both as amusement and as training for battle. In the jousts, two knights attempted to unseat one another from their horses with blows from lances and by skill in horsemanship. In tournaments many knights were utilized in a program designed to exhibit the skill and showmanship that the knights had gained during their long period of training. They were lined up as two teams at each end of the lists, as the grounds were called, and upon a signal they attempted to unseat the members of the opposing team. This meleé kept on until one team was declared the victor. Many of the knights wore their lady's colors on their armor and attempted with all their strength and skill to uphold her honor. During these tournaments death often resulted for many participants. It was during these exhibitions that a knight had the oppor-

tunity to display his personal bravery, skill, prowess, strength, and courage.

Physical education played a major part in preparing for chivalry. The objective of physical education, however, was for the purpose of self-preservation only. There were no objectives as worthy as those in Greece, which collectively aimed at total individual development. Before the invention of gunpowder and while there was no centralized government, men had to depend on physical strength, endurance, stamina, and skill to keep them alive. Consequently, physical education was a contributing factor to their day-to-day living.

PHYSICAL EDUCATION DURING THE RENAISSANCE

The transitional period in history between the dark years of the medieval period and the beginning of modern times, the fourteenth to sixteenth centuries, was known as the period of the Renaissance and was an age of great progress for mankind.

During the medieval period men lacked originality. Individuality was a lost concept, and interest in the hereafter was so prevalent that men did not enjoy the present. The Renaissance caused a change in this way of life. There was a revival or rebirth of learning, a belief in the dignity of man, a renewed spirit of nationalism, an increase of trade among countries, and a period of exploration. Scientific research was used to solve problems; books were printed and thereby made available to more people; and there was a renewed interest in the classics. This period is associated with such names as Petrarch, Boccacio, Michelangelo, Erasmus, da Vinci, da Gama, Columbus, Galileo, and Harvey.

The Renaissance period also had an impact upon physical education. With more attention being placed on enjoyment of the present and the development of the body, asceticism lost its hold on the masses. During the Renaissance the theory that the body and the soul were inseparable, that they were indivisible, and that one was necessary for the optimum functioning of the other became more popular. It was believed that learning could be promoted through good physical health. A person needed rest and recreation from study and work. The body needed to be developed for purposes of health and for preparation for warfare.

Some outstanding leaders in the Renaissance period who were responsible for spreading these beliefs concerning physical education are mentioned briefly.

Vittorino da Feltra (1378–1446) taught in the court schools of northern Italy and was believed to be one of the first teachers to combine physical and mental training in a school situation. He incorporated daily exercises in the curriculum, which included dancing, riding, fencing, swimming, wrestling, running, jumping, archery, hunting, and fishing. His objectives of physical education emphasized that it was good for disciplining the body, for preparation for war, and for rest and recreation and that good physical condition helped children learn other subject matter much better.

Pietro Vergerio (1349–1428) of Padua and Florence wrote a treatise entitled *De Ingenius Moribus,* in which the following objectives were emphasized: physical education is necessary for the total education of the individual, as preparation for warfare, to better undergo strain and hardship, as a means of fortifying the mind and body, as an essential for good health, and as a means of recreation to give a lift to the spirit and the body.

Pope Pius II's (1405–1464) objectives of physical education were good posture, body health, and aid to learning.

Sir Thomas Elyot (1490–1546) of England wrote the treatise on education entitled *The Governor,* which elaborated on such objectives of physical education as recreation and physical benefits to the body.

Martin Luther (1483–1546), the leader of the Protestant Reformation, did not preach asceticism as a means of salvation. He saw in physical education a substitute for vice and evil pursuits during leisure hours such as gambling and drinking, a means of obtaining elasticity of the body, and a medium of promoting one's health.

François Rabelais (1490–1553), a French educational theorist, emphasized the objectives of physical welfare, the fact that physical education is an important part of education and aids in mental training, and that it is good preparation for warfare.

Roger Asham (1515–1568), professor at Cambridge in England, proclaimed the value of physical education as a preparation for war and as a means of resting the mind.

John Milton (1608–1674), the English poet, expressed his views on physical education in his *Tractate on Education.* In this treatise he discussed how physical education helps in body development, is a means of recreation, and is good preparation for warfare.

John Locke (1632–1704), famous English philosopher and a student of medicine, supported physical education in a work entitled *Some Thoughts Concerning Education.* His objectives could be summed up under health as a means of meeting emergencies involving hardships and fatigue and as a means of having a vigorous body at one's command.

Michel de Montaigne (1533–1592), a French essayist, stressed that physical education was necessary for both body and soul and that it was impossible to divide an individual into two such components, since they are indivisible and together comprise the human being being trained.

John Comenius (1592–1671), a Bohemian educational reformer, and *Richard Mulcaster* (1530–1611), an English schoolmaster, had as their objectives of physical education a means of maintaining health and physical fitness and a means of obtaining rest from study.

Jean Jacques Rousseau (1712–1778), a French writer, in his book *Emile* points out what he considers to be an ideal education. In this education, physical education would contribute to the objectives of health and a vigorous body. He stressed that the mind and body are an indivisible entity in man and that both are bound together.

The Renaissance period helped to interpret the worth of physical education to the public in general. It also demonstrated how a society that promotes the dignity and freedom of the individual and recognizes the value of human life will also place in high respect the development and maintenance of the human body. The belief became prevalent that physical education is necessary for health, as a preparation for warfare, as a means of developing the body, and as a means of providing recreation for the wealthier classes. However, at that point in history, society failed to recognize universally, to any degree, the important contributions that physical education can make to the esthetic, social, and moral life of society.

SOME POPULAR SPORTS AND THE COUNTRIES OR CULTURES MOST OFTEN CREDITED WITH THEIR ORIGIN OR MODERN FORM OF PLAY

Sport	Origin
Archery	England
Badminton	India
Baseball	United States
Basketball	United States
Billiards	Egypt
Bowling	Egypt
Boxing	Sumeria
Cricket	England
Croquet (roque)	France
Curling	Scotland
Fencing	Germany
Field events	Greece
Field hockey	Greece and Persia
Fives (handball)	Ireland
Football	England
Golf	Scotland
Gymnastics	Greece
Horseracing	England
Horseshoes	Greece
Hurling	Ireland
Ice hockey	Canada
Ice skating	Scandinavia
Jai alai	Spain
Judo	Japan
Jujitsu	China
Lacrosse	North American Indians
Lawn bowls	England
Paddle tennis	England

Sport	Origin
Platform tennis	United States
Polo	India
Quoits	England
Shuffleboard	Persia
Skiing	Scandinavia
Skin diving	South Sea Islands
Soccer	Rome
Softball	United States
Speedball	United States
Squash rackets	England
Squash tennis	United States
Surfing	Polynesia
Swimming	England
Table tennis	England
Target rifle shooting	British Isles
Tennis	France
Track events	Greece
Volleyball	United States
Water polo	England
Water skiing	France
Weight lifting	Egypt and Japan
Wrestling	Sumeria
Yacht racing	England

ORIGINS OF WORDS AND TERMS COMMONLY USED IN PHYSICAL EDUCATION*

Although our language and speech comes from all over the world, it is very interesting how various terms and words have entered the field of physical education. Many words and terms have passed through languages from all corners of the globe before reaching the United States. It is hoped that the reader will find the origins of these words and terms useful as well as interesting reading and study. For further information, consult the references at the end of this chapter.

Amateur (ăm á tûr; ăm á tur). Amateur comes from the Latin meaning lover *(amator)*. The term was first used to indicate those athletes who won events in the Olympic games but refused to capitalize commercially on their fame. The present Anglo-Saxon spelling was given to the word in the late eighteenth century. The term was used to distinguish "Gentleman Jack Jackson" from the fighters of his

---

*I am indebted to Robert N. Kasper, teacher of health and physical education at Macomb's Junior High School, New York, New York, for his research concerning the origin of the words and terms listed.

time who fought for money. He was an amateur since he would not fight for profit.

Archer (är' chor). From the Latin *arcus,* or bow, referring to a person who uses a bow and arrow.

Arena (à rē'na). Arena is the Latin word for sand. There was so much bloodshed in the gladiatorial contests in the Roman amphitheaters that sand was liberally distributed on the ground to soak up the blood. The place of combat obtained its named from the sand.

Athlete (ăth'lēt). *Athlos* referred to a Greek contest and *Athlon* to a prize. An athlete was one who contended for a prize in a contest. The meaning for this term, therefore, has been used since the time of the Greeks and the Olympic games.

Ball (bôl). Originally, a voter put a black or white ball into a special box when he cast a secret ballot. Now the word refers to any spherically shaped object and is derived from the Middle English word *bal.*

Bowl (bōl). A bowl is a weighted ball that is used for the game called bowling. The phrase "to throw" refers to the release of the spherical object known as a bowl.

Box (bŏks). This word is derived from the Greek *pyxos,* or box tree. In the sport of boxing, the ring is box shaped, and the clenched fist blows of the combatants are "boxes" or cuffs.

Canoe (kà'nōō'). The canoe was used in China, Polynesia, Africa, and other places. It did not originate with the American Indian. Some of the members of Christopher Columbus' crew borrowed the word from the Haitian *kanoa* and took it back to Spain. The term came to America from Spain and originally referred to a dugout made from a hollowed log.

Coach (kōch). The word *coach* comes from the vehicle also called coach. The maker of the first coach vehicle lived in a town in Hungary called Koszi or Kocsi. The word comes from the name of this town. A coach in the sports sense is one who carries the athlete along.

Contest (kŏn'test). The word *contest* comes from the Latin *contestari,* meaning to call witness. When we break this down further, we have (*con* + *testari,* to be a witness). When you have witnesses arraigned on both sides, you have a contest.

Circus (sûr kus). The word *circus* comes from the Latin *circulus,* meaning a small ring. The Romans had a very large building in Rome that housed a large ring. This structure was called the Circus Maximus. The great shows and spectacles were held in the Circus Maximus during Roman times. The enclosure had a track or large ring laid out for chariot races, games, and other activities.

Drill (drĭl). It is through a pun on the word *bore*

that the word has been applied to the exercises in which soldiers engage. The word is derived from the Dutch *drillen,* meaning to pierce or to bore. All drills turn round and round and bore, as do soldiers in many of their exercises turn in various formations.

Exhibition (ĕk'sĭ bĭsh'ŭn). The word exhibition is from the French and Latin *exhibeo: ex,* meaning out, and *habeo,* meaning hold. This takes its meaning from the fact that at exhibitions the artist holds out his pictures so that others may see them.

Exercise (ĕk'ser sīz). To exorcise is to chase out the demons, and to exercise is to let out the animals (to keep them at work). This is from the Latin *ex,* meaning out, and *arcere,* meaning to confine, enclose. The original sense of the word is expressed in the statement "Don't get exercised" or all worked up.

Fan (făn). A *fan* is one who goes into a frenzy about a particular sport or interest. He is an ardent admirer and devotee. During Roman times some priests were so inspired by religious frenzy that they would tear their robes aside and cut their bodies so that blood spurted in all directions. These priests were believed to be so inspired because of the goddess who worshiped in the fane or temple. This zeal was referred to by the Romans as *fanaticus.* Our word *fanatic* is derived thus. The literal meaning is "inspired by the fane."

Forfeit (fôr'fĭt). The word originates from the French. It is a compound of the French words *fors,* meaning outside, and *fait,* meaning done. It means that it is something that is done outside the law. In early days in England and France *forfaite* was a crime, and a person was arrested when he was so discovered. Today, it refers to a penalty applied in games and sports.

Game (găm). The old English term *gamen* meant fun. It had a very broad meaning, embracing all forms of amusement. Today, it relates primarily to a contest.

Gymnast (jĭm năst). **Gymnasium** (jĭm nā'zĭ-ŭm). These terms come from the Greek words *gymnos,* meaning naked, and *gymnazo,* meaning to train naked. A literal interpretation of gymnast is the performer who is naked while performing, and of gymnasium, a place where such a performance takes place. A custom in ancient Greece was to exercise in the nude since the body was considered to be a thing of beauty and something that should be exhibited for all to see.

Three intellectual centers of Athens in ancient Greece were the Academy where Plato resided, the Lyceum, attended by Aristotle, and Kynosarge, attended by Antisthenes. The gymnasium was a place where much learning also took place and where a person attended when he achieved manhood.

Intramurals (in'trà mūrals). The word is derived from the Latin *intra,* meaning within, and *murus,* meaning wall. In this sense it means sports that are played within the walls or a school, not with other schools.

Marathon (mār'a thŏn). Marathon comes from the time in 490 B.C. when the Athenians defeated the Persians at the battle of Marathon. Since that time it has been used to name a long-distance running event over a course approximately 26 miles long.

March (märch). The word comes from the French *marcher,* meaning to walk. Originally the word had a slightly different meaning and included treading or tramping.

Match (măch). This word is derived from the Anglo-Saxon *gemaecca,* referring to husband and wife or male and female animal. The German influence added the meaning "to bring together."

Net (nĕt). Net comes from the Latin word *nassa,* which meant a fishnet. Our tennis net and other sports nets such as in volleyball and badminton resemble the fishnet.

Novice (nŏv'ĭs). Novice comes from the French *novice* and the Latin *novititius* or *novus,* meaning new. A person just taking up a game or sport is a novice or somebody just beginning —new to the game.

Olympiad (o lĭm'pĭ ăd). This was the period of 4 years between the celebrations of the Olympic games. It started out this way in Greece and has been passed down from 776 B.C.

Olympic games (o lĭm'pĭk). This was the name given to the most widely known of the four sacred festivals held in ancient Greece. The Olympic games were held at Olympia every fourth year in the month of July. The festival began with sacrifices and included racing, wrestling, and other contests and ended on the fifth day with processions, sacrifices, and banquets to the victors, who were given olive leaves to wear as garlands to symbolize their victory.

Racket (rak'et). The word *racket* is originally from the Arabic *rahat,* meaning palm of the hand. A racket is usually held in the palm of the hand and is used in many games, including tennis, badminton, and squash.

Race (rās). The word *race* comes from the Old English word *raes,* meaning hurry or rush. A race is an event in which the contestants hurry as fast as they can to cross a goal or reach some other objective.

Relay (rē'lā). The word *relay* comes from the French verb *relayer,* meaning to lose the hounds. As it was originally used, a relay meant to hold some fresh hounds in reserve during a hunt. These fresh hounds were re-

leased at the strategic moment so that the scent was not lost. Of course, as it is used today it means a number of runners or contestants who relieve another group in a track event or other activity.

Score (skōr). The word *score* comes from the word *scoru,* which was borrowed by the English from the Old Norse *skor,* meaning notch. This was the way a score of a game was recorded—by making notches on a stick. The same practice was followed in American history by pioneers who notched their guns. Items are still scored by marking them with grooves, cuts, and other designs.

Scout (skout). The word *scout* comes from the Old French *escoute,* meaning a person who was a spy or an eavesdropper. It is now used in sports to refer to one who watches another team to obtain information of importance to his own team.

Shuttlecock (shŭt'l kŏk'). The Anglo-Saxon word *scytel,* referring to the back-and-forth motion of a weaver's tool gave rise to the word *shuttlecock,* now a cork and feather object that is batted back and forth.

Ski (skē). In Norwegian, the word *ski* means snowshoe or a slender wooden runner that is used in snow, the modern ski.

Sport (spŏrt). The word *sport* is derived from the Latin words, *des,* meaning away, and *porto,* meaning carry. In other words, in its original meaning it meant to carry away or to carry away from one's work or business. It also is an abbreviation of the word *disport,* meaning to amuse oneself.

Strategy (străt'e jĭ). The word *strategy* comes from the Greek word *strategos* or general, which broken down combines *stratos,* army, + *agein,* to lead. This refers to the plan or strategy by which the general leads his forces to victory.

Stunt (stŭnt). The origin of the word *stunt* is rather cloudy. Some persons trace its origin to a trick done by a stunted acrobat, as opposed to a full-sized acrobat. Others suggest it comes from the word *stint,* meaning a task, and also from the German *Stunde,* meaning an hour or period of time. As part of early college athletic slang, it was used to refer to any feat or performance.

Team (tēm). The derivation of this term is very interesting since the earlier form was the Old English *tem,* which pertained to a set, a brood, or litter, or a number of animals harnessed in a row. From this early beginning it gradually became associated with a closely associated group of individuals or animals, such as a team of horses or a basketball team.

Tournament (tŏur'na ment). The derivation dates back to the Old French and the words *tournoi* and *tournament,* referring to its basic concept

—to turn. The English used it as *tourney* and *tournament*, particularly in the days of feudalism when knights dressed in armor rode away from each other and then turned and charged each other.

Trophy (trō fy). The word *trophy* comes from the Greek word *trope,* meaning putting to flight or a turning point in a battle or contest. The word *tropaion* referred to a monument that was erected at the exact spot where the enemy was stopped and turned back. It later came to mean any monuments that were erected. A trophy now means a cup or other ornament conferred for winning a contest or to signify some other accomplishment.

Umpire (ŭm′pīr). The word *umpire* originates from the Latin words *non per,* meaning not equal, that is, uneven or third person. This means that the umpire is an odd man who decides the dispute.

Varsity (vär′sĭ tĭ). Varsity refers to a shortened form of university, for example, varsity baseball team; the varsity team selected to represent a college or a school.

Volley (vŏl′ĭ). The Latin word *volare,* "to fly," gives rise to volley, or keeping a ball in motion without allowing it to strike the ground.

Yacht (yŏt). A yacht is now a pleasure craft that is often used for racing. The Dutch word *jagt,* to speed or hunt, gave the yacht its original purpose. It was used by privateers to quickly hunt and overtake other ships to raid.

Specific activities

Badminton (băd mĭn′tn). In India badminton was known as *Poona.* This was where the game was first observed by English army officers in the 1860's. It was adopted by the English and formally introduced at a party given in 1873 by the Duke of Beaufort at his country place, which was called "Badminton in Gloucestershire." The game was referred to after this as "The Game at Badminton." As a result, *badminton* became the official name.

Baseball (bās′bâl). It is believed that baseball originated from the fifteenth century game of prisoners' base; prisoners' base was originally known as prisoners' bars, but the letter "r" was later dropped.

Cricket (krĭk′ĭt). The Old French word *criquet* referred to a curved bat. Now, the game of cricket is played by two teams of eleven men each.

Curling (kûr′lĭng). The Middle English word *crul,* which described the curving path of a stone, gave rise to this word. The game of curling is played on ice, and heavy smooth stones are pushed toward a marker for score.

Golf (gŏlf). The origin of *golf* is somewhat obscure. However, most scholars believe it comes from the Dutch word *kolf. Kolf* is the term used for a club used in such games as hockey and croquet. Although most of the early accounts of the game of golf are associated with Scotland, many persons feel it is a Dutch game and to prove their point show that the Scotch imported their best golf balls from the Dutch.

Hockey (hŏk′ĭ). The word *hockey* probably took its name from the Old French word *hoquet,* meaning a crook or shepherd's staff. Hockey is a very old game, having been played by the Greeks and the Persians.

Hurling (hûr′ling). This is the Irish name for a game that is almost identical to field hockey. It comes from the Old French word *houler,* to hurl.

Jujitsu (jōō jĭt′ sōō). The word *jujitsu* originally comes from the Chinese word *jiu-shu,* meaning to defeat an opponent by using his own strength and size against him, rather than resorting to weapons.

Lacrosse (là kros′). The Indians played this game called baggataway, with sometimes hundreds of players on a side. The French formalized the game and named it from the stick used which they asserted resembled the "crozier's staff" (Old French *crossier,* meaning bearer of the crosse, bishop's crook).

Polo (pō′lō). The Tibetan word *pulu* means ball. This game was invented by an Englishman living in India and resembles hockey played on horseback.

Quoits (kwoits). The verb "to quoit" means to make an object slide. In its early form the game of quoits was a sliding rather than a throwing game. It comes from the Anglo-French word *jeu de coytes.*

Soccer (sŏk′er). The game soccer is sometimes called association football. It is claimed that the word *soccer* originated by shortening the word *association* to *assoc* and then eliminating the first two letters of the latter term, leaving "soc." The game is very popular in England.

Tennis (tĕn′ĭs). Some scholars suggest that the word *tennis* comes from the city of Tinnis in the Egyptian Delta, which during the Middle Ages was noted for its fine linen and where the best tennis balls were made.

Tumbling (tŭm′blĭng). The word *tumbling* comes from the Anglo-Saxon word *tumbian,* which meant to dance.

QUESTIONS AND EXERCISES

1. Discuss in approximately 500 words the history of physical education from the time of primitive man until the start of the modern European period.

2. From the physical point of view, why was the need for a planned physical education pro-

gram not as great in the time of primitive man as it is today?

3. What was the attitude toward physical education in ancient China?

4. What are the forces that directly or indirectly drive men into physical activity?

5. What was the effect of Hinduism upon physical education in ancient India?

6. Contrast the attitude toward physical education in ancient China and India with that in Egypt, Assyria, Babylonia, Syria, Palestine, and Persia.

7. Describe the routine you would have followed if you had grown up in Persia during the reign of King Cyrus.

8. How do many countries utilize physical education for destructive purposes?

9. Compare physical education in ancient Greece with that prevalent today in the United States.

10. What were the objectives of physical education during the "golden age" in ancient Greece?

11. Compare the roles of physical education in the city-states of Sparta and Athens.

12. What were the palaestra and the gymnasium? What kind of activities did each provide?

13. What were the names of some of the outstanding national festivals in Greece and what gods did they honor?

14. Describe the games held at Olympia, bringing out the following points: (a) requirements for contestants, (b) events, (c) rewards, and (d) attitude of Greeks toward these games.

15. What was the attitude of each of the following toward physical education: (a) Socrates, (b) Plato, (c) Aristotle, and (d) Xenophon?

16. Compare the Greeks and the Romans in their attitudes toward physical education.

17. In approximately 250 words discuss the statement: American is going the way of the Romans.

18. What were the Dark Ages? Was this a dark period in history for physical education? Explain.

19. Discuss asceticism and scolasticism and show how they still exist in many forms in twentieth-century society.

20. What was the influence of the feudalistic period upon physical education?

21. How did each of the following contribute to physical education: (a) da Feltra, (b) Vergerio, (c) Pope Pius II, (d) Sir Thomas Elyot, (e) Martin Luther, (f) Rabelais, (g) Asham, (h) John Milton, (i) Locke, (j) Comenius, and (k) Rousseau?

Reading assignment

Bucher, Charles A., and Goldman, Myra: Dimensions of physical education, St. Louis, 1969, The C. V. Mosby Co., Reading selections 27 to 29.

SELECTED REFERENCES

Abbott, E. A.: Society and politics in ancient Rome, New York, 1909, Charles Scribner's Sons.

Barnes, H. E.: The history of western civilization, New York, 1935, Harcourt, Brace & Co., Inc.

Bauer, L.: Chinese dances for children, Journal of Health and Physical Education 4:22, 1933.

Bennett, Bruce L.: Improving courses in the history of physical education, Journal of Health, Physical Education, and Recreation 37:26, 1966.

Botsford, G. W., and Sihler, E. G.: Hellenic civilization, New York, 1915, Columbia University Press.

Bowra, C. M.: Xenophanes and the Olympic games, American Journal of Philology 59:257, 1938.

Brink, D. B., and Smith, P.: Athletes of the Bible, New York, 1914, Associated Press.

Bucher, Charles A.: Are we losing the Olympic ideal? Sports Illustrated, August 8, 1955.

Bucher, Charles A.: Let's put more sportsmanship into the Olympics, Reader's Digest, September, 1955.

Bucher, Charles A.: Scorekeepers vs. first principles, Journal of Health, Physical Education, and Recreation 35:26, 1964.

Butler, A. J.: Sport in classic times, London, 1930, Ernest Benn, Ltd.

Buttree, J. M.: The rhythm of the Redman, New York, 1930, A. S. Barnes & Co.

Caillois, Roger: Man, play, and games, New York, 1961, The Free Press of Glencoe, Inc. (translated from the French).

Carcopino, J.: Daily life in ancient Rome (translated by E. O. Lorimer), New Haven, 1940, Yale University Press.

Chryssafis, J.: Aristotle on kinesiology, Journal of Health and Physical Education 1:14, 1930.

Chryssafis, J.: Aristotle on physical education, Journal of Health and Physical Education 1:3, 1930.

Clark, Ellery H.: The Olympic games and their influence upon physical education, Journal of Health, Physical Education, and Recreation 35:23, 1964 (reprinted from The American Physical Education Review).

Coomaraswamy, A.: The dance of Siva, New York, 1918, Sunrise Turn.

Dulles, Foster Rhea: A history of recreation—America learns to play, New York, 1965, Appleton-Century-Crofts.

Falkener, E.: Games ancient and oriental and how to play them, London, 1892, Longmans.

Fuld, L. F.: Physical education in Greece and Rome, American Physical Education Review 12:1, 1907.

Gardiner, E. N.: Athletics of the ancient world, Oxford, 1930, Clarendon Press.

Genasci, James E., and Klissouras, Vasillis: The delphic spirit in sports, Journal of Health, Physical Education, and Recreation **37**:43, 1966.

Gray, J. H.: Physical education in India, American Physical Education Review **24**:373, 1919.

Hackensmith, C. W.: History of physical education, New York, 1966, Harper & Row, Publishers.

Hoh, G.: Physical education in China, Shanghai, 1926, Commercial Press.

Lee, J.: Play in education, New York, 1922, The Macmillan Co.

Leonard, F. E., and Afflect, G. B.: A guide to the history of physical education, Philadelphia, 1947, Lea & Febiger.

Lucas, John A.: Coubertin's philosophy of pedagogical sport, Journal of Health, Physical Education, and Recreation **35**:26, 1964.

Means, Richard K.: A history of health education in the United States, Philadelphia, 1962, Lea & Febiger.

Monograph IV: Quest, The National Association for Physical Education of College Women and The National College of Physical Education Association for Men, April, 1965.

Rice, Emmett A., Hutchinson, John L., and Lee, Mabel: A brief history of physical education, ed. 5, New York, 1969, The Ronald Press.

Schleppi, J. R.: Architecture and sports, The Physical Educator **23**:123, 1966.

Trekell, Marianna: Speaking to the future, Journal of Health, Physical Education, and Recreation **37**:29, 1966.

Van Dalen, Deobold B., and Bennett, B. L.: A world history of physical education, ed. 2, New York, 1971, Prentice-Hall, Inc.

Weston, Arthur: The making of American physical education, New York, 1962, Appleton-Century-Crofts.

Woody, Thomas: The fair sex in Greek society, Research Quarterly **10**:57, 1939.

Woody, Thomas: Life and education in early societies, New York, 1949, The Macmillan Co.

References for word origins

Brewer, Ebenezer: Dictionary of phrase and fable, New York, 1952, Harper & Brothers.

Funk, Charles E.: Thereby hangs a tale, New York, 1950, Harper & Brothers.

Funk, Wilfred: Word origins and their romantic stories, New York, 1950, Wilfred Funk, Inc.

Holt, Alfred H.: Phrases and word origins, New York, 1961, Dover Publications, Inc.

Menke, Frank G.: The encyclopedia of sports, New York, 1961, A. S. Barnes & Co.

Shipley, Joseph T.: Dictionary of word origins, New York, 1945, The Philosophical Library, Inc.

Weekley, Ernest: Concise, etymological dictionary of modern English, New York, 1952, E. P. Dutton & Co., Inc.

12/Changing concepts from beginning of modern European period to present

A study of physical education in the modern European period shows many reasons why special programs in this area were established and the nature of such programs in the various countries of Europe. The spirit of nationalism and the necessity of being prepared for warfare were two leading causes for instituting programs of physical activity on the European continent. Physical education was increasingly being recognized for its therapeutic value. Stress was placed on physical education as a science, requiring study in anatomy, physiology, and other foundational sciences. There was a trend toward a games and sports program to supplement the rigid and formal type of gymnastics. The public was becoming cognizant of a need for incorporating a planned program of physical activity in the schools. It was being more fully recognized that the physical and the mental go hand in hand and give support to each other and that exercise is necessary for optimum growth and development. It is interesting to note in passing that the potentialities of physical education as a means of developing acceptable social and moral traits still were not fully realized. Education *of* the physical was to a great extent the predominant objective, with less regard for education *through* the physical.

PHYSICAL EDUCATION IN EUROPE

A study of the various men and countries that influenced physical education during the modern European period shows what each contributed to the growth and advancement of this field.

Germany

Physical education in Germany during the modern European period is associated with such names as Basedow, Guts Muths, Jahn, and Spiess.

Johann Bernhard Basedow (1723–1790) was born in Hamburg and early in life went to Denmark as a teacher. Here he witnessed physical education in practice as part of a combined physical and mental training program. After gaining a wealth of experience in Denmark, he went back to Germany and decided to spend all of his time in the reform of educational methods. In 1774 he was able to realize his objective of establishing at Dessau a school that he called the Philanthropinum. In this model school physical education played an important part in the daily program of all students. The activities included such items as dancing, fencing, riding, running, jumping, wrestling, swimming, skating, and marching. This was the first school in modern Europe that admitted children from every class in society and that offered a program where physical education was a part of the curriculum. Such an innovation by Basedow did much to influence the growth of physical education in Germany as well as in the rest of the world.

Johann Christoph Friedrich Guts Muths (1759–1839) brought his influence to bear upon the field of physical education through his association with the Schnepfenthal Educational Institute, which had been founded by Christian Gotthilf Salzmann (1744–1811). Guts Muths succeeded Christian Carl Andre as the instructor of physical education at this institution and remained on the staff for 50 years. His beliefs and practices in physical education were recorded for history in various books, two of which are of special importance, *Gymnastics for the Young* and *Games*. These books give such information as illustrations of various exercises and pieces of apparatus, arguments in favor of physical education, and the relation of physical education to educational institutions. Because of his outstanding contributions, Guts Muths is often referred to as one of the founders of modern physical education in Germany.

Friedrich Ludwig Jahn (1778–1852) is a name associated with the Turnverein, an association of gymnasts that has been in evidence ever since its innovation by Jahn. Jahn's incentive for inaugurating the Turnverein movement was love of his country. It was during his lifetime that Napoleon overran Germany and caused it to be divided into several independent German states. Jahn made it his life's work and ambition to help in bringing about an independent Germany free from foreign control. He felt that he could best help in this movement by molding German youth into strong and hardy citizens who would be capable of throwing off this foreign yoke.

To help in the achievement of his objective, Jahn accepted a teaching position in Plamann's Boys School. In this position he worked regularly with the boys in various outdoor activities. He set up an exercise ground outside the city called the Hasenheide. Before long Jahn had erected various pieces of apparatus, including equipment for jumping, vaulting, balancing, climbing, and running. The program grew in popularity; soon hundreds of boys were visiting the exercise ground or turnplatz regularly, and more apparatus was added.

Jahn's system of gymnastics was recognized throughout Germany, and in many cities Turnvereins were formed, using as a guide the instructions that Jahn incorporated in his book *Die Deutsche Turnkunst*. When Jahn died, his work carried on and turner societies became more numerous. In 1870 there were 1,500 turner societies, in 1880 there were 2,200, in 1890 there were 4,000, in 1900 there were 7,200, and in 1920 there were 10,000. Turnvereins are still in existence in many parts of the world.

The objectives of Jahn's work in physical education were tied up with his desire for an independent Germany. He believed that through physical education his country could be made strong. Despite the over-

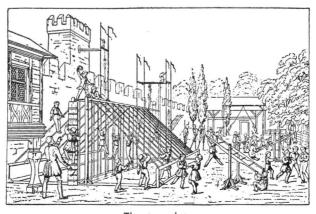

The turnplatz.

whelming political motive, Jahn saw in physical education a means of aiding the growth and development of children, social equality, and its importance in the curriculum of the school. Many persons have disagreed with Jahn's gymnastics. They argue that they were not founded on the sciences of physiology and anatomy, were too heavy for children, were too rigid and formal, and did not provide a program for the women.

Although there may be some disagreement as to Jahn's motives and methods, he has had a great influence on physical education in Germany, as well as throughout the world. He instilled in the German people a love for gymnastics that has been passed down for several generations.

Adolph Spiess (1810–1858) was the founder of school gymnastics in Germany, and, more than any other man in German history, he helped to make physical education a part of school life. Spiess was proficient in physical education activities himself and was well informed as to the theories of such men as Guts Muths and Jahn. His own theory was that the school should be interested in the total growth of the child—mental, emotional, physical, and social. Physical education should receive the same consideration as the important academic subjects such as mathematics and language. It should be required of all students, with the possible exception of those a physician would excuse. There should be provisions for an indoor as well as an outdoor program. Elementary school children should have a minimum of 1 hour of the school day devoted to physical education activities, which should be taught by the regular classroom teacher. The upper grades should have a progressively smaller amount, which should be conducted by specialists who were educators first but who were also experts in the field of physical education. The physical education program should be progressive, starting with simple exercises and proceeding to the more difficult. Girls as well as boys need an adapted program of physical activity. Exercises combined with music offer an opportunity for the individual to express himself more freely. Marching exercises aid in class organization, discipline, and posture development. Formalism should not be practiced to the exclusion of games, dancing, and sports.

Many of Spiess' theories and practices have been incorporated in school programs of physical education the world over. Spiess recognized the valuable contribution physical education could make in the education of boys and girls. He appreciated the values of such a program in developing the body and in developing an individual socially and morally.

There are other outstanding individuals in modern German history who have influenced physical education, including Eiselen, Koch, Hermann, and Von Schenckendorff. However, the names of Basedow, Guts Muths, Jahn, and Spiess stand out as the ones who, in large part, have influenced physical education the most.

Sweden

The name of *Per Henrik Ling* (1776–1839) is symbolic of the rise of physical education to a place of importance in Sweden. The "Lingaid," held at Stockholm, in which representatives of many nations of the world participate, is a tribute to this great man.

Ling's greatest contribution is that he strove to make physical education a science. Formerly physical education had been conducted mainly on the premise that people believed it was good for the human body because it increased the size of one's musculature; contributed to strength, stamina, endurance, and agility; and left one exhilarated. However, many claims for physical education had never been proved scientifically. Ling approached the field with the mind of a scientist. Through the sciences of anatomy and physiology, he examined the body to determine what was inherent in physical activity to enable the body to function in a more nearly optimum capacity. His aims were directed at determining such

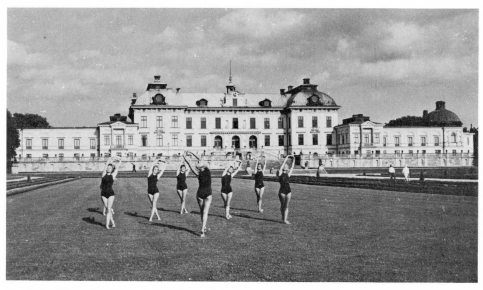

The Idla Girls, the famous Swedish group of amateur women gymnasts, displaying their graceful program in front of the seventeenth-century Royal Palace of Drottningholm.

things as the effect of exercise on the heart, the musculature, and the various organic systems of the body. He felt that through such a scientific approach, he would be better able to understand the human body and its needs and would be better able to select and apply physical activity intelligently.

Ling is noted for establishing the Royal Central Institute of Gymnastics at Stockholm, where teachers of physical education received their preparation in one of three categories—educational gymnastics, military gymnastics, or medical gymnastics.

Ling believed that physical education was necessary for the weak as well as the strong, that exercise must be prescribed on the basis of individual differences, that the mind and body must function harmoniously together, and that teachers of physical education must have a foundational knowledge of the effects of exercise on the human body.

Ling's objectives for physical education included the desire to see each person develop his body to the fullest extent, to restore health to individuals with weaknesses and afflictions, and to make the country strong against aggressors.

In 1839 *Lars Gabriel Branting* (1799–1881) became the director of the Royal Central Institute of Gymnastics upon the death of Ling. Branting spent the major part of his time in the area of medical gymnastics. His teachings were based on the premise that activity causes changes not only in the muscular system of the body but also in the nervous and circulatory systems as well. Branting's successor was *Gustaf Nyblaeus* (1816–1902), who specialized in military gymnastics. An innovation during his tenure was the inclusion of women in the school.

The incorporation of physical education programs in the schools of Sweden did not materialize as rapidly as many leaders in the field had hoped. As a result of the teachings of Ling and other leaders, a law was passed in 1820 requiring a course of physical education on the secondary level. More progress was made in education when the values of physical education to the growth and development of children became apparent in Sweden. To *Hjalmar Fredrik Ling* (1820–1886), most of the credit is due for the organization of educational gymnastics in Sweden. He was

Synopsis of the theory of the Swedish Educational Gymnastics of

The basis of Swedish Gymnastics	Philosophical progression.	Classification according to gymnastic effects.	Aim.	Contents.	Types.	Physical.
Contents of a table of exercises, or the progression within each lesson.	Movements for general effects.	1. Introductions.	Transition from mental to physical activity.	True: movements of {Order, Rhythm} Transitory {Regular, Irregular.}	Head-movements. Correct base. Respiratory exercises. Leg-movements. Lateral trunk-movements. Double-arm-extension. Preparation to jumping.	Induce equilibrium. Review [save time]. Prepare for stronger movements.
		2. Arch-flexions.	To cultivate extensibility of expiratory muscles, i.e. to supple the chest.	False: [excentric contraction] {Sagittal. Lateral.} True: [passive extension]	Grasp arch st. 2 Heel elev. Oblique gr. arch st. 2 Heel elev.	Widen inferior chest. Straighten dorsal spine. Flatten shoulderblades. Draw up viscera.
		3. Heaving-movements.	To cultivate contractility of inspiratory muscles: to elevate the chest.	Introductory {Head-Flex. Head-rot.} False: natural apparatus. True {mov. & extension} Suspension, {" & contraction} Resistance.	2 A. ext. sidew. Horiz. travels} Lateral ex. 2 A. ext. upw.} Vertical} pansion Vertical travel	Expand pectoral chest. Internal elevation. Develop muscular arm. Elongate spine. Increased afflux in thorax and arms. Increase intra-cardiac pressure.
		4. Balance-movements	To cultivate equilibrium in ordinary positions and correct general posture.	movements of standing and walking.	movements from Standing, half-standing and Falloutst. positions.	Develop extensors of body. [Lessen blood-pressure.]
	Movements for special (local) effects.	5. Shoulder-blade-movements.	To increase the sphere of activity of shoulder-joint and skill of hand.	Movements of arms with isolation of chest and head.	2 Arm-flinging: expansion 2 Arm-elevation: localization.	Correct localization of shoulder. Widening of pectoral chest. Straightening of dorsal spine. Widening of shoulder-girdle. Broadening of back. Equal development of cerebral halves
		6. Abdominal exercises.	To improve digestion & support viscera.	Contractions of the vertical group of abdominal muscles.	Stoopfalling pos. Knee st. I. backw Flex.	Flatten abdomen. Accelerate flow in mesenteric veins. Drive viscera up. Straighten lumbar spine.
		7. Lateral trunk movements.	To affect large vessels & develop waist-muscles.	Rotations and Sideways Flexions of the trunk. {I. rot. I. sidew Flex. Oblique arch Flex " sidew. " Leg-elev. sidew.}	Trunk-rotation. Trunk-sideways-Flex.	Accelerate flow in vena cava. Widen the chest. Produce internal elevation. Develop nature's corsets. Improve portal circulation.
	Movements for general effects.	8. Slow leg-movements.	Diminish arterial pressure. Equalize circulation.	Movements increasing the capacity of the vessels of the leg.	Knee-Flexion. Trunk Forw. Flex.	Decrease quantity of blood in chest. Increase vis-a-fronte in veins. Decrease heart-beat. Lessen cerebral pressure.
		9. Leaping. [running, jumping & vaulting]	Develop general coordination, control & speed.	Jumping. Vaulting.	Jumping with whole, half or double start. Vaulting with whole, double or half start.	Develop elasticity. " extensors of legs. Increase blood-pressure. " peristalsis.
		10. Respiratory exercises.	Produce normal respiration. Remove venous congestion.	Movements of respiration accompanied by some arm-movement.	2 Arm-flinging. 2 Arm-elevation.	Lessen blood-pressure. Increase elasticity of air-cells. " respiratory power.

Copyright 1893 by

Pehr Henrik Ling, elaborated by Baron Nils Posse.

EFFects.		Progression.	Limitations.	Relations.
Physiological.	**Psychological.**			
Circulatory revulsion: change current from intellectual to motor cells.	Connect origin of exercise with its means:— teachers mind with pupil's mind; pupils " " " muscles.	Depend on class from which they are borrowed.	Few for short lesson. Many " long " Gentle " easy " Strong " hard "	Every exercise is an introduction to the next harder of same class.
As of thoracic aspiration. Better oxygenation.	—	False to true to False. wlk. c. st. | close st. " b " | turn st. turn wlk. a st. st. " stride " | turn close st. " wlk. b " | stride st.	Quality (power) should correspond to the heaving - movement of the same lesson.	1. Prep. for the heav⁹ mov⁵ 2. Depend for progression on shoulderblade - mov⁹ 3. Resemble abdom: exer. 4. Prep for vaulting 5. Merge into heav: mov⁵ ⁷ vault.
Increase the respiratory power. Accelerate the heart-beat and respiration. Relieve congestion of the head ⁷ spine.	Consciousness of power. Repose.	Mainly individual. Hanging. | Bend-hang Fall-hang | Stoop- " Climb-hang | Crook- " Balance-hang | Arch-hang	Quality:— Proportioned to the arch-flex. of same lesson. Quantity:— Two or more for advanced pupils	1. Regulate progression of arch-Flexions. 2. Delay use of abdom. exercises 3. Can be substituted by shoulderblade movements ⁷ lateral trunk movements. 4. Transitory forms { arch-flex. should-mov⁹ abdom. exers cont. J. moves
Improve respiration. " metabolism. " cerebration.	Localization of cerebral effort. Automatic coordination. Consciousness of power. Repose.	Double heel-elevation. " knee-Flexion. Leg-elevation.	Quality:— should correspond to mental ability.	1. Follow heaving-mov⁵ 2. Improve all free exercises. 3. Become introductions ⁷ slow leg-movements. 4. Much needed by children, less " " adults.
Improved action of organs in chest and abdomen.	Localization of thought. Concentration of mind. Symmetrical development of faculties.	Standing | Forw. lying. Stoop st. | Turn fallout st. Fallout st. | Foot grasp " " Horizontal ⁷ st.	Quantity:— Two or more in one lesson. Quality:— Expansion before localization.	1. Substitutes for heaving-movements. 2. Regulate progression of arch-Flexions. 3. Regulate progression of respiratory exercises.
Increase intestinal absorption. Induce peristalsis. Increase intestinal elimination.	[Improved digestion makes a more cheerful disposition]	Lying Stoop Falling. Knee-standing. Foot-grasp - sitting. Half knee-standing. Foot-grasp half standing.	Quantity:— Begin late, use easy ones for children " stronger " adults.	1. Compare arch-flexions. 2. Prepare for certain heaving-movements and vaulting.
Increase activity of liver. " capillary osmosis from intestines. " elimination from alimentary tract.	—	Rotation. | Sidew. flex. Turn st. ⁷ st. ext. | Turn st. side. flex. Turn st. backw. flex | Leg-elev. sidew. Turn arch ⁷ st. ext. | Sidew. hang.	Rotation precedes sidew. flex. in same lesson.	1. Substitutes for heaving mov⁵ 2. Complete effects of abdom. exer 3. Merge into heaving - mov⁵ 4. " " vaulting. 5. " " games ⁷ sports.
Ease respiration. Remove fatigue.	Mental revulsion even to cessation of attention.	None especially. Strength depends on preceding exercises.	Used when preceding exercises are strong, otherwise not. Too many will weaken the heart.	1. Derived from balance-movements. 2. Follow after any movement, whenever necessary.
Increase exhalation. Elimination of CO_2. Increase metabolism. Improve cerebral localization.	Courage. Appreciation of { space { time } effort. Presence of mind. Exhilaration.	Standing } { Jump. Running } { Vault.	Can never be introductions. Quantity ⁷ quality should be proportioned to rest of lesson.	1. Evolution of all others in same lesson and from lesson to lesson. 2. Merge into heaving-mov⁵ 3. " abdom. exercises. 4. " arch-flexions. 5. " lateral J. mov⁵ 6. Hopping = continuous balance-movement.
Improved oxygenation of tissue. Elimination of CO_2 ⁷ H_2O. [stir] Lessened temperature [evapor] " Fatigue [and need of sleep].	Exhilaration. Repose.	Dependent on progression of shoulder-blade-mov⁵	Abnormal forms:— holding the breath, while exercising; forcible exhalation.	1. Prep. by arch-flexions and heaving-mov⁵ 2. Evolution from should-mov⁵ 3. Occur at end of lesson. 4. " " begin. " 5. " " any part " "

Baron Nils Posse.

largely responsible for physical education becoming an essential subject in all schools for both boys and girls and on all institutional levels. Today, most schools in Sweden require a period a day for physical education, which is devoted to a program of games and Swedish exercises.

Denmark

Denmark has been one of the leading European countries in the promotion of physical education. *Franz Nachtegall* (1777–1847) was largely responsible for the early interest in this field. He had a direct influence in introducing physical education into the public schools of Denmark and in preparing teachers of this subject.

Franz Nachtegall had been interested in various forms of physical activity since childhood and had achieved some degree of skill in vaulting and fencing. He began early in life to teach gymnastics, first to students who visited his home and then in 1799 in a private outdoor gymnasium, the first to be devoted entirely to physical training. In 1804 Nachtegall became the first director of a Training School for Teachers of Gymnastics in the Army. For a time, only service personnel were allowed to pursue the course; later, however, civilians were also given permission. The need was great for instructors in public schools and in teachers' colleges, so that graduates readily found employment. In 1809 the secondary schools and in 1814 the elementary schools were requested to provide a program of physical education with qualified instructors. It was shortly after this that Nachtegall received the appointment of Director of Gymnastics for all Denmark.

The death of Nachtegall in 1847 did not stop the expansion of physical education throughout Denmark. Some of the important advances since his death have been

Danish performers at New York University.

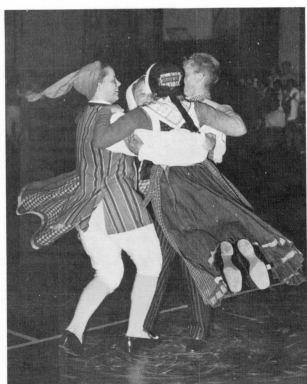

the organization of Danish Rifle Clubs or gymnastic societies, the introduction of the Ling system of gymnastics, complete civilian supervision and control of programs of physical education as opposed to military supervision and control, greater provision for teacher education, government aid, the incorporation of sports and games into the program, and the work of Niels Bukh.

One of the innovations in the field of physical education has been the contribution of Niels Bukh with his "Primitive Gymnastics." Patterned to some extent after the work of Ling, they attempted to build the perfect physique through a series of exercises performed without cessation of movement. His routine included exercises for arms, legs, abdomen, neck, back, and the various joints. In 1925 he toured the United States with some of his students, demonstrating his "Primitive Gymnastics."

Great Britain

Great Britain is known as the home of outdoor sports, and her contribution to this field has influenced physical education the world over. When other European countries were utilizing the Ling, Jahn, and Guts Muths systems of gymnastics, England was utilizing a program of organized games and sports.

Athletic sports are a feature of English life. As early as the time of Henry II, English youth were wrestling, throwing, riding, fishing, hunting, swimming, rowing, skating, shooting the bow, and participating in various other sports. The games of hockey and quoits, for example, were played in England as early as the fifteenth century, tennis as early as 1300, golf as early as 1600, and cricket as early as 1700. Football is one of the oldest of English national sports. Games were played in all

Danish gymnastic team performing at New York University.

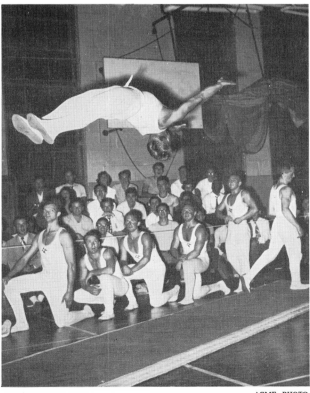

ACME PHOTO.

parts of England from the earliest of times.

In addition to outdoor sports, England's chief contribution to physical education has been through the work of *Archibald Maclaren* (1820–1884). Maclaren at an early age enjoyed participating in many sports, but especially fencing and gymnastics. He also studied medicine and was eager to make a science of physical training. In 1858 he opened a private gymnasium where he was able to experiment. In 1860 Maclaren was designated to devise a system of physical education for the British Army. As a result of this appointment, he incorporated his recommendations in a treatise entitled *A Military System of Gymnastic Exercises for the Use of Instructors*. This system was adopted by the military, and Maclaren undertook the responsibility of training a cadre of Army and Navy men in his system of exercises.

Maclaren contributed several other books to the field of physical education. Some of these were *National Systems of Bodily Exercise, A System of Fencing, Training in Theory and Practice,* and *A System of Physical Education*. In his works he points out that the objectives of physical education should take into consideration that health is more important than strength; that the antidote for tension, weariness, nervousness, and hard work is physical action; that recreative exercise as found in games and sports is not enough in itself for growing boys and girls; that physical exercise is essential to optimum growth and development; that physical training and mental training are inseparable; that mind and body represent a "oneness" in man and sustain and support each other; that exercises must be progressive in nature; that exercises should be adapted to an individual's fitness; that physical education should be an essential part of any school curriculum; and that physical education should be organized and administered effectively so that all of its potentialities will be realized.

Since the time of Maclaren the Swedish system of gymnastics has been introduced into England and has been well received. Many ideas were also imported from Denmark. Leaders came from Denmark and Sweden in the persons of Knudsen, Langkilde, and Osterberg. Training schools for teachers were established, and educational laws were passed promoting physical education in the schools. There was more emphasis on the health movement, and laws were passed providing for health services, healthful school living, and health instruction.

Probably one of the major contributions of England to physical education has been "movement education," which is discussed at length in Chapter 13.

• • •

Germany, Sweden, Denmark, and England have led Europe in the promotion of physical education. Other countries of Europe as a rule imported the various systems of Jahn, Guts Muths, and Ling. There are persons from other countries who have also contributed much to the field of physical education and who should be mentioned. From Switzerland, Pestalozzi with his educational theories, Dalcroze and his system of eurythmics, and Clias did a great deal to advance the field of physical education. Colonel Amoros from France inaugurated a system of gymnastics, and Baron Pierre de Coubertin was instrumental in reviving the Olympic games in 1896 at Athens. Johann Happel from Belgium was outstanding in physical education and was director of a normal school of gymnastics. Dr. Tyrs from Czechoslovakia organized the first gymnastic society in his country.

The dates of origin in history of some common sports are given in Table 12-1.

PHYSICAL EDUCATION IN AMERICA

Physical education in America has experienced a period of great expansion from the colonial period, when little regard was had for any planned program of activity, until today, when programs are required in the public schools of most of our states

Table 12-1. Chronological distribution of established dates of origins*

Sport	Date of origin†	Sport	Date of origin†
Wrestling	(2160) 1788 B.C.	Soccer	1859
Boxing	(2160?) 850 B.C.	Squash racquets	1859
Field events	(900 B.C.?) 776 B.C.	Swimming	(1530) 1859
Track events	(900 B.C.?) 776 B.C.	Roller skating	1863
Hunting	(2357) 400 B.C.	Trap shooting	1866
Kite flying	(1121) 221 B.C.	Field trials	1866
Coursing	7 A.D.	Bicycle racing	1868
Cock fighting	77	Badminton	1870
Angling	200	Skiing	(1750) 1870
Falconry	350	Target pistol shooting	1871
Horse racing	(648 B.C.) 1174	Model sailboat racing	1872
Tennis	1230	Lawn tennis	1873
Lawn bowls	1366	Football (American)	1874
Quoits	(450 B.C.) 1409	Dog racing	(1810?) 1876
Golf	(1380?) 1457	Roque	1879
Target rifle shooting	1498	Ice hockey	(1810) 1880
Fencing	1517	Rodeo	(1830) 1880
Hurling	1527	Judo	1882
Shuffleboard	1532	Tobogganing	(1837?) 1883
Archery (target)	(1530) 1585	Water polo	1885
Billiards	(1520?) 1590	Field hockey	(B.C.?) 1886
Fowling	(2475 B.C.) 1596	Birling	1888
Polo	(475?) 1596	Table tennis	1889
Curling	1607	Darts	(1850?) 1890
Ice skating	(500) 1659	Rope spinning	(1850?) 1890
Cricket	(1600) 1744	Squash tennis	1890
Fives	1746	Basketball	1891
Yacht racing	(1675) 1775	Automobile racing	1895
Pedestrianism	(1610) 1792	Volleyball	1895
Racquets	(1555) 1799	Jai alai	1896
Horseshoes	(1750?) 1801	Paddle tennis	1898
Coaching	(1590) 1807	Motorcycle racing	1902
Steeplechasing	(1740) 1810	Corkball	1904
Mountaineering	(1780?) 1811	Motorboat racing	1904
Gymnastics	(1790) 1816	Model airplane flying	1905
Pigeon racing	(1800) 1818	Airplane flying	1907
Harness racing	1825	Soaring	1909
Sculling	(1715) 1839	Speedball	1920
Lacrosse	(1400) 1839	Softball	(1890) 1923
Rowing	1839	Miniature golf	(1860) 1927
Bowling (ten pins)	(1600) 1840	Soapbox racing	1927
Croquet	1840	Six man football	1933
Handball	(1500?) 1840	Skin diving	1934
Baseball	(1750) 1846	Miniature auto racing	1936
Rugby	1846	Water skiing	1939
Iceboating	(1720) 1850	Skish	(1880?) 1939
Weight lifting	(1720) 1854	Flickerball	1948
Canoe racing	(1790?) 1859		

*Eyler, Marvin H.: Research Quarterly **32**:484, 1961.

†The date given after each sport is that of the earliest documented evidence of its origin in organized form. Dates shown in parentheses are those of documented evidence of previous existence, as unorganized or noncompetitive activity. A date in parentheses with a question mark indicates that reputed evidence previous to this date may not actually refer to this specific sport.

and when physical education is becoming a respected profession.

Colonial period

During the colonial period in America conditions were not conducive to organized physical education programs. The majority of the population lived an agrarian existence and felt that they received enough physical exercise working on the farms. Also, there were few leisure hours during this period that could be devoted to various forms of recreational activities. In certain sections of the country, such as New England, religious beliefs were contrary to participation in play. The Puritans, espe-cially, denounced play as the work of the devil. Participation in games was believed just cause for eternal damnation. Pleasures and recreation were banned. Stern discipline, austerity, and frugality were thought to be the secrets to eternal life and blessedness.

People of some sections of the nation, however, brought with them from their mother countries the knowledge and desire for various sports. The Dutch in New York liked to engage in such sports as skating, coasting, hunting, and fishing. However, the outstanding favorite was bowling. In Virginia many sports were popular, such as running, boxing, wrestling, horse racing,

Origins of contemporary sports. **A,** Percentage distribution of place of origin for ninety-five sports. **B,** Percentage distribution of activities from which the ninety-five sports evolved.

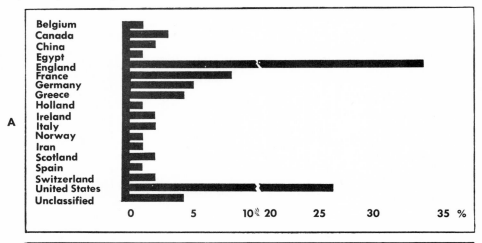

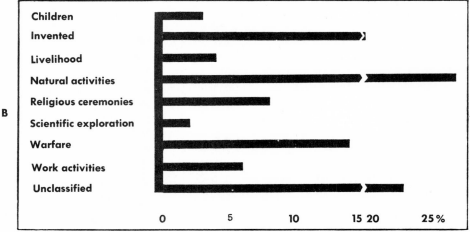

FROM EYLER, MARVIN H.: RESEARCH QUARTERLY
32:483. 1961.

cockfights, fox hunts, and later cricket and football.

During the colonial period little emphasis was given to any form of physical activity in the schools. The emphasis was on the three R's on the elementary level and on the classics on the secondary level. The teachers were ill prepared in the methodology of teaching. Furthermore, on the secondary level students were prepared mainly for college, and it was thought that physical activity was a waste of time in such preparation.

National period*

During the national period of the history of the United States, physical education began to assume an important place in American society.

The academies, as many of the secondary schools were called, provided terminal education for students; instead of preparing for college, they prepared for living. These educational institutions utilized games and sports as after-school activity. They had not reached the point, however, where they thought its value was such that it should occupy a place in the daily school schedule. They encouraged participation during after-school hours on the premise that it promotes health and rest from the mental phases of school life.

The U. S. Military Academy was founded in 1802 and gave physical training an important place in its program of activities. Through history, this training school has maintained such a program, and today it is considered one of the best in existence.

It was during the national period that German gymnastics were introduced to America. Charles Beck introduced Jahn's ideas at the Round Hill School at Northampton, Massachusetts, in 1823; and Charles Follen introduced them at Harvard University and in Boston. Both Beck and Follen were turners and proficient in

---

*The period from the American Revolution to the Civil War.

the execution of German gymnastics. Their attempt to introduce German gymnastics into the United States, however, was not successful at this time. A few years later they were introduced with more success in German settlements located in such cities as Kansas City, Cincinnati, St. Louis, and Davenport. Turnverein associations were organized, and gymnastics were accepted with considerable enthusiasm by the residents of German extraction. As for native Americans, the majority of them felt that the formal type of gymnastic program was not suitable for their purposes.

The Turnverein organizations spread, and by 1852 there were twenty-two societies in the North. The oldest Turnverein in the United States, which flourishes to the present day, is the Cincinnati Turnverein, founded November 21, 1848. The Philadelphia Turnverein, one of the strongest societies today, was founded on May 15, 1849. A national organization of Turnvereins, now known as the American Turnerbund, was established in 1850 and held its first national turnfest in Philadelphia in 1851. Societies from New York, Boston, Cincinnati, Brooklyn, Utica, Philadelphia, and Newark were represented. There were 1,672 turners in the United States in 1851. At the outbreak of the Civil War there were approximately 150 Turnverein societies and 10,000 turners in the United States. After the Civil War these organizations continued to grow and exercised considerable influence on the growing physical education profession. The Turnverein organizations were responsible for the establishment of the Normal College of the American Gymnastic Union. Many outstanding physical education leaders graduated from this school.

There were notable advances in physical education prior to the Civil War. In 1828 a planned program of physical education, composed mainly of calisthenics performed to music, was incorporated by Catherine E. Beecher in the Hartford Female Seminary in Connecticut, a famous institution of higher learning for women and girls. The introduction of the Swedish Movement

Cure in America, the building of gymnasiums in many large cities, the formation of gymnastic and athletic clubs by many leading institutions of higher learning, and the invention of baseball were all events of importance in the progress of physical education in America during this period.

Physical education in America from Civil War until 1900

Many outstanding leaders and new ideas influenced physical education in America in the period from the Civil War to 1900.

After the Civil War the Turnverein societies were established for both boys and girls. The members of these associations gave support to various phases of physical education and especially encouraged the program in the public schools. The objectives of the Turners were notable. They disapproved of too much stress being placed on winning games and professionalism. They felt that the main objectives should be to promote physical welfare and to provide social and moral training. The opposed military training in the schools as a substitute for physical education and supported the playground movement.

From 1859 to the early 1870's, Dr. George Barker Winship gained considerable publicity by emphasizing gymnastics as a means of building strength and large muscles.

In 1860 Dr. Dio Lewis devised a new system of gymnastics and introduced it in Boston. As opposed to Winship, Lewis was not concerned with building muscles and strength. He was more interested in the weak and feeble persons in our society. Instead of large muscles, he aimed at developing agility, grace of movement, flexibility, and improving one's general health and posture. He also stressed that teachers should be well prepared, and in 1861 he established a normal school of physical education in Boston for training teachers. Lewis opposed military training in our schools. He felt that sports in themselves would not provide an adequate program but that gymnastics should also be included. Through lectures and written articles, Lewis became a leading authority on gymnastics used in the schools and the public in general. He is noted for advancing physical education to a respected position in our society. Several leading educators, after hearing Lewis, set up planned physical education programs in their school systems.

In the 1880's the Swedish Movement Cure was made popular by Hartvig Nissen, head of the Swedish Health Institute in Washington. This system was based on the Ling or Swedish gymnastics so well known in Europe and recognized in America for inherent medical values. Also in the 1880's Mrs. Hemenway and Amy Morris Homans

The wand drills were an important part of program activities in the 1890's.

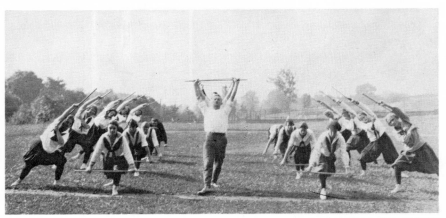

Exhibition on the parallel bars by the men's physical education class.

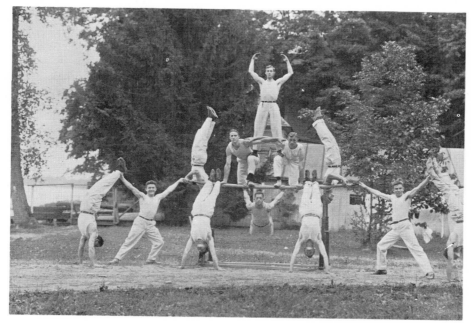

COURTESY HAROLD L. RAY, WESTERN
MICHIGAN UNIVERSITY, KALAMAZOO, MICH.

The staff and first normal class in physical education of the Chautauqua school, dated 1886. Pioneers in the field who taught this first operational summer school of physical education are identified by numbers, as follows: *1,* Dr. Eliza M. Mosher, Brooklyn; *2,* Dr. Jay W. Seaver, Yale; *3,* Hope Narey, Holyoke; *4,* Dr. Julius King, Cleveland; *5,* Dr. Claes Enebuske, Boston; *6,* Dr. Henry Boice, Trenton; *7,* Henry S. Anderson, Yale and Brooklyn; *8,* Emily M. Bishop, Jamestown and New York City; *9,* Dr. William G. Anderson; *10,* Lee Pennock, Jamestown and New York City; *11,* Dr. Louis Collin, Boston; *12,* Gertrude Jeffords, Jamestown, accompanist. Those persons not identified by numbers were students.

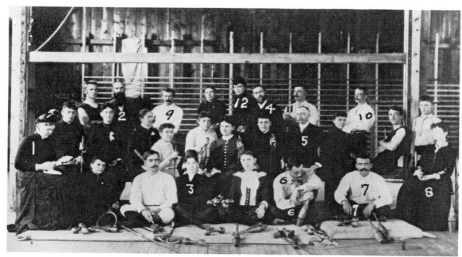

COURTESY HAROLD L. RAY, WESTERN
MICHIGAN UNIVERSITY, KALAMAZOO, MICH.

added their contributions to physical education. They stimulated the growth of Swedish gymnastics; founded a normal school for teachers at Framingham, Massachusetts; contributed to the school children of Boston, Massachusetts, by offering courses of instruction in Swedish gymnastics to schoolteachers; and influenced the establishment of the Boston Normal School of Gymnastics.

In the 1890's the Delsarte System of Physical Culture was introduced by Francois Delsarte. His system was based on the belief that by contributing to poise, grace, beauty, and health certain physical exercises were conducive to better dramatics and better singing.

During this period American sports began to achieve some degree of popularity. Tennis was introduced in 1874, and in 1880 the United States Lawn Tennis Association was organized. Golf came to America in the late 1880's and in 1894 the United States Golfing Association was formed. Bowling had been popular since

the time of the early Dutch in New York, but it was not until 1895 that the American Bowling Congress was organized. Basketball, one of the few sports originating in the United States, was invented by James Naismith in 1891. Some of the other sports that became popular during this period were wrestling, boxing, volleyball, skating, skiing, lacrosse, handball, archery, track, soccer, squash, football, and swimming. In 1879 the National Association of Amateur Athletics of America was developed. The American Athletic Union developed out of this organization.

Physical education has played a large part in the Young Men's Christian Association, an organization that is worldwide in scope and that is devoted to developing Christian character and better living standards. Robert J. Roberts was an outstanding authority in physical education for the YMCA in the late 1800's. In 1885, an International Training School of the YMCA was founded at Springfield, Massachusetts. Roberts became an instruc-

Dr. Rich's Institute for Physical Education.

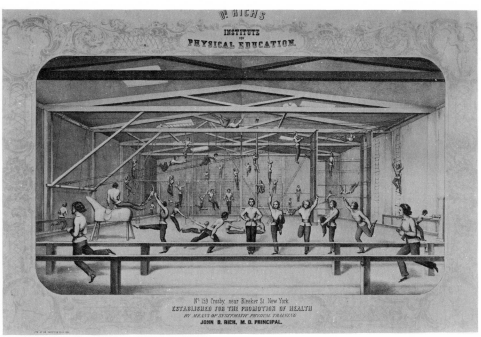

FROM THE J. CLARENCE DAVIES COLLECTION, MUSEUM OF THE CITY OF NEW YORK.

To the members of the Athletic Club:

MISGUIDED MORTALS—Dwell as I do in the atmosphere of piety with which my father's home is always pervaded, and separated as I am from the vanities of this wicked world, it is not often that I receive tidings from the valley of worldliness which stretches out far below me.

But I have been made acquainted with that zeal for a fleshly gospel, and for a merely muscular grace, which has unhappily broken out in our once religious village.

It was a sufficiently mournful token of the decay of Zion that so many professors fell from their allegiance and built that temple to Baal, which, I think, you call a Club House—an edifice erected to frivolity, and unconsecrated by one prayer or psalm.

But my cup of spiritual grief was filled, when I learned that even the handmaidens of our village are also bowing down to this pagan fashion, and are learning the unscriptual practice of gymnastics, and having heard that you are this night to discuss formally the subject of women's part in your gymnasium, I write unto you this letter of counsel, warning, and re-proof. Where in the Bible can you find the least authority for gymnastics? Echo answers, where?

That pagan name does not occur anywhere in the sacred volume, from Genesis to Revelation. But while gymnastics are not mentioned by name, they are referred to, and that with the severest censure. The Apostle Paul (I Tim. iv. 7, 8) says to Timothy: Exercise thyself rather unto Godliness. For bodily exercise profiteth little; but Godliness is profitable unto all things.

Also, is it not a great shame and a scandal, that young ladies should be so negligent of propriety as to take part in diversions which must cause an unseemly exposure of their feet, and even of their ankles?

The Apostle Paul would not allow women to appear in public with their heads uncovered. What would he have said to you who are willing not only to show your heads, but your ——————? I am too much shocked to finish the sentence.

The Scripture teaches also that woman was intended to be weak. But your gymnastics oppose the will of Providence, and the words of Scripture, by making woman strong.

It is the duty of woman to stay at home and comfort her husband (here there were smiles and profuse whisperings among the ladies) and take care of his house. But how can she properly discharge this duty if she goes to the gymnasium?

We are also told in the Scripture that it is the will of God that the great duty of woman should be attended with suffering; "In sorrow shall thou bring forth children." But so profane has the world grown, that you gymnastic people openly boast that woman can be so strengthened as to bear children without great pain, and thus thwart the righteous will of Heaven. Need I say more to prove to you the error of your present course? I pray that you may see the wickedness of your way, and turn your unscriptural Club House into a temple of the living God.

Yours sorrowfully,
"JERUSHA SNIPP"

Excerpt from the Brawnville Papers
by Moses Coit Tyler
(Fields, Osgood & Co., Boston, 1869)

A letter written in the 1860's reflects how some people felt about physical education.

tor there, as did Luther Gulick, who later became Director of Physical Training for the New York City Public Schools. After Gulick left Springfield, Dr. McCurdy became head of the physical education department.

The first Young Women's Christian As-sociation was founded in Boston in 1866 by Mrs. Henry Durant. This organization is very similar to the Young Men's Christian Association in nature and has a broad physical education program for its members.

Physical education made major advances

in colleges and universities with the construction of gymnasiums and the development of departments in this area. Two of the great leaders in physical education during the last half of the nineteenth century were Dr. Dudley Allen Sargent, who was in charge of the physical education work at Harvard, and Dr. Edward Hitchcock, who was head of the physical education department at Amherst. Sargent is known for his work in teacher preparation, remedial equipment, exercise devices, college organization and administration, anthropometric measurement, experimentation, physical diagnosis as a basis for activity, and scientific research. Some of the schools that constructed gymnasiums were Harvard, Yale, Princeton, Bowdoin, Oberlin, Wesleyan, Williams, Dartmouth, Mt. Holyoke, Vassar, Beloit, Wisconsin, California, Smith, and Vanderbilt. Intercollegiate sports also began to play a prominent part, with the first intercollegiate meet in the form of a crew race between Harvard and Yale in 1852. Williams and Amherst played the first intercollegiate baseball game in 1859, and Rutgers and Princeton the first football game in 1869. Other intercollegiate contests in such sports as tennis, swimming,

basketball, squash, and soccer were soon to follow.

Organized physical education programs as part of the curriculum began to appear early in the 1850's in elementary and secondary schools. Boston was one of the first communities to take the step under the direction of Superintendent of Schools, Nathan Bishop. The cities of St. Louis and Cincinnati followed soon afterward. During the next two decades there were only a few instances in which physical education was made part of the school program. However, in the 1880's there was a renewed drive in this direction, with the result that physical directors were appointed in many of the larger cities, and many more communities recognized the need for planned programs in their educational systems.

In 1885, in Brooklyn, the American Association for the Advancement of Physical Education was organized with Edward Hitchcock as the first president and Dudley Sargent, Edward Thwing, and Miss H. C. Putnam as vice-presidents. William G. Anderson was elected secretary and J. D. Andrews, treasurer. This association later became the American Physical Education Association and at the present time is

An early physical education program.

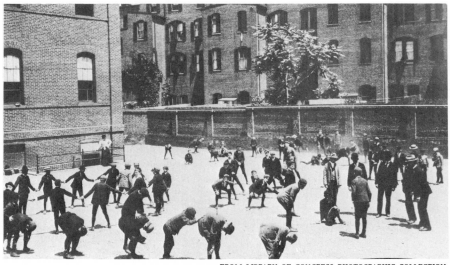

A SCHOOL PRINCIPAL'S INSTRUCTIONS TO HIS TEACHERS IN THE YEAR 1872

1. Teachers each day will fill lamps, clean chimneys, and trim wicks.
2. Each teacher will bring a bucket of water and scuttle of coal for the day's sessions.
3. Make your pens carefully. You may whittle nibs to the individual tastes of the pupil.
4. Men teachers may take one evening each week for courting purposes, or two evenings a week if they go to church regularly.
5. After ten hours of school, the teachers should spend the remaining time reading the Bible or other good books.
6. Women teachers who marry or engage in other unseemly conduct will be dismissed.
7. Every teacher should lay aside from his pay a goodly sum of his earnings for his benefit during his declining years so that he will not become a burden to society.
8. Any teacher who smokes, uses liquor in any form, frequents pool or public halls, or gets shaved in a barber shop will give good reason to suspect his worth, intentions, integrity, and honesty.
9. The teacher who performs his labors faithfully and without fault for five years will be given an increase of twenty-five cents per week in his pay providing the Board of Education approves.

---

known as the American Association for Health, Physical Education, and Recreation. The purpose of this organization is to keep the standards of the profession high, interpret physical education to the public, promote physical education so as to secure adequate programs for the entire country, and provide well-trained teachers.

A struggle between the Swedish, German, and other systems of gymnastics developed in the 1890's. Advocates of each system did their best to spread the merits of their particular program and attempted to have them incorporated as part of school systems. In 1890 Baron Nils Posse introduced the Swedish system in the Boston schools, where it proved popular, and it was later adopted throughout the schools of Massachusetts. The Swedish system had more popularity in the East, and the German system was more prevalent in the Middle West. A survey in the 1890's points out not only the prevalence of the various systems of gymnastics but also the prevalence of physical education programs in general throughout the country. It was reported, after a study of 272 cities, that eighty-three had a director of physical education for their school systems; eighty-one had no director, but teachers were responsible for giving the exercises to the students; and in 108 cities the teachers could decide for themselves whether exercises should be a

part of their daily school programs. A report on the dates the physical education programs were established in the schools surveyed show 10% were established before 1887, 7% from 1887 to 1888, 29% from 1889 to 1890, and 54% from 1891 to 1892. In respect to the system of gymnastics used, the report showed 41% used the German type of gymnastics, 29% Swedish, 12% Delsartian, and 18% eclectic.* Only eleven cities had equipped gymnasiums. It was not long, however, before there was greater expansion in gymnasiums, equipment, trained teachers, and interest in physical education. Ohio in 1892 was the first state to pass a law requiring physical education in the public schools. Other states followed, and there were thirty-three in 1925. Today there are only a very few that have not provided such legislation.

Developments affecting physical education at the turn of the century

Many new developments were taking place at the turn of the century in the area of general education that were to leave their impact upon physical education.

PROFESSIONAL EDUCATION WAS GIVEN INCREASED ATTENTION. Teachers College, Columbia University, was organized. A

---

*A combination of the various systems of gymnastics.

Skating in Central Park, New York, 1885.

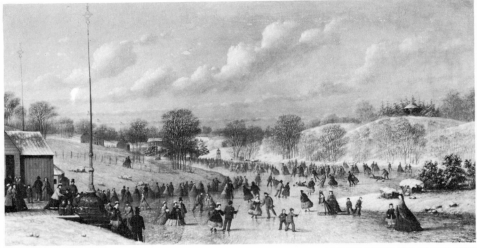

FROM THE J. CLARENCE DAVIES COLLECTION, MUSEUM OF THE CITY OF NEW YORK.

Boating on Lake Chautauqua.

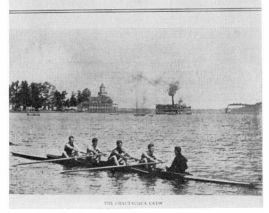

RECREATION AND STUDY

Chautauqua Affords Opportunity for Instruction Under the Best Instructors, Together with Abundant Outdoor Recreation and an Attractive Program of Concerts, Popular Lectures and the Best Entertainments.

THE CHAUTAUQUA CREW

COURTESY HAROLD L. RAY, WESTERN
MICHIGAN UNIVERSITY, KALAMAZOO, MICH.

Photographs of the Chautauqua institution—early showcase for physical education in the late 1800's and early 1900's. It was located on Lake Chautauqua in southwestern New York State. William G. Anderson, founder of the American Association for Health, Physical Education, and Recreation, was active at this institution.

School of Education was established at the University of Chicago, and a Graduate School of Education came into being at Harvard. The first junior college was founded in Joliet, Illinois, in the year 1902.

PSYCHOLOGY WAS INFLUENCING EDUCATIONAL THINKING. In 1878, *Wilhelm Max Wundt* (1832–1920), a German physiologist, founded a psychological laboratory in Leipzig that many American students attended. Wundt's studies in the area of the play interest of animals and humans stimulated much interest at home and abroad. *William James* (1842–1910), a follower of Wundt, proclaimed many pragmatic theories and was known particularly for his research into such things as habit formation, mental discipline, transfer of training, and instincts. *E. L. Thorndike* (1874–1949), who studied under William James, a specialist in the area of educational psychology, made contributions in such areas as the learning process, mental testing, and child psychology. He was particularly well known for his introduction of the stimulus–response (S–R) theory of learning.

SOCIOLOGY WAS INFLUENCING EDUCATIONAL THINKING. *George H. Mead* (1863–1931), expounded on the theory that man is the product of his social interaction with other men. *John Dewey* (1859–1952) interpreted the impact of industrial and social changes upon education.

THE IMPORTANCE OF CHILD STUDY GAINED GREAT EMPHASIS. *G. Stanley Hall* (1845–1924) was the leader of the Child-Study Movement and advocated the "Recapitulation" theory of play (see Chapter 18). Hall was particularly interested in play and games as a means of fulfilling the health needs of children and youth. Much of the emphasis upon rhythms and dancing, he felt, should take place during the adolescent period. He stressed that informal play and games were superior to the formal calisthenic type of exercise. *John Mason Tyler* (1851–1929), a biologist, stressed the need to know the biological characteristics of children in order to prescribe the physical activities best suited to their needs.

He stressed gymnastics as well as play and games.

YOUTH-SERVING PROGRAMS WERE INITIATED IN GREATER NUMBER. Scouting, Camp Fire Girls, Girl Scouts of America, playground activities, and outdoor activities were given much greater attention by the American public and educators in general.

PHYSICAL EDUCATION PROGRAMS IN SCHOOLS AND COLLEGES GAINED MOMENTUM. As a result of these and other developments, a survey by the North American Gymnastic Union of physical education programs in fifty-two cities showed that gymnastic programs averaged 15 minutes in the elementary schools and two periods weekly in the secondary schools. Cities that were surveyed showed 323 gymnasiums in existence and many more under construction. Extensive interscholastic programs also existed, as a survey of 290 high schools in 1907 showed that 28% of the students engaged in one or more sports. The controversy over interscholastic athletics for girls was very pronounced, with such people as *Jessie Bancroft* and *Elizabeth Burchenal* stressing the importance of intramural games for girls rather than interscholastic competition. A majority of colleges and universities had departments of physical education, and most institutions of higher learning provided some program of gymnastics for their students. A survey by *Thomas D. Storey* in 1908 gave information concerning leadership in physical education. It showed that of the institutions surveyed, 41% of the directors of physical education possessed medical degrees, 3% of the directors held doctor of philosophy degrees, and the remaining possessed a bachelor's degree. Intercollegiate athletics were brought under more rigid academic control as the abuses mounted. Intramural athletics gained in prominence as the emphasis on athletics for all gained momentum.

Physical education in the early twentieth century

Some of the great names that should be mentioned in any discussion of the history of physical education during the early part of the twentieth century will be discussed.

Thomas Dennison Wood was one who made an outstanding contribution to the field of physical education. A study of his career shows that he attended Oberlin College, was the first director of the physical education department at Stanford University, and later became associated with Teachers College, Columbia University. He believed there should be more emphasis on games and game skills and introduced his new program under the name "Natural Gymnastics."

Clark Hetherington is also well known to physical educators. His thinking was influenced by his close association with Thomas D. Wood, who chose Hetherington as his assistant while he was at Stanford. Hetherington's contributions resulted in a clearer understanding of children's play activities in terms of survival and continued participation. This was also true of athletics and athletic skills. Hetherington became head of the physical education department at New York University and, along with his successor, *Jay B. Nash,* was responsible for its becoming one of the leading teacher training schools in the nation.

Robert Tait McKenzie, a physical educator, surgeon-scientist, and artist-sculptor, served distinguished periods at McGill University and the University of Pennsylvania. He was known for his great contribution to sculpture, for his dedication to helping physically underdeveloped and atypical individuals overcome their deficiencies, and for his writings of such books as *Exercise in Education and Medicine,* published in 1910.

Jessie H. Bancroft, a woman pioneer in the field of physical education, taught at Davenport, Iowa, Hunter College, and Brooklyn and New York City Public Schools. She greatly influenced the development of physical education as a responsibility of homeroom teachers in elementary schools. She also contributed much to the field of posture and body mechanics, was the first living member of the AAHPER to receive the Gulick Award, and was well known for her book *Games for the Playground, Home, School, and Gymnasium.*

Delphine Hanna, an outstanding woman leader of physical education, developed a department of physical education at Oberlin College, which sent outstanding graduates all over the country. She was instrumental in motivating not only many outstanding leaders in the female ranks but also encouraged such outstanding men as Thomas Wood, Luther Gulick, and Fred Leonard to follow illustrious careers in physical education.

James H. McCurdy studied at the Training School of Christian Workers at Springfield Medical School of New York University, Harvard Medical School, Springfield College, and Clark University. He was closely associated with Springfield College, where he provided outstanding leadership in the field of physical education. He published such works as *The Physiology of Exercise* and was editor of the *American Physical Education Review.*

Luther Gulick, born in Honolulu, was director of physical education at Springfield College, principal of Pratt High School in Brooklyn, Director of Physical Education for Greater New York City Public Schools, and president of the American Physical Education Association. He taught philosophy of play at New York University, helped to found and was the first president of the Playground Association of America (later to become the National Recreation Association), was associated with the Russell Sage Foundation as director of recreation, and was president of Camp Fire Girls, Inc.

Health education and recreation, branches of what were formerly phases of the physical education program, grew during the early twentieth century to the extent that specialists and programs distinct and separate from those of physical education were utilized in many communities. Health education proved its value in educating the public about available health services, in respect to scientific health knowledge, and in respect to healthful living. Recreation came to the front in helping the public better

Physical education costumes for American women in previous years.

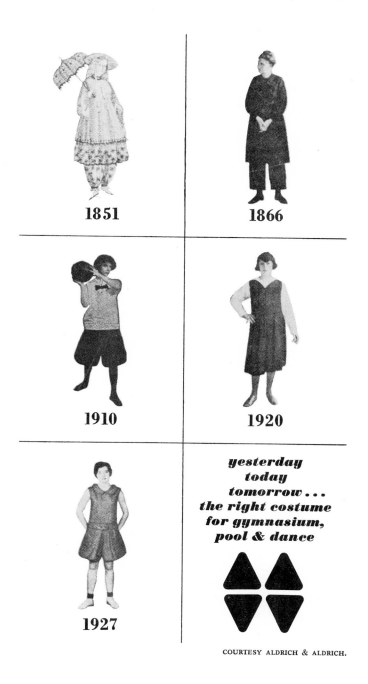

1851   1866

1910   1920

1927

*yesterday
today
tomorrow...
the right costume
for gymnasium,
pool & dance*

COURTESY ALDRICH & ALDRICH.

utilize their increased leisure, which resulted from a higher standard of living. Through programs that dealt with such activities as arts and crafts, athletics, dramatics, and music, mental and physical dividends resulted for many persons.

The playground movement had a rapid period of growth after the first sand garden was set up in 1885 in Boston. In 1888, New York passed a law that provided for a study of places where children might play out of doors. In New York the name of Jacob A. Riis was symbolic of the playground movement in that city. In Chicago a playground was managed by Hull House. In 1906 the Playground and Recreation Association of America was established to promote the development of rural and urban playgrounds, with Dr. Gulick as president. Since that time playgrounds have been established in many cities and smaller communities throughout the country.

In the field of teacher education in physical education, higher standards were established and better trained leaders were produced. The 2-year normal school became a thing of the past, with 4 years of preparation being required. The trend in professional preparation required of students a broad general education, a knowledge of child growth and development and the psychology of learning, and specialized training in physical education, including a knowledge of the foundational sciences, curriculum materials, and methodology.

Physical education progressed in the early twentieth century to a point where it was increasingly recognized as an important part of American culture, with several new trends in evidence. Sports, athletics, and team games became more important, with broad and extensive programs being established in schools, recreational organizations, and other agencies. The National Collegiate Athletic Association, National Association of Intercollegiate Athletics, and other leagues, organizations, and associations were formed to keep a watchful eye on competitive sports. Nevertheless, the emphasis on gate receipts and winning

games resulted in many problems. The struggle between the formal and informal types of physical education programs continued to exist.

During the early twentieth century a new physical education started to evolve. Using a scientific basis, it attempted to discover the physical needs of individuals and the part that a planned physical education program can play in meeting these needs. It recognized that education is a "doing" process and that the individual learns through doing. It stressed good leadership, in which exercises and activities are not a matter of mere physical routine but, instead, are meaningful and significant to the participant. It stressed a varied program of activities that included the fundamental skills of running, jumping, climbing, carrying, throwing, and leaping; camping activities; self-testing activities; "tag" and "it" games; dancing and rhythmical activities; dual and individual sports; and team games. It stressed the need for more research and investigation into what type of physical education program best serves the needs of children and adults. It stressed the need for a wider use of measurement and evaluation techniques to determine how well objectives are being achieved. Finally, it provided a program that better served to adapt individuals to the democratic way of life. Other significant events during this period included the following:

The Athletic Research Society was founded in 1907 by Dr. Sargent and Dr. Gulick.

Football was abolished in New York City Public Schools in 1910 because of unfavorable conditions.

The Athletic Research Society, backed by the American Physical Education Association, established a committee to aid in the development of intramural sports within the schools.

The American Physical Education Association provided time for dance sessions at annual meetings—folk dancing was stressed.

The American Physical Education Association established sections in their organization for anthropometry, elementary schools, normal schools, college directors, nonschool groups, private secondary schools, and medical gymnastics.

The Girls' and Women's Section of the Ameri-

OUR PRESIDENTS ARE SPORTSMEN

George Washington was a master woodsman and horse lover.

John Quincy Adams was an expert in billiards.

Andrew Jackson was fascinated by horse racing and owned several thoroughbreds.

John Tyler was playing marbles when he received the news that Benjamin Harrison had died and that he was now President.

Abraham Lincoln was an excellent wrestler.

Ulysses Grant was a gifted horseman.

Grover Cleveland enjoyed fishing and hunting.

Theodore Roosevelt developed skill in riding, wrestling, and boxing.

Woodrow Wilson coached football.

Warren G. Harding's forte was golfing.

"Silent Cal" Coolidge was a fisherman and a horseman.

Herbert Hoover possessed expertise in fishing. President Hoover pointed out on one occasion that "Presidents have only two moments of personal seclusion, one is prayer. The other is fishing—and they can't pray all the time."

Franklin D. Roosevelt enjoyed fishing.

Harry Truman went swimming and also fished.

Dwight D. Eisenhower established himself as the best golfer among presidents.

John F. Kennedy participated in many sports, including golf, swimming, and sailing.

Lyndon B. Johnson enjoys riding.

Richard M. Nixon sails, golfs, and swims.

---

can Physical Education Association was recognized for the first time on a convention program in 1914.

District associations of the American Physical Education Association came into being.

National headquarters of the American Physical Education Association was transferred from Boston to New York.

There were forty-seven foreign members of the American Physical Education Association by 1910.

World War I (1916-1919)

World War I started in 1914, and America's entry in 1918 had a critical impact on the nation and education. The Selective Service Act of 1917 called to service all men between the ages of 18 and 25 years. Health statistics gleaned from Selective Service examinations aroused considerable interest in the nation's health. Discussions were held on the most feasible manner for achieving top physical condition.

Social forces were also at work during this period. The Eighteenth Amendment was passed, which had to do with the prohibition of selling alcoholic beverages. This opened up the period of the "rum runners" and "speakeasies." Out of this movement came the Anti-Saloon League and the Woman's Christian Temperance Union, which were in later years to have a great impact on the introduction of health teaching into the schools. The emancipation of women was furthered by passage of the Nineteenth Amendment. Women also began to show interest in sports and physical education, as well as in other fields formerly considered to be "off limits."

During World War I many physical educators provided leadership for physical conditioning programs for the armed forces and also for the people on the home front. Such persons as Dudley Sargent, Luther Gulick, Thomas Storey, and R. Tait McKenzie contributed their services to the armed forces. The Commission on Training Camp Activities of the War Department was created, and Raymond Fosdick was named as the head of this program. Joseph E. Raycroft of Princeton University and Walter Camp, the creator of "All-Americans," were named to head the athletic divisions of the Army and the Navy, respectively. Women physical educators were also active in conditioning programs in communities and in industry at home.

After the war was over and the public had an opportunity to study the medical examiner's report for the men who had been called to military duty, pressure built up for the government and education to do something about the fact that one-third of

our men were found physically unfit for armed service and that many more were physically inept. Also, a survey by the National Council on Education in 1918 showed that children in the elementary and secondary schools of the nation were woefully

---

Fifty Years Ago in the Journal

The currently controversial issue of sex instruction in the schools was a topic of concern to members of the American Physical Education Association in March 1919. "Sex Instruction in Connection with Physical Training in High Schools" was the subject of a meeting in Connecticut, at which statements of policy were agreed to by participants, who represented both college and high school physical education programs. The document was published in full in the Journal of fifty years ago, and the quotations below show that while some of the arguments are still pertinent, the developing role of the school health educator has brought about a new perspective on sex education in today's schools.

"The necessity for sex education in high schools is plain and apparent. Since, however, investigations show that knowledge of sexual matters comes to children before high school age the desirability of sex education in grammar and primary grades is established. At the present time, however, it may be more practical to confine sex education to high school pupils. . . .

"Physical training holds a unique position in this respect [as an agency to communicate the facts to all high school students] for all high school pupils no matter what courses they might elect come for physical training. This is the first advantage of the physical training teacher. All teaching is so much more effective if it can be linked up with life itself and if it can be made practicable. In this respect physical training has once more unusual opportunities.

"The practice of physical education in a high school makes necessary certain precautionary measures in regard to both sexes so that no harm may come to the sexual apparatus by exercise. This means for the female to be made acquainted with the facts underlying menstruation and the effect of exercise thereon. This matter must be broached to every female student in a high school and might as well be made then the basis of further sex instruction which will come in as a matter of course. In dealing with the males, advice as to the wearing of protective appliances so as to prevent harm to the testes in physical training practice is likewise necessary and opens the way for general sex instruction. . . .

"Physical work in itself is an antidote against undue manifestations of sexual life in the young. . . . The selection of individuals for games gives occasion to point out that sexual development is closely allied with the development of not only physical properties but also mental and moral ones as evidenced especially in the different physiques and mentalities in domestic animals. where unsexing is practiced. The advantage of continence to preserve fitness for certain games, the unfitting influence of premature sexual indulgence, can be readily brought to the attention of especially the male in the high school.

"With all this advantage of physical education one thing must be insisted upon that such knowledge gained by formal and informal instruction will be no help unless character building is coupled with it. The demand then for character building through physical education must be reiterated in this connection."

FROM JOURNAL OF HEALTH, PHYSICAL EDUCATION, AND RECREATION **40**:47, 1969.

---

50 Years Ago in the Journal

The February 1919 issue of the *American Physical Education Review* was the "Western District Convention Number." It contained the two-day program details on one and a half pages of its 6″ x 9″ format. In contrast with one of today's district meetings, the program consisted of general sessions only, seven in number, plus three demonstrations (swimming, dance, and calisthenics). Both morning and afternoon schedules had "community singing" breaks, evidently a welcome moment of relaxation since the second day's program began with a display of calisthenics by the cadets of the School of Military Aeronautics (University of California, Berkeley) at 6:20 a.m.

The impact of World War I on the theory, philosophy, and curriculum of physical education is evident in the titles of the main articles for the issue—"Physical Education in the Light of the Present National Situation," "American Athletics Versus German Militarism," and "The Influence of the War Upon Physical Education"—and the notes, which included a synopsis of the practical guide used by the French centers of military and physical re-education.

Of special interest is the description of a new game invented by James Naismith. Called Vrille (or Vree) Ball, its underlying principle was "to be simple enough so that it could be played by the novice and yet require such skill as to interest the expert," but it never gained the popularity of the other game Naismith created. Played on a rectangle 24′ x 24′ by two teams of three men each, the game involved batting a ball back and forth so that on each exchange it bounced off a rectangular wood or cement target on the ground in the middle of the field. The regulation ball was a leather covered rubber bladder 12″ in circumference and it was hit with the hands. Like basketball, it was invented by Naismith to fit certain requirements demanded by the physical education instructional program. It was designed to give many of the benefits of handball or tennis, providing exercise, developing skills, and combining recreation with competition. It was economical of expense and space; elastic enough to be played on almost any kind of grounds; and capable of being played when only two could get together but flexible enough to accommodate several. Perhaps in attempting to meet too many special requirements, it failed to meet a basic need of maintaining enthusiasm. We would be interested in knowing if any teacher is still using Vrille Ball in his physical education classes.

FROM JOURNAL OF HEALTH, PHYSICAL EDUCATION, AND RECREATION **40**:42, 1969.

subpar physically. The survey indicated that as many as three-fourths of them could be placed in this category. The result was the passing of much legislation in the various states to upgrade physical education programs in the schools. The following states listed laws enacted between 1917 and 1919: Alabama, California, Delaware, Indiana, Maine, Maryland, Michigan, Nevada, New Jersey, Oregon, Pennsylvania, Rhode Island, Utah, and Washington. To provide supervision and leadership for the expanded programs of physical education, state departments of public instruction established administrative heads for their states in many sections of the country.

Significant events during this period also included the following:

Fourteen states enacted laws regarding physical education.

Draft statistics aroused popular interest in health and physical education.

New York appointed the first state director of physical education.

Many colleges established departments of physical education.

Dr. William Burdick, President of the American Physical Education Association, appointed a Committee on Women's Athletics.

Dr. Elmer Mitchell helped to develop intramural sports.

Seven "cardinal principles" of education developed.

Ernest H. Arnold of the New Haven Normal School was active in the work of the American Physical Education Association as president and in other positions.

The National Recreation Association established the National Physical Education Service.

Golden 20's (1920-1929)

The "golden" or "roaring" 20's ushered in a period when people wanted to relax, have a good time, and forget the tragic war that had just passed. The period was an opportune moment for the growth of "big-time" athletics and an era of spectator sports.

The 20's showed the way for a "new physical education" advocated by such leaders as Hetherington, Wood, Nash, and Williams. The move away from the formal gymnastic systems of Europe was well received. The temperament of the times seemed to emphasize a less formal type of program. More games, sports, and free play were the order of the day.

The feeling that physical education had greater worth than building strength and other physical qualities, as incorporated in the thinking of the "new physical education," aroused much discussion. Franklin Bobbit, a University of Chicago educator, commented: "There appears to be a feeling among physical educationists that the physical side of man's nature is lower than the social or mental, and that . . . they, too, must aim primarily at those more exalted nonphysical things of mental and social type." William Burnham, of Clark University, felt that physical education could contribute to the whole individual. Clark Hetherington felt that physical education had different functions in a democratic society than in Europe, where some the the gymnastic systems prevailed. Jesse Feiring Williams stressed the importance of physical education in general education.

Thomas D. Wood, Rosalind Cassidy, and Jesse Feiring Williams published their book, *The New Physical Education,* in 1927; it stressed the biological, psychological, and sociological foundations of physical education.

Another development during this period included the stress on measurement in physical education by such persons as David K. Brace and Frederick Rand Rogers, as a means of grouping pupils, measuring achievement, and motivating performance.

Programs of physical education continued to expand in schools and colleges. The elementary school program of physical education stressed mainly formal activities. The secondary school program also felt the influence of the formalists. In addition, there were periodic lectures on hygiene. Interscholastic athletics continued to grow in popularity, with the need being felt to institute controls. The National Federation of High School Athletic Associations was established in 1923. At the college and university level a study by George L. Meylan reported in 1921 that of 230 institutions surveyed, 199 had departments of physical education presided over by administrative heads and an average of four staff members per institution. Many of the staff members had professorial rank. More than three-fourths of the institutions required physical education for their students, with the most general requirement being for 2 years in length. The 20's also saw a boom in the area of stadium construction.

Many problems arose in respect to college athletics. As a result, the Carnegie Foundation provided a grant in 1923 for a study of intercollegiate athletics in certain institutions in the south by a Committee of the Association of Colleges and Secondary Schools. Later, a study was conducted of athletic practices in American colleges and universities. The report of this study was published in 1929 under the title *American College Athletics*. The report denounced athletics as being professional rather than amateur in nature and as a means of public entertainment and commercialization. Problems such as rcruiting and subsidizing athletics also were exposed.

During this period there was an increase in the intramural athletic programs in colleges and universities. Women's departments of physical education also showed a greater growth over the previous period discussed. Women's programs experienced an increase in the number of staff, hours required for student participation, activities offered, and physical education buildings in use.

Some other significant happenings during this period were the following:

A spectator boom in athletics was observed.
The "new physical education" was accepted.
Social education was recognized as an objective of physical education.
Intramural programs were expanded.
Growth of the recreation and playground movements was encouraged.
More emphasis was placed on sports that could be played in adult life.
Dancing was introduced into many school programs.
The number of institutions preparing physical education personnel was increased from twenty in 1918 to 139 in 1929.

Corrective physical education was made a part of many university programs.
Laws regarding physical education were enacted by more than twenty states.
The National Federation of State High School Athletic Associations was established.
The Women's Division of National Amateur Athletic Federation was established.
Doctoral programs were offered at Teachers College, Columbia University, and New York University.

Depression years (1930-1939)

The 1929 stock market crash ushered in the Great Depression, which affected education. The golden 20's had seen an era of plenty. Now unemployment and poverty reigned. Health and physical education had a difficult time surviving in many communities. The numbers on the unemployed list brought about the program of leisure-time education. This was also the era when the government subsidized the Works Progress Administration and other agencies in constructing recreation and other facilities.

During the period of the economic depression in the United States, many of the gains achieved by physical education in the schools of the nation were lost. Budgets were cut back and programs in many cases were either dropped or downgraded. In the 1932-1934 period an estimated 40% of the physical education programs were dropped completely. There were legislative moves in several of the states, such as Illinois and California, to do away with the physical education requirement.

Another development during the depression years was that the physical educator became more involved in recreation programs in the agencies and programs concerned with unemployed persons. These later programs were being subsidized through special governmental assistance. The national association, taking cognizance of the increased interest in recreation, voted to change its title to include the word *recreation*—the American Association for Health, Physical Education, and Recreation.

A new interest captivated many physical educators, namely that of facilities concerned with programs of physical education, athletics, and recreation. Several publications appeared before the end of the 1920's on this subject.

The trend in physical education programs was away from the formal type to an informal games and sports approach. Also, what constitutes an acceptable program of physical education at various school and college levels was outlined by William R. LaPorte of the University of Southern California in his publication *The Physical Education Curriculum—A National Program*, published in 1937. This publication, which is still in use today, left a deep imprint upon elementary and secondary physical education programs.

Interscholastic athletic programs continued to grow and in some situations dominated physical education programs and created many educational problems. The collegiate athletic program received a temporary setback from the Carnegie Report but then started to grow again. The National Association of Intercollegiate Basketball was established in 1940 for the purpose of providing an association for the smaller colleges. It later changed its name to National Association of Intercollegiate Athletics in 1952. In 1937, representatives of the Junior Colleges of California met for the purpose of forming the National Junior College Athletic Association.

Intramural athletics continued to grow in colleges and universities. Women's athletic associations also increased in number. The principles that guided such programs were established largely by the National Section on Women's Athletics, now called the Division of Girls and Women's Sports.

Some significant happenings during this period are as follows:

The objective of leisure-time education became important to the field of physical education.

Civilian Conservation Corps was used for recreation projects.

WPA proved a boost for recreation.

Many more states added state directors to their rosters.

Women's Athletic Section of APEA was organized.

Health and Recreation were added to the title of the American Physical Education Association.

Educational Policies Commission formulated educational objectives.

APEA became a department of the National Education Association.

First woman president of national association, Mabel Lee of the University of Nebraska, was elected.

First issues of *Journal of Health and Physical Education* and the *Research Quarterly* were published.

Physical education in the mid–twentieth century

Physical education has made great strides in the middle of the twentieth century. The period from the start of World War II until the beginning of the 70's has seen many changes in regard to the role and preparation of physical educators, student involvement, curriculum reform, growth of sports, women's liberation, and international involvement. The more significant historical happenings for physical education in the middle twentieth century period will be discussed here.

IMPACT OF WORLD WAR II

The country was jolted from depression by World War II. Physical education received an impetus as physical training programs were established under Gene Tunney in the Navy, Hank Greenburg in the Air Force, and sports leaders in other branches of the armed forces. Schools and colleges were urged to help develop physical fitness in the youth of the nation. A return to more formalized conditioning programs resulted.

The need for a national program of physical fitness was evident as a result of Selective Service examinations and other indications that American young people were not in good physical shape. Several steps were taken in this direction. President Roosevelt appointed John B. Kelly, of Philadelphia, National Director of Physical Training. In 1941, Mayor Fiorello LaGuardia, of New York City, was appointed by President Roosevelt as Director of Civilian Defense in Charge of Physical Fitness, and a National Advisory Board was established. William L. Hughes, of the national association, was appointed chairman. In 1942, a Division of Physical Fitness was established in the Office of Defense, Health, and Welfare Services. In 1943, John B. Kelly was appointed chairman of a Committee of Physical Fitness within the Office of the Administrator, Federal Security Agency.

The war years had their impact on programs of physical education in schools and colleges of the nation. In many instances, elementary school physical education classes met daily, and secondary and college classes also were increased in number. The program of activities took on a more formal nature with the purpose of physically conditioning the children and youth of America for the national emergency that existed. Such activities as running, jumping, throwing, climbing, and tumbling were stressed. Girls and women as well as boys and men were exposed to these programs.

Some significant happenings in this period were the following:

> Broad physical training programs were established in the armed forces.
> Physical reconditioning programs were provided for injured returnees.
> Obstacle courses and other devices to condition youth were developed in schools.
> Interest in physical education and health was stimulated as a result of Selective Service medical statistics.
> Need for better interpretation of the meaning of physical education was stressed as sports leaders rather than professionals were selected to head physical training programs.

THE PHYSICAL FITNESS MOVEMENT

In December, 1953, an article was published in the *Journal of the American Association for Health, Physical Education, and Recreation* entitled "Muscular Fitness and Health." The information contained in this article was to have major implications for physical education. The article discussed the physical deficiencies of American children in contrast with European children

and brought to the attention of the American people the deplorable physical condition of the nation's youth. As a result, a series of events followed that may be called the physical fitness movement.

James B. Kelly of Philadelphia and Senator James Duff of Pennsylvania called the information discussed in this article to the attention of the President of the United States. In July, 1955, President Eisenhower convened a group of prominent sports figures in Washington to explore the fitness problem. Later, he called a Youth Fitness Conference at the Naval Academy in Annapolis. About 150 leaders in the fields of sports, education, youth programs, recreation, health, and related areas met for 2 days and discussed the fitness problem in detail. At the conclusion of the conference President Eisenhower issued an executive order establishing a President's Council on Youth Fitness and appointed Dr. Shane MacCarthy as executive director. Following this, a President's Citizens Advisory Committee on Fitness of American Youth was appointed.

As a result of President Eisenhower's decrees, fitness became a national topic for consideration. Several states, including California and Illinois, established their own committees on physical fitness. Such cities as Flint and Detroit developed special projects. The YMCA, Amateur Athletic Union, and other organizations put forth special efforts to promote fitness. Several business concerns became involved, such as General Mills, which established the Wheaties Sports Foundation. The magazine *Sports Illustrated* devoted regular features to fitness. The National Research Council of the AAHPER authorized the testing of American children in regard to their physical fitness. The College Physical Education Association for Men published a special report entitled "Fit for College." Operation Fitness USA was inaugurated by the AAHPER to promote fitness, leadership, public relations, and research. The project established motivational devices such as certificates of recognition, achievement

Twentieth-century physical education stresses a varied program of activities.

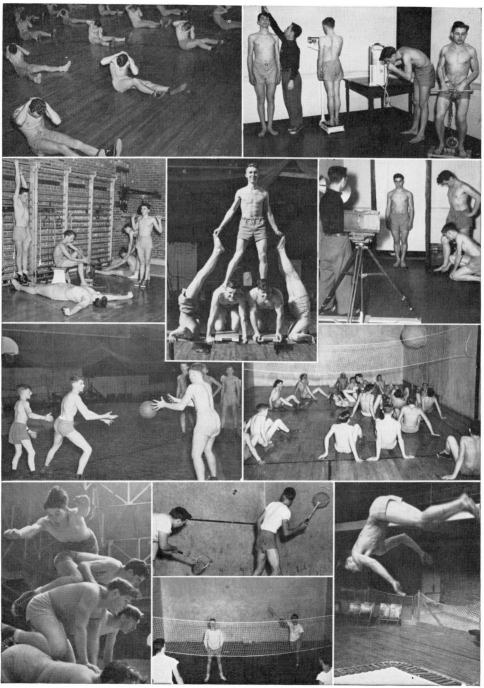

GOULD ACADEMY, BETHEL, MAINE.

awards, and emblems for students at various levels of achievement.

When John F. Kennedy became President of the United States, he appointed Charles "Bud" Wilkinson of Oklahoma to head his council on youth fitness. The name of the Council was changed to the President's Council on Physical Fitness. The council introduced its "Blue Book" with suggestions for school-centered programs.

President Kennedy released a statement on health and physical fitness in which he outlined the following program:

Identify the physically underdeveloped pupil and work with him to improve his physical capacity.

Provide a minimum of 15 minutes of vigorous activity each day for all pupils.

Use valid fitness tests to determine pupils' physical abilities and evaluate their progress.

When President Lyndon Johnson became president he appointed Stan Musial to head his Council on Physical Fitness. Later, when Stan Musial resigned this position, he appointed Captain James A Lovell, Jr., U.S.N., to replace him. The council's name was again changed to the President's Council on Physical Fitness and Sports.*

PROFESSIONAL PREPARATION

The war and postwar teacher shortage represented a critical problem for the nation. During the war 200,000 teachers left jobs and 100,000 emergency certificates were issued. Many of those who left did not return and the inadequately trained replacements were hired. The critical shortage forced administrators to discard their standards in selecting teachers. In the physical education field there was a need for reinterpreting the meaning and objectives of physical education and a rededication of teachers to prewar ideals, along with the desire of teachers to improve their professional status.

Professional preparation programs increased in number during this period, with over 600 colleges and universities partici-

pating in such programs. Some of the larger institutions developed separate professional programs for health, physical education, and recreation personnel, whereas many of the smaller institutions concerned themselves with only physical education. A trend developed to have evaluative criteria utilized so that the standards for such programs could be upgraded.*

SPORTS

There were four significant developments in respect to the development of sports during the mid–twentieth century period of history. There was a renewed interest in girls' and women's sports, intramurals, lifetime sports, and sport programs for boys and girls below the high school age.

GIRLS' AND WOMEN'S SPORTS. In 1962, the Division for Girls' and Women's Sports and the Division of Men's Athletics of the AAHPER held their first joint conference so that the views of both men and women in the profession could be expressed. Two years later, the first National Institute on Girls' Sports was held for the purpose of promoting sports for girls and women. In 1965 a study conference met to discuss and develop guidelines needed in the area of competition for girls and women. In addition to these steps that were taken to promote girls' and women's sports, additional moves included the development of a liaison with Olympic Games officials as a part of the Olympic development movement, the publication of guidelines for girls and women in competitive sports by the DGWS, and the exploration of the social changes in society that had implications for sport programs for women. All of these steps represented a new departure toward providing greater opportunities for girls and women to engage in competitive sports at both the high school and college levels.

INTRAMURALS. As sports became more

---

*For more information on the President's Council see Chapter 16.

*See Chapter 21 for a discussion of various conferences held during this period of the undergraduate and graduate preparation of physical education teachers.

and more popular at various educational levels, there was a renewed interest in providing sports competition for all students, not just the skilled elite. A meeting that helped to spur this movement was held in 1956 when the National Conference on Intramural Sports for College Men and Women met in Washington, D. C. Its purpose was to consider intramural programs for college men and women, to formulate principles, to recommend administrative procedures relating to current and future programs, and to provide greater opportunity for more young men and women to participate in healthful recreational activities. The intramural movement continued to grow, with leadership being provided by the National Intramural Association. More play areas and facilities were constructed for intramural programs.

LIFETIME SPORTS. This period saw a stress on the sports that can be played during a person's entire lifetime. Giving leadership to this movement was the establishment of the Lifetime Sports Foundation in 1965. Its purpose was to promote fitness and lifetime sports and to give assistance to groups engaged in these areas. This same year, the AAHPER approved the Lifetime Sports Education Project, an adjunct of the Lifetime Sports Foundation. School and college physical education programs reflected the influence of such projects, with greater emphasis being given to the teaching of such activities as bowling, tennis, golf, and badminton.

SPORT PROGRAMS FOR BOYS AND GIRLS BELOW THE HIGH SCHOOL LEVEL. Considerable controversy was generated during this period concerning sports for children below the high school level. In 1953, a National Conference on Program Planning in Games and Sports for Boys and Girls of Elementary School Age was held in Washington, D. C. It was the first time that organizations representing medicine, education, recreation, and other organizations serving the child had ever met with leaders of organizations who promote highly organized competitive activities for children. Two of the

recommendations to come out of this conference were: (1) that programs of games and sports should be based on the developmental level of children and that there should be no contact sports for children under 12, and (2) that competition is inherent in the growth and development of the child and will be harmful or beneficial depending upon a variety of factors. Regardless of these recommendations, the field of sports competition for youngsters grew rapidly. Little Leagues and competition of a varsity pattern for children were inaugurated in many communities and schools. Educators continued to ask, however, whether highly organized forms of sports were in the best interests of children and young people below the high school age.

INTERNATIONAL DEVELOPMENTS

International meetings of leaders of health, physical education, and recreation from various parts of the world were initiated in the mid–twentieth century in order to improve their status and programs. Conferences were held and joint projects conducted. Furthermore, the Peace Corps recruited many physical educators to work in selected countries of the world.

World seminars in physical education were held, such as the one in Helsinki in 1952. The first International Congress in Physical Education was held in the United States in 1953 and considered such topics as recreation, sports, correctives, dance, and tests and measurements. Approximately 100 world leaders in physical education from over forty different countries attended this meeting.

In 1958, at the annual meeting of the World Confederation of Organizations of the Teaching Profession, the WCOTP appointed a committee to make plans for a World Federation of National and International Associations of Health Education, Physical Education, and Recreation. The purpose was to provide a way in which to unite representatives from all associations of these fields in a worldwide organization.

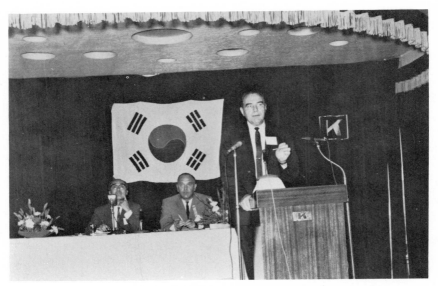

The secretary-general of ICHPER addressing the delegate assembly.

The following year the WCOTP established the International Council of Health, Physical Education, and Recreation (ICHPER). This organization has been active on the world scene and meets annually to consider problems of global interest.

In addition to these international meetings, many other steps have been taken internationally, including Pan-American Institutes and People-to-People Sports Committees. Physical educators found that much can be learned and accomplished through involvement with their colleagues in other lands.

THE HANDICAPPED

The mid–twentieth century saw a realization develop on the part of physical educators that their field of specialization could make a contribution to the handicapped student, including the mentally retarded, the physically handicapped, the poorly coordinated, and the culturally disadvantaged. One of the events that accented this movement was a grant from the Joseph P. Kennedy, Jr. Foundation in 1965, which enabled the AAHPER to establish the Project on Recreation and Fitness for the Mentally Retarded for the purposes of research, program development, and leadership training.

Adapted physical education programs received increasing attention, with special programs being included in professional preparation institutions to provide leadership for this area. Furthermore, governmental grants of funds enabled greater stress to be placed on this particular phase of the physical education program.

RESEARCH

The need for research in physical education grew to much greater importance in the eyes of physical educators than it had heretofore. The Research Council of the AAHPER was established in 1952 as a section under the General Division. Its functions and purposes included that of promoting research along strategic lines, developing long-range plans, preparing and disseminating materials to aid research workers in the field, and synthesizing research materials in areas related to the professional fields.

As a result of the increased recognition of the importance of research, studies were conducted in such areas as exercise physiology, motor learning, sociology of sport, and teaching methods.

FACILITIES AND EQUIPMENT

With the growth of physical education programs and the construction of new facilities to accommodate these programs, meetings, research, and interest were generated regarding facilities and equipment for physical education.

In 1947 a grant was made by the Athletic Institute to help sponsor a National Facilities Conference at Jackson's Mill, West Virginia. Fifty-four outstanding education, park, and recreation leaders met with architects, engineers, and city planners to prepare a guide for planning facilities for health, physical education, and recreation programs. Facilities conferences have been held periodically in various parts of the United States since 1947.

The Council on Equipment and Supplies of the AAHPER was formed in 1954. Its purpose was to allow manufacturers, distributors, buyers, and consumers of materials used in the areas of health education, physical education, and recreation to work together on problems of mutual concern.

The great amount of monies expended for facilities and equipment in physical education, including sports programs, has been responsible for continued interest in this area so that these monies may be expended in the most profitable manner possible.

SIGNIFICANT CURRENT DEVELOPMENTS HAVING IMPLICATIONS FOR PHYSICAL EDUCATION

Education is undergoing a period of change, and physical education, as a part of education, is also undergoing change. The teacher's and coach's roles are changing as the needs of society change, student activism raises many questions as to the administration and conduct of our programs, curriculum reform is widespread as the old way of doing things is found to be outmoded, the stress on sports continues to increase but with it comes many problems, the women's liberation movement is affecting physical education, and new types of facilities are being utilized. Each of these

current developments will be discussed in more detail in this section.

Teachers, coaches, paraprofessionals

More concern is being expressed by educators and the public alike about the teacher—his qualifications, competencies, and preparation. Discussed here are some significant new developments that should command the attention of every physical educator because of the implications they have for his field of work. These new developments are not discussed here from the standpoint of whether they are desirable or undesirable. Instead, they are recorded here as historical happenings in education and in physical education.

THE PUBLIC WANTS TEACHER ACCOUNTABILITY. According to a recent Gallup Poll, the public is beginning to question educators as to whether American education is doing a good job. This sentiment is also reflected, as Gallup suggests, in the many school bond issues and budgets that fail to be passed by the voters. Also related to this problem is the desire on the part of many adults for national student achievement tests so that school systems may be compared and thus evaluated as to what kind of teaching job is being done. Furthermore, these same adults suggest that teachers should be paid in accordance with the work they do rather than according to the present seniority system.

Teacher accountability has also given strong impetus to the growth of *performance contracting,* where local schools contract with private companies for part of their teaching load. For example, one school system in the Midwest (Gary, Indiana) contracted with Behavioral Research Laboratories to operate one of its elementary schools for 4 years. The company reorganized the Banneker Elementary School and receives $800 per student annually. The agreement provides that the company will bring the students' levels of achievement up to or above national norms in basic curriculum areas. If the company fails to do this, it will be required to refund to the city the fees paid for each child who does not achieve the desired level. The government is also subsidizing some performance contracting, as evidenced by the action of the U. S. Office of Education awarding in May, 1969, a $270,000 grant to the Texarkana, Arkansas, school district and to the Liberty Eylau school district of Texarkana, Texas, for a 5-year dropout prevention program.

Although performance contracting has arguments both pro and con, it is being utilized more and more in educational circles as the public seeks to obtain the desired results from their school systems and teachers. This has implications for every subject and every teacher in our schools and colleges today, including physical education.

PARAPROFESSIONALS ARE PLAYING MORE IMPORTANT ROLES IN PHYSICAL EDUCATION. There is a growing trend to use paraprofessionals, or adults who can assist a teacher of physical education in nonteaching tasks involved in the teaching-learning process. The value of the paraprofessional, it is pointed out, is that he can free the trained physical education teacher from many clerical and other routine tasks and thus enable this teacher to devote more time to his students, to the teaching process, and to research. The duties of the paraprofessional might include such duties as handling audiovisual aid equipment, keeping records, ordering and issuing uniforms and supplies, providing certain additional safety measures in the conduct of physical education activities, helping in locker room assignments, selling tickets, assisting in the testing program, and other duties that normally utilize the teacher's time. It is maintained that such an assignment would require careful screening of applicants, a preliminary period of orientation and training, and some consideration whereby paraprofessionals might pursue a career in this field.

Questions have been raised about the role of paraprofessionals. Can the profession be assured that if paraprofessionals are utilized for ordering and issuing uniforms and supplies, for example, their duties will stop with these nonteaching assignments? Or, in the interest of economy, is it possible that a school system might find some assignments for these persons that enables the board of education to reduce the professional staff? A second question is concerned with how the physical educator utilizes the time that accrues as the result of hiring of the paraprofessionals. It is recommended that guidelines and assurances be established to ensure that physical educators utilize such time in a manner that will enhance the contribution of physical education to the rank and file of the student body.

PROFESSIONAL PREPARATION OF COACHES IS STRONGLY RECOMMENDED. An estimated one-fourth of all head coaches in secondary schools throughout the United States do not have any professional preparation for this particular function. Many coaches obviously are not trained in the field of physical education. Recognizing the important responsibility that coaches have for the sound physical education and safety of their players, this represents a critical problem. Some coaches, for example, know nothing whatsoever about first aid and thus when injuries occur are at a loss to know what should be done to ensure the health of the injured player.

The lack of preparation of coaching personnel has resulted in a determined effort on the part of many educators, including physical education personnel, certification officials, the AAHPER Division of Men's Athletics, and others, to require coaches to have at least minimum preparation in this field. The AAHPER points out that such preparation should include such areas as *medical aspects of athletic coaching,* which includes a knowledge of medical examinations, protective equipment and facilities, training, injuries, and safety problems; *principles and problems of coaching,* including such areas as personal qualities of the coach, organization for athletics, training rules, and coaching ethics; *theory and techniques of coaching,* including educational implications of athletics, scouting, and rules and regulations; *kinesiological foundations of coaching,* including knowledge of the human anatomy and mechanics of movement; and *physiological foundations of coaching,* including exercise physiology factors, nutrition, drugs, and conditioning. As a result of this national effort a few states have instituted some requirements to ensure better qualified coaches.

There have also been significant new developments in the preparation of teachers of physical education (see Chapter 21) and placing the responsibility for the certification of teachers upon the college and university from which the person graduates (see Chapter 23).

Student activism

Student unrest is characteristic of the times. Students have spoken out on many public issues, rioted on the nation's campuses, criticized the older generation, burned their draft cards, rebelled against authority, marched on Washington, voiced strong opposition to the war, and proclaimed that they want to be involved.

Student unrest has penetrated most of the nation's college and university campuses, and more than 2,000 high schools have also experienced sit-ins, boycotts, and other forms of student protest. Some of the things "bugging" students include having no participation in forming policies to which they must conform, being required to take courses in school with which they cannot identify, listening to educators whose teaching is not relevant to the times, and having no active involvement in the educational process.

Student unrest must be carefully considered. School administrators need to make concessions, the avenues for communication between the generations must be opened, rigid rules should be carefully reviewed and in many cases eliminated, curriculums should be reviewed, students should be invited to participate in planning, and disciplinary actions must be just and meaningful.

The nation and the nation's schools and colleges in particular are going through times that make it imperative to listen to the views of young people. The various student types cannot all be viewed or treated in the same way. The activists, conservatives, antisocials, hippies, joiners, drug addicts, women's libs, gay boys, grinds, goofoffs, and other types must be understood and not classified as all members of the same group. To think of them as a group rather than as individuals might very well result in a polarization of adults and youth, which would do more harm and widen the generation gap.

Many educational institutions are making is possible for the student to assume more responsibility for his own learning. For example, in the traditional system many of a student's courses are required and what he studies in any given course is prescribed by the teacher. Now, some schools and colleges are giving youth more freedom in shaping their own individual learning programs, with faculty help, and working independently. There is a trend toward independent and interdisciplinary study. Students are going from the classrooms in many cases to test theory against reality. At the University of California at Santa Cruz, for example, the entire process of undergraduate education has been changed, with the stress on individual freedom and responsibility in planning and pursuing a course of study.

Physical education must recognize the importance of involving the student in the program, decision making, and conduct of his own education. In keeping with this philosophy the AAHPER has established a Student Action Council that is open to all undergraduate and graduate students enrolled in health, physical education, or recreation in professional preparation institutions who are members of this national organization. This council has been established to develop a better means of communication between the generations, to conduct student leadership conferences, to hold meetings, and to work on projects related to their interests, such as preservation of their environment.

Student involvement should not be limited to the national professional organizational level. It should become a common practice wherever physical education programs exist at all educational and agency levels.

Curriculum reform movement

A recent survey by the Educational Testing Service of Princeton, New Jersey, found more important changes in school curriculums and teaching methods in the last 10 years in the United States than in any previous decade. Innovations were reported to have affected the teaching of mathematics, foreign languages, science, and other subjects.

SELECTED CURRICULUM PROJECTS

Although the curriculum reform movement has not affected physical education on a national scale to any large degree, there have been some significant curriculum projects that need to be identified.*

BATTLE CREEK, MICHIGAN. A cooperative curriculum development project in Battle Creek combines the efforts of members of the physical education staff of the Battle Creek Schools and members of the faculty of Michigan State University. The major objectives of the project are to identify the essential elements of a curriculum model, organize the content of this model in terms of objectives and philosophy, and then develop a physical education program based on this model.

DAYTON, OHIO. The Dayton program involves an approach to motor perceptual problems as related to underachievement in elementary school children. Dayton's Body Management Program, largely motivated through the efforts of psychologist Newell Kephart, utilizes such aids as balance and walking boards, trampolines, and simple

---

*Many of these curriculum projects, as well as other significant curriculum developments, are identified and discussed in AAHPER publications. For example, see AAHPER: Promising practices in elementary school physical education, Washington, D. C., 1969, The Association.

exercises to train children in basic readiness skills that normal children have already achieved before coming to school.

DEKALB, ILLINOIS. A program of movement education involves DeKalb Schools and the women's physical education department of Northern Illinois University. This cooperative program is aimed at demonstrating the values of movement experiences for children, providing a medium for the pre- and in-service education of teachers, establishing a laboratory for observing and recording children's behavior, and providing a center for the preparation and distribution of pertinent instructional materials.

DES MOINES, IOWA. A cooperative project in Des Moines combines the efforts of Drake University and the Johnston Elementary School designed to develop, utilize, and evaluate teaching-learning materials involving both cognitive and psychomotor concepts. The project is aimed at helping children understand basic concepts relating to their physical education experience.

ELLENSBURG, WASHINGTON. A project called "Broadfront" represents an attempt to provide a comprehensive program of health, physical education, and recreation for all students in the Ellensburg school system. Utilizing physical education, health, community school, camping and outdoor education, and special education experiences closely integrated with other aspects of the school program, the program purports to contribute maximally to the health and education of all students from kindergarten through grade twelve.

NEW ORLEANS, LOUISIANA. A curriculum project funded by the Ford Foundation in the New Orleans public schools is designed to determine whether classroom teachers can be adequately trained to conduct meaningful movement education programs in the elementary school.

PLATTSBURG, NEW YORK. A funded program in the Plattsburg school system utilizes movement education as a key part of the total physical education program. The development of a curriculum guide for movement education in the elementary school was an important objective of this program.

PULLMAN, WASHINGTON. A cooperative project between the Pullman schools and Washington State University is aimed at improving the elementary school physical education programs in Pullman. The project consisted of, first, designing an elementary school physical education program incorporating ideas from other countries such as England, Germany, and the Scandinavian countries and, second, determining the effect these innovations had on the physical fitness, motor ability, and social behavior of the children.

SONOMA COUNTY, CALIFORNIA. An inter–school district curriculum project in Sonoma County was designed to better achieve such objectives of physical education as skill development, physical fitness, and social-emotional development in elementary, intermediate, and high school students.

SUWANEE COUNTY, FLORIDA. A curriculum project in physical education involves six rural counties and is designed to improve elementary school programs.

PROGRAMS FOR THE HANDICAPPED

One of the encouraging curriculum developments in recent years has been the attention devoted to the handicapped, with the realization that physical education can make a major contribution to this important segment of our population. A cursory review of the articles in professional journals in the last few years will find a discussion of subjects that reflect only in small measure the contribution that physical education can make to the handicapped: "The Forgotten Student in Physical Education," "Adapted Table Tennis for the Physically Handicapped," "Referral Forms for Adapted Physical Education," "Dance and the Deaf," "Recreational and Leisure-Time Activities of Blind Children," "Motor Performance of Visually Handicapped Children," "Physical Education: A Substitute for Hyperactivity and Violence," "New

Horizons in the Administration of Adapted Physical Education."

The AAHPER is active in programs for the handicapped and has a full-time specialist on the staff devoting his efforts to improving programs in this area. Aspects for which services and materials are either available or are being developed include:

1. Deprivation (cultural, economic, and social)
2. Hearing impairments (deafness and hard of hearing)
3. Illness and infirmed conditions
4. Low physical fitness and specific motor deficiencies
5. Mental retardation (mild, moderate, severe, and profound)
6. Neurological impairments and brain damage
7. Physical and orthopedic handicaps
8. Special health problems (cardiac, multiple sclerosis, and muscular dystrophy)
9. Serious maladjustments, emotional disturbances, and social maladjustments
10. Visual handicaps (blindness and partial sightedness)

The program of the New Trier Senior High School in Illinois is an example of a school system that has incorporated an outstanding adapted physical education program into its physical education curriculum. Developed several years ago, the program is designed to provide a meaningful program of physical education for students who are permanently or temporarily handicapped and who can benefit from corrective exercises and/or activities recommended by the student's physician. In addition, other students who are found to be lacking in such qualities as strength and coordination are provided a special program of activities to alleviate these deficiencies.

Another project of note is the Buttonwood Farms Project, which involves a specially designed physical education–recreation program for emotionally disturbed and mentally retarded children. The Buttonwood Farms Project of Temple University utilizes physical conditioning, fundamental movement, sports skills, and recreational activities to help in the development of body control, with additional benefits such as improved body image, self-concept, and self-confidence.

PROGRAMS FOR INNER CITY YOUTH

The culturally, economically, and educationally disadvantaged youths who inhabit the inner cities of our nation represent a significant challenge to physical education programs. Physical activity, sports, games, and dance often appeal to these youths and consequently represent an avenue of contact that may impel youngsters to become more involved with other subjects in the curriculum. Although there has been much conjecture as to what type of physical education program is best for the inner city, few if any outstanding models have been developed. The National Conference of City and County Directors devoted their annual meeting in December, 1969, to this subject.*

Growth of sports and related problems

No greater truism exists than that sports fascinate Americans. Billions of dollars are spent every year in its name. As much as $200,000 is charged for 1 minute of advertising when a Super Bowl football game is being played. The *New York Times* devotes more space to sports than it does to art, books, education, television, or the theater. Schools, colleges, youth-serving agencies, and many other institutions sponsor sports programs for their constituency.

The great growth of sports in recent years has brought with it attendant problems, three of which will be discussed here as being currently significant.

THE BLACK ATHLETE

Over the course of history in sports it has been commonly regarded that athletics represent a setting where prejudice and dis-

---

*Proceedings of the conference are available from NEA Publications-Sales, 1201 Sixteenth Street N.W., Washington, D. C. The report is entitled "Preparing Teachers for a Changing Society." The reader will find many helpful suggestions for the physical education curriculum for inner city youth.

crimination have been effectively solved. It has been said, for example, that "sports are color blind" and that on the playing field the person is recognized for his ability alone; reward is given without regard to race or class. Yet many black athletes claim that much racial discrimination exists today. They claim that quota systems exist for Negro players in some professional leagues and that coaches, managers, and front office personnel are never blacks.

Sports have produced a major arena for the world to see the plight of oppressed people. For example, the Olympic boycott by black athletes and the refusal of black athletes to compete with citizens of the Republic of South Africa helped to publicize the struggle the blacks are waging against the white man.

In school and college circles black athletes have brought attention to the authoritarianism on the part of coaches, to schools that fail to schedule teams who have black participants, and to discriminatory conditions that athletes face as part of a school or college team. The point is made that too often the black athlete's job in college is to compete in sports, not to get an education.

Efforts are being made on the part of educators and coaches to resolve the problem of the black athlete. To do this all players must be treated equally, and there must be open avenues of communication for all to voice their complaints and feelings. The blacks must be recruited not only because they are good athletes but also because they are good scholars. Every attempt must be made to let them fulfill *all* of their educational goals. The role that the black athlete has played in American sports has been an inspiration to all, black and white alike. In the future physical education can serve as a vehicle to better understand the nature of the black athlete and his contribution to our society.

AMATEURISM

The growth of sports in America and other cultures of the world and the acclaim given those nations and athletes who excel have contributed to a significant change in the concept of the amateur in sports. Although traditionally the amateur did not receive money or have active government support for demonstrating his athletic prowess, today he is frequently given financial remuneration in terms of expenses and in other forms, and he receives government support in some nations of the world.

According to *Time* magazine (June 2, 1967): "Amateur tennis players receive $9,000 a year from the United States Lawn Tennis Association for playing on the Davis Cup team and track and field stars compete for merchandise in the form of phonographs and television sets." What is true in the United States exists to an even greater extent in some nations abroad. It is common knowledge that the governments of the Soviet Union, Hungary, and Czechoslovakia, to mention only three, subsidize their athletes.

Many reasons have been suggested for the changing concept of what constitutes an amateur in sports. One important consideration is that times have changed. When the ancient Olympic games were staged, the

Sports have become "big time."

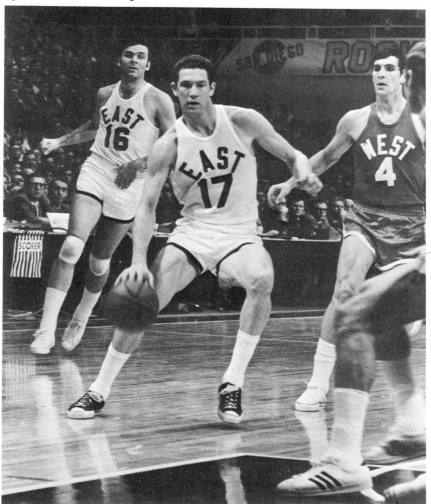

concept of national sports programs did not exist. When the Olympics were revived in 1896 by de Coubertin, there were very few professionals. The stress was upon individual performance.

As has been mentioned, probably one of the most significant reasons for the changing concept of amateurism is that it affects a nation's image. Historically, we know this to be true. An example is the feats of Jesse Owens in the 1936 Olympics in Berlin and his snub by Hitler. Many people felt that American prestige was enhanced as a result of Owens' winning the gold medals. A nation's image is affected by how well its athletes perform in the Olympics and other international contests. Consequently, which athletes are eligible to represent a nation has implications for how effective the performance of that nation will be in the athletic contests in which they participate.

The eligibility of athletes is determined to a great extent in the way the word *amateur* is interpreted. The definition of amateurism adhered to in the United States, according to many public figures, works against the best interests of this country and the prestige of the United States in world affairs. Therefore, these persons argue, it is important to carefully review the whole matter of international athletics in light of the concept of amateurism that exists in the countries of the world. The fact that some social systems do not distinguish, as we do, between the professional and the amateur places some countries at a disadvantage when they hold to traditional concepts that have become outdated.

ANTIATHLETICS AND ANTI–PHYSICAL EDUCATION MOOD

Throughout the country high school and college students are demanding a stronger voice in the educational process. Many students at present are complaining that the money spent on big-time college athletic programs and high school sports cannot be justified. Newspaper reports indicate that some California college students have urged

that the money given annually to athletic departments can be spent in a manner more broadly representative of all students. In addition, these students criticized the construction of a $550,000 press box on the football stadium. In Texas, students protested the spending of several millions of dollars on an addition to the football stadium, while much less money was being spent on a new humanities research center.

Some students and faculty complain that athletics are too authoritarian and militaristic. Others say they cannot be justified because too few students benefit from the program. A Gallup Poll indicates that in a survey of 1,061 students interviewed at sixty colleges, a declining interest in sports was definitely noticeable. Of the students interviewed, 57% in the East indicated that they were less interested in sports, 44% in the Far West were in this same category, and 35% of the students in the South were in this category. Students feel they should devote more of their time to the social causes of the day rather than to athletics.

Along with the antiathletic mood, there is also some evidence of a broader anti–physical education mood. This is evident in the Education, Training, Market Report publication, which pointed out that 40 million children are being cheated out of a well-rounded physical education program because of the emphasis upon the skilled athlete. An article in *Family Health* in September, 1970, carried a similar story. The October 18, 1970, *New York Times* gave further support to the fact that many students despise physical education and that many programs have little value for youth. Furthermore, reports indicate that the voting down of school budgets has resulted in curtailment of programs, facilities, and personnel.

Women's liberation movement

The women's liberation movement represents another significant change in our society having implications for physical education. Basically, the women's liberation movement rests upon the premise that women should have a voice in the decisions that control their destiny. Betty Friedan, author of *The Feminine Mystique,* was responsible for forming the National Organization for Women (NOW), which has as its primary objective the gaining of equal rights for women, including their rights in respect to the political and legal processes of this country. More militant groups advocating such bizarre notions as manless societies and the abolition of the family unit have also emerged.

The women's liberation movement is leaving its imprint upon physical education. Girls' rules have been changed in such sports as basketball to allow more freedom and more similarity to men's rules. Girls now play on the entire basketball court, and guards as well as forwards are permitted to shoot for the basket. The liberation movement has helped to do away with many of the old taboos. Femininity and athletic skill and fitness are viewed as complementary to one another. Budgets in physical education departments are being carefully scrutinized and equated to see that the financial needs of girls' and women's programs are adequately met. In such noncontact sports as tennis and golf, girls are playing on varsity school teams along with the boys. In some communities in New Jersey and New York, girls who have been denied the right to play in such sports have appealed their cases to proper authorities. Now that they are becoming more active in athletic programs, women are beginning to question the quality of educational interscholastic programs. They are also raising questions as to whether a man or woman is best qualified to coach some teams.

The field of physical education is faced with the opportunity to totally educate the individual, and this means both men and women. In some cases the girls' and women's programs have suffered because of lack of staff, budget, facilities, and other essentials. From now on, as a result of the women's liberation movement, there will be a greater consideration of all students, both men and women.

Facilities

There are many new trends in facilities for physical education programs. New paving materials, new types of equipment, improved landscapes, new construction materials, new shapes for swimming pools, partial shelters, and synthetic grass are just a few of the many new developments. Combination indoor-outdoor pools, physical fitness equipment for outdoor use, all-weather tennis courts, and lines that now come in multicolors for various games and activities are other new developments.

In gymnasium construction some of the new features include the utilization of modern engineering techniques and materials. This has resulted in welded steel and laminated wood modular frames; arched and gabled roofs; domes providing areas completely free from internal supports; exterior surfaces of aluminum, steel, fiber glass, and plastics; different window patterns and styles; several kinds of floor surfaces of nonslip material; prefabricated wall surfaces; and better lighting systems with improved quality and quantity and less glare. Facilities are moving from use of regular glass to either plastic and fiber glass panels or to an overhead skydome. Lightweight fiber glass laminated over an aluminum framework is proving popular. This requires no painting, the cost of labor and materials is lower, there is no need for shades or blinds to eliminate glare, and the breakage problem is reduced or eliminated.

Locker rooms and service areas are including built-in combination locks with built-in combination changers to permit the staff to change combinations when needed. There is more extensive use of ceramic tile because of its durability and low-cost maintenance. Wall-hung toilet compartment features permit easier maintenance and sanitation with no chance for rust to start from the floor. Odor control is being effectively handled by new dispensers. New thin-profile heating, ventilating, and airconditioning fan coil units are now being used.

Other new developments that are proving popular are the geodesic fieldhouse, bubble tops for swimming pools, air-supported structures, partial shelters, new artificial turf, rubber-cushioned tennis courts, sculptured play apparatus, rubberized all-weather running tracks, and many types of auxiliary gymnasiums.

Other new developments

Many significant new developments in physical education have been discussed at length in other parts of this text and so are not included here. Some of these are movement education (see Chapter 13) and international relations (see Chapter 14).

QUESTIONS AND EXERCISES

1. Identify the following: Basedow, Guts Muths, Jahn, Spiess, Ling, Branting, Nachtegall, Nyblaeus, Bukh, Maclaren, Beecher, Delsarte, Homans, Sargent, Anderson, Hetherington, Wood, and Gulick.
2. In approximately 250 words describe the changing conceptions in regard to physical education that occurred during the modern European period.
3. Describe the growth of the Turnverein movement in Germany and in the United States. To what extent has it affected physical education in this country?
4. What were some of the principles of physical education as established by Adolph Spiess? Compare these with the principles of modern-day physical education.
5. What were some of the contributions to physical education made by Per Henrik Ling?
6. What has been the role of physical education in Denmark during the modern European period?
7. How has Great Britian influenced education in the United States?
8. Compare the attitude of most school administrators in colonial times in America with the attitude of most school administrators today.
9. Why were the Puritans opposed to play? What is the relationship between puritanism and asceticism?
10. Describe the growth of physical education in the United States during the national period.
11. What type of physical education has been evolving during the twentieth century?
12. To what extent do you feel that physical education has progressed from ancient times to the present? Document your answer.
13. Identify the following: Philanthropinum, Turnplatz, Royal Central Institute of Gymnastics, Primitive Gymnastics, American Turnerbund, Dio Lewis, Winship, American Association for Health, Physical Education, and Recreation, and National Gymnastics.
14. What are three significant new developments in physical education?

Reading assignment

Bucher, Charles A., and Goldman, Myra: Dimensions of physical education, St. Louis, 1969, The C. V. Mosby Co., Reading selections 30 to 33.

SELECTED REFERENCES

Ainsworth, Dorothy S.: The history of physical education in colleges for women, New York, 1930, A. S. Barnes & Co.

Bennett, Bruce L.: Improving courses in the history of physical education, Journal of Health, Physical Education, and Recreation 37:26, 1966.

Bucher, Charles A.: Little League baseball can hurt your boy, Look, Aug. 11, 1953.

Caillois, Roger: Man, play, and games, New York, 1961, The Free Press of Glencoe, Inc. (translated from the French).

Coaching Certification Committee, Illinois Association for Professional Preparation in Health, Physical Education, and Recreation: A survey of special certification requirements for athletic coaches of high school interscholastic teams, Journal of Health, Physical Education, and Recreation 41:14, 1970.

Dulles, Foster Rhea: America learns to play, New York, 1966, Appleton-Century-Crofts.

English, Fenwick: Questions and answers on differentiated staffing, Today's Health 58:53, 1969.

Esslinger, Arthur A.: Certification for high school coaches, Journal of Health, Physical Education, and Recreation 39:42, 1968.

Hackensmith, C. W.: History of physical education, New York, 1966, Harper & Row, Publishers.

Leonard, Fred E., and Affleck, George G.: A guide to the history of physical education, Philadelphia, 1947, Lea & Febiger.

Lucas, John A.: Coubertin's philosophy of pedagogical sport, Journal of Health, Physical Education, and Recreation 35:26, 1964.

McIntosh, Peter C.: Physical education in England since 1800, Toronto, 1952, Clarke, Irwin & Co.

Means, Richard K.: A history of health education in the United States, Philadelphia, 1962, Lea & Febiger.

Metzner, Henry: A brief history of the North American Gymnastic Union, Indianapolis, 1911,

The National Executive Committee of the North American Gymnastic Union.

Randall, Martin W.: Modern ideas on physical education, London, 1952, G. Bell & Sons.

Ridini, Leonard, M.: An experimental design for the training of paraprofessionals in physical education, Journal of Health, Physical Education, and Recreation **41:**23, 1970.

Schwendener, Norma: A history of physical education in the United States, New York, 1942, A. S. Barnes & Co.

Seventy-fifth Anniversary of the AAHPER, Journal of Health, Phyical Education, and Recreation, vol. 31, April, 1960.

Shadduck, Ione G.: Johnston research project—a curriculum based on concepts, The Physical Educator **27:**107, 1970.

Van Dalen, Deobold B., and Bennett, B. L.: A world history of physical education, New York, 1971, Prentice-Hall, Inc.

Weaver, Robert B.: Amusements and sports in American life, Chicago, 1939, The Chicago University Press.

Wells, H. G.: The outline of history, New York, 1931, Garden City Publishing Co., Inc.

Weston, Arthur: The making of American physical education, New York, 1962, Appleton-Century-Crofts.

13/Movement education—a developing concept in physical education

Today, a relatively new concept is being introduced into our schools that may prove helpful in enhancing the worth of physical education programs. The concept is known as movement education. Movement education is not new, for England has long been involved in education for movement. Many books, articles, and pamphlets have been and are being written on movement education. The writers come from diverse groups and include, among others, kinesiologists, dance educators, researchers, and physical educators on all levels of instruction. With all the written material on movement education, one thing remains clear—there is no one common definition of movement education. It seems to be both a philosophy of method in physical education as well as a teaching approach.

Movement experiences provide a person with information about himself and the environment in which he lives. Many centuries ago, the Greek philosopher Socrates expressed the need for man to move about in order to have an understanding of himself. It also appears that early experiences in movement form a sturdy foundation for the later learning of more sophisticated sports skills.

To better understand the movement education trend, it is necessary to first describe the nature of movement education.

NATURE OF MOVEMENT EDUCATION

Movement is integral to the human being. Everything that man does, whether he is re-acting to his environment or simply expressing himself, involves movement of some sort. Movement in itself is thus a tool of life; the more efficiently man moves, the more meaningful his life is.

Movement is a means of communication oftentimes called preverbal language. It is through movement that one can express his feelings without using spoken language. Dance educators have long advocated that it is almost impossible to communicate the emotions of a dance by using language, but, through the body, the imagery of a dance can be conveyed.

Movement experiences can be extremely beautiful, and a knowledge of movement will contribute to a richer appreciation of such experiences. Being aware of the gracefulness of a skier as he glides down the slopes or the well-controlled movements of the gymnast as he performs on the parallel bars can make these events a more worthwhile and richer experience for the viewer. Of course, the experience derived by the individual performer yields the greatest rewards of all.

It is through movement that physical education proceeds. It is through movement education that physical educators seek to develop the fullest potential in their students.

Movement educators seek not only to have the individual understand and appreciate the movement of which he is capable but also to appreciate the varieties of movement of which others are capable.

Programs of movement education are not

conducted haphazardly. Rather, they are structured on a problem-solving basis, leaving the individual free to relate to force, time, and space through his particular use of balance, leverage, and technique. Movement educators hold that numerous activities have common elements, all of which are based on a comprehensive knowledge of movement fundamentals. The better the individual is able to perceive movement patterns, they feel, the more ease there will be in developing skills, for these skills will tend to develop as a concomitant of learning to move.

Movement education strives to make the individual aware of the movement of his entire body and to become intellectually as well as physically involved. The challenge set by a problem in movement is first per-ceived by the intellect and then solved by the body moving through space, reacting to any obstacles within that space and to the limitations and existing restrictions. Learning accrues as the individual accepts and attempts to solve increasingly difficult problems. Inherent in this is the concept of individual differences. There may be numerous ways to solve a stated problem, and the individual chooses the method that best suits his abilities and capacities. Individual rather than group development is the basic premise of movement education.

Thus, movement education may be defined as individual exploration of the ability of the body to relate and react to the physical concepts of the environment and to factors in the environment, be they material or human.

An old bicycle tire becomes a piece of physical education equipment for an elementary school student in a movement exploration program.

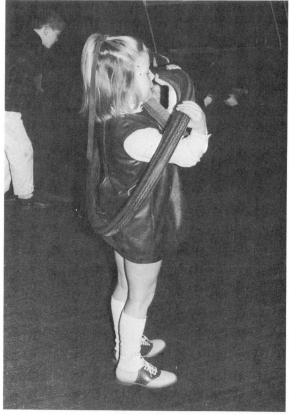

BROADFRONT PROGRAM, ELLENSBURG PUBLIC SCHOOLS, ELLENSBURG, WASH.

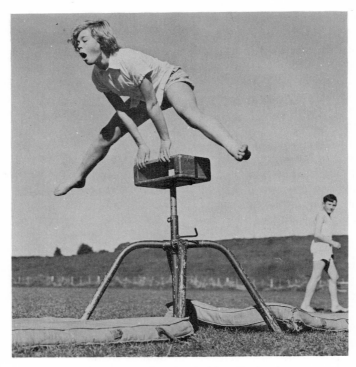

Movement education in New Zealand.

ORIGINS OF MOVEMENT EDUCATION

The roots of movement education may be traced back to the theories of Rudolf Laban, a dancer, and to the effect his theories had on modern-day physical education in England. Laban fled Germany during World War II and eventually settled in England, where he established the Laban Art of Movement Center, an institution that has trained many movement educators.

Laban stressed the fact that man's body is the instrument through and by which he moves and that each individual is endowed with certain natural kinds of movement. Laban believed strongly in exploratory movement and in a spontaneous quality in movement. He was opposed to the rigidity of set series of exercises that left no room for creativity or self-expression. Laban was a movement analyst, and as such he believed that man could not only learn to move efficiently and effectively but could also develop a strong kinesthetic awareness of movement.

During World War II, England revised its entire educational structure and restated its philosophy of education. Where physical education had once been little more than formal gymnastics, now the freedom of bodily movement, creativity, and expression were stressed. Laban's principles were freely employed. Over the course of the years these principles have been expanded and broadened into the concept of movement education as it is carried on in England today.

In England, the classroom teacher is in charge of physical education in the elementary schools, and both boys and girls, beginning in the first grade, are educated in movement. In the secondary schools the movement education program is continued for girls under the guidance of a trained physical educator. The program is based on problem solving. The teacher sets the problem, then guides, assists, and suggests, but in no way dictates a solution. There is no teacher demonstration, and thus no imitation, leaving the child free to establish his own patterns of movement, set his own tempo, and make wise use of space.

Within the last 15 years, a trend toward concentrated movement education has developed in the United States, based on the English programs. Unlike England, however, where movement education is concentrated in the early school years, in the United States movement education first received its impetus in the college and university physical education programs for women. These programs have attempted to develop movement patterns as the dancer's vehicle of expression. A working definition of movement education terms was introduced in 1956 by the National Association for Physical Education of College Women in order to more effectively communicate with each other.

In recent years movement education programs have become a part of elementary schools in the United States. The leaders in the field of movement education are in agreement that this concept should play a vital role in determining the future direction of physical education, particularly in the lower grades.

SCHOOLS OF THOUGHT

Despite varied viewpoints concerning movement education, it is generally agreed that movement education is activity centered rather than verbal centered, and thus the movement itself, the awareness of the body, and its range of abilities are very important. Rather than a force to be overcome, the body becomes the prime tool through which all movement takes place.

It is necessary at this point to take a look at the various schools of thought in movement education in order to gain greater insight as to why the leaders in the field believe it will play an important role in the future of physical education.

Dance educators have long used the philosophy of educating for movement. As early as 1914 a dancer named Diana Watts published, in the United States, a book entitled *The Renaissance of the Greek Ideal*. The book was her philosophy of movement, drawn from her research into early Greek statues and paintings of athletes in motion. Modern-day dance educators often describe dance as nonverbal communication. Dance is viewed as creative and expressive movement in time and space through the instrument of the body. Dance educators have also expressed the belief that movement by the body has important academic implications. They feel that through movement the child is given the opportunity to develop judgment and curiosity and thus become more resourceful and creative.

The kinesiologists are students of human movement and view it as an academic discipline. They look at physical education as a process whereby human movement is studied and refined as an educational procedure. The kinesiologists contend that the student who has a knowledge of how his body moves will not only learn skills more readily but also perform more effectively and efficiently. They agree with the movement educators that movement education utilizes physical activity predominantly and that activity is also the end result of the process of movement education.

Physical educators have used many of the concepts of movement education, often without cognition. In physical education, the student can be guided toward development only if the body is put to use, for movement of the body is the basic tool of physical education. However, in many physical education programs, intellectual awareness of the body is not developed, and thus there is no understanding of how the body moves through time and space. As physical educators are becoming more aware of the applications and implications of movement education, many are beginning to provide experiences in movement for their students and are guiding them into an understanding of, and an appreciation for, these experiences.

On the college level, particularly in programs for women, courses variously called by such titles as movement education, foundations of movement, or body mechanics are now being offered. These courses allow for exploration of the capacities of the human body and for the discovery and increased understanding of its movement abilities.

Physical educators are becoming increasingly concerned with the development of the individual and are making more allowances for individual differences in rate of skill learning. The intellect and body are increasingly viewed as interactive and interdependent. Those who have made a study of motor learning state that movement problems must be meaningful. That is, the student must understand the fundamentals of movement before he can successfully attempt the learning of a complex skill. It is up to the instructor to set the problem, ascertain whether the student understands it, and then observe and guide the learning in relation to the abilities, capacities, and needs of that student.

TRADITIONAL APPROACH VERSUS MOVEMENT EDUCATION

The traditional approach to physical education needs little explanation. Syllabuses, or course outlines, specify several weeks of one activity followed by several weeks of another, often unrelated. In the elementary schools in the United States, games of low organization, folk and square dances, tumbling and gymnastics, and lead-up games often comprise the major part of the program. Later school years, for both boys and girls, are devoted to the learning of specific sport skills. Rhythmics, or fundamental movement, is sometimes included, but as a minor phase of the program.

The movement education approach to physical education is founded on an entirely different premise. Movement education is not a gap-filler of several lessons but an on-going method of teaching physical education beginning with the earliest school years. Movement education does not abandon or fully supplant the traditional approach as we know it. Rather, it forms a firmer foundation for more meaningful skill learning, for increased pleasure in the skillful use of the body, and for the development of life-long physical effectiveness and efficiency.

To understand the full meaning of movement education, it is necessary to identify and compare its various key concepts. In so doing it will be possible to see it as a part of the whole that is physical education. Table 13-1 gives a comparison of movement education concepts and traditional physical education concepts that will prove useful in differentiating between these two approaches to the teaching of physical education.

KEY CONCEPTS OF MOVEMENT EDUCATION

Movement education has been widely accepted by physical educators because of certain basic concepts that emphasize its importance in educational programs.

Movement education is individual exploration

Through individual exploration each student is encouraged to find his own solution to a problem involving physical movement. Although there may be various ways to solve the problem, the child chooses the method that best suits his abilities. Furthermore, this individual exploration is concerned with the natural movements of childhood. Children enjoy running, jumping, climbing, leaping, and other physical movements, and they tend to perform these movements of their own volition. Movement educators seek to capitalize on these natural movements of childhood as they guide the child through an individual exploration of the many varieties of these movements.

Formalized physical education programs tend to stress conformity to stylized patterns of movement. Through movement education it is felt the child's individualized patterns of movement can be reinforced and retained. Movement education classes provide an unlimited opportunity for children to explore

Table 13-1. A comparison of movement education and traditional physical education concepts

Movement education	Traditional physical education
A. The program	
1. The program is activity centered.	1. The program is verbal centered.
2. The program is student centered.	2. The program is teacher centered.
3. The program attempts to develop an intellectual awareness of the body.	3. The program attempts to develop skills oftentimes lacking in intellectual comprehension.
4. The program places an emphasis on the problem-solving method, which includes exploration and discovery, based on the individual needs of the student.	4. The teacher serves as a model to be imitated by the students, and the method includes lecture and demonstration based on the needs of the group.
5. Repetition of problems leads to a greater variety of solutions.	5. Repetition of drills leads to an improved performance in motor skills.
6. Syllabus develops as each class period uncovers the needs of the individual that must be explored.	6. Syllabus often unrelated to previous learning experiences is presented to the students.
B. Role of the teacher	
1. In the learning process the teacher educates his students.	1. In the learning process the teacher trains his students.
2. The teacher is imaginative and creative in the methods he uses.	2. The teacher utilizes the traditional methods of teaching.
3. The teacher guides his students in the activities in which they are participating.	3. The teacher leads his students in the activities in which they are participating.
C. Role of the student	
1. Motivation for learning comes from inner self.	1. Motivation for learning comes from the teacher.
2. The student experiences the joy of his own natural movements and unique style.	2. Individual body types are not considered.
3. The student demonstrates his ability to reason logically and intelligently.	3. The student demonstrates his ability to take orders and follow directions.
4. The student demonstrates independence.	4. The student often lacks independence.
5. The student faces each new situation in an enthusiastic and intelligent manner.	5. The student oftentimes exhibits difficulty when confronted with new situations.
6. The student evaluates his own progress.	6. The teacher evaluates the student's progress.
7. The student develops at his own rate of progress.	7. Rate of progress is dependent upon the norm of the student development within the class.
8. Success is based on the student's goals.	8. Success is based on the teacher's goals.
9. The student competes with himself.	9. The student competes with his fellow classmates.
D. Class atmosphere	
1. There is an informal class atmosphere.	1. There is a formal class atmosphere.
2. Varied formations are used.	2. Set formations are used.
3. The teacher exhibits permissive behavior.	3. The teacher exhibits strict behavior.
4. Individual needs of the students are the determining factor in the allotment of time to be spent in any activity.	4. The completion of the subject matter is the determining factor in the allotment of time to be spent in any activity.
E. Facilities and equipment	
1. The facilities are considered secondary to the need for a resourceful and creative teacher.	1. Facilities are of prime importance, although the need for a resourceful and creative teacher is recognized.
2. The equipment is created to meet the needs of the individual.	2. The individual must adjust to the equipment used.
3. The equipment is used in many different situations.	3. The equipment is limited in its use.

the uses of their bodies for movement in ways that are creative and self-expressive.

There are many patterns used for the exploration process, two of which are the locomotion and balance patterns. In the locomotion pattern the child moves about from one area to another. For example, a child may be asked to walk around a room without colliding with other children or with walls or apparatus. This is the beginning of learning to use space wisely and controlling the body within the confines of an area. Through the various locomotor patterns such as running, jumping, and hopping the child is encouraged to analyze the differences between these movements and the concept known as walking. The child who is given the opportunity to participate in such experiences will soon become aware of how the movements of one part of the body influence the other parts. For example, the child who runs around in a circle will become aware of how his body leans toward the center as he performs this movement pattern. Through individual exploration the child is encouraged to discover what his body can and cannot do while he is walking, running, or jumping.

Through individual exploration the child is also given the opportunity to participate in experiences that will help him understand the concept known as balance. Through the various balance patterns in which the child participates, he will become more fully aware of the mechanisms involved in maintaining the same position in space. One of the basic balance patterns is the standing position. Through individual exploration the child, by changing the position of his feet or by moving his head, will become aware of the position that must be maintained if proper balance is to result. For example, the child who places all of his body weight on his toes will soon realize that he is not standing in the proper position, and by exploring other foot positions he will become aware of the fact that his weight must be concentrated on the whole foot if he is to experience proper balance.

Through individual exploration the child

is given the opportunity to be creative. As he participates in various movement patterns he discovers what movements his body can make, in what directions his body can move, and what parts of the body are involved in executing a specific movement. Individual exploration is an extremely important concept of movement education. Physical education teachers should motivate their students and encourage them to participate in experiences that will aid them in creating various movement patterns. Hopefully, through individual exploration the student will discover his own abilities and the solution to his particular problems.

Movement education is student centered

Whereas traditional physical education has been concerned with the role of the teacher in the learning process and has focused much attention on the teacher, movement education looks to the student as the center of the learning process. In movement education the individual needs of each student have priority. In movement education the motivation for learning comes from the student's inner self rather than from the teacher. The teacher is not a model to be imitated by the students. It is the task of the teacher to guide, observe, and set the tone of each class. In movement education the student is given the opportunity to experience the joy of his own natural movements and unique style. The student who participates in movement programs does not merely take orders and follow the teacher's directions, but instead he demonstrates his own independence and ability to reason logically and intelligently. Students are challenged to discover their own unique methods and techniques for solving problems in movement or in a skill performance. No one method is assumed to be the only acceptable answer, leaving students free to use their own bodies in an individually suitable manner.

The teacher should be creative and imaginative. The teacher in movement education programs should guide students to success by helping them to evaluate and refine their movements and by providing encouragement. For example, if a child is experiencing difficulty in attempting to jump onto a platform, the teacher might ask: "Can you use your arms in any way to help you jump higher?" After the student has received this information from the teacher, he will still be encouraged to perform the movement and discover by his own exploration whether or not his arms help him to jump higher. Thus he becomes resourceful and is better able to face new problems with the confidence that he can solve them.

Any student can participate meaningfully in the movement education program regardless of his size or athletic abilities. The individual student can work on his own needs and progress at his own pace. The student competes with himself rather than with the group as a whole. He looks to his own abilities to provide the solutions to problems.

In movement education programs it is frequently apparent that while some children are working on a simple movement, others in the class are working on a more complex movement. The answers that the children find to the solution of their own problems will be different, but all are acceptable because success is measured in respect to the particular movement and the abilities of the participants in performing that movement.

Movement education involves problem solving

Movement education begins with simple problems. Learning accrues as the student solves these problems and then seeks to solve increasingly more complex ones. Repetition of various problems is aimed at obtaining a greater variety of solutions. If children are first asked to walk around a room without colliding with each other and perform successfully, building upon this the movement educator may then ask the children to run or hop or jump around the room again without colliding. By beginning with the simple, natural skills of childhood, the movement educator is adhering closely to the known facts of child growth and development, that is, that it is the large muscles and gross motor skills that develop first. The movement educator seeks to enhance this development to pave the way for the later development of the finer motor skills and coordinations.

A child who is becoming educated in movement begins with the walking, running, twisting, and falling problems. As the child solves the initial problem of walking without colliding, he may then be asked to express a mood or feeling, to change direction at will, to change direction at a signal from the teacher, or to walk while using his hands and arms in different ways. Music may be added to lessons. As a specific lesson progresses, games may be played encompassing the problem that has been set. A lesson in hopping or leaping may include a game of modified tag. At the conclusion of a lesson, there may be a period of demonstration by the children so that the movements they have created may be evaluated and discussed by the entire class. In this way, a depth of understanding is reached concerning the movements.

As apparatus is added, the problem facing the child may be to move along a horizontal ladder in any way he wishes. As facility is gained, the problem may be made more complex by specifying that the child move along using his hands only, or using the outside rails only. With other equipment, the same procedure is used. General movement precedes more advanced problems such as mounting, vaulting, and dismounting. This approach allows each child to succeed, since no patterns of movement are required or specified. As the child experiences success, he is motivated to improve on his performance.

The problem-solving method allows the child to be less dependent on the teacher, thus forcing the child to use his own thought processes. In such a manner the child will be developing the ability to be independent. Students who merely imitate the actions of the teacher will not benefit as much as those who attempt to discover various solutions to problems by themselves. The educated student is one who has developed the ability to critically analyze each new situation that he is faced with in an intelligent and logical manner. Teachers should not be models for students, for the best education will only result when the student discovers the meaning to questions by utilizing his own thought processes and resources.

The child learns to intellectually perceive the position of each segment of his body prior to attempting any physical skill performance. Through the utilization of the problem-solving approach, the child begins to think about what his body can do and how he can best utilize his body. The understandings that result help to give the child insight into individual differences in skill performance. They also help him to develop confidence in the capabilities and capacities of his own body for movement. Time, space, force, and flow of movement are key words. The child learns to intellec-tually consider these factors as the core of the movements he executes.

Movement education is less formal than traditional physical education

In movement education class organization does not follow the formalized patterns of traditional physical education. Lines, circles, and set formations are avoided. For the sake of safety, penalties may be imposed for collisions or needless use of space or equipment. Interaction is encouraged and frequently the individual may work with a partner or in small groups, depending on the nature of the problem. Since the determining factor in deciding what problems are to be presented to the class are based on the needs of the individuals within the group, rather than the group as an entity, most instructions by the teacher are given on an individual basis rather than to the class as a

The balance beam provides a medium for movement experiences.

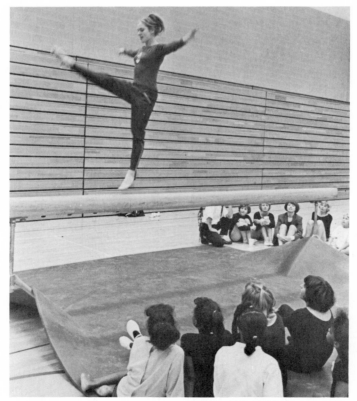

FLINT PUBLIC SCHOOLS, FLINT, MICH.

whole. For example, the teacher will instruct a student who is working on the balance beam to discover "what he can do," "where he can move," and "how he moves." Furthermore, in movement education there are no formal drills or highly organized classes of activities. The learning climate is intentionally informal so that the child will be free to express himself as an individual rather than as an instrument who moves to the command of the teacher.

At the same time, movement education is highly organized and structured in the sense that it has definite objectives that must be met, classes follow a logical sequence, and progression exists that leads to the realization of program objectives and goals. In addition, these programs are not lacking in discipline. Much of the discipline in movement education classes come from the activity and from the inner direction of the children themselves. Movement education classes demand much of the teacher in regard to a concrete philosophy, sound objectives, logical progressions, the understanding of proper techniques and methodology, and liberal amounts of imagination and creativity.

Movement education facilitates the learning of many skills

The natural movements of childhood form the basis for future motor skill development. These movements will tend to develop haphazardly, and future skill performances will be inefficient unless the body is effectively educated in movement.

The ability of the child to perceive his body as an entity helps to promote physical skill development. Children who are retarded in physical skill development often do not have the insight to consider their bodies as wholes. They tend to be concerned first with the individual segments, and thus they attempt to correct performance errors by altering the position or action of a single arm or leg and fail to measurably improve their performance. Movement educators feel that the experience will be most meaningful to the child if he learns to consider the inter-

action of all parts of his body before skill performance is significantly improved. Movement educators recognize the need to learn specific sports skills, such as the strokes of swimming, the methods of pitching or batting a softball, the thrusts and parries of fencing, or the ways to trap and kick a soccer ball. The English have found that many of these specific skills must be taught by traditional methods, and they allot time in their physical education programs in order to accomplish these tasks. However, they have found that prior experience in the solving of problems in movement gives the child a vast store of knowledge on which to build, so that specific skill learnings in the context of their application to a game are made easier. For example, a problem-solving experience in using the feet or legs to stop a rolling ball will help the child in learning the fundamentals of a soccer trap. Solving a problem in propelling the body across a shallow pool will help the child discover how his body reacts in water and give him confidence in learning some strokes in swimming.

Movement education seeks to produce a feeling of satisfaction in movement

Movement educators seek to produce a feeling of satisfaction in the movement experiences engaged in by students. Through emphasis on individual exploration, it is hoped that students will participate in meaningful and pertinent activities. By making the child the explorer in the educational process, it is hoped that he will be encouraged to try new activities and to discover new insights in his relationships to other persons. By utilizing the problem-solving method, it is hoped that the child will select a solution to the problem based on his own particular abilities and therefore meaningful to him. By emphasizing an informal class atmosphere where students are given instructions based on their individual needs, it is hoped that students will better understand their own physical movements. By not emphasizing competition, movement educators feel that children will be free from the tensions that can be aroused by participating in highly competitive activities. Movement educators believe that when such a learning environment is established, students will derive meaning from the activities in which they are participating and a feeling of satisfaction will result.

Movement education encourages an analysis of movement

Traditional physical education gives little instruction to students in the analysis of movement. Movement education provides an opportunity for students to observe and analyze themselves and others in the process of movement. At the conclusion of a lesson, there may be a period of demonstration by the students so that the movements in which they have been involved can be evaluated and discussed by the entire class. Greater understanding of movement is an outcome of this process. For example, demonstrations at the end of the lesson may show that one child vaults higher than another because he has learned that the use of his arms will aid his jump. Discussion of this point by the class will give helpful information to those children who find their own vaults inadequate but have not been able to discover why. Through an analysis of their own and the movements of other children, they will better understand what needs to be done in order to achieve the best performance.

Movement education involves equipment

Many of the pieces of apparatus and equipment found in a regular physical education class can be used in movement education classes. At times, the teacher will have to devise various pieces of equipment to fit the needs of a particular lesson. When apparatus or equipment is used, rules of safety, space, and appropriateness of use need to be stressed. Equipment and apparatus used must conform to the age and size of the child. Balls should be easy to grasp, and paddles should fit the hand of the child. Heavy apparatus such as vaulting

boxes and climbing ladders must be scaled to the size most appropriate to the children using them.

Movement education programs must be constantly evaluated

The need for program modifications and adaptations are frequent in movement education. The need for revision will be noted only if programs are objectively evaluated periodically to see whether the goals that have been set are being achieved.

DEVELOPING A MOVEMENT EDUCATION PROGRAM IN THE ELEMENTARY SCHOOL*

The elementary school child requires a wide variety of experiences in basic movement and movement patterns. Common movement elements help the educator to devise a movement education program that moves toward its objectives in a logical progression.

IN THE EARLY ELEMENTARY SCHOOL GRADES, KINDERGARTEN TO GRADE THREE, THE MAJOR EMPHASIS SHOULD BE ON THE NATURAL MOVEMENTS OF CHILDHOOD. The locomotor movements—including running, walking, jumping, skipping, hopping, and sliding—and the nonlocomotor movements —including pulling, pushing, lifting, twisting, and stretching—should be emphasized.

BEGINNING WITH GRADE FOUR, THE TECHNIQUES OF HANDLING IMPLEMENTS MAY BE A PART OF THE PROGRAM. In grades four to eight locomotor and nonlocomotor movements should still continue to receive stress, but in a more sophisticated form. The child may also be introduced to the handling of such implements as softball bats and field hockey sticks and to such skills as soccer-type kicks and traps that can be used in lead-up game situations.

THE MOVEMENT EDUCATOR MUST HAVE A THOROUGH UNDERSTANDING OF EACH SKILL

---

*Parts of this section have been taken from Bucher, Charles A., and Reade, Evelyn: Physical education and health in the elementary school, New York, 1971, The Macmillan Co.

BEFORE PRESENTING IT TO THE CHILDREN IN A PROBLEM-SOLVING SITUATION. The teacher must understand the mechanics involved in a skill before a child's performance of this skill can be evaluated. Furthermore, the teacher must know the end result desired from the performance of this or another skill or combination of skills.

PROBLEMS MUST BE PROPERLY DEVISED AND SET BY THE TEACHER SO THAT THE DESIRED END RESULT CAN BE ACHIEVED. If, for example, the teacher has planned a lesson in walking for a first-grade lesson, certain specifications must be made so that the children will achieve the desired response. Proper use of space, force, timing, and flow of the movement should be considered and presented to the children as parts of the problem before beginning any physical movements.

VARIETY MUST BE PLANNED INTO EACH MOVEMENT EDUCATION CLASS. On any given day a movement education class should include a review of problems solved previously, and new challenges should be presented in a progressive order. After new problems have been explored the class may conclude with a noncompetitive game that incorporates many of the skills the children have already learned or are currently practicing.

SKILLS MUST BE PROGRESSIVELY TAUGHT FROM GRADE TO GRADE. While a class of first-grade children may concentrate their efforts on a unit of running involving the correct performance in the execution of the skill, a second-grade class might progress to running with a partner or running through obstacle courses that require starting, stopping, and changes of direction.

STANDARDS OF SKILL PERFORMANCE MUST RELATE TO THE INDIVIDUAL CHILD. Each child in a movement education class must be evaluated on the basis of individual performance. The exploratory nature of movement education demands that individual rather than group standards be set. A single common standard of performance cannot be demanded or expected.

THE PROGRAM MUST HELP THE CHILD TO GAIN CONFIDENCE IN HIS OWN PERFORM-

ANCE. Satisfaction in meeting basic and simple challenges will help the child to gain confidence. More difficult problems in tumbling, for example, such as cooperating with a partner in Eskimo rolls and pyramid building, should be introduced only after the children have gained control of their own bodies and have confidence in the use of their bodily skills.

A SOUND FOUNDATION OF BASIC MOVEMENT SKILLS SHOULD PRECEDE THE INTRODUCTION OF GAMES OF LOW ORGANIZATION. Many games of low organization can be adapted to use on any age and grade level. For example, games of the tag type can be introduced as soon as the children have learned the skills essential for that activity. Low organization games that contain elements unfamiliar to the children in a particular class should not be incorporated into the program for that class until the children are thoroughly ready for them.

A SOUND FOUNDATION OF BASIC MOVEMENT SKILLS SHOULD PRECEDE THE INTRODUCTION OF SPECIFIC SPORT SKILLS. In traditional physical education programs on the elementary school level, such games as kickball and softball are often mainstays of the program. Frequently, children play these games without having had adequate instruction and practice in the highly specific skills involved. Introduction of these activities as a concomitant of a sound movement education experience helps place them in their proper perspective in the elementary school physical education program.

An example of an outstanding program in movement education exists in DeKalb, Illinois. The DeKalb, Illinois, public schools have served as one pilot center for movement education programs in the United States. The DeKalb philosophy places emphasis upon the development of the individual for all the possible movement situations that might be faced, whether they be in the classroom or out on the playing fields. The teachers in DeKalb desire their students to have a greater understanding of how their bodies move and the reasons why this is possible.

The DeKalb public schools provide an environment that increases the students' interest and desire to learn. The learning environment includes ropes, ladders, balance beams, tables and benches for jumping off and on, and mats for rolling. Emphasis is on the individual—"self-directed activity" is the key phrase in the program. Each child is given the opportunity to explore at his own rate. The teachers in DeKalb encourage their students to select a task that is within their reach. They do not want students to select tasks that are not appropriate to their level of development, because such tasks will probably not be solved successfully. Movement programs are created to give all children the opportunity to succeed, because this increases their joy and pleasure in movement. In accord with the informal atmosphere that exists in movement education programs, flexible scheduling is an important part of the DeKalb movement education program. Classes are arranged to provide students with the opportunity to participate in as many experiences as possible.

GUIDELINES FOR THE MOVEMENT EDUCATION PROGRAM*

Because movement education is new and still in the experimental stage in the elementary schools of the United States, no set procedures or standardized methodologies have as yet been developed for the country as a whole. The unique nature of movement education may indeed preclude its standardization. A movement education curriculum must meet the needs of the children concerned, and the teaching approach and methodology must also be directly concerned with the children to be served.

The folowing guidelines for specific grade groupings are intended as a general outline

---

*Taken from Bucher, Charles A., and Reade, Evelyn: Physical education and health in the elementary school, New York, 1971, The Macmillan Co.

only and are not inclusive of all of the activities that may be offered in a program. Specific activities can only be appropriately chosen by the teacher after the specific needs, interests, and abilities of the children in a particular program have been determined.

Program for kindergarten to grade three

Basic locomotor and nonlocomotor skills should form the program emphasis in these grades. Locomotor skills to be practiced may include:

Walking	Leaping
Running	Hopping
Skipping	Jumping
Sliding	Falling

Nonlocomotor skills to be practiced may include:

Lifting	Twisting
Pulling	Stretching
Pushing	Bending
Swinging (of parts of the body)	Turning

Balance in performing a locomotor or nonlocomotor skill should be emphasized, as well as the use of the different parts of the body in performing a skill. In walking, for example, the use of the arms for momentum and the position of the trunk and head are as essential as the action of the legs.

After skills have been practiced as entities at different speeds, with various forces (a hard or soft step, for example), with free or restricted movement and in limited or unrestricted spaces, two or more skills may be combined. For example, children may be asked to combine various patterns of leaps and hops, or runs and skips, or twists and stretches, or they may be asked to perform these movements with a partner.

Many locomotor movements may incorporate obstacles. For example, children may be given a problem that involves running along an inclined plane, hopping over a low rail, and finally jumping on and off a low platform. Nonlocomotor skills may be combined into similarly imaginative patterns devised by the children under the guidance of the teacher. Locomotor and nonlocomotor skills may be combined in infinite variations and patterns.

Rhythmical skills may also be introduced during these early years. Many movement education classes can and should be conducted to a musical accompaniment. Children enjoy music and relate and react well to it.

Games of low organization incorporating the locomotor and nonlocomotor skills learned and practiced by the children are especially adaptable to movement education. A few of the many games suitable for kindergarten to grade three include:

Brownies and Fairies
Red Light
Squirrel in the Tree
Cat and Mouse
Crows and Cranes
Thief O Thief
Three Deep

Odd Couple Out
Streets and Alleys
Steal the Bacon
Numbers Change
Simple Tag and
    variations

Simple tumbling stunts such as forward and backward rolls, animal walks, basic ball throwing and catching skills, and physical fitness skills may also be parts of the program.

Program for grades four to eight

In these grades work on the basic locomotor and nonlocomotor skills should be continued. However, more advanced challenges, such as running more sophisticated obstacle courses, encouraging the child to perform varied movements and combinations of movements are important. Also, the children should gain additional experience in working with a partner or with several other children.

During these years the use of the vaulting box, parallel bars, vaulting horses, and bucks can be introduced, and by the end of the elementary school movement education experience the children should be able to perform simple routines on this equipment.

Sport skills, such as dribbling a basketball or soccer ball, can be developed as concomitants of the movement education program. The use of striking implements such as softball bats and hockey sticks can be properly introduced.

As adeptness and confidence in the use of the body as a tool for movement increases, tumbling and gymnastics skills of intermediate and advanced level may be included in the curriculum.

QUESTIONS AND EXERCISES

1. What is meant by movement education?
2. Trace the history of movement education in Europe and the United States.
3. What are the various schools of thought regarding movement education?
4. How does movement education differ from the traditional approach in physical education?
5. What are the key concepts of movement education?
6. What are the essential elements that must be taken into consideration when creating a movement education program?
7. Read one reference on movement education and give a report to the class.

Reading assignment

Bucher, Charles A., and Goldman, Myra: Dimensions of physical education, St. Louis, 1969, The C. V. Mosby Co., Reading selections 34 to 36.

SELECTED REFERENCES
Allenbaugh, Naomi: Learning about movement, NEA Journal 56:48, 1967.

Barham, Jerry N.: Toward a science and discipline of human movement, Journal of Health, Physical Education, and Recreation 37:65, 1966.

Braley, William T.: The Dayton program for developing sensory and motor skills in three, four, and five year old children, perceptual-motor foundations: a multidisciplinary concern, Washington, D. C., American Association for Health, Physical Education, and Recreation, pp. 109-111.

Brown, Margaret C.: The English method of education in movement gymnastics, The Reporter of the New Jersey Association for Health, Physical Education, and Recreation, January, 1966, p. 9.

Bucher, Charles A.: Administrative dimensions of health and physical education programs, including athletics, St. Louis, 1971, The C. V. Mosby Co.

Bucher, Charles A.: Methods and materials for secondary school physical education, ed. 3, St. Louis, 1970, The C. V. Mosby Co.

Godfrey, Barbara B.: Movement—the fundamental learning process, presented at the Physical Education Division Special Interest Meeting, AAHPER National Convention, Washington, D. C., 1964. Mimeographed.

Godfrey, Barbara B., and Kephart, Newell C.: Movement patterns and motor education, New York, 1969, Appleton-Century-Crofts.

Hackett, Layne C., and Jenson, Robert G.: A guide to movement exploration, Palo Alto, California, 1966, Peek Publication.

Howard, Shirley: The movement education approach to teaching in English elementary schools, Journal of Health, Physical Education, and Recreation, 38:31, 1967.

Kiphard, Ernst J.: Behavioral integration of problem children through remedial physical education, Journal of Health, Physical Education, and Recreation, 41:47, 1970.

Kleinman, Seymour: The significance of human movement: a phenomenological approach, National Association of Physical Education for College Women Report, 1962, p. 123.

Locke, Lawrence F.: Movement education—a description and critique. In Brown, Roscoe C., Jr., and Cratty, Bryant J., editors: New perspectives of man in action, Englewood Cliffs, New Jersey, 1969, Prentice-Hall, Inc.

Locke, Lawrence F.: The movement movement, Journal of Health, Physical Education, and Recreation 37:26, 1966.

Lockhart, Aileene: Conditions of effective motor learning, Journal of Health, Physical Education, and Recreation, 38:36, 1967.

Ludwig, Elizabeth A.: Basic movement education in England, Journal of Health, Physical Education, and Recreation, 32:18, 1961.

Ludwig, Elizabeth A.: Toward an understanding of basic movement education in the elementary schools, Journal of Health, Physical Education, and Recreation 39:28, 77, 1968.

Metheny, Eleanor: Movement and meaning, New York, 1968, McGraw-Hill Book Co.

National Association of Physical Education for College Women and National College Physical Education Association for Men: Quest (Monograph II), Tucson, Arizona, 1964.

Smith, Hope M.: Implications for movement education experience drawn from perceptual motor research, Journal of Health, Physical Education, and Recreation 41:32-33, 1970.

Smith, Hope M.: Introduction to human movement, Reading, Massachusetts, 1968, Addison-Wesley Publishing Company.

Tillotson, Joan: A brief theory of movement education. Mimeographed.

Ulrich, Celeste: No harbor, North Carolina Association of Health, Physical Education, and Recreation Journal, November, 1966, p. 3.

14/International physical education in our contemporary world

International education has become a major consideration in institutions of learning and among governmental and civic-minded officials and persons. It represents the key to a peaceful and prosperous future for all of mankind.

WHAT IS INTERNATIONAL EDUCATION?

INTERNATIONAL EDUCATION IS A TERM USED TO DESCRIBE THE MANY TYPES OF EDUCATIONAL RELATIONS AMONG COUNTRIES OF THE WORLD. It applies to the ways various governments and people of the world communicate with each other through such means as individuals and materials. It is also the study that goes on in order to achieve a better understanding of the many peoples of the world. The aim of international education is to promote better cooperation and harmony among nations.

INTERNATIONAL EDUCATION IS A TERM THAT CONTRIBUTES TO THE GOAL OF MAN LIVING PEACEFULLY WITH HIS COUNTER-PARTS IN ALL SECTIONS OF THE WORLD. It involves knowledge and human behavior that transcends cultures, boundaries, and nationalism and recognizes the dignity of man and his interdependent relationship with other men wherever he lives.

INTERNATIONAL EDUCATION IS A TERM THAT RECOGNIZES THE UNIQUENESS OF INDIVIDUALS AND CULTURES. International education recognizes that various peoples have customs, traditions, and beliefs that differ from other countries and cultures.

These ways of thinking and behaving are a part of a way of life that should be recognized and accepted for their own worth without any attempt from the outside to change these ways of behaving. Each culture has a right to live according to its own belief and standard of values.

INTERNATIONAL EDUCATION TRIES TO CORRECT INTERNATIONAL MISUNDERSTANDING AND ILL WILL. International education is aimed at the study of nations, the forces that cause misunderstandings, and the control of these forces through peaceful educational means. It attempts to present true and accurate facts as a means of countering propaganda and information that distort and erroneously describe a culture, country, or its people.

SOME HISTORICAL MILESTONES IN INTERNATIONAL EDUCATION

1. In the seventeenth century, John Comenius, the Moravian bishop and educator, suggested an international Pansophic College as a means of advancing international understanding. He was called "the teacher of nations."

2. Marc-Antoine Jullien wrote his *Esquisse et Vues Preliminaires d'un Ouvrage sur l'Education Comparée* in 1817 in which he proposed the development of an educational commission for the purpose of collecting information on education in Europe and disseminating it to interested parties.

3. Educators like Rousseau, Pestalozzi, Herbart, Froebel, Montaigne, and Kant envisioned international education as a means of accomplishing world peace.

4. The nineteenth century saw many plans for and creation of international educational organizations, international fairs, and student federations.

Students started to study in foreign universities, and history textbooks critically evaluated the glorification of war.

5. The Council of the League of Nations in 1921 created a Committee on Intellectual Cooperation. In 1925, the Council established the International Institute of Intellectual Cooperation.

6. In 1925, the Bureau Internationale d'Education was founded in Geneva and published various comparative educational studies.

7. In 1938, H. G. Wells proposed a World Encyclopedia for the purpose of unifying knowledge toward international understanding.

8. In 1942, the Conference of Allied Ministers of Education met to plan and develop an educational and cultural program. The United States joined the conference in 1944 and submitted a draft of a constitution for the establishment of an Educational and Cultural Organization of the United Nations. This was later to become the Constitution for UNESCO. This famous paragraph was included in the constitution: "Since wars begin in the minds of men, it is in the minds of men that the defense of peace must be constructed."

9. In 1945, UNESCO, the United Nations Educational, Scientific, and Cultural Organization, was formed. It has concerned itself with such functions as textbook improvement, cultural interchange, mass communications, and international cooperation in the natural sciences.

10. In 1946, the Fulbright Act, named after its sponsor, Senator J. William Fulbright of Arkansas, started the first major international exchange program for students, teachers, and scholars. It was financed from foreign currency funds derived from the sale of surplus U. S. war materials overseas. The Smith-Mundt Act in 1948 and Fulbright-Hays Act of 1961 have helped to provide money for the program and consolidate the program under the sponsorship of the State Department. In 1948, there were twenty-two nations and eighty-four grant recipients. Presently, the program involves approximately 136 nations and more than 5,100 grantees. Since its inception, the Fulbright Program has been responsible for more than 82,500 persons receiving exchange grants. Of this number, 29,000 Americans have studied abroad and about 53,000 foreign students and scholars have studied in this country.

11. Today, there are nearly 100,000 foreign students in the United States. More than 8,000 foreign interns and residents are employed in American hospitals.

12. The International Education Act of 1966, passed by the U. S. Congress, provides for the strengthening of American educational resources for international studies and research. In passing the Act, the Congress declared that a knowledge of other countries is of utmost importance in promoting mutual understanding and cooperation between nations, that American educational resources form the base for promoting understanding between the United States and other countries, and that opportunities would be made available for all U. S. citizens to learn more about other countries, peoples, and cultures. The Act provides for:

a. Graduate centers to be established as a setting for national and international research studies and training in international affairs.

b. Institutions of higher learning to be given grants to assist them in developing programs to improve undergraduate education in international studies. Grants could also be given for such projects as faculty planning, training of faculty members in foreign countries, expansion of foreign language courses, work in humanities related to international studies, student study and travel programs, and programs where foreign teachers and scholars could visit institutions of higher learning as visiting faculty or resource persons.

EDUCATION—A FORCE IN INTERNATIONAL RELATIONS*

On the main campus at the University of the Philippines in Quezon City is the "Oblation" statue. This majestic sculpture symbolizes the belief of Dr. Rizal, a former Filipino leader, when he proclaimed that youth is the hope of the motherland, and therefore young people must be provided with an excellent educational program. The world traveler soon realizes that what is true of the Philippines is true everywhere— all eyes are focused on youth and education.

Schools and colleges represent the road to success for the son of the owner of the rattan factory in Cebu City in the Philippines, they provide hope for a prosperous free China and for the woman on her knees in the terraced rice fields of Taiwan, they symbolize the tools for effective self-government for the people in the struggling new countries of Africa, they signify honor for the family whose history has been closely linked to industry in Osaka, Japan, and they represent the path to leadership roles in many walks of life for aspiring young

---

*Parts of this section have been adapted from Bucher, Charles A.: Health and physical education in other lands, Journal of Health, Physical Education, and Recreation **33:**14, 1962.

people in the countries of Europe. Although war clouds, great military machines, and spaceships to the moon are in the news, there is confidence among the peoples of the world that education will help human beings to better understand the importance and means of achieving true and lasting peace.

In contrast to America, many countries have national programs of education. The educational standards, courses of study, time allocations, attendance, and even facility requirements in some cases are outlined by a national ministry of education or other agency. Therefore, in these countries there is great uniformity in the educational programs. It is sometimes difficult for the people in other countries to comprehend our system of individual state responsibility for education.

Americans should have a sense of pride and accomplishment in the manner in which their educational system has captured the imagination of the people of the world. Our educational system greatly impresses foreigners because America provides an education adapted to the needs of the poor man's

son as well as the rich man's daughter, the student who wants to be a plumber as well as the one who wants to be a scientist, and the girl with the IQ of 90 as well as the one with an IQ of 140.

A comment made by a Chinese student still lingers clearly in my thoughts. After a lecture in southern Taiwan, the boy sadly commented: "What I wouldn't give to study in America." I have heard this remark repeated many times over by boys and girls throughout the world who look to America as a land of educational opportunity and the country that can provide the leadership for helping people to live a more peaceful, healthful, and prosperous existence. This remark undergirds a deep faith in America. In turn, it clearly shows the responsibility each American has to further educational excellence and to learn as much as possible about the cultures of the world.

HEALTH AND PHYSICAL EDUCATION AROUND THE WORLD

Fitness and physical well-being are important objectives that concern all peoples. Individuals the world over are interested in

Physical education programs in the Republic of China.

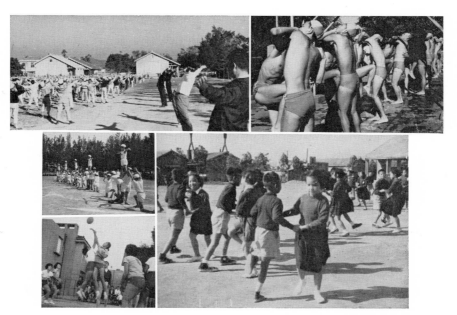

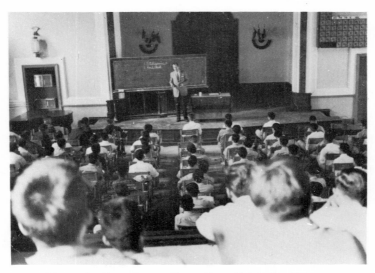

The author lecturing at Cheng Kung University, Taiwan.

sports, games, and other physical education activities. Physical education and the various gamut of activities that comprise the profession represent an interest common to people of all countries. A tennis match at Forest Hills or Wimbledon often includes players from Australia, Brazil, Spain, and France. The British Open Golf Tournament attracts enthusiasts from all over the world. Specialists in winter sports from many countries display their prowess at Saint Moritz. The Olympic festival is, of course, the greatest and most famous sports gathering, bringing together athletes from many nations. Through these international events, physical education has potentialities as one medium by which international understanding may be reached and by which people of various countries may be brought closer together.

Through such activities as Olympic festivals; competition in such sports as tennis, golf, crew, polo, soccer, and hockey; seminars on physical education and health; international conferences; and relations between educational institutions, other agencies, and individuals of various lands, good will can be promoted and the people of many cultures can come to better understand each other. The emphasis in all of these activities, however, must be on friendly com-

petition, sociability, and the desire to meet the needs of people. The stress cannot be on athletic dominance, winning at any cost, and interest in selfish personal desires and ambitions.

Leadership

The five most important things to the Chinese, in order of priority listing, are heaven, earth, government, family, and teacher. The teacher is very important to the Chinese way of life, and this is also true in many countries of the world.

There are many dedicated leaders in the professional fields of physical education, health, and recreation in other countries. These outstanding leaders, whether in Europe, Africa, Australia, Asia, or elsewhere, render a great service to students and citizens of their country and place their profession on a respected level in schools and colleges. Many of them feel their field of work is not regarded as important as some of the academic subjects such as science, mathematics, language, and history. But they are not discouraged and are working hard to gain status.

A foreigner in their midst is likely to be aware that in some Oriental countries, for example, there are many medical doctors on physical education staffs, few women teachers compared to the number in America, and a lower pay scale.

The students majoring in physical education, health, or recreation in professional preparation institutions in many countries stimulate a traveler's interest. Their eagerness to know about world developments in their professional fields, the enthusiasm they display for the games and sports in which they engage, and the keen sense of humor they possess make it a joy to be with them. One realizes that there is a rich reservoir of leadership in their respective nations for the years ahead. The professional preparation programs vary in length and content from less than 1 year to 4 years and from one course in skills to much the same type of curriculum our students experience in this country.

Facilities

Few nations can compare their health and physical education facilities to those in America. In some foreign schools and colleges and in some sections of a country, province, or city, there are beautiful and modern facilities that compare favorably with or are better than ours. However, assessing facilities in the world as a whole, America is much more richly blessed with good facilities on a broad scale than are other nations. The eyes of many foreign health and physical education teachers would open wide if they could see some of our indoor swimming pools, spacious gymnasiums, health suites, and playground facilities. The Japanese teacher, for example, would notice the green grass on playfields compared to the dirt he has to contend with and the showers our athletes take after a workout compared with the cold sponge baths some of his sports participants must endure.

But with all our facilities, equipment, and supplies, the question arises as to whether they are used as advantageously in America as the foreigner uses his. To see the rooftop playgrounds and the corridors on the outside of school buildings jammed with physical activity in Hong Kong, to look into the judo halls and see the muscular action taking place on the tatami mats in Japan, and to observe the games being played out-of-doors even during inclement weather in China makes one wonder if, with all our facilities, a better job could be done.

Activities

The activities that constitute the health and physical education programs in other countries are varied and interesting. In the Far East, for example, one is impressed to see more basketball being played in the Philippines than in America, the dexterity with which young and older persons alike kick the rattan ball in the game of sipa, and the beautiful folk dances that play such an important part in the Philippine culture.

The many sports and game activities in Hong Kong are a carryover from England because of the British influence. More high school boys play field hockey than do girls. Cricket is engaged in by various clubs but not to any degree in the schools. Track and field events are very popular.

In Japan, judo, kindo (fencing), Japanese tennis, as well as many of the typical activities offered in American programs, are popular. But in traveling throughout Japan it is interesting to note the great amount of formal activity, such as calisthenics, apparatus, and stunts. Even in the elementary schools there is considerable use of apparatus activities.

The activities that young men engage in and the way these activities are taught are significant. American high school boys should see their counterparts in the Philippines doing folk dances and in Hong Kong playing field hockey. It is interesting to see these rugged, masculine boys engaging in what Americans view mainly as girls' activities. The use of textbooks and discussion groups in physical education in some schools also shows the importance placed on getting at the "why" of physical activity as well as the activity itself.

Athletic clubs in many different activities exist in some foreign schools, colleges, and communities. These clubs sponsor and provide for instruction and participation in many sports and other activities. Students and adults engage in apparatus, riding, dance, tennis, soccer, basketball, or other activities on a voluntary basis.

Physical fitness

Physical fitness is a frequently discussed subject throughout the world. Of course, much of this interest has been sparked by the physical fitness movement in America and the comparative tests that have been administered in various parts of the globe. There is some concern in other countries as to whether the American children and youth are as inferior physically as the test results indicate. Many of the people abroad, especially those who have traveled throughout our country, question the results of these tests and doubt whether their boys and girls are in any better physical condition than ours. .

The future

A person who travels abroad, whether in Europe, Africa, South America, or some country in the Far East or other part of the world, cannot help but be impressed with the efforts being put forth by physical education, health, and recreation leaders to upgrade and improve their professional fields. They are dedicated people who, in order to improve, are forming professional associations within their countries. As one meets with these professional people, attends their meetings, and talks with students majoring in the field, he is firmly convinced that Americans should work closely with them. There is an urgent need for a strong professional association that binds together and helps each to progress a little more rapidly than he could alone.

GUIDELINES FOR INTERNATIONAL RELATIONS IN PHYSICAL EDUCATION

America is deeply involved in international affairs. If it is to occupy a position of leadership in the world, if it is to render a service to humanity over the face of the globe, and if it is to be a dynamic force for international peace, it must promote many facets of relatonships to establish common bonds among peoples everywhere. One of these common bonds is physical education. Through sports and physical activities a medium is offered to further international relationships.

The work of the World Confederation of Organizations of the Teaching Profession; International Council on Health, Physical Education, and Recreation; International Association of Physical Education and Sports for Girls and Women; and the People-to-People Sports Committee will be discussed later in this chapter. These organizations and many others are making outstanding contributions. In addition, the American Association for Health, Physical Education, and Recreation, through its International Relations Section, is also contributing. Some of these contributions include the following:

1. *Consultant services*—To domestic groups within the profession, professional groups in other countries, and in other ways
2. *Program services*—Developing and presenting programs at national and international meetings
3. *Newsletter*—Concerning international affairs and distributed to officers and interested persons
4. *Book project*—Books and professional publications collected within the United States and sent to other countries
5. *Hospitality*—Orienting, socializing with, and in general making guests from other countries feel at home and benefiting from their visit to the United States.

The work of international cooperation, however, must not stop at the national level but must extend into the schools located in villages, towns, and cities from coast to coast. According to the Committee on International Relations, National Education Association, some ways by which the schools can meet the challenge are as follows*:

1. *Education for adaptability.* Education

---

*National Education Association, Committee on International Relations: Local association activities, Leaflet No. 12, Washington, D. C., July, 1962, The Association.

must seek to help people develop qualities of flexibility and adaptability to meet changing societal conditions. In physical education attempts should be made to help participants understand the role of sports and games in the various cultures of the world and the way such activities can help in promoting international understanding.

2. *Education for cultural empathy.* Education must seek to help people understand that cultures and countries are different. Folkways, mores, and ways of doing things vary as a person crosses borders. Physical education can help to show and educate people about the various games and sports of other nations, the uniforms they wear, their standards of sportsmanship, values, and other aspects that influence physical education around the world.

3. *Education for ideological clarity.* Education must make human beings aware of the principles democracy stands for and that are essential to the survival of our way of life. Since sports and games represent democracy in action, participants in sports can show respect for the other fellow, the necessity of playing by the rules, the best sports behavior in Olympic competition, and the ways physical education activities should be conducted in order to further the cause of humanity.

4. *Education for patience.* Education must teach people that deep differences do exist between the communist and democratic countries and that these differences will not be ironed out for many years to come. Therefore, for those who believe in democracy there must be constant goals of fitness and preparedness so that this way of life may be preserved for generations to come.

5. *Education for knowledge of the world.* This is a "one world" era. Therefore, it is important to understand other peoples and other countries—the way they live, their customs, and their strong and weak points. Only as people know these facts will they understand why each person behaves as he does. Physical education can help to promote knowledge and understanding. Through an appreciation of the sports and games played by people in other countries, a better understanding of the culture develops.

6. *Education for responsibility.* Each person must come to recognize that he has a stake in international relations. It is not limited to a few. As each person contributes to other people and countries, peace will have a much better chance of becoming a reality. Physical education should impress upon each student this responsibility.

OPPORTUNITIES FOR SERVICE AT HOME

The physical educator does not need to travel to other countries in order to further good international relations. There is much work to be done in this country—at home. Some opportunities that are open to each physical educator on the home front are as follows:

1. *Teach national and cultural backgrounds of dances and games in physical education classes.* Sports, dances, and games should not be conducted in a vacuum. Boys and girls should understand their origin and the role they play in the various cultures of the world. Our physical education classes can play a dynamic part in furthering international understanding by orienting students about other countries through the medium of physical activities.

2. *Welcome foreigners.* Many physical educators, sports enthusiasts, and athletes visit and travel throughout the world. Each physical educator should be hospitable, make the person or persons welcome, and act as a guide to show and tell them about our programs. These courtesies will help to cultivate new friends for our profession and countries.

3. *Send books, CARE playground kits, and sports equipment to other countries.* People in other countries want information about our physical education programs. They welcome books, periodicals, and other literature that describe our programs, methods, and teaching techniques. An important service can be rendered by contributing literature to this worthy cause. Other countries are also interested in receiving sports equipment.

4. *Join international associations.* Physical educators should become involved in professional association work in international relations. The American Association for Health, Physical Education, and Recreation and many state associations have active sections or divisions in this area. In addition, such organizations as the International Association of Physical Education and Sports for Girls and Women are seeking members to help to carry out their objectives.

5. *Be knowledgeable about international affairs.* The physical educator should become acquainted with happenings on the international scene, world events that are taking place, and the work of such organizations as the United Nations. The physical educator should read and subscribe to some foreign publications.* As the physical educator becomes better informed about international happenings, he will be more qualified to give students such information.

International dates of special interest

Physical educators should be aware of international dates of special interest and the opportunities these days afford for planning special activities to contribute to international understanding. A few dates are:

Columbus Day—second Monday in October
United Nations Day—October 24
Thanksgiving—fourth Thursday in November
Human Rights Day—December 10
Bill of Rights Day—December 15
Christmas—December 25
Brotherhood Week—February
Easter—March or April
World Health Day—April 7
Pan American Day—April 14
Flag Day—June 14

Resources

The National Education Association also lists the following resources for those who wish to contribute to international education:

1. *Information about pen pals, classroom, and school affiliation may be obtained from:*
School and Classroom Department, People-to-People, Inc.

---

*One excellent resource of international information is *Other Lands and Other Peoples: a country-by-country fact book,* a publication of the Committee on International Relations of the National Education Association.

2401 Grand Avenue
Kansas City, Missouri 64141
2. *Materials on Asia may be obtained from:*
Asia Society
112 East 64th Street
New York, New York 10021
3. *Materials on Latin America may be obtained from:*
Department of Public Information
Pan American Union
Washington, D. C. 20006
4. *Periodicals*
INTERCOM—Foreign Policy Association
345 East 46th Street
New York, New York 10017
INTERCOM is an invaluable resource publication for teachers. It is perhaps the most complete, reliable, and useful available.

OPPORTUNITIES FOR SERVICE ABROAD

For the physical educator who is interested in serving abroad there are many opportunities to make this desire come true. A selected few are as follows:

1. *Student and teacher exchange programs.* Each year more than 7,000 persons representing over 100 countries are exchanged to teach, study, lecture, and engage in research or in other educational or cultural activities through programs sponsored by the Department of State. For more information write Teacher Exchange Section, Bureau of International Education, U. S. Office of Education, Washington, D. C.

2. *Peace Corps.* On September 21, 1961, the Peace Corps Act was passed by the U. S. Congress. Today there are thousands of Peace Corps volunteers serving in foreign assignments. Many physical educators are a part of the Peace Corps, and the American Association for Health, Physical Education, and Recreation is working closely with this organization. Applicants may obtain Peace Corps questionnaires from the American Association for Health, Physical Education, and Recreation, post offices, or from the Peace Corps, Washington, D. C. 20525.

The Peace Corps and VISTA have merged into a new agency called ACTION, the citizens' service corps. Under the new arrangement volunteers can be assigned either in developing countries or in cities and other locations in this country.

A few foreign countries and areas where health and physical education and recreation specialists have been used are the Ivory Coast, Tunisia, Ceylon, Iran, Thailand, Colombia, and Indonesia. According to the American Association for Health, Physical Education, and Recreation, the criteria used in respect to physical education and athletic programs include obtaining volunteers who are graduates from accredited institutions with a physical education major or a physical education minor with a recommendation from the college, athletes who have graduated from college and are recommended by the physical education department, and individuals trained in physical education or outstanding athletes strongly recommended by professional people in the field.

3. *Teach Corps.* The National Education Association has established a Teach Corps, which utilizes the services of experienced American teachers in providing summer in-service training for teachers in foreign lands. For further information write Committee on International Relations, National Education Association, 1201 16th Street, N.W., Washington, D. C. 20036.

4. *United Nations Educational, Scientific, and Cultural Organization.* UNESCO seeks teachers to serve in developing countries around the world. It has an international fellowship and travel study program in war-devastated or underdeveloped countries. Write to UNESCO, Department of Exchange of Persons, 19 Avenue Kleber, Paris 16, France, or to Office of International Administration, U. S. Department of State, Washington, D. C. 20520.

5. *Armed forces.* Bases operated overseas by the armed forces have teaching positions available for elementary and secondary school teachers. For details write to branch of service, chief of personnel of the particular branch of service in which interested.

6. *World Health Organization.* For physical educators with competencies in the area of health, opportunities exist in various parts of the world. Write to Personnel Office, World Health Organization, 1501 New Hampshire Avenue, N.W., Washington, D.

C., or to United Nations, 777 United Nations Plaza, New York, N. Y. 10017.

7. *Fulbright grants.* An avenue for foreign service for those with advanced education and degrees may be available through the Fulbright program. This program has been in operation for several years and has been very popular for those interested in lecturing or teaching abroad for a year. If interested, write Conference Board of Associated Research Councils, Committee on International Exchange of Persons, 2101 Constitution Avenue, Washington, D. C.

8. *United States Agency for International Development (AID).* The AID program exists in such areas of the world as Asia, Africa, Far East, Near East, Greece, and Turkey. Most positions are at the teacher training level, with 2 years considered to be the minimum length of assignment. For more information write to AID, U. S. Department of State, Washington, D. C. 20520.

9. *The Association of Commonwealth Universities.* This Association has vacancies for recently graduated students from colleges and universities. The address is 36 Gordon Square, London W.C. 1, England.

10. *Central Bureau for Educational Visits and Exchanges.* This bureau serves as an office and clearinghouse for information on educational travel and official exchanges. It is located at 91 Victoris Street, London S.W. 1, England.

11. *Council on International Exchange.* This council, which serves as a clearinghouse for information on exchange programs and travel throughout the world, has its offices at 777 United Nations Plaza, New York, N. Y. 10017.

12. *Institute of International Education.* The Institute conducts educational exchange programs for colleges, universities, foundations, corporations, foreign governments, and other organizations. Write to the Institute, 809 United Nations Plaza, New York, N. Y. 10017.

13. *Overseas Educational Service.* This organization helps American scholars who have problems on extended overseas service and recruits faculty and administrators to

fill new or vacant positions. Write to Overseas Education Service, 522 Fifth Avenue, New York, N. Y. 10036.

14. *Pan American Health Organization.* This organization considers applications in such fields as nursing, public health, and medical fields. It has its office at Pan American Sanitary Bureau, 525 23rd Street, N. W., Washington, D. C. 20037.

15. *Schools in outlying areas.* Such places as the Panama Canal Zone, Territory of Guam, American Samoa, Trust Territory of the Pacific Islands, and the Virgin Islands offer teaching opportunities in elementary and secondary schools and in colleges. For more information write to the area of interest.

16. *Binational centers.* Private organizations have established binational centers in many countries in order to bring about better understanding between the United States and these countries. Binational centers are presently located in the Near East, Europe, and the Far East. Classes are offered at all educational levels. For more information write to the U. S. Department of State, Washington, D. C. 20520.

17. *Schools in the Middle East, Far East, Africa, and Europe sponsored through the International Schools Service.* A wide range of educational services are offered through this independent, nonprofit organization concerned with international programs of technical aid, diplomacy and industrial efficiency. For more information write International School Services, 392 Fifth Avenue, New York, N. Y. 10018.

18. *Schools in Latin American republics through the Inter-American School Service.* American-sponsored administrative and teaching positions exist in Latin American through the Inter-American Schools Service. For more information write to the U. S. Department of State, Washington, D. C. 20520.

19. *Church-sponsored schools.* Protestant-, Catholic-, and Jewish-sponsored schools and colleges in many countries of the world offer teaching opportunities for those who are interested. For more informa-

tion write to The Religious Education Association, 545 West 111th Street, New York, N. Y. 10025.

20. *Schools operated by American firms overseas.* Some American business and industrial concerns operate elementary and secondary schools in several countries of the world for the children of American employees. Teaching opportunities exist in these schools.

Several international areas in which physical educators may utilize their talents have been pointed out. Any student who has a sincere interest in physical education, possesses a degree of skill in the various physical activities, has qualities that make for good leadership, and possesses the initiative and drive to get ahead will never have to worry about finding a place for his talents in one of these settings.

SELECTED INTERNATIONAL COMPETITIONS
Olympic games

The First Olympiad was held in 776 B.C. at Olympia, Greece. It was originally a 5-day event held every 4 years during the month of August. The earliest Olympics honored the Greek god Zeus. The facilities for these contests were open fields, and spectators lined the sides or sat on convenient slopes. An early Christian emperor named Theodosius termed the Olympics decadent and abolished them in 394 A.D. In 1896, the Olympics were revived by the Baron Pierre de Coubertin and were held in Athens. The United States participated that year, the Asian nations joined in 1932, and Russia entered for the first time in 1952. The first modern Olympics included competition in track and field, weight lifting, wrestling, swimming, cycling, tennis, gymnastics, fencing, and shooting. The scope of competition now includes, in addition to the above, boxing, rowing, yachting, water polo, canoeing, field hockey, basketball, the modern pentathlon, riding, soccer, handball, and judo. Tennis is no longer part of the Olympics.

The winter Olympic games were first

initiated in 1924 and were held in Chamonix, France. They are now held in the same year as the summer Olympics, but they need not be held in the same country. Events in the winter Olympics include the luge, ice hockey, speed and figure skating, skiing, and bobsledding.

The International Olympic Committee is responsible for the conduct of the games.

Asian Games

The Asian Games were first held in Manila in 1913. The participating countries of China, Japan, and the Philippines held what they called the First Oriental Olympic Games in that year. After 1921, the competition was renamed the Far Eastern Championships. Ceylon, India, Indonesia, Malaya, and Thailand were invited to join but were prevented from doing so by financial difficulties. A political dispute ended the competition between the three original nations in 1934. At that time, India invited Ceylon, Afghanistan, and Palestine to compete in the West Asiatic Games. War ended the competition after the first year. The First Asian Games were held in New Delhi, India, in 1951 under the sponsorship of the Asian Games Federation. Initially, competition was to be held every 3 years, but it is presently held every 4 years. In 1954, eighteen countries participated, and nineteen competed in 1958. By 1962, twenty-two nations were involved. Objectives of the Asian Games include the setting of new Asian Game records and the breaking of as many Olympic and world records as possible. Competition for men includes boxing, cycling, field hockey, soccer, basketball, riflery, water polo, weight lifting, and wrestling. Men and women compete in their own divisions in badminton, swimming and diving, table tennis, track and field, volleyball, and tennis.

Pan-American Games

The Pan-American Games, initiated in 1951, are limited to nations of the western hemisphere, including, among others, such nations as the United States, Canada, Argentina, Mexico, Bolivia, and Brazil. Presently, about twenty-four nations compete in these games, which are held every 4 years, between Olympics. The Pan-American Sports Organization administers the same guidelines set down for Olympic competition.

Men compete in many of the same activities that are included in the Olympics, with the addition of tennis and baseball. Women compete in Olympic events and also include basketball, tennis, and synchronized swimming in their schedule of events.

British Empire and Commonwealth Games

This competition is limited to member nations of the British Empire. The games began in 1930 and are held every 4 years in a non-Olympic year. The British Empire and Commonwealth Games Federation administers the competition in which approximately forty nations join. The events are of an individual rather than a team nature and include badminton, boxing, cycling, fencing, shooting, swimming and diving, track and field, weight lifting, and wrestling.

World Maccabiah Games

These games were initiated in 1931, and are held in Israel every 4 years. They are limited to Jewish athletes. The International Maccabiah Games Committee administers the games on the Olympic pattern. Presently, about twenty-five nations participate. Men compete in many of the Olympic events plus golf, bowls, and table tennis. Women also compete in Olympic-type events and add golf and table tennis to their list of activities.

World University Games

The International Federation of University Sports has conducted this competition since 1947. It is held every 2 years during an odd-numbered year. Approximately thirty-five countries send university students to participate in the games. Events included are track and field, basketball, soccer, gymnastics, tennis, fencing, and swimming and diving.

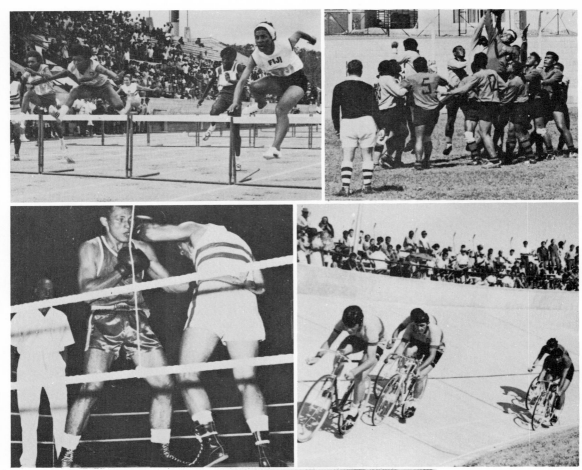

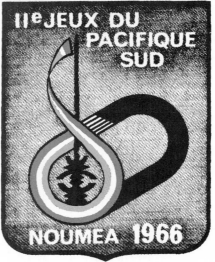

South Pacific Games.

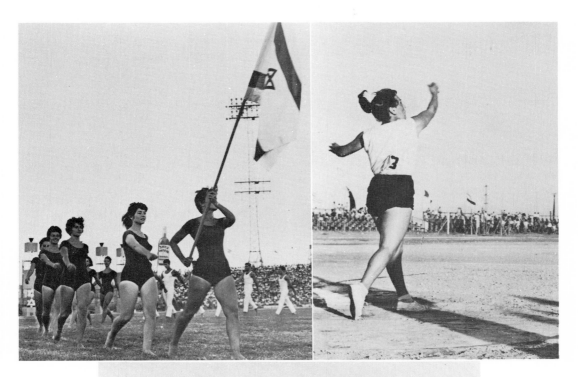

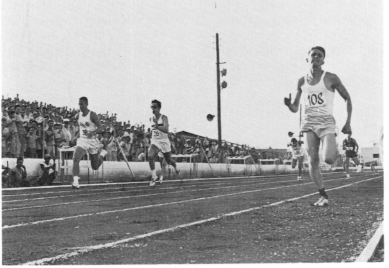

The Maccabiah Games.

Table 14-1. Spectator sports and popular dances of other countries*

Country	Sport	Dance
Australia	Soccer, cricket, boxing, swimming, tennis	Modern, ballet
Belgium	Soccer, cycling, tennis	Ballet, folk
Canada	Hockey, football, baseball, basketball, skiing	Modern, ballet
Denmark	Soccer, gymnastics, handball, swimming, track and field	Modern, ballet
Dominican Republic	Baseball, tennis	Folk
England	Football (soccer), boxing, cricket, tennis	Modern, ballet
France	Soccer, tennis, cycling, boxing	Ballet
India	Soccer, cricket, field hockey, tennis, badminton	Folk
Mexico	Bullfighting, soccer, baseball, jai alai	Modern, folk
Norway	Skiing, soccer, skating, track and field, swimming	Modern, folk
Peru	Soccer, bullfighting, boxing, track and field	Folk
Russia	Soccer, track and field, gymnastics, hockey	Ballet

*From Wessel, Janet: Movement fundamentals, Englewood Cliffs, New Jersey, 1961, Prentice-Hall, Inc., p. 271.

SELECTED MAJOR INTERNATIONAL COMPETITIONS IN SELECTED AMATEUR SPORTS

BADMINTON. The International Badminton Federation sponsors international competition in this sport. The Thomas Cup for men was initiated in 1940 and the Uber Cup for women in 1956. Competition is held every 3 years.

CHESS. The first World Chess Championships were held in 1851, under the sponsorship of the International Chess Federation. This organization continues to host this competition on a yearly basis.

CYCLING. The Tour de France, sponsored by the International Cycling Union, is a yearly event.

GOLF. The Americas Cup Golf Match, between the United States, Mexico, and Canada, has been held every 2 years since 1952. The Ryder Cup Match, first held in 1922, matches the United States against Great Britain every 2 years. The World Cup golf matches involve players from around the globe.

ICE SKATING. The World Figure Skating Championships have been held yearly since the late 1870's. The World Speed Skating Championships have been a yearly event since 1893. Both are under the sponsorship of the International Skating Union.

RIDING. The International Horse Show is held on a yearly basis.

ROWING. The Royal Yacht Club has sponsored the Henley-on-Thames Royal Regatta yearly since 1839.

SHOOTING. The National Rifle Association each year sponsors several international postal matches under the rules set down by the International Shooting Union: the International Free-Pistol Postal Match, the Mayleigh Cup International Smallbore Rifle Postal Match for Women, and the International Smallbore Rifle Three-Position Postal Match. International outdoor postal matches are held for Smallbore Rifle Prone and three-Position, Free-Rifle Three-Position, Free-Pistol, and Center-Fire Rifle.

SKIING. The International Federation of Skiing sponsors the World Ski Championships every 3 years.

SOCCER. Every 4 years the International Federation of Soccer sponsors the World Cup Matches.

SWIMMING. The International Amateur Swimming Federation sponsors the World Swimming Championships every year.

TENNIS. The United States Outdoor Tennis Championships have been sponsored yearly since 1881 by the U. S. Lawn Tennis Association. Under the guidance of the International Lawn Tennis Association, committees of the nations involved have sponsored the Wimbledon Championships since 1877; the Davis Cup for men since 1900; and the Wightman Cup for women of the United States and England since 1923.

YACHTING. About every 3 years since

1851, the New York Yacht Club has sponsored the America's Cup in cooperation with the yachting body of the challenging nation.

SELECTED INTERNATIONAL ORGANIZATIONS

There are many organizations concerned with physical education in international affairs. These organizations render an invaluable service to humanity. In a "one world" era it is not only important for the physical educator to be acquainted with professional organizations active on the domestic scene but also those that play active roles on the international scene. A few of the outstanding international professional organizations with which the physical educator should be familiar are as follows.

World Confederation of Organizations of the Teaching Profession

The World Confederation of Organizations of the Teaching Profession (WCOTP) was founded at Copenhagen, Denmark, in 1952. It is composed of 140 national members and sixty-five associate members, who represent 5 million teachers in ninety countries around the world.

The purposes of the WCOTP include providing an organization in which professional teachers at all educational levels can utilize education for furthering international understanding and world peace, teachers can unite their efforts to upgrade their educational policies and practices throughout the world, and international educational policies can be molded by the associated effort of teachers from all the countries represented in the organization.

Although membership in WCOTP consists largely of associations and institutions, interested persons may subscribe for and receive its publications. Membership consists of national members (educational or teachers' associations), associate members (regional, provincial, state, and local teachers' associations and institutions), and international members (international educational organizations).

The WCOTP is governed by an assembly of delegates, the highest governing body; an executive committee, which carries out the work of the confederation for the assembly of delegates; and a secretary general, who executes the decisions of the assembly and executive committee.

WCOTP has three international members concerned with specialized phases of education: the International Council on Health, Phyical Education, and Recreation (ICHPER), the International Council on Education for Teaching (ICET), and the International Reading Association (IRA).

WCOTP conducts conferences and seminars throughout the world for leaders of teacher organizations and other educators on various educational problems. Conferences and seminars have been held in such places as Ceylon, United States, Costa Rica, Vietnam, Nigeria, Peru, Colombia, and Indonesia. The WCOTP also works closely with the United Nations, especially with such organizations as the World Health Organization, Economic and Social Council, and the Food and Agriculture Organization.

WCOTP publishes an annual report and, in addition, such periodicals as *Panorama: Teaching Throughout the World* and *Echo*. These publications appear in many different languages.

International Council on Health, Physical Education, and Recreation

At the annual meeting of the WCOTP in Rome in 1958, a special committee discussed and formulated a statement of the purposes and functions of organizations of health, physical education, and recreation. The committee drafted a constitution and presented it to the WCOTP assembly of delegates for approval. Then, in 1959, at the annual meeting of the WCOTP in Washington, D. C., an official decision was made to form an International Council on Health, Physical Education, and Recreation (ICHPER). WCOTP approved this organization in August, 1959.

The purposes of ICHPER include helping WCOTP to accomplish its objectives; encouraging, developing, and upgrading programs of health, physical education, and recreation throughout the world; working

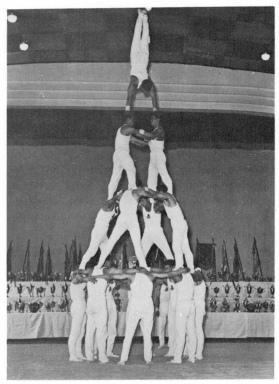

ICHPER conference in Seoul, Korea. Members of the Kyung-Hee University gymnastic team performing before the delegates of the congress.

closely with other international organizations concerned with these special fields; improving the professional status of teachers; supporting, encouraging, and sponsoring the exchange of research findings and information for the profession; and promoting the exchange of teachers and students among the countries of the world.

The groups throughout the world who are eligible to join ICHPER are international organizations in health, physical education, and recreation, national organizations, and regional or geographical area organizations. The aim of the Council is to bring representatives from countries into this one organization so that it can be the official world spokesman for the professions. Through such representation it hopes to promote better school programs in health, physical education, and recreation. More specifically, it will do this by attempting to improve teaching methods, training teachers, providing

materials for teaching, and doing research. It is anticipated that ICHPER will plan and conduct conferences, seminars, courses, world congresses, lectures, demonstrations, exhibits, and many other experiences to carry out its objectives.

The administration of the Council rests with an assembly of delegates appointed by member organizations or the executive committee and an executive committee composed of officers of the Council and members elected by the assembly of delegates. The officers of the Council include the president, the vice-president, and the secretary-general. The president and vice-president are elected for 3-year terms, and the secretary-general is appointed by the executive committee. ICHPER has met in such cities as, Washington, Amsterdam, New Delhi, Stockholm, Rio de Janeiro, Paris, Addis Ababa, Seoul, Vancouver, and Dublin.

Materials and information on ICHPER

can be secured by writing to this organization at 1201 16th Street, N.W., Washington, D. C. 20036.

There are six types of membership, with annual fees as follows: individual, $10; institutional, $10; contributing, $25 or more; international, $10; national, $10; and regional, $5. Membership each year provides four issues of *ICHPER Bulletin,* a four-page newsletter reporting significant professional developments and activities, four issues of *Gymnasion,* Proceedings of the International Congress of ICHPER, and research reports.

In the years ahead it is expected that ICHPER will be very active on the international scene, making recommendations to governments, advising on equipment and facility needs, exchanging personnel, assisting member organizations, supporting recreational activities, and providing leadership in many ways for the fields of health, physical education, and recreation.

International Association of Physical Education and Sports for Girls and Women

Women in physical education, feeling the need to know about and participate in sports in other countries and to solve common problems, prompted the foundation of the International Association of Physical Education and Sports for Girls and Women. Membership is open to women who engage in physical education work at any of the educational levels, elementary through college, as well as leaders in adult programs. Members can participate in the congresses that are held, usually every fourth or fifth year, in one of the fifty-one countries that participate in the Association. Meetings have been held in such cities as Stockholm, Paris, London, Washington, D. C., Cologne, and Tokyo. There are two types of membership: *individual* membership with dues of $3 per year, and *national* membership (for national and international organizations) with dues of $5 per year. Aims of the Association are as follows:

1. To promote closer working relationships among women physical educators in various countries of the world.

2. To work closely with various organizations that render services to women.
3. To afford opportunities through congresses and meetings to discuss and help in the solving of mutual problems.
4. To encourage research and exchange of persons and ideas and to promote other activities related to physical education and sports for women.

For more information write to the Association, c/o Dr. A. Gwendolyn Drew, Washington University, St. Louis, Missouri 63130.

International Amateur Athletic Federation

On July 17, 1912, representatives from the athletic associations of sixteen countries met in Stockholm, Sweden, with the aim of establishing an international organization devoted to amateur athletics. The first official meeting of the IAAF took place in Berlin in 1913.

Some of the objectives of the International Amateur Athletic Federation are:

1. To attempt to eliminate racial, political, and religious discrimination from athletics
2. To foster friendship and cooperation between members of the Federation
3. To prevent any country or individual being denied the right to participate in international athletics on racial, religious, or political grounds
4. To establish rules and regulations governing international competition in amateur athletics
5. To help in the organization of the Olympic Games
6. To establish standards for the establishment of World and Olympic records

The organization is governed by a President, an Honorary Secretary, and a fifteen-member council, which is composed of representatives from each of the following area groups: Africa, Asia, Australasia, Europe, North America, and South America.

The National Governing Body for Amateur Athletics in any country or territory is eligible for membership in the International Amateur Athletic Federation. The dues range from 5 pounds (British) to 100 pounds.

The principal publications include: *IAAF*

Handbook (in English and French); *IAAF Bulletin,* three issues per year; *IAAF World, European, and Olympic Record Supplements* (from 1959); and IAAF Scoring Table for Men's and Women's Track and Field.

The address of the IAAF is 162-164 Upper Richmond Road, London S.W. 15, England.

International Federation of Physical Education

The International Federation of Physical Education (FIEP) was founded in 1923 in Brussels. The home office is now located in Lisbon, Portgual. The aims of this organization are to promote health, wholesome recreation, and the social adaptation of the individual. The Federation is concerned with the scientific, technical, pedagogical, and social aspects of physical education and sport. It communicates with responsible people and organizations of world physical education such as teachers of physical education, school and sport physicians and scientists, official departments and agencies, International Councils of physical education, schools of physical education, and research institutes.

Its bulletin is printed quarterly in five languages and carries articles related to research in the areas of science and exercise, book reviews, and international views of physical education. Its publications are the *FIEP Bulletin,* the *International Chronicle,* and a bibliographic bulletin called *Books and Magazines.*

International Council of Sport and Physical Education

The International Council of Sport and Physical Education (ICSPE) was founded in 1956 in Melbourne, Australia. The General Assemblies have been held in such countries as Iran and Mexico.

The aims of this organization include acting as a clearinghouse for international cooperation in sports and physical education, promoting the social good of sports and physical education, and promoting research

and the exchange of ideas and assistance between countries. The ICSPE cooperates closely with the UNESCO, ICHPER, and other related organizations such as the International Olympic Committee.

Publications of ICSPE include *ICSPE Newsletter, Revue Analytique d'Education Physique et Sportive* (published by the Bureau of Documentation and Information), *Who's Who in Physical Culture, Declarations on Sports* (published in English, French, Spanish, Arabic, and German), and reports of seminars and study meetings.

International Recreation Association

The International Recreation Association (IRA) was founded in 1956 in Philadelphia. This organization seeks to advance recreation on an international basis by aiding various countries in need of assistance, by answering inquiries, by placing qualified teachers and leaders in youth agencies, and by distributing information.

The IRA has made significant contributions in the following areas:

1. Organizing and conducting exchange programs for governments, foundations, and recreation agencies, enabling more than 300 leaders from fifty countries to observe and study recreation in the United States
2. Recruiting and training volunteers who have served in more than eighty countries
3. Arranging for an exchange of recreation leaders from various countries

The IRA publishes the *IRA Bulletin,* which is sent regularly to 3,500 leaders in ninety-nine countries. The IRA also distributes helpful information about recreation to affiliated agencies and informs leaders of government, business, and professions of the importance of planning for leisure. The IRA also distributes a hospital recreation guide, *On the Mend.* The address of the IRA is 345 East 46th Street, New York, N. Y. 10017.

International Bureau of Education

The International Bureau of Education (Bureau International d'Education—BIE) was founded in 1925 in Geneva and serves as an international educational information center for all countries. In 1946, after the founding of UNESCO, that organization joined the BIE in setting up a common program. Subsequently, an agreement was reached by the two organizations whereby the BIE transferred its resources and functions to UNESCO. In November, 1968, the General Conference of UNESCO adopted statutes establishing the BIE as an integral part of the organization.

This organization publishes research studies on educational organizations and an international bulletin printed in English and French. The Ministries of Education in member countries send an educational progress report each year that is incorporated into an educational yearbook. An Intergovernmental Conference on Public Education is sponsored each year. The Bureau also maintains an extensive library of education textbooks, journals, and legislative documents pertaining to education. The address of the Bureau is Palais Wilson, 1211 Geneva 14, Geneva, Switzerland.

International University Sports Federation

The International University Sports Federation (Fédération Internationale de Sport Universitaire—FISU) was established in 1948 in Luxembourg. The purposes of the Federation are:

1. To encourage the development of physical education among students of all countries by exchanging information on university sports
2. To sponsor international sports meetings
3. To promote the moral value of sports on an amateur basis

The FISU is composed of national organizations, National University of Sports Organizations, or National Union of Students, in fifty-six countries. The Federation holds a General Assembly every 2 years. The Executive Committee is composed of President, Vice-President, Secretary, Treasurer, and assessors. It has one paid and four voluntary staff members. The languages of the Federation are French and English. The membership dues are $100 in Swiss francs.

FISU has sponsored biennial World Student Games in summer and winter sports (Universiades) in such places as Sofia, Porto Alegre, Budapest, Tokyo, Chamonix, Villars, Sestriere, and Innsbruck.

In addition to Universiades, the Federation has sponsored sports days in such places as Macolin, Obertraum, London, and Grunewald.

The Federation publishes the *FISU Bulletin* and numerous brochures in French and English. All correspondence to FISU should be directed to FISU Secretariat, BP 75, Leuven 1, Belgium.

International Sports Organization for the Disabled

The International Sports Organization for the Disabled was established March 26, 1961, in Paris under the auspices of the World Veterans Federation. Some of the activities of the organization include sports meetings, training courses for coaches, seminars, and exhibitions. The aims of the organization are:

1. To promote sports for the handicapped or disabled on an international level
2. To coordinate all international functions of member organizations

The membership of the International Sports Organization for the Disabled is composed of national associations for the disabled in seventeen countries. The organization holds an annual General Assembly. It has an Executive Board and several technical-medical committees. The staff of the organization is voluntary. The languages of the organization are English, German, and French. The address of the organization is Franklin Moore House, 185-187 High Road, Chadwell Heath, England.

International Federation of Sports Medicine

The International Federation of Sports Medicine (Fédération Internationale de Medicine Sportive—FIMS) was founded in St. Moritz in 1928. The aims of the Federation are:

1. To improve physical and moral health by

sporting activities, particularly physical education, gymnastics, games, and other sports

2. To make scientific studies of the effect of participating in sporting activities

The FIMS membership includes national federations in thirty-eight countries. Its members are persons interested in research, teaching, coaching, and medical aspects of sports. They concern themselves with the physiological aspects of sports as well as the prevention and care of injuries incurred in sports.

People-to-People Sports Committee

The People-to-People Sports Committee is one of the forty-one people-to-people programs established in 1956. It has as its main purpose the involvement of Americans in the conduct of international affairs through sports. The membership consists of more than 500 individuals in the United States who are prominent in the field of sports or its promotion. Its headquarters is at 277 Park Avenue, New York, N. Y. 10017.

It is a nongovernmental, nonprofit, membership corporation that has engaged in such projects as tours of the United States by basketball teams from other countries and sending boys' basketball teams from California to Japan and Korea. Its key to success has been its ability and willingness to get individual and business help in defraying expenses for foreign visitors and in helping American athletes go overseas. The key persons responsible for the Committee's work are a director, a secretary, and a chairman. They work closely with the U. S. Department of State in carrying on their work.

PHYSICAL EDUCATION IN SELECTED COUNTRIES AROUND THE WORLD
Australia

The island continent of Australia, composed of six states, is approximately the same size as the mainland United States. The population of Australia is almost totally made up of people of British descent, although many European immigrants have re-

cently settled there. Manufacturing, commerce, building, construction, and farming are the major sources of income.

EDUCATIONAL STRUCTURE. Education is compulsory between the ages of 6 and 15, except in Tasmania, where the upper age is 16. The six state governments are responsible for the progress of education in their own states. A director of education heads the state education department in each capital city, and under him are the directors of the specific educational areas. Each state has a state director of physical education.

PHILOSOPHY OF EDUCATION. The Australian educational system seeks to accomplish such goals as preparing its students to be well-rounded individuals, satisfying the needs and abilities of each individual, and giving vocational preparation.

PHILOSOPHY OF PHYSICAL EDUCATION. Physical education is required in all elementary and secondary schools and in all teacher-training curriculums in colleges and universities. It seeks to develop physical fitness in students by promoting proper growth and by building adequate amounts of strength, endurance, and coordination. Social and emotional development and the learning of recreational skills are also primary aims.

PHYSICAL EDUCATION IN INFANTS' SCHOOLS. These schools are attached to the primary schools, and children may enter when they are 5. Physical education is the responsibility of the classroom teacher and is a phase of the total program. The emphasis is on creativity, self-expression, and the acquisition of skills needed in later school years. Dancing and rhythmics make up the bulk of the physical education activities.

PHYSICAL EDUCATION IN ELEMENTARY SCHOOLS. This educational level accepts children from the age of 8 until they have completed the work of the seventh grade at age 12 or 13. Physical education is the responsibility of the classroom teacher, who may call upon physical education resource people attached to the state education department. In grades one through four, approximately 1 hour a week is devoted to physical education, while grades five through seven have approximately 2 hours of physical education a week. The activities included in the program are games, marching, stunts and tumbling, gymnastics, track and field, and lead-up games for such sports as tennis, softball, and basketball. Where a pool is available, swimming is taught.

PHYSICAL EDUCATION IN SECONDARY SCHOOLS. Australia has four kinds of secondary schools: 5- or 6-year college preparatory high schools; 3- to 4-year junior high schools for those students entering vocations; 2- to 5-year home science schools for girls planning to become teachers or nurses or who will enter other service occupations; and 3-year agricultural schools. All secondary schools have physical education specialists, although two schools may share the services of a single specialist. Up to 3 hours a week, including participation in the intramural program, are devoted to physical education. Dancing, rhythmics, the skills of various sports, gymnastics, games, track and field, and swimming are all parts of the program.

PHYSICAL EDUCATION IN HIGHER EDUCATION. Physical education is required only for those planning to enter the teaching profession.

PHYSICAL EDUCATION FACILITIES. Indoor facilities, especially gymnasiums, are generally poor, but many indoor facilities are currently under construction. Equipment is generally inadequate. Outdoor facilities are more than ample.

TEACHER TRAINING. Professional programs in physical education are offered at the state universities in three states and through the state education department in conjunction with the universities in the remaining three states. A diploma course lasts 3 years and a degree course from 4 to 5 years, depending on the amount of part-time study the prospective teacher engages in.

Brazil

Brazil is a tropical country. The Amazon Basin being a typically hot, tropical climate, while the Highlands, which includes roughly half of the total area, are subtropic.

EDUCATIONAL STRUCTURE. The responsibility for public education is divided among federal, state, and municipal governments. State and local governments have almost exclusive control over elementary and secondary school, and the responsibility for higher education is in the federal ministry of education. The federal government, through the Federal Council of Education, advises the state ministries of education and also helps coordinate various educational programs on the state level.

PHILOSOPHY OF EDUCATION. In general, Brazilians, through their schools, seek to eliminate illiteracy and to provide a high standard of education that will increase productivity and improve life standards of the country.

PHILOSOPHY OF PHYSICAL EDUCATION. The physical education programs of Brazil have been influenced by those foreign countries that have made significant contributions in the area of physical education. Brazil seeks to utilize the best methods and systems of physical education in order to develop the psychophysical potentialities of pupils. Emphasis is placed on the physiological, the sociological, and the psychological development of the individual.

PHYSICAL EDUCATION IN ELEMENTARY SCHOOLS. In grades one through five, the classroom teacher is responsible for instruction in physical education. In many schools physical education classes are conducted for 40 to 45 minutes twice a week, while some special groups receive daily programs of 20 to 30 minutes in order to improve their physical and mental-moral-social condition. The activities included in the program are games, natural activities, stunts and tumbling, recreational gymnastics, rhythmical activities, and sports.

PHYSICAL EDUCATION IN SECONDARY SCHOOLS. The National Education Law permits the states to create their own systems of education. The physical education programs of Brazil vary greatly from state to state. Each state is composed of several educational districts. Each district has a physical education supervisor who receives guidance from the physical education department of each state. In some schools, the program consists of two parts, namely, a service program (regular classes in gymnastics, games, and sports, stunts and tumbling, and dance) and an interschool program (extraclass activities such as intramurals, intercollegiate gymnastics, and dance demonstrations).

PHYSICAL EDUCATION IN HIGHER EDUCATION. Physical education as a subject is not included in the curriculums of Brazilian universities, nor is there any emphasis on extraclass physical education activities.

PHYSICAL EDUCATION FACILITIES. Because of rapid population growth and meager school budgets, only the most pressing educational needs are being given top priority. As a result, physical education facilities are very often poor or entirely lacking in the schools of Brazil.

TEACHER TRAINING. There are eleven physical education schools in Brazil that train teachers of physical education. Rio de Janeiro's Federal University has a Physical Education Sports School in which studies are completed in 3 years.

Brazil has postgraduate courses for physicians and physical education teachers, as well as graduate courses for physiotherapists.

Canada

Canada is the second largest nation in square miles in the world. Both the French and English languages are spoken there. Agriculture is a leading industry, but mining, forestry, and fishing are leading occupations.

EDUCATIONAL STRUCTURE. Each of the ten Canadian provinces controls and administers its own schools. Thus, although the compulsory entry age for school is 6 years nationwide, the age that youth may leave the schools may be from 14 to 16, depending on the particular province. Likewise, some elementary schools include only the first six grades, while in other provinces the first seven or eight grades are part of the elementary school. Canada has many church-supported schools that set individual policies free of any provincial controls.

PHILOSOPHY OF EDUCATION. General education in Canada has been strongly influenced by the philosophies of the United States, Great Britain, and Europe. The provision of an adequate education for all and preparation for a vocation are primary educational concerns.

PHILOSOPHY OF PHYSICAL EDUCATION. The attainment of physical fitness, basic skills needed for life and leisure, and social and emotional fitness are major objectives. The development of recreational skills has always been of major importance. Canada also places great emphasis on educating for movement and is considered to be a leader in the area of movement education.

PHYSICAL EDUCATION IN ELEMENTARY SCHOOLS. A general shortage of trained elementary school physical educators has placed the classroom teacher in the role of responsibility for physical education on this level. In general, three 15-minute periods of physical education a week are given. The activities included are movement skills, sport skills, and activities designed to increase physical fitness.

PHYSICAL EDUCATION IN SECONDARY SCHOOLS. In general, two 35-minute periods a week are conducted by a trained physical educator. The activities of the elementary school are continued, and dance, gymnastics, tumbling, basketball, volleyball, and other team and individual sports are added. Where a pool is available, swimming instruction is included in the program. In some schools, the program is much like that found in high schools in the United States, but sports particularly enjoyed by Canadians, such as rugby, curling, and ice hockey, are parts of the program.

PHYSICAL EDUCATION IN HIGHER EDUCATION. Physical education on the college and university levels is limited. Where programs and requirements are in effect, football, hockey, basketball, swimming, tennis, and badminton are among the activities offered.

PHYSICAL EDUCATION FACILITIES. Although most elementary schools have play-rooms rather than gymnasiums, facilities in general are good and improving. There is much continuing construction of gymnasiums. Qualified staff for all school programs is a goal of professional associations in Canada.

TEACHER TRAINING. The length of the program, the specific courses offered, the degree conferred, as well as the standards that must be met for certification, vary from province to province. Common courses required of all teachers are methods, history, and philosophy of physical education, educational psychology, and student teaching. Because of particular provincial standards, a teacher certified in one province may not be eligible for certification in another.

England

The people of England are urbanized and engage mainly in the manufacture of steel and other commodities. Shipping and boatbuilding are large industries. The rural areas are dotted with small farms, but these do not produce enough of the marketable items needed.

EDUCATIONAL STRUCTURE. England has a dualistic educational structure, made up of state-supported and independent schools. Although there is a ministry of education, all state schools are autonomous. They form their own educational syllabuses and establish their own curriculums.

PHILOSOPHY OF EDUCATION. English schools attempt to accomplish such goals as helping their students become individuals capable of thinking and acting independently. An environment is provided in which the child can develop socially and individually, grow mentally and physically, learn to live a good and useful life, and learn to become a worthy citizen.

PHILOSOPHY OF PHYSICAL EDUCATION. Although there is no common syllabus for physical education, both the state and the independent schools attempt to help the child gain a joy and appreciation of bodily movement, to develop and maintain fitness, and to gain the skills, attitudes, and appreciations he needs to enjoy his leisure and work productively.

PHYSICAL EDUCATION IN ELEMENTARY SCHOOLS. Education in England is compulsory from the age of 5. At that time, the child begins an almost daily program of physical education under the guidance of his classroom teacher. Four times a week, for about 40 minutes each time, the child engages in vigorous outdoor sports and games. He runs, climbs, jumps, throws, and explores all the varieties of movement. As he progresses through elementary school, he begins to learn some of the skills of gymnastics, apparatus, and dance and the fundamentals of such dual sports as boxing and tennis, and he engages in track and field events. He is introduced to basketball, soccer, rugby, cricket, lacrosse, and hockey.

PHYSICAL EDUCATION IN SECONDARY SCHOOLS. The secondary schools have a specialist in physical education on the staff, although the classroom teacher may often supplement and help the work of the specialist. The program for boys and girls is separate and is heavily weighted with gymnastics. The skills of the elementary grades are improved on, and swimming is often added to the curriculum. Physical education is offered four periods a week. Two periods are instructional, and the other is a double period once a week where a single game or sport is played, often competitively.

PHYSICAL EDUCATION IN HIGHER EDUCATION. There is no required program in physical education except for those preparing to teach in the elementary schools. Facilities, equipment, and personnel are available if the student wishes to participate in physical activities.

PHYSICAL EDUCATION FACILITIES. The quality and quantity of facilities vary widely. Playing fields are abundant at all schools, but few elementary schools have gymnasiums. School camp facilities are often provided, and athletic clubs often make their facilities available to the schools.

TEACHER TRAINING. There are no specialists in physical education in the elementary schools. Elementary classroom teachers must take courses in physical education and handle this part of the program. Teacher training for grades above the elementary level is accomplished through programs ranging from 1 to 3 years in length. College graduates who wish to teach physical education must take a 1-year specialized course. There are seven colleges for women and two for men that offer a 3-year program in physical education exclusively. England at present is experiencing a shortage of well-qualified physical educators.

India

India is densely populated, and the population continues to grow faster than India can produce food for her people. The large cities of Calcutta, Madras, and Bombay are overpopulated. India's climate is hot and there is a long rainy season.

Many Indians are engaged in farming but cannot grow much more than what they personally need. The chemical, steel, and engineering industries employ most of the urban population.

EDUCATIONAL STRUCTURE. The state controls education through its ministry of education, with an elected education minister. The ministry is departmentalized and includes a department of physical education. Each state has its own director of physical education who serves in an administrative and supervisory capacity. Education is compulsory from the age of 6 through 14.

PHILOSOPHY OF EDUCATION. The aim of education in India is to provide an opportunity for the individual to reach his full potential, culturally, vocationally, and personally.

PHILOSOPHY OF PHYSICAL EDUCATION. Physical education in India seeks to help the individual develop physically, mentally, and socially; to learn skills that have a recreational value; and to reach his full potential as a person.

PHYSICAL EDUCATION IN ELEMENTARY SCHOOLS. In grades one through five, physical education is the responsibility of the classroom teacher. Physical education is offered each day in most schools, for a total of 2 hours each week. Calisthenics, games, and stunts make up a major part of the program.

PHYSICAL EDUCATION IN INTERMEDIATE SCHOOLS. In grades six through eight, physical education is taught by a specialist. Four classes are held each week, each class being about 30 minutes in length. Activities offered are calisthenics, rhythmics, games, gymnastics, track and field, and marching.

PHYSICAL EDUCATION IN SECONDARY SCHOOLS. This is a 3-year school, and essentially the same activities are offered as are given in the intermediate school, but in greater depth. Depending on the school, there may be from one to four physical education periods a week.

PHYSICAL EDUCATION IN HIGHER EDUCATION. Although many colleges and universities have a 2-year requirement, the lack of facilities and personnel often makes the program difficult to carry out. When the program is operable, 2 hours a week of physical education are offered. The activities included in the programs vary widely from gymnastics and team and individual sports to combative activities, and the student is largely allowed to elect his activities.

PHYSICAL EDUCATION FACILITIES. Although most schools have outdoor play areas, the lack of gymnasiums and playgrounds severely hampers the program, particularly in the lower grades.

TEACHER TRAINING. There are fifty schools that train physical education instructors exclusively. India also has more than 2,000 teachers' colleges and two universities that train physical educators. There is a 1-year program that leads to a certificate, a 2-year program that leads to a diploma, and a 3-year program that leads to a bachelor's degree.

Israel

Only about a third of the population of Israel is native born. Immigrants from Asia, Africa, and Europe make up most of the population. Hebrew is the official language of the country, but English is frequently

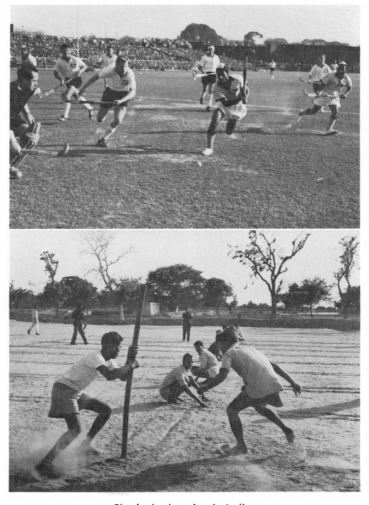

Physical education in India.

spoken. The people engage in farming, shipping, industry, and science and technology. Military training is compulsory for all men and women for 2 years beginning at the age of 19.

EDUCATIONAL STRUCTURE. Education is free and compulsory between the ages of 5 and 14. Beyond the age of 14, tuition is charged in the public schools. The Ministry of Education and Culture is responsible for all phases of primary and secondary education.

PHILOSOPHY OF EDUCATION. Education is geared toward developing a citizenry who can contribute to the advancement of the country. Toward this end, school programs are heavily weighted with courses in Hebrew culture and literature. The schools also strive to help their students develop as individuals and seek to give them practical training for vocations.

PHILOSOPHY OF PHYSICAL EDUCATION. Physical education is conducted under the guidance of an Authority for Sports and Physical Education, a state arm that is responsible for the coordination of all physical education. Physical education is devoted primarily to increasing and maintaining

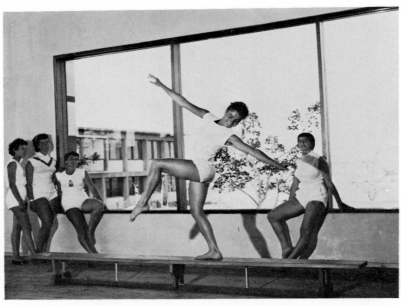

Students engaging in physical education activity at Wingate Institute for Physical Education, Israel.

physical fitness and to providing instruction in leisure-time pursuits.

PHYSICAL EDUCATION IN KINDERGARTENS. Although school need not be started by children until the age of 5, these schools are provided for students from the ages of 3 through 5. Physical education is required for a period of 2 hours each week. The program includes dances, rhythmics, games, and native activities.

PHYSICAL EDUCATION IN ELEMENTARY SCHOOLS. This school terminates with the eighth grade. Physical education is required 2 hours each week, and the program of the kindergarten is continued through grade three. Beginning with the fourth grade, the skills of such sports as soccer and basketball are added, and specialists are in charge of the program.

PHYSICAL EDUCATION IN SECONDARY SCHOOLS. In addition to the 2-hour physical education requirement, there is a 2-hour pre-military training period weekly, based on physical education activities. The programs, taught by specialists, include rhythmics, wrestling, handball, table tennis, swimming,

track, soccer, gymnastics, apparatus, volleyball, and basketball.

PHYSICAL EDUCATION IN HIGHER EDUCATION. Except in programs of teacher training, physical education is not offered or required.

PHYSICAL EDUCATION FACILITIES. Facilities are extremely poor according to American standards, both indoors and out-of-doors. In many areas, the school building itself is inadequate even for the process of general education.

TEACHER TRAINING. The Physical Education Teachers College at Wingate Institute and the related Institute of Education for Movement at present offer a 2-year professional program in physical education.

There is an acute shortage of well-trained physical education teachers, especially women, but the training program is now being enlarged and improved.

Italy

The people of Italy are striving toward a more industrialized and modern economy. The vast majority of the people are employed in industry: automobiles, business machine manufacture, steel, oil, wine production, and handicrafts. Those persons who are in agriculture are mostly grape growers, but their number is decreasing.

EDUCATIONAL STRUCTURE. A national minister of education is responsible for control of the various school curriculums and for the supervision, organization, administration, and coordination of all education. A higher council of public education serves as a central advisory committee on the national level. Each provincial government has advisory committees on education that include primary and secondary education sections as well as a director of physical education. On the local level, there are inspectors and supervisors of education, as well as school boards. These boards are staffed by teachers and are advisory rather than policy-making bodies.

PHILOSOPHY OF EDUCATION. Education in Italy is compulsory from the age of 6 through 14. The aim of education is to produce a worthy, law-abiding citizen who is prepared to labor for the good of society, his country, and himself.

PHILOSOPHY OF PHYSICAL EDUCATION. The militaristic prewar aims of physical education have given way to the objectives of helping each individual reach his potential physically, morally, and mentally.

PHYSICAL EDUCATION IN ELEMENTARY SCHOOLS. The elementary schools encompass grades one through five. Physical education is taught by the classroom teacher during four 35-minute periods each week. Activities included are those that help to increase balance and coordination, fundamentals of movement, lead-up games, and rhythmics.

PHYSICAL EDUCATION IN INTERMEDIATE SCHOOLS. In grades six through nine, physical education is taught by a specialist for two 1-hour periods each week. Rhythmics, apparatus and tumbling, calisthenics, winter sports, water sports, fencing, track and field, and soccer make up the program.

PHYSICAL EDUCATION IN HIGH SCHOOLS. Depending on choice of career, an Italian child may select a 4- or 5-year high school. Physical education follows the same content as that of the intermediate school.

PHYSICAL EDUCATION IN HIGHER EDUCATION. Physical education is not offered or required in the colleges and universities of Italy.

PHYSICAL EDUCATION FACILITIES. Italy has, in general, excellent facilities for physical education, particularly for outdoor activities. At present, many facilities are in the planning stage or are nearing completion.

TEACHER TRAINING. Only the University of Rome presently offers a teacher-training program in physical education. This is a 3-year course heavily weighted in the sciences and the development of skill proficiency. Before being licensed, a prospective teacher must meet high standards of physical fitness, pass a practical test of skill proficiency, and take a written cultural examination.

Teachers of physical education are in very short supply and do not enjoy the status or prestige of other educators.

Japan

Japan has a large population and shows one of the highest rates of population increase in the world. Many of Japan's workers are engaged in agricultural trades, but a recent and continuing employment trend is toward industry.

EDUCATIONAL STRUCTURE. The ministry of education and local school boards help to advance the progress of Japanese education. The ministry of education, however, is a liaison agency rather than a controlling one. Its functions are to give guidance to educational and research institutions, aid with procurement and disbursing of educational funds and materials, and coordinate many of the educational services. The school boards serve the same function as do those in the United States.

PHILOSOPHY OF EDUCATION. The aim of Japanese general education is to develop a well-rounded individual who will be a patriotic, responsible, and moral citizen.

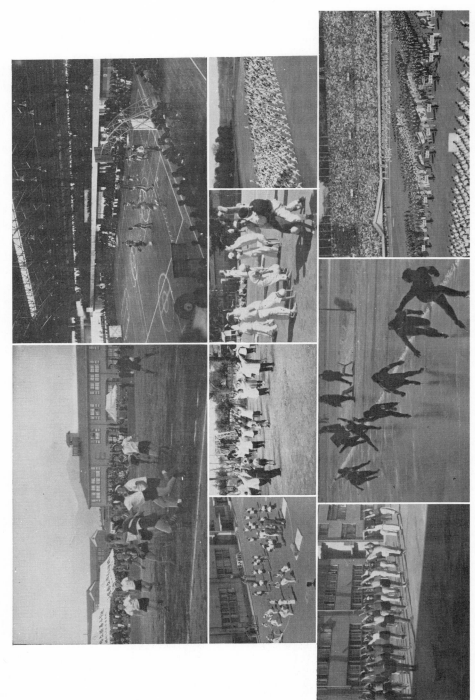

Japanese physical education programs.

COURTESY S. EBASHI, UNIVERSITY
OF TOKYO, TOKYO, JAPAN.

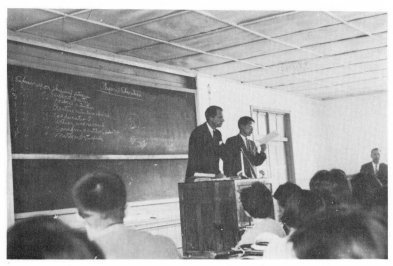

The author meets with Japanese students. Professor Ebashi, of the University of Tokyo, is the interpreter.

PHILOSOPHY OF PHYSICAL EDUCATION. Physical education is compulsory from elementary school through college. The aim is to develop sound and fit minds and bodies, to imbue a spirit of democracy in sports and life, and to develop a healthy and health-knowledgeable individual.

PHYSICAL EDUCATION IN ELEMENTARY SCHOOLS. The ministry of education publishes a course of study that is followed in the elementary schools. All of the children have three 45-minute periods of physical education each week, and in addition they may participate in intramurals. The activities covered are rhythmics, apparatus, gymnastics, calisthenics, track and field, and various ball games. The skills of swimming, skiing, and skating are often included, and physical performance tests are administered periodically.

PHYSICAL EDUCATION IN UPPER ELEMENTARY SCHOOLS. This level covers grades seven through nine. In the seventh grade, physical education classes are held three times each week. In grades eight and nine, one period of health and two of physical education are offered. The activities of the lower elementary school are continued, but the boys also receive instruction in judo, kindo, and sumo, while the girls have additional instruction in dance and rhythmical exercise. Performance tests are also given at this school level.

PHYSICAL EDUCATION IN SECONDARY SCHOOLS. The basic elementary program is continued for all students, with the addition of such team sports as basketball, softball, and volleyball. Individual and dual activities include tennis, badminton, and advanced instruction in swimming and diving.

PHYSICAL EDUCATION IN HIGHER EDUCATION. The activity program of the secondary schools is carried over to the colleges and universities. All students are required to take two university credits in activity courses and two additional credits in physical education theory courses. Electives among the latter include kinesiology, physiology, the history of physical education, and the administration of physical education.

PHYSICAL EDUCATION FACILITIES. Japan has inadequate facilities in many of its elementary schools and few parks for recreation. It lacks research facilities and adequate laboratories for major students in colleges and universities. Some public schools do have adequate gymnasiums, and many have substantial outdoor play areas.

TEACHER TRAINING. There are three private schools, fifty-four state colleges and universities, one private university, and five junior colleges that offer courses in teacher preparation. The private schools and universities prepare teachers for the secondary schools in a 4-year program. The junior colleges offer a 2-year program geared toward those students who are preparing to teach in the elementary schools.

Mexico

The climate of Mexico varies according to altitude and rainfall. The most densely populated areas of Mexico are in the cool zone, above 6,000 feet, with a mean temperature of 63° F. Most of Mexico is deficient in rainfall.

EDUCATIONAL STRUCTURE. Each of the twenty-nine states in Mexico controls and administers its own schools. Education in the territories and the federal district is administered by the federal government. Primary schooling, grades one through six, is free and compulsory. The secondary schools are designed so that a student may prepare himself to enter a teacher-training institute, vocational or commercial school, or university.

PHILOSOPHY OF EDUCATION. In a plan entitled "Education and National Development," the ministry of education has set forth educational aims that illustrate the philosophy of education in Mexico. These aims are: (1) the well-balanced development of the pupil from the intellectual, physical, and moral point of view, (2) the development of pupils' manual skills, and (3) the acquisition of an objective concept of modern life.

PHILOSOPHY OF PHYSICAL EDUCATION. Physical education in the schools of Mexico is administered by a national office in the ministry of education. This office establishes standards and policies, issues directions, and oversees personnel.

The major objectives of physical education include the development of the human body; the development of physical, intellectual, and moral qualities; and the training of the individual so that he can be most productive.

At present in Mexico there is a growing awareness of the educational value of sports. The student is allowed to select his own activities. One important aspect of girls' physical education is the inclusion of rhythmical activities, with the emphasis on folk and regional dances. Physical education classes are scheduled twice a week for 50 minutes throughout the student's school years, except at the university level.

PHYSICAL EDUCATION IN ELEMENTARY SCHOOLS. Physical education in the elementary schools of Mexico is similar to that of the United States, with emphasis on rhythmical activities, games of low organization, gymnastics, and various traditional Mexican games (rondas).

PHYSICAL EDUCATION IN SECONDARY SCHOOLS. Physical education in the secondary schools is mainly concerned with the six "basic" sports—track, basketball, soccer, swimming, volleyball, and gymnastics—with the choice of these activities left to the student.

Although there are no regular school-sponsored sports competitions as known in the United States, some schools have teams and belong to sports leagues. Competition in these leagues is intense, with great numbers of participants and spectators.

PHYSICAL EDUCATION IN HIGHER EDUCATION. Physical education at the university level is not uniformly required. Whether or not it is offered depends upon the attitude of the administration. In some universities, physical education is not required because the administration feels that it is not as important as the academic subjects.

PHYSICAL EDUCATION FACILITIES. Because of the limited space around the schools in urban areas, both physical education and recreational programs suffer. However, these limited areas will be supplemented with facilities, where available, developed by the Social Security Institute and other agencies.

TEACHER TRAINING. Upon graduating from the secudaria (grade nine), those students who wish to become physical education teachers enter one of the four schools of physical education for a period of 3 years.

The main emphasis in these schools is on skills, with less attention being given to theory and a background of general education.

Netherlands

The Netherlands has a maritime climate with cool summers and mild winters.

EDUCATIONAL STRUCTURE. Private schools outnumber public schools at all levels of instruction in the Netherlands. Freedom of choice in education is guaranteed by the constitution and private as well as public schools are subsidized by the government. The minister of education, in whom the power resides for all schools, nevertheless has delegated considerable power to the local school administrators.

School attendance is compulsory between the ages of 6 and 15.

PHILOSOPHY OF EDUCATION. Education in the Netherlands is based on the philosophy that all children should be free to have an education that is in harmony with their way of life and their religious beliefs.

PHILOSOPHY OF PHYSICAL EDUCATION. Physical education in the Netherlands is based on a "Basic Teaching Plan" that defines the role of physical education in the education of the child. This plan offers a list of various activities that should be offered at all grade levels. Some of the specific objectives of physical education as stated in the "Basic Teaching Plan" are:

1. The maintenance and improvement of health
2. The development and organic strength, muscular strength, and agility
3. The development of good posture
4. The development of creativity and self-expression
5. The development of desirable social behavior

PHYSICAL EDUCATION IN ELEMENTARY SCHOOLS. Physical education has been a required subject in Dutch elementary schools since 1890. Since available space is at a premium, however, many schools suffer from a lack of facilities and space as well as from a lack of trained personnel. Physical education is taught by the elementary classroom teacher.

PHYSICAL EDUCATION IN SECONDARY SCHOOLS. Physical education is a required subject in all secondary schools, with 3 hours a week being allotted in the lower grades and 2 hours a week in the upper grades. Unlike American high schools, Dutch secondary schools have no athletic budgets, no athletic directors, and no coaches.

The emphasis is on the educational aspects of sports. Participation by all is encouraged and is accomplished by numerous clubs and teams throughout the country. Large numbers of people participate in sports clubs and organizations after graduating from school. The largest such organization is the Royal Dutch Soccer Union with 500,000 members.

PHYSICAL EDUCATION IN HIGHER EDUCATION. Physical education is not required at the university level. The six universities stress academics, with emphasis on law, medicine, theology, humanities, and the physical and behavioral sciences. In recent years, because of the great interest shown in recreational sports, new facilities have been built for sports activities. The Dutch government is also actively supporting the building of such facilities. All schools have sports clubs and teams, but their aim is mainly recreation. There is some interschool competition among the clubs of the various schools, but there are no collegiate leagues or conferences.

PHYSICAL EDUCATION FACILITIES. Since space is at a premium in the Netherlands, there is a great shortage of adequate gymnasiums, swimming pools, and outdoor facilities. Sometimes private business and government join forces to sponsor the building of sport centers.

TEACHER TRAINING. Secondary school physical education teachers receive their training at the academies of physical education. There are five such 4-year academies at the present time. The entrance requirements at these schools are very stringent. Upon graduating from these academies, the prospective teachers are ready to take the government-regulated examinations for teacher certification. These examinations are comprehensive and require a student to demonstrate a high degree of proficiency in various skills as well as knowledge in the theoretical and scientific aspects of physical education.

New Zealand

In general, the climate of New Zealand is temperate. The Maori's, a Polynesian people, make up a very small segment of the population. Most New Zealanders are of British birth or descent. The nation is irregular and mountainous to the extent that many children cannot travel to school, and must study at home by radio or through correspondence courses.

EDUCATIONAL STRUCTURE. Education is compulsory from the age of 7 through 15. The state education department controls all education, including syllabuses, but delegates much of its authority to local educa-

tion boards. The secondary schools are run by boards of governors. Parent committees help to run the primary schools. The education department has a division of physical education.

PHILOSOPHY OF EDUCATION. Education is provided free for everyone up to the age of 19. Individualism is stressed, as is mental, social, and physical development.

PHILOSOPHY OF PHYSICAL EDUCATION. The schools of New Zealand believe strongly in physical fitness and its maintenance, in the development of lifetime sports skills, and in striving to help the individual become a thinking, mature, and responsible adult.

PHYSICAL EDUCATION IN ELEMENTARY SCHOOLS. In grades one through six, the classroom teacher, at times aided by a physical education specialist, is responsible for instruction. Three 30-minute instructional periods a week are supplemented by a single 30-minute game period each week. This latter period is highly organized. Basic movement skills, dances, games, and the

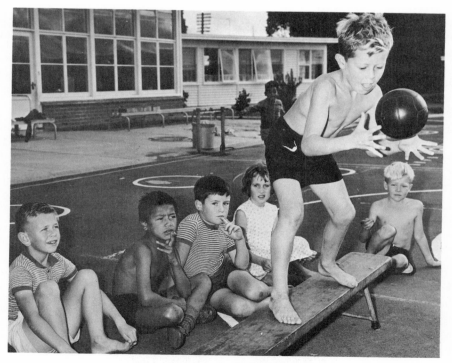

New Zealand physical education.

sport skills of volleyball, cricket, gymnastics, apparatus, and swimming are included in the program.

PHYSICAL EDUCATION IN SECONDARY SCHOOLS. A physical education specialist is available in the secondary schools, but the classroom teacher continues to give instruction in physical education. Two 40-minute instructional periods and a 30-minute game period are standard in most schools. The elementary school skills are continued, and winter and summer sports, leisure-time activities, and track and field are added to the program. Physical education is not compulsory after the tenth grade.

PHYSICAL EDUCATION IN HIGHER EDUCATION. Physical education is not offered or required in the colleges and universities of New Zealand.

PHYSICAL EDUCATION FACILITIES. The elementary schools have good outdoor facilities but have limited or no indoor facilities. However, swimming pools are available on a wide scale. The secondary schools often have an indoor gymnasium-type room available and adequate equipment for the program.

TEACHER TRAINING. The School of Physical Education of the University of Otago is the only school that trains physical educators exclusively. Nine teachers colleges and five universities also train physical educators. The courses vary in length from 2 to 3 years, depending on whether the preparation is for the elementary or secondary school level.

Philippines

The Republic of the Philippines consists of an archipelago of approximately 7,100 islands.

EDUCATIONAL STRUCTURE. The law requires all children between the ages of 7 and 10 to attend elementary school through fourth grade. Many children complete the full 6-year elementary school and then go on to the 4-year high school. Public elementary school education is free, but students pay a small tuition fee in the government-operated high schools.

PHILOSOPHY OF EDUCATION. The Filipinos strive, through their schools, to educate the whole child through physical, mental, social, and emotional development. It is believed that the individual capabilities, interests, readiness, and motives of the child should guide the teacher in teaching him in all areas of school work.

PHILOSOPHY OF PHYSICAL EDUCATION. The Philippine society stresses physical activity with the aim of developing motor fitness. There is a growing emphasis in physical education on human development, with the ultimate goal of enhancing the individual's self-concept.

PHYSICAL EDUCATION IN THE ELEMENTARY SCHOOLS. At the nursery and kindergarten levels there is no definite time allotment given to physical education. However, in grades one through four physical education, together with art and music, is allotted 40 minutes per day, and in grades five and six, 50 minutes per day. Calisthenics, simple stunts and tumbling, rhythmics, games, and dance are a part of the program.

PHYSICAL EDUCATION IN SECONDARY SCHOOLS. The Filipino secondary school is a 4-year school designed for both college- and vocation-bound students. One period of 40 minutes per day is allotted for physical education. In addition, there is Philippine military training during each semester of the third and fourth years in the college preparatory program. Those students in the vocational training program receive only one-half period per day. During the first and second years of high school, physical education is allotted a double period (80 minutes) per day. High school physical education stresses competitive athletics, big-muscle activity, and sports skill development. There is also much stress on Philippine folk dances.

PHYSICAL EDUCATION IN HIGHER EDUCATION. On the college level physical education is prescribed as a requirement for graduation. At least four semester units of physical education are required. These units comes from such courses as natural movement, gymnastics, rhythmical activities, and fundamental skills and athletics.

PHYSICAL EDUCATION FACILITIES. Since most of the Philippines' physical education is conducted outdoors, these facilities are adequate. However, indoor facilities are often poor or entirely lacking.

TEACHER TRAINING. A minimum of four semester units of physical education is required by the board of national education in the teacher education curriculums of all colleges and universities. This minimum number of credits is needed to satisfy general education requirements, and an additional eighteen units is needed to fulfill the requirements for a concentration in physical education.

Sweden

The people of Sweden populate most heavily the large cities and towns of the south. They engage in such occupations as

Philippine folk dances.

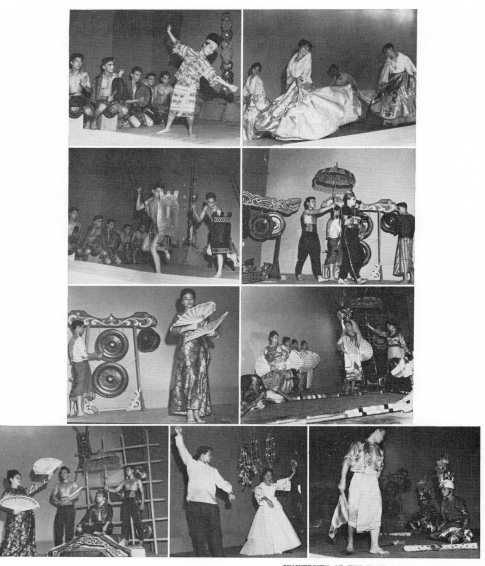

UNIVERSITY OF THE EAST, MANILA, PHILIPPINES.

steel production, shipbuilding, farming, mining, fishing, and forestry.

EDUCATIONAL STRUCTURE. The Royal Board of Education oversees and administers the schools of Sweden but delegates much of its authority to the provincial school boards. Education is compulsory through the ninth grade.

PHILOSOPHY OF EDUCATION. The aim of Swedish education is primarily to help in-

dividuals realize their full potential as independent and reliable adults who are sound in both mind and body.

PHILOSOPHY OF PHYSICAL EDUCATION. Physical education in Sweden has as its major objective the all-around development of each individual, both physiologically and psychologically.

PHYSICAL EDUCATION IN ELEMENTARY SCHOOLS. In grades one through five, boys

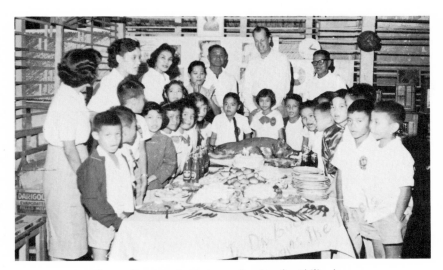

The author at a party in a school in the Philippines.

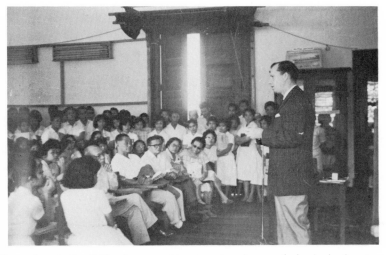

The author in the Philippines speaking to an audience of physical educators.

and girls are taught together by the classroom teacher. They have two or three physical education classes a week for a total of 1½ hours. Folk dance, rhythmics, games, and winter sports make up the program.

PHYSICAL EDUCATION IN INTERMEDIATE SCHOOLS. The intermediate school encompasses grades four through six. The physical education classes are still taught by the classroom teacher and the program is the same as that of the elementary school.

PHYSICAL EDUCATION IN SENIOR SCHOOLS. In grades seven through nine, physical education is taught by a specialist. The program includes folk dance, gymnastics, games, track and field, swimming, winter sports, and orienteering. The classes are held three times a week for a total of about an hour and are conducted out-of-doors whenever possible.

PHYSICAL EDUCATION IN SECONDARY SCHOOLS. The secondary school is a 3-year school designed for the college- or university-bound student. Physical education is conducted from 1 to 4 hours a week, depending on the individual school. The program parallels that of the senior school.

PHYSICAL EDUCATION IN HIGHER EDUCATION. Physical education is not required in the colleges and universities of Sweden, but ample facilities and equipment are available for those who wish to participate in activity.

PHYSICAL EDUCATION FACILITIES. All Swedish schools have a gymnasium, a playroom, and an outdoor play area. There are also many parks, swimming pools, and private and public athletic clubs with ample facilities.

TEACHER TRAINING. The Royal Central Gymnastic Institute and twenty teacher-training schools offer 2-year teacher preparation courses. Besides a broad range of activities including gymnastics, dance, and mountaineering, prospective teachers also must take such science courses as anatomy and physiology, first aid, history of physical education, courses in methods and materials, and student teaching.

Thailand

Thailand has a tropical climate, and for much of the country there are three distinct seasons: the hot season from March through May, the rainy or wet season June through October, and the cool season November through March.

EDUCATIONAL STRUCTURE. Education is compulsory for children 7 to 15. The schools of Thailand are controlled by the ministry of education. In February, 1955, the ministry of education enlarged the educational program and established a teacher-training department. A department of physical education was also formed.

The Toledo schools teach Philippine dances.

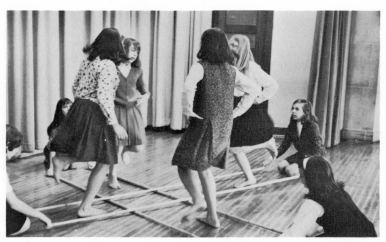

TOLEDO PUBLIC SCHOOLS, TOLEDO, OHIO.

PHILOSOPHY OF EDUCATION. The primary aim of education in Thailand is to lower the illiteracy level of its people and to teach the cultural heritage of Thailand.

PHILOSOPHY OF PHYSICAL EDUCATION. The Thais feel that physical education has a strong contribution to make to the total welfare of each student. As a result, there are many fine physical education programs throughout the kingdom. Some of the objectives of physical education programs in Thailand are:

1. To develop each student's physical and mental health

2. To foster cooperation and mutual respect among students
3. To inculcate habits of good citizenship, good health, and accident prevention
4. To instruct students in the proper use of leisure time

PHYSICAL EDUCATION IN ELEMENTARY SCHOOLS. Physical education in elementary grades (primary education level) is very similar to the programs in the United States. For the lower grades, activities include simple games (games of low organization), rhythmical activities, stunts and tumbling, and story plays.

In the middle elementary grades com-

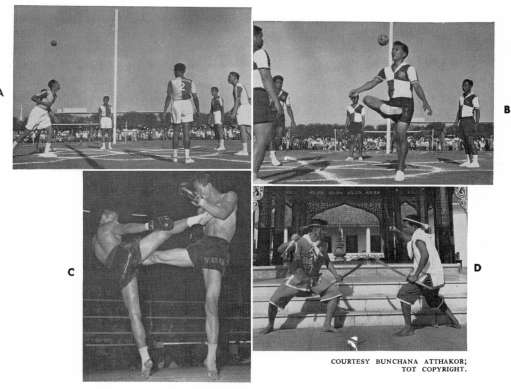

COURTESY BUNCHANA ATTHAKOR;
TOT COPYRIGHT.

Sports in Thailand. **A** and **B,** Takraw is played with a ball of woven wicker. The object is to keep the ball in motion, hitting it with any part of the body—instep, heel, knee, shoulder, or forearm. It sounds simple, but actually the game calls for skill and stamina. **C,** Thai-style boxing. Thai boxing is completely different from boxing in other parts of the world. A player opens the bout, followed by a preliminary display of each boxer's skill and style; all this and the fight are accompanied by the music of two drums and a pipe. Although the bouts appear to be rough-and-tumble affairs, really they are exhibitions of scientific skill and split-second timing. **D,** Traditional Thai-style sabering. Each sword-fighter uses two Thai-style sabers, holding one in each hand. It is now an art as well as a sport, whereas in the old days it was also one of the actual combat weapons in warfare.

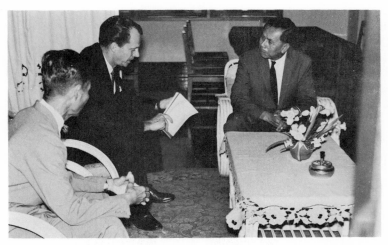

The author in Bangkok with the head of physical education in Thailand.

petitive activities are introduced in the form of lead-up games, running, and relay races. In the upper primary grades (students 10 to 14 years) team and individual sports as well as folk and national dancing comprise the physical education program.

PHYSICAL EDUCATION IN SECONDARY SCHOOLS. The activities offered in secondary schools are similar to the ones offered at the junior high school level in the United States. The aim is to raise the pupils' skill level to the point where they can participate reasonably well in various sports.

Level II (preuniversity, ages 18 to 20) has no required physical education program. The physical education requirements depend on the administration of each school. In general, if a sport or physical education is offered, it is conducted after classes are over. Thus the sport programs in Thai secondary schools are very much like the intramural sports programs in the United States.

PHYSICAL EDUCATION IN HIGHER EDUCATION. At this level physical education is not required. The emphasis here is on recreation.

PHYSICAL EDUCATION FACILITIES. Physical education facilities by American standards are poor. Outdoor facilities are somewhat more numerous, but the real need lies in indoor facilities and equipment, of which there is a great shortage.

TEACHER TRAINING. Thailand has a 2-year college of physical education where no degrees are awarded but a teacher's certificate and a diploma are bestowed upon its graduates. A 4-year degree program in physical education has recently been initiated at Chulalongkorn University, where graduates of the college of physical education may work toward a Bachelor of Education degree.

Union of South Africa

South Africa is a multiracial country that operates on the principle of apartheid, or the separation of races. There are two official languages, English and Afrikaans.

EDUCATIONAL STRUCTURE. The Union Department of Education supervises, coordinates, and administers special and technical high schools and universities for white residents. In each province, a department of education administers its own public schools and teacher-training colleges. Each of these major departments also has a division of physical education. The Department of Bantu Education administers the schools for the nonwhite population.

PHILOSOPHY OF EDUCATION. The schools of South Africa seek to develop a sound and responsible citizenry, whether black or white.

PHILOSOPHY OF PHYSICAL EDUCATION.

Physical education is compulsory throughout the public school system. It seeks to develop individuals who are mentally and physically fit, have good health habits and knowledge, have good social behavior, and have developed an interest in recreational pursuits.

PHYSICAL EDUCATION IN ELEMENTARY SCHOOLS. A trained physical educator, often aided by the classroom teacher, gives each child a half-hour period of physical education three times a week. Movement skills, rhythmical activities, folk dancing, games, calisthenics, and apparatus are all part of the program.

PHYSICAL EDUCATION IN SECONDARY SCHOOLS. In the secondary schools, physical education classes are conducted once or twice a week for 30 minutes each time. These classes are taught by a physical education teacher and include the activities of the elementary school plus track and field, gymnastics, volleyball, and swimming, if a pool is available.

PHYSICAL EDUCATION IN HIGHER EDUCATION. Physical education is not required or offered in the colleges and universities of South Africa.

PHYSICAL EDUCATION FACILITIES. Facilities are generally poor according to American standards. Gymnasiums are lacking, although construction is continuously going on. The schools do have outdoor fields and, in some cases, all-weather outdoor facilities.

TEACHER TRAINING. Five universities and fourteen teachers colleges offer preparation in physical education. In general, the universities require 3 years of general university work plus a year of specialization in physical education to teach on the secondary level. A 2-year general education course, plus a year of specialization in physical education, satisfies the elementary level teaching requirement. The teachers colleges offer 2-year courses.

Union of Soviet Socialist Republics

Much of the population of Russia is urban. The Russian people come from more than 200 ethnic groups that speak at least 150 languages. The Russian-speaking people make up half the population. This diversity of culture and language affects the schools: over the country as a whole, forty languages are used in the instructional programs, with the Russian language itself a common elective subject.

EDUCATIONAL STRUCTURE. The process and progress of education in Russia are directly controlled by the state through its ministry of higher education and the ministry of culture, a subordinate body. Within each of the fifteen Soviet republics, there is also a ministry of education that is responsible to the state.

Physical education in Russia is also under state control. Subordinate to the Presidium of the Central Committee is the Republic Sports Committee and, under it, the fifteen regional sports committees. Most aspects of physical education, from teacher placement to sports clubs, to curriculum and the publishing of journals, are controlled, organized, and scrutinized by the Central Committee.

PHILOSOPHY OF EDUCATION. The purpose of Soviet education is to prepare the student, both physically and mentally, to serve the state. The goals of the state take precedence over any personal goals the student may have. The student is expected to become a selfless, willing, and highly productive worker; to consider the needs of society above his own personal needs; and to devote his life to the improvement of society.

PHILOSOPHY OF PHYSICAL EDUCATION. The purpose of physical education in the Soviet Union is to build a nation of superbly physically fit individuals. The Soviets regard physical fitness as the key to the survival and progress of their nation. Physical education is compulsory for all students until the completion of their second year in a university, vocational, or technical school. Great emphasis is placed on physical activity as a recreational pursuit for all citizens, and there are many mass activities provided for everyone, regardless of age. The spectator is not regarded as a productive citizen.

PHYSICAL EDUCATION IN PRESCHOOLS.

The ministries of health and education provide and supervise preschool institutions. A child may be accepted into one of these schools beginning at 2 months of age. For those old enough to participate, the physical education program is essentially one of basic movement. Children are taught and encouraged to run, climb, jump, throw, and play games of low organization.

PHYSICAL EDUCATION IN ELEMENTARY SCHOOLS. At the age of 7, Soviet children begin their years of compulsory schooling. In the first and second grades, the emphasis in physical education is on rhythmical activities, gymnastics, and active games. At the third-grade level, skiing and track and field are added to the program. Through the fourth grade, the child is taught by his classroom teacher. Throughout his elementary school years, the child receives 45 minutes of physical education instruction at least twice a week, along with supplementary activity periods at the discretion of the teacher.

PHYSICAL EDUCATION IN SECONDARY SCHOOLS. Secondary education includes grades five through eleven, and physical education is taught by a specialist. Although the major emphasis is still on gymnastics, such activities as basketball, soccer, volleyball, and water sports are also stressed. The skills of skiing and track and field continue as part of the program. Unless the weather interferes, the program is an outdoor one, and coeducational. The classroom teacher continues to provide periods of vigorous activity over and above the biweekly 45-minute instructional periods. It is at this level that the lifelong concept of intense competition is introduced.

PHYSICAL EDUCATION IN HIGHER EDUCATION. Physical education is required in the first 2 years of university-level education. Students are given a variety of activities to choose from, but all must learn to swim and all are required to pass physical fitness tests.

PHYSICAL EDUCATION FACILITIES. The facilities provided for physical education are excellent. There are parks set aside specifically for recreational and cultural pursuits.

There are many camps, sports clubs, and youth groups, all with their own facilities. Beyond this, there are special sports schools devoted to giving intensive instruction to children. Between the ages of 12 and 18, a child with a high degree of facility in a sport is recommended for acceptance at one of these schools. Here, outside of school hours, he receives concentrated coaching twice a week for 2 hours each time. This system has helped to develop many of the Russian champion athletes.

TEACHER TRAINING. The Soviet Union prepares its physical educators to be either teachers or coaches. The coaches concentrate on one particular sport and work in the sports clubs. The teachers who go into the schools are trained intensively in gymnastics. They also concentrate, although less than the coaches, on a particular game or sport.

Graduates of 11-year secondary schools may enter one of the sixteen training institutions for physical educators or go to one of the fifty colleges or universities, or one of the more than twenty other specialized schools of physical education. Prospective teachers and coaches must be highly proficient in the skills of physical education and have taken specific background courses in sciences and Russian studies. If accepted, they enter a 4-year program that, in the academic areas, closely parallels the programs in the United States.

West Germany

The population of the German Federal Republic, which is almost entirely urban, includes many refugees from East Germany. These people are mainly white-collar workers or skilled artisans. The small segment of rural dwellers is engaged in the raising of stock, while the urban workers are employed in the iron, coal, steel, auto, and optical industries.

EDUCATIONAL STRUCTURE. Each of the ten states of West Germany has its own ministry of education, which is directed by a minister of education. The ministries are responsible for the administration of the

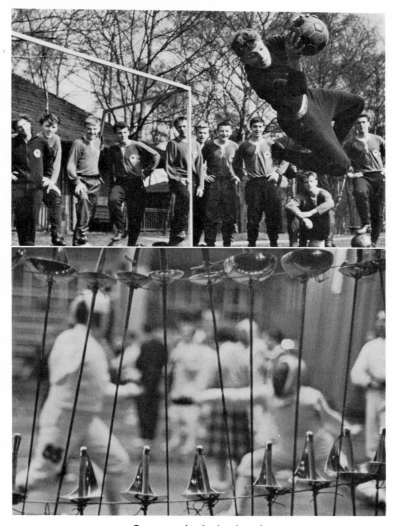

German physical education.

public schools in each state and for introducing new legislation pertaining to the schools.

PHILOSOPHY OF EDUCATION. Following the division of Germany after World War II, the German schools were reorganized to eliminate the militaristic aspects. West Germany, the United States, England, and France cooperated to achieve the reorganization. Thus, in philosophy, the schools of West Germany became much like those of the Allied countries. At the present time, general education is compulsory from the age of 6 through 14. The aim of general education is to produce a well-rounded, moral, and responsible individual. German schools are structured to suit individual needs. Thus, those students who complete the 4-year elementary school may go on to the terminal intermediate school or to a secondary school. The intermediate school is designed for those who will enter an occupation or go on to technical training following the completion of grade ten. The secondary school is designed for the college- or university-bound student and terminates with grade thirteen, the equivalent of the first year of college.

PHILOSOPHY OF PHYSICAL EDUCATION. The aim of the program is to contribute to the total development of the individual through activity and participation. Sought-after goals are the development of physical fitness, a love of movement, creativity, and a sense of fair play.

PHYSICAL EDUCATION IN ELEMENTARY SCHOOLS. During the first 4 years of schooling, classes in physical education are held two or three times a week for a total of 1 hour. Activities included are basic movement skills, such as running, jumping, throwing, and climbing; gymnastics; tumbling and apparatus; games of low organization; and swimming.

PHYSICAL EDUCATION IN INTERMEDIATE SCHOOLS. This school includes grades five through ten. Physical education is offered two or three times a week for a total of about 1 hour. The program of the elementary school is continued in the intermediate school with the addition of track and field, soccer, volleyball, and basketball.

PHYSICAL EDUCATION IN SECONDARY SCHOOLS. This school division encompasses grades five through thirteen. Physical education is taught three times a week for a total of 1 hour. The program is essentially the same as that of the intermediate school, but in some schools rowing, skiing, ice skating, and hiking are added to the curriculum.

PHYSICAL EDUCATION IN HIGHER EDUCATION. West German universities have departments of physical education, and some training is compulsory for all students. However, the program is limited at the university level both by equipment and facilities and the lack of sufficient status of these departments in the educational structure.

PHYSICAL EDUCATION FACILITIES. West Germany has a severe shortage of facilities and well-qualified teachers of physical education.

TEACHER TRAINING. West Germany has two schools solely devoted to training teachers of physical education. These schools have a 3-year course that students may enter after spending 1 year in another teacher-training institution. These schools also train teachers for all three levels of public instruction. Germany has three teacher-training colleges and twenty-six universities that offer degree courses in physical education. Students electing a 3-year course teach on the elementary level. To teach on the intermediate or secondary level, a 4-year course is mandatory.

QUESTIONS AND EXERCISES

1. Do a comparative study of physical education in one country in each of five continents.
2. What role does education play in the lives of other countries in the world?
3. Trace the history of ten sports, showing the country that was responsible for its origin.
4. Do a research paper on the Peace Corps and how physical education is helping to promote international good will through this organization.
5. What are three outstanding international organizations in health, physical education, and recreation? What are the objectives of each?
6. Write an essay of approximately 500 words on the history of the Olympic games.
7. Prepare a plan for students majoring in physical education to follow in promoting good international relations within their college.
8. Invite a foreign person to your class to discuss the role of sports and physical education in his country.

SELECTED REFERENCES*

American Council on Education: Universities of the world outside the U.S.A., 1875 Massachusetts Avenue, N.W., Washington, D. C. 20036.

Institute of International Education: Handbook on international study, 1 East 67th Street, New York, New York.

International Council of Health, Physical Education and Recreation (assorted publications), 1201 16th Street, N.W., Washington, D. C. 20036.

Johnson, William, editor: Physical education around the world, Monographs Nos. 1, 2, and 3, Indianapolis, 1966, 1968-1969, Phi Epsilon Kappa Fraternity.

Publications of the World Confederation of Organizations of the Teaching Profession: *Panorama: teaching throughout the world* and *Echo*.

---

*Information on the various international organizations and countries discussed in this chapter was taken from these publications.

(Also assorted publications, 1201 16th Street N.W., Washington, D. C. 20036.)

VanDalen, Deobold, and Bennett, Bruce: A world history of physical education, Englewood Cliffs, New Jersey, 1971, Prentice-Hall, Inc.

*International organizations**

International Amateur Athletic Federation Yearbook, 1969-1970, International Amateur Athletic Federation, 162-164 Upper Richmond Road, London S.W. 15, England.

International Association of Physical Education for Girls and Women Constitution (revised), January, 1969.

International Bureau of Education Leaflet, February, 1970.

International Federation of Physical Education Leaflet, 1969.

International Federation of Physical Education: Statutes.

International Recreation Association Brochure, 1970.

People-to-People Sports Committee Brochure, 1970.

World Confederation of Organizations of the Teaching Profession Brochure, 1969-70.

*Information on the various international organizations and countries discussed in this chapter was taken from these publications.

Yearbook of International Organizations, ed. 12, Union of International Associations, Brussels, Belgium, 1968-1969.

Other countries

Barron, Louis, editor: Worldmark encyclopedia of nations: Americas, New York, 1967, Harper and Row, Publishers.

Barron, Louis, editor: Worldmark encyclopedia of nations: Australasia, New York, 1967, Harper and Row, Publishers.

Barron, Louis, editor: Worldmark encyclopedia of nations: Europe, New York, 1967, Harper and Row, Publishers.

Datoc, Salud C.: Physical education in the Philippine schools, Asian Journal, International Council of Health, Physical Education, and Recreation, June, 1969.

Education in Brazil, brochures.

International Council of Health, Physical Education, and Recreation Q'Aire Report no. 1: Physical education and games in the curriculum, Washington, D. C., The Council.

International Yearbook of Education, International Bureau of Education, vol. XXIX, 1967.

World Book Encyclopedia: Philippines, vol. XV, Chicago, 1970, Field Enterprises Education Corp.

PART FIVE

Scientific foundations of physical education

15/Biological makeup of man
16/Biological fitness
17/Psychological interpretations of physical education
18/Sociological interpretations of physical education

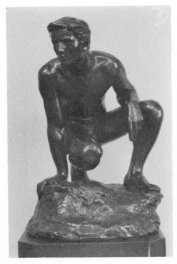

WORK OF R. TAIT MCKENZIE.
COURTESY JOSEPH BROWN, SCHOOL OF
ARCHITECTURE, PRINCETON UNIVERSITY.

15/Biological makeup of man

To A Physiology Professor*

Wise is the one

> who can dissect
> with uncommitted facts
> pounding heart longings
> sucking lung desires

> who can analyze
> with principled laws
> muscle-sculptured action
> gravity-bound patterns

> who can understand
> with humbled reason
> thinking eye thoughts
> feeling brain sight

> who can communicate
> with child-like rapture
> passion-filled flesh pittings
> undaunted human aspiration

He combines seeing with the seen.

BETTY WILLIS BROOKS

Better to hunt in fields, for health
Unbought, than fee the doctor for a
Nauseous draught. The wise, for cure,
On exercise depend; God never made
His work for man to mend.

JOHN DRYDEN

Today, physical education is based on scientific facts and principles. As such, its program is developed as a result of systematized knowledge based on verifiable general laws. This knowledge covers many areas of learning. The physical education program is established with respect to the biological, psychological, and sociological

*Quest (Monograph III), December, 1964.

aspects of growth and development. It aims to develop youth into citizens who have the capacity to enjoy a happy, vigorous, and interesting life. To accomplish this task, it is necessary to know the individual, how his physical body functions, how he learns, why he acts as he does, and his relation to the group, society, and world of which he is a part. Furthermore, the human being represents a unified whole, each part being necessary to the successful functioning of every other part. The individual reacts as a "whole" organism and not just in parts. Therefore education should be concerned with whether or not activities benefit the "whole" individual and not just one part. When a child swims, there should be concern not only for the physical development that ensues from this experience but for the social, mental, and emotional aspects as well.

In Chapters 15 through 18 an attempt is made to point out some of the scientific knowledge that has a bearing on physical education and the "whole" individual from the standpoint of biology, psychology, and sociology. Such knowledge will help to clarify the role of physical education in our society.

MAN'S BIOLOGICAL HISTORY

This chapter will be devoted to the fundamental scientific interpretations of physical education that are biological in nature.

Man's potential—and his performance

Dr. Joseph W. Still spent many years studying human physical and intellectual behavior. The illustration shown below depicts his research into the physical growth and ages and the psychic growth and ages of man.

A study of these charts will show that not more than 5% of the population follow the upper success curves (dotted line). The failure curve in regard to physical growth shows the physical development of people today to be lacking. They are exposed to very little physical exercise; they eat, drink, and smoke too much; and they decline rapidly after 30 years of age. It will also be noted that four sections are identified where peak performance in various sports occurs. The psychological growth chart also shows an emphasis on the failure type of performance. Mental traits excel at different stages of development. Memorizing ability is great in youth, creative imagination reaches its height in the twenties and thirties, skill in analysis and synthesis of subject matter reigns in the middle years, and the age of philosophy characterizes the later years. Dr. Still raises the question: "How can we prevent these failures?" He goes on to point out: "As a starter, everyone should say: If I want respect as a human being I have the

The physical and psychic growths and ages of man—possibility and performance. The upper lines indicate the physical and psychological potentials of normal people, with peak periods for various activities. The lower lines indicate how most people fail to measure up.

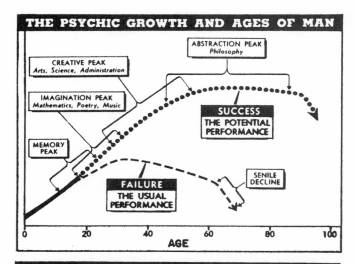

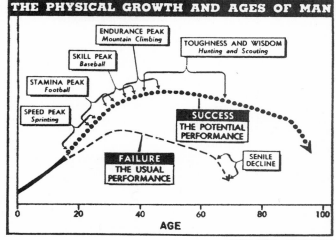

FROM STILL, JOSEPH W.:
THE NEW YORK TIMES MAGAZINE,
NOV. 24, 1957.

obligation to respect and care for and develop my body and mind."* I am sure we would all agree that this is a good philosophy for successful living.

Biologically, man is designed to be an active creature. Although changes in civilization have resulted in his decreasing the amount of activity needed in accomplishing the basic tasks associated with living, man's body has not changed. Therefore man must become well informed as to the health requirements that his biological base demands and recognize the importance of vigorous physical activity in his life. If he does not, his health, productivity, and effectiveness in life will suffer. Being physically educated is essential to proper functioning in life. Furthermore, it is closely tied in with man's mental powers, as well as with his emotional, social, and spiritual powers.

If man is to survive as a productive creature living a vigorous and interesting life, there must be a recognition of the biological requirements placed upon him. Physical education is essential to the life he lives. Physical activities can contribute much to his effectiveness. Skills, health knowledge, and protective services are necessities.

Evolution

A study of the evolution of man points to the necessity for physical activity. Evolution refers to the development of a race or of a species, during which period of development a series of changes take place and morphological and physiological characteristics are acquired that distinguish a particular species or group.

The evolution of man shows that he has made great progress in developing himself from a lower form of life. If a person studies the history of mankind, it will be discovered that man has gradually evolved. Evidence shows that there have been many eras of growth. During the first era there existed only one-celled plants and animals. Next came the era of the invertebrates,

when forms of life such as sponges and starfish existed without a spinal column. Then followed the age of fishes, amphibians, reptiles, dinosaurs, mammals, birds, *Homo sapiens,* and, finally, historic man. Thus man has evolved.

Physical education must help to develop a higher and better plane of living as its part in this "evolving" process if it is to justify its worth. A study of evolution shows that man should not follow a sedentary existence but, instead, should be active, should exercise the various parts of his body, and should spend more time in the out-of-doors. Therefore physical education has many potentialities. To train youth successfully nature's methods should be followed. This holds true also in regard to the activities in which man engages. Primitive man obtained his food, provided shelter, and protected himself against a hostile environment through activities that involved walking, running, hopping, climbing, throwing, carrying, leaping, and hanging. These are consistent with the evolutionary process. These activities have formed the basic movements for man throughout his long history. They are a part of his inheritance. The games, dances, and other physical education activities that are utilized today have as a basis these racially old activities. For example, basketball is running and throwing, and dancing is walking, leaping, stretching, and hopping. Man, in his attempt to evolve into a higher and higher plane of living, should follow a physical education program based on these fundamental activities rather than one that does not conform to such standards. These activities will best serve the purposes of developing a body with a strong framework and adequate motor mechanism. They will aid in enabling man to move with freedom, with rhythm and grace, and with less utilization of energy.

Biological defects of man in light of his structure

Biologically, the "evolving" process in man has resulted in many advantages and also many disadvantages. Today man has

---

*Still, Joseph W.: New York Times Magazine, November 24, 1957.

a high standard of living. He has automobiles, trains, and jet planes to take him wherever he wants to go, television and radio sets to see and hear world events, highly mechanized machinery to manufacture goods for every need and desire, beautiful houses and buildings in which to live and congregate, and other conveniences and luxuries to please and entertain him. However, there is another side to the picture. Are all of these devices, inventions, and luxuries that are characteristic of his mode of life helping him biologically? Hickman, an expert on physiology, points out some interesting facts in respect to the highly specialized and artificial life that man leads. These are summarized in the following paragraphs.

In this "evolving" process man has changed his means of locomotion from a quadruped to a biped position. This has had implications for his health. It is believed man originally walked on all fours.* An upright position has influenced adversely man's digestive and circulatory systems. It has compressed his large intestine with resulting conditions of constipation and colitis. This position has caused an irregular distribution of blood as a result of the heart's being below several parts of the body. It is a contributing cause of fainting. Hemorrhoids and varicose veins are caused to some degree by the increased blood pressure in lower regions of the body. An upright posture has increased the difficulty of balance, and consequently many postural problems have developed. In a report to the National Academy of Sciences, S. W. Briton, University of Virginia scientist, pointed out that the upright position was the result of the development of a superior brain in man, but that at the same time such a position resulted in fallen arches, varicose veins, and possibly sinus and heart trouble.

*According to the April 3, 1950, issue of Life Magazine, there is now evidence to show that primitive prehumans stood erect. Raymond Dart, famed anthropologist from South Africa, discovered the pelvis of an early ape man that indicated an erect posture.

He also reported that such a position resulted in major adjustments on the part of the circulatory and nervous systems.

The problem that arises as a result of man being placed in a biped position can be alleviated through physical education activities that stress standing, walking, jumping, leaping, and other fundamental movements. It is important to compensate for this position by developing in each child a strong trunk musculature to house the vital organs and nerve centers. It is important to strengthen the abdominal muscles so that the viscera is in proper position. Furthermore, the elements of body mechanics must be recognized so there is proper body balance as man carries himself on his legs.

Man has a very complex nervous system that has difficulty adapting to present-day living. Evidence of this is the high rate of insanity and mental disorders that prevail. As the demands for a college degree increase and as the pressures of college life grow, it is apparent that more and more students are turning to psychiatrists for help. University psychiatrists have reported an increase in students utilizing their services. The type of competition wherein man is continually striving to get ahead of his fellow men has resulted in several nervous maladjustments that have their effect on the entire human mechanism. Diseases such as angina pectoris may be to a great degree the result of conditions that involve worry and sorrow. Seven hundred thousand people die each year of heart disease, which many individuals feel is at least partially related to the nervous tension involved in modern-day living.

As a result of the fast pace man follows, he is placing more and more reliance on drugs and narcotics as a means of enjoyment, stimulation, and escape. Tobacco, coffee, tea, alcohol, LSD, and marijuana are good examples. Many other drugs and narcotics are used as sedatives and to eliminate pain. The result of all this indulgence and self-medication has meant mental and physical deterioration to many users. It has also resulted in more suicides on our nation's campuses. Instead of aiding and helping to cure man's maladjustments, they have frequently tended to aggravate the situation.

Tobacco, drugs, colds, and respiratory diseases are blunting man's sense of taste and smell to the point where they are now greatly inferior to those of other animals. Close work, writing, and the like have been detrimental to man's eyesight. The noise from jet planes, the screeching of subway trains, and the blare of automobile horns have helped to deaden man's hearing. Man is losing some of the senses that have been of great assistance over the years in interpreting his environment.

It has been stated that individuals in the United States are the best fed of those anywhere in the world but at the same time are the most undernourished. This is very true for a broad segment of the population. Today it is common practice to prepare foods that tickle the palate. Steaks, chops, and other choice cuts of meat taste good but are lower in nutritional content than many of the lower-priced cuts, such as liver and kidneys. Many people also eat an over-abundance of rich sweets and pastries, to the neglect of selecting their diet from the four basic groups of food. Such practices have led to dental caries and possibly to disorders of the stomach, such as ulcers, tumors, and cancer. Furthermore, a great amount of the food lacks bulk, and consequently the alimentary tract does not function satisfactorily.

Man has evolved into a hairless animal, which necessitates the wearing of clothing and provision for shelter. These artificial devices for protection against the elements have resulted in irregular body surface temperatures, with greater susceptibility to cold. Furthermore, clothing prevents the body from absorbing the healthy rays of the sun. This is conducive to rickets, tuberculosis, and other maladies.

Originally the purpose of the sex drive was to procreate the race. When not used for this purpose the sex drive was latent in man and did not cause many of the social problems that exist today. Society has evolved to a point where the sex instinct has to be curbed through will power or other outlets found for it. In weaker members of the population, outlets are sought in the form of perversion and other means considered anti-social. This has resulted in crime, mental disorders, and venereal disease. Unhappiness, pain, and shame have been visited upon many families as the result of promiscuity in sex relations.

Man spends more and more of his time indoors. His work, recreation, and living are mainly confined to offices, buildings, houses, and modes of transportation that are overheated, lack fresh air, and are not conducive to good health. In following the line of least resistance, man finds it much easier to settle back in a chair where it is warm and comfortable than to face the elements where he might have to exercise a bit to get the blood circulating. As man grows older, he is no longer motivated to be as active as he once was. He spends a great deal of time watching others perform. Modern man has fallen prey to the disease known as "spectatoritis."

Along with less outdoor life, man is congregating in cities where hundreds of people live in one block and breathe germs into each others' faces. Man's early existence was in the wide open spaces where he developed a strong and sturdy body and a nervous system that was adapted to his needs. The changeover to an urban, indoor existence has been so rapid in his history that adaptation is far from being realized at the present time.

The maxim "survival of the fittest" has become a thing of the past. Present-day humanitarian values decree that the unfit should be protected and allowed to endure, as well as the fit. Therefore the unfit, as well as the fit, are allowed to procreate the race. This results in many undesirable strains being continued from generation to generation. The humanitarian outlook on such a practice is understandable. However, in viewing this condition from a purely biological viewpoint, it can be seen that the race is thereby weakened, not only from the standpoint of resistance to disease but also in regard to perpetuating many factors that will make disease more imminent.

A perusal of the facts just mentioned would tend to encourage one to believe that man is living a decrepit, weak, and unhealthy existence and is degenerating to the point where he may become extinct. The facts do set one's mind to thinking in this direction. Whether or not man can adapt himself to a highly industrialized, urban, inactive existence remains to be seen. At the present time, the facts in regard to

his mental and physical deterioration sound a warning. The great advances made by the medical profession in combating infectious diseases have been outstanding. These diseases are rapidly being brought under control. But what about such maladies as nervous disorders, heart disease, and cancer? What are the solutions to these scourges of mankind? Is man attempting to change too rapidly from an existence characterized by out-of-door living, simple diet, active pursuits, and quiet living to one characterized by an indoor existence, choice food, fast living, and inaction? Is man's nervous system adequate to meet such a rapid change? The answers lie in the future.

Major causes of death in the United States.

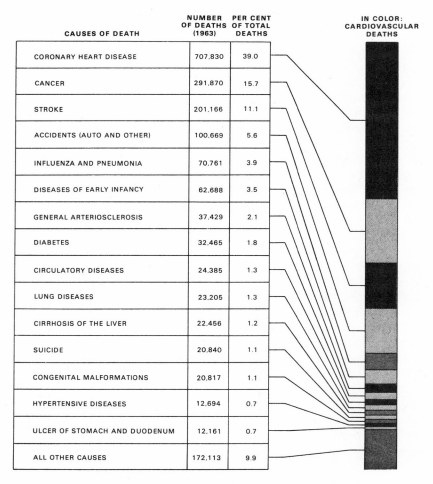

CAUSES OF DEATH	NUMBER OF DEATHS (1963)	PER CENT OF TOTAL DEATHS
CORONARY HEART DISEASE	707,830	39.0
CANCER	291,870	15.7
STROKE	201,166	11.1
ACCIDENTS (AUTO AND OTHER)	100,669	5.6
INFLUENZA AND PNEUMONIA	70,761	3.9
DISEASES OF EARLY INFANCY	62,688	3.5
GENERAL ARTERIOSCLEROSIS	37,429	2.1
DIABETES	32,465	1.8
CIRCULATORY DISEASES	24,385	1.3
LUNG DISEASES	23,205	1.3
CIRRHOSIS OF THE LIVER	22,456	1.2
SUICIDE	20,840	1.1
CONGENITAL MALFORMATIONS	20,817	1.1
HYPERTENSIVE DISEASES	12,694	0.7
ULCER OF STOMACH AND DUODENUM	12,161	0.7
ALL OTHER CAUSES	172,113	9.9

FROM TIME-LIFE BOOKS SPECIAL REPORT: THE HEALTHY LIFE, NEW YORK, 1966, TIME, INC.

HEALTH OF THE NATION

The United States ranks very high in regard to the health of its people when compared with the other nations of the world. However, in analyzing the health statistics of this country, it can readily be seen that disease and ill health are prevalent in great numbers in the population and that much of this disease and ill health are preventable. Although we have the best facilities and personnel in the world for combating disease, there is still room for improvement. One of the important government agencies working toward improved health conditions is the U. S. Public Health Service.

Some health statistics that show where improvements can be made in the health of the nation are as follows:

1. One out of ten college students will have emotional conflicts of sufficient severity to warrant professional help.
2. The number of suicides is going up, and three times as many suicide attempts are made by females as by males. The most common age for both sexes is 19 years.
3. There are approximately 10 million overweight teen-age boys and girls in the United States, and from 15% to 20% of all adolescents are overweight to the point where it is a medical problem.
4. An estimated 1 billion unfilled dental cavities exist in men, women, and children throughout the United States.
5. Venereal disease rates are going up with more than 600,000 cases a year among young people ages 15 to 24.
6. More than $8 billion is spent each year on tobacco.
7. Nearly 200 million Americans breathe polluted air, detrimental to their health.
8. An estimated one out of four hospital beds throughout the world is occupied by a person suffering from disease caused by polluted water.
9. The American public is defrauded of over $100 million a year through the mails, much of which is concerned with health matters.
10. Estimated costs of sick-leave payments in industry exceed $2 billion annually.
11. Of the draftees not qualified for military service, about one-half are turned down for medical reasons.
12. Six out of every ten Americans use laxatives frequently.
13. There are more than 5 million men and women alcoholics in the United States.
14. A majority of drug addicts are between 18 and 20 years of age.
15. At least 5,000 lives could be saved annually if occupants were not thrown from vehicles in accidents. If used, seat belts would cut down on these fatalities.
16. Each year over 325,000 people die whose deaths should have been prevented.
17. Nearly 5 million man-years of work are lost each year as a result of bad health.
18. From 30% to 60% of all patients seeking doctors' advice today have emotional disorders.
19. Approximately 250,000 to 400,000 children under 18 years of age appear in courts each year.

In respect to young people, health statistics show that, as a result of better nutrition, boys and girls in the United States are taller and heavier than their parents. At the turn of the century fewer than four out of 100 men attained a height of 6 feet or more. Today more than twenty-five out of 100 are this tall. Women are also increasing in height, with many now reaching 5 feet, 7 inches. College statistics of young people tell a similar story. In 1885 the average Yale freshman was 5 feet, 7½ inches tall and weighed 136 pounds. Only about 5% of the class stood more than 6 feet tall. Today the average freshman is more than 3 inches taller and 20 pounds heavier, and better than 30% of the class is over 6 feet tall. Young women at Vassar and Smith colleges are about 2 inches taller and 10 pounds heavier than were comparable girls at the turn of the century. Girls are also maturing earlier, as indicated by the onset of menstruation, which has dropped from the age of 14 in 1900 to 12.8 years of age today. However, an estimated 10% to 15% of American teen-agers are too fat and have poor eating habits. Many of them are physically inactive. The statistics indicate, however, that the stamina and skill of teen-agers in the United States is improving.

Young people enjoy an unprecedented freedom from infectious diseases because of antibiotics. They learn more at an earlier age than did their parents because of new educational techniques.

Although the draft statistics have shown that overall rejection rates from the armed services have climbed from 22.7% in World War II to 23.6% during the Korean War to an estimated 44% in 1965, military statisticians note that part of this increase is because mental testing has been more discriminating. On the positive side it has been noted by the Army Surgeon General's Office that the recruit of today is 1.2 inches taller and 18 pounds heavier than the recruit of World War I, and ½ inch taller and 7 pounds heavier than the recruit of World War II.

In spite of some encouraging signs modern-day man continues to be a victim of many preventable defects and diseases. Industrial life, with its concentration of people in urban areas, air pollution, sedentary pursuits, routine work, unemployment, and other evils, may be listed as contributing factors. Despite the fact that the United States has the highest standard of living in the world, many of its citizens are still living a second-class existence. In the ghetto areas of our nation's cities, poverty and disease are widespread. A child who is born of poor parents has a much greater risk of dying earlier in life than the child of a wealthy family. Research has indicated that the poor suffer from more chronic conditions than other citizens. The diseases that take the lives of most ghetto residents are tuberculosis, pneumonia, and influenza. In many of our poverty-stricken areas venereal disease and drug abuse are also widespread. The tension associated with modern-day living and the fear, hate, and worry that contribute to many mental disorders are other factors. Man was not intended to live an existence characterized by fear of atom and hydrogen bombs; hate for people of other races, creeds, and nationalities; and worry over his security. There is a need for a greater number of doctors, nurses, and psychiatrists and for more facilities to aid in the prevention and cure of disease. Furthermore, there should be more measures established to cross the chasm between medical services and low incomes.

Physical education cannot prevent or treat many of the defects and diseases found in human beings today. However, it can contribute to a healthy populace in many ways. It can provide a source of pleasure and a substitute for worry, hate, and fear among many persons suffering with mental disorders. Our modern industrial age has contributed markedly to weak physiques and to insufficient strength. Physical education can help in developing strength, stamina, endurance, and a state of physical fitness in the individuals who are lacking in these important characteristics. It can also help by

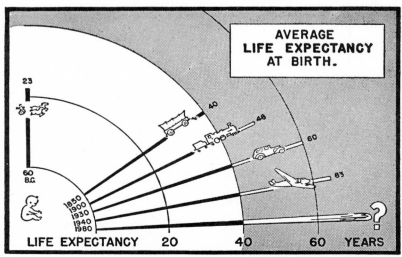

FROM ADULT HYGIENE AND GERIATRICS,
INDIANA STATE BOARD OF HEALTH.

providing a means of relaxation after long hours of work. Physical education can develop in the children of today the skills, interests, and attitudes that will ensure them many enjoyable moments during their leisure time. Physical education can also help in developing the "whole" individual so that a healthier, more stable, and more peaceful world can be built.

MAN'S ORGANIC FOUNDATIONS
Biological basis of life

The cell of the human body is the biological basis of life. The human body starts from one cell and, as a result of many divisions and redivisions, many thousands of cells are formed. Many of the cells are formed into units that function as the organic systems of the body. Every part of the body has cells—the brain, liver, stomach, and arms and legs included. One estimate has been made that there are 400 billion cells in the body and approximately 5 million cells in a small drop of blood.

The cells of the body are alive. They take in food and oxygen and give off waste material. In order to keep alive, the organism must have food and oxygen and must eliminate wastes. The cells perform this function. They are bathed in a liquid called lymph that carries food and oxygen to the cells and takes away wastes.

The muscles of the body are made up of cells. In the evolutionary process these muscle cells developed from rather simple to complex structures. The muscular system developed before many of the other systems of the body. As the muscle cells became more specialized, other units of cells were needed to carry food and oxygen to the various parts of the body and to carry away wastes. Thus began the excretory, digestive, respiratory, and circulatory systems. These systems developed in response to a need that was stimulated and initiated by the muscular system. They develop in a human body and grow strong in response to the work placed upon them by the muscular system. Therefore, muscular work increases capacity of the individual for performance.

Makeup of the human body

The human body is a very intricate mechanism, the makeup of which should be familiar to every physical educator. As the Old Testament states about the human body: "I am fearfully and wonderfully made." The student of physical education will study the human body in detail during his training. The following discussion will be concerned with only a brief review of some of the aspects of the human mechanism that have special implications for the bio-logical interpretations of physical education.

THE SKELETON. The skeleton of the human body can in many ways be compared to the framework of a building under construction. The framework represents the foundation or outline on which the building will be constructed. It represents the size, shape, and contour of the building. The skeleton also performs this function for the human body. It is a framework that protects the various bodily systems.

The bones that make up the skeleton in older persons have less animal matter than do the bones of children. Therefore an elderly individual's bones are brittle, break easily, and heal slowly. In children small amounts of mineral matter make bones more flexible, and consequently they can be bent in various shapes. This has implications for a child's posture. The child's skeleton is very flexible; therefore, such practices as habitual standing and sitting in a stooped position for long periods of time may result in abnormal posture.

The skeleton is made up of joints that make movement possible. There are three main kinds of joints: the *synarthroses,* or immovable joints; the *amphidiarthroses,* or slightly movable joints; and the *diarthroses,* or freely movable joints. Diarthrotic joints are the ones with which physical educators should be most concerned. Basically there are two kinds of diarthrotic joints with which the physical educator should be especially concerned: the ball and socket and the hinge. Examples of the ball and socket are the shoulder and hip, and examples of the hinge joint are the elbow, knee, or fingers. The joints of the body are essential to movement. Some of the more important movements that the physical educator should be aware of are the following: *flexion* (movement that reduces the angle between the bones, as in bending fingers to close the hand), *extension* (movement that increases the angle between bones, as in straightening the fingers to open the hand), *abduction* (movement away from the midline of the body, as in moving the arm straight out to the side), and *adduction* (movement toward the midline of the body, as in returning the arm back to the side of the body).

Physical educators should be well informed as to the action of the joints in various activities, the care and training needed to develop and strengthen these areas and the common disorders of the skeletal system. One disorder is *rickets*. Rickets is a disease of the bone resulting from a deficiency of vitamin D and of sunlight. A physical educator must become familiar with some of the common signs of this disease if he is to recognize it in his students. Children with rickets are usually irritable, weak, and restless and appear to have deformities such as knock-knees and bowlegs. Physical educators can play an important part in recognizing such deformities and can thus inform the individual's family of their findings, which will hopefully lead to the necessary medical treatment.

MUSCULATURE. The musculature of the human body is an essential to movement; consequently, the physical educator should be familiar with its composition and action. In studying anatomy and kinesiology he will discover in detail the various muscles and how they function in body movement. He will discover how important muscles are to the human body; how they provide for locomotion, give form to the body, produce body heat, and make breathing, circulation, and other vital movements possible.

There are three types of muscles in the human body: *skeletal* muscle, *smooth* muscle, and *cardiac* muscle. Skeletal muscles are voluntary and under the control of our conscious will. They are attached to the bones and make it possible to move about during our daily activities. It is skeletal muscles with which the physical educator should be most concerned.

Two principles with which every physical educator should be familiar are *muscle tonus* and *reciprocal innervation*. *Muscle tonus* means the constant, partial contraction of the muscles of the body. It has to do with the elasticity of muscle. This is essential to good posture and to the efficient functioning of some of the organic systems. This slight contraction on the part of muscles makes it possible for them to react to stimuli within the space of a very short time. Such a phenomenon makes muscle contraction possible with a minimum expenditure of energy. A state of muscle tonus is essential to good body health.

Reciprocal innervation refers to the part that antagonistic muscles play in performing coordinated movements. This principle works on the theory that whenever a group of muscles contracts to perform a movement, the antagonistic muscles relax, so that a coordinated, smooth, rhythmical movement results. A good example of this principle is the movement of flexing the arm. The biceps contracts and the antagonistic muscle, or triceps, relaxes, resulting in free and easy action. When a person is a novice in a game, he quite often performs in an awkward and uncoordinated manner because his antagonistic muscles do not relax and allow for free and easy movement. The proper coordinations between the muscle groups have not been established.

CIRCULATORY SYSTEM. The circulatory system of the body carries food and oxygen to and brings wastes from the multitude of cells that make up the organism. These elements are transported by means of blood through a system of tubes called blood vessels. The blood is kept flowing as a result of heart action.

There are two sets of blood vessels—the *arteries* that carry the blood from the heart and *veins* that carry the blood to the heart. Arteries divide into smaller and smaller branches called capillaries, which connect with the cells. The capillaries unite with veins and then the veins, with various small tributaries, unite into larger veins going to the heart.

The heart has four chambers, the two upper chambers being the auricles and the two lower chambers the ventricles. The veins send blood to the auricles, the walls of the auricles contract, and the blood then goes to the ventricles. The ventricles contract, sending blood to the various parts of the body. After forcing the blood into the arteries, the heart relaxes for a moment and rests. Then the process is repeated. There are two valves between the auricles and the ventricles and two at the mouths of the arteries. The valves prevent the blood from flowing backward.

The blood follows a definite route through the heart. The right side of the heart sends blood to the lungs, where the blood picks up oxygen and then goes back to the left side of the heart. On the left side of the heart, the blood is forced into the arteries and to the entire body. After nourishing the cells and picking up the wastes, it goes back to the right side of the heart. The entire process consumes less than 1 minute.

The composition of the blood is interesting to examine. The liquid part is known as plasma. Within the plasma float millions of little red and white corpuscles. The red corpuscles carry oxygen from the lungs to the various cells throughout the body, and the white corpuscles kill disease germs that enter the body. About nine-tenths of the blood is plasma; the rest is dissolved food and other materials such as wastes. The capillary walls are very thin, and as the blood goes through them, the plasma escapes and becomes lymph surrounding the cells. Oxygen breaks loose from the red corpuscles and passes into the lymph and to the cells. Waste materials pass through the lymph into the blood. The lymph acts as a middleman between the cells and the blood as it passes oxygen and food to the cells and wastes to the blood. In addition to the blood capillaries, there are also lymphatic capillaries that take the impure lymph from among the cells and carry it to the blood.

The machine that is the center of the circulating system is the heart. Its action results in nourishment being sent to the millions of cells throughout the body. It beats continuously day and night. It is essential to life. Nothing should be done to harm this delicate piece of machinery. The body should be protected against disease germs that might impair its use. Exercise should be adapted to an individual's needs so as not to place too much of a strain on the heart. This is especially true of adults who have passed middle life. However, it should be remembered that the heart is a muscle, and like all muscles, it becomes stronger with use. This has implications for the physical educator in providing activities for children of school age. If a child's heart is normal and healthy, it cannot be injured through exercise. There is considerable evidence to support this tenet. This should not preclude, however, that physical educators should determine through an examination of health records and consultations with physicians whether a child has a rheumatic fever history or some other cardiac disturbance that might make strenuous exercise questionable. Furthermore, the physical educator should be cognizant of the fact that even though the normal heart tissue of children cannot be damaged by exercise, very strenuous exercise can do damage to other parts of the body besides the heart. For example, overfatigue has implications for a child's emotional health.

RESPIRATORY SYSTEM. The respiratory system consists of air tubes leading into billions of microscopic permeable air sacs in the lungs. It has two main functions—taking oxygen into the body and giving off carbon dioxide.

In respect to oxygen, the body leads a hand-to-mouth existence. Oxygen cannot be stored; it must be taken in as needed. The body takes in oxygen every minute of the day and night. If the organism stops breathing, it will die within the space of a very short time. Carbon dioxide is given off through the respiratory system. It is formed in the cells and carried by the blood to the lungs and then escapes into the air.

The chest cavity, where the lungs and also the heart are located, is protected by the sternum or breast bone and the ribs. In breathing, the ribs lift upward and outward, and the diaphragm is pulled downward. The air passes to the lungs through the trachea, which is kept open by rings of cartilage. The trachea divides, with a branch going to each lung. Within the lungs these branches divide again and again and end in little air sacs. The branches of the trachea are called bronchial tubes. The walls of the air sacs are very thin, and the blood flows in them through capillaries. Oxygen passes into the blood through the walls of the air sacs. Carbon dioxide passes into the sacs and out of the lungs. The air in the lungs gives off oxygen and takes on carbon dioxide.

One important point should be clear to the physical educator in interpreting the respiratory system for his work. So-called "breathing exercises" are not beneficial to the human mechanism. They should be discounted because it is a physiological fact that oxygen cannot be stored up for future use but is taken in as needed. The respiratory system supplies enough oxygen in normal activity for body needs. The amount of oxygen used by the cells is determined by the needs of the tissues and not by the oxygen that is available. Except for corrective therapy, breathing exercises have no value for the human body.

NERVOUS SYSTEM. The nervous system is the "boss" of the human body. It issues the orders and controls and regulates everything the organism does. It controls the organs and other parts of the body; acts as an organ of the mind; regulates body heat, secretion of digestive juices, and excretion of wastes; and controls every movement that is made. The nervous system is composed mainly of the brain, spinal cord,

nerves that go out from the brain and spinal cord to various parts of the body, and ganglia or masses of gray tissue found in inner organs of the body.

The fundamental unit of the nervous system, the nerve cell or neuron, is found in all the various parts of the nervous system and especially in the brain and spinal cord. It is of gray color. It is through the neuron that messages are carried between the receptors or cells that receive the impulses to the effectors or cells that react to the impulses, such as found in a muscle or gland. The nerve fibers that connect nerve cells with various parts of the body are white in color (gray in the center) and form the machinery that carries the messages or impulses. The gray core of the fiber is a branch of a nerve cell.

Three kinds of neurons are found in the nervous system: (1) the *sensory* neuron, (2) the *motor* neuron, and (3) the *intermediate* neuron.

The sensory or afferent neuron carries impulses into the central nervous system. These impulses may be carried from the skin, eye, ear, and various other parts of the body to the brain. These impulses are responsible for feeling, seeing, hearing, and understanding the condition of the body at all times. The motor or efferent neuron sends messages from the spinal cord to the muscles and results in muscular action. The intermediate neuron lies entirely within the central nervous system itself and has no contact with the outside.

The brain, a vital part of the nervous system, is located within the cranial cavity and weighs approximately 50 ounces. It has three principal divisions. The first division is the *cerebrum* or major part of the brain. The gray outer layer of the cerebrum or the *cortex* is the seat of intelligence. It thinks and feels, decides what individuals will do, and governs the whole body. The second section, the *cerebellum,* is located under the back lobes of the cerebrum. It assists in controlling muscles of locomotion, balance, and equilibrium. The third division, the *medulla oblongata,* is the enlarged upper end of the spinal cord and is composed in large part of fibers that connect various parts of the body and brain, some of which are sensory and some motor fibers. The medulla also has centers that control the heart and lungs. When the medulla is injured, death results. The heart stops beating and breathing stops.

The nervous system controls the body to a great degree unconsciously or involuntarily. This is called *reflex action.* An example of this can be seen after striking an individual just below the kneecap. Involuntarily the leg will move upward. Practically all control of the internal organs is carried on by reflexes. These are natural reflexes, and the organism is born with them.

Another set of reflexes, different from the natural ones, consists of those that can be developed through practice. A swimmer does not think of how he is going to swim, how he is going to move his arms or his legs in the crawl stroke. Instead, it becomes automatic with him as a result of practice. An important part of education is concerned with developing the right kind of reflexes. In physical education such social reflexes as fair play, respect for the individual, courtesy, and the like are important. As a result of practice, these attributes become a reality without thought to one's actions. In a sense these habits can be viewed as reflexes formed by repetition of acts. Physical educators should remember that this type of reaction is most readily formed in youth and that many situations exist in the playground, gymnasium, and swimming pool where they can be most readily practiced.

The nervous system needs good care if it is to serve the individual. Adequate sleep is an essential for a well-ordered nervous system. Continual loss of sleep will make one irritable, cross, and upset. Fresh air and exercise are an antidote for people who find themselves getting a "case of nerves." Finally, a peaceful mind free from worry, fear, and hate is conducive to an existence free from emotional strife and an upset nervous system.

DIGESTIVE SYSTEM. The digestive system is responsible for preparing foods for absorption so that they may be transported to cells throughout the body. The absorption of food is important because foods supply the energy that the body needs while it builds and repairs tissue and controls the various metabolic processes essential to a healthy life. The organs of the *alimentary canal* are the prime components of the digestive system. They include the *mouth, tongue, teeth, pharynx, esophagus, stomach, small intestine,* and *large intestine.* There are accessory glands that also play an important part in digestion, namely, the *liver* and *pancreas.*

In the digestive process, the first step takes place in the mouth, where *mastication* reduces the food to small particles and mixes it with saliva. *Deglutition* follows mastication. There is now a formation of a *bolus* of food and a subsequent propelling of the bolus from the mouth through the pharynx and the esophagus to the stomach. In the stomach the food is churned, mixed with gastric juices, and converted to a substance known as *chyme.* In the small intestine, bile from the liver and pancreatic juices combine with the chyme. Foods are then broken down into amino acids, simple sugar, and fatty acids, which are used by the cells for energy. The waste materials that are not absorbed by the cells for energy are carried into the large intestine to be excreted.

Basically speaking, the digestive system has little, if any, function during actual exercising. However, it is important to follow a proper diet in order to have the necessary energy that most activities require. Irregular meals can interfere with the orderly propulsion of food through the digestive system, and too many sweets can result in an overweight condition that can lead to obesity. These deficiencies can interfere with the normal functioning of the digestive system and can limit the amount of energy needed for normal functioning. Physical educators should educate their students regarding foods that are the best energy producers. Physical education teachers, including coaches, should also provide their students with information about weight control. Proper exercise programs together with knowledge of proper nutrition can help students achieve a higher level of fitness.

EXCRETORY SYSTEM. Wastes produced by the cells and picked up by the bloodstream must be eliminated from the body. This is accomplished by four widely separated organs. The *lungs* eliminate the carbon dioxide as previously explained. Water, salts, and small amounts of other wastes are eliminated by the *perspiration glands* in the skin. The *kidneys* extract water, salts, and urea, which is the waste produced from the use of certain foods by the cells. The *liver* helps in the process of removing wastes from the bloodstream.

The large intestine is often classified as an organ of excretion, although it has little to do with getting rid of the wastes produced by the body cells. The large intestine eliminates undigested food.

ENDOCRINE SYSTEM. There are two general classes of glands in the body that manufacture substances or secretions to be used by the body. The glands with ducts or passageways pour their secretions into another organ like the salivary glands and the liver. There is a second type of gland called an *endocrine* or *ductless gland,* which produces substances that are absorbed directly into the bloodstream and carried throughout the entire body. These substances contain important chemicals known as hormones, which have far-reaching effects on body growth, development, and function.

Examples of endocrine glands are the *thyroid,* which produces a hormone that regulates the rate of metabolism or the chemical changes that take place in cells to produce energy; the *pituitary,* the so-called "master gland" that manufactures several hormones of great importance in physical growth and development; and the *gonads,* which are responsible for the bodily changes in boys and girls at adolescence.

The work of the endocrine glands is so interrelated that it is hard to assign a specific function to a specific gland. The hormones work together to stimulate and regulate many body characteristics such as size, shape, and appearance and many body functions such as metabolic rate.

INTEGUMENTARY SYSTEM. The skin and membranes of the body are grouped together to form the integumentary system. Their major task is protection of underlying tissues.

The skin covers the surface of the body and provides a tough layer of protection from bacteria, dirt, mechanical injury, and temperature. It also contains glands that produce oil, to keep the skin pliable, and perspiration, which is of importance in regulating body temperature.

The internal organs of the body are lined with membranes that also serve as protection to underlying tissues. Many of these membranes secrete lubricating substances, such as mucus, which among other things keeps tissues moist.

REPRODUCTIVE SYSTEM. The continuation of the race is accomplished through the reproductive systems of men and women. The sex organs of male and female unite to produce gametes that form the zygote and eventually a new human being. The reproductive glands are known as *gonads.* In the male they are called testes and produce sperm. In the female they are called ovaries and produce eggs, or ova. In addition to the ovaries the reproductive system of the female includes the uterus and a passageway from the uterus to the outside of the body. In the male there are tubes leading from the testes to the outside of the body.

The impact of heredity

The difference in growth rates as well as the differences in the physical makeup of human beings is the result of heredity. Heredity is the process by which certain physical and mental characteristics are transmitted from parents to their children. Not all personal characteristics are inherited. Other factors, such as education and environment, influence one's characteristics. Heredity does give a person the color of his eyes, the color and texture of his hair, the size and shape of his facial features, the color of his skin, and his basic body build.

Some physical defects may be inherited from parents. These include such things as color blindness, deafness, and extra fingers and toes. Scientists are still uncertain about the role heredity plays in intelligence, but reliable evidence suggests that both high and low levels of intelligence run in families.

A person is the result of a complex biological process in which each of his parents contributed certain characteristics to his makeup, as they in turn, and all others in their family back through time, were produced by the same random selection of characteristics from their parents. Each person as he produces children will similarly pass on certain characteristics, but neither he nor his parents nor their parents before them had any control over the characteristics transmitted to the next generation. So it is that the body build, hair color, skin color, and so on that make up a person are individual in nature. Unless he is an identical twin, he will find that the other members of his family may differ markedly from him in size and appearance.

CHROMOSOMES AND GENES. As you already know, your existence as a human being is the result of the union of a male germ cell (sperm) with a female germ cell (ovum) to form a single cell or fertilized egg. Over approximately a 9-month period, the fertilized egg divides and subdivides and grows in size until a human being is formed.

Within each of the male and female germ cells are tiny structures called *chromosomes*. There are forty-six such chromosomes in the nucleus of each human cell. Each of these chromosomes, in turn, carries thousands of additional structures called *genes,* which determine the characteristics that are inherited by human beings.

Genes are arranged in rows of fine fibers within the chromosome, looking much like a string of beads when examined under a microscope. (Genes, by the way, are so small—some scientists believe them to be the size of viruses—that until the development of the electron microscope in recent years, study of them was very difficult.) Genes exist in pairs within the cells of each human being. During the union of the male germ cell with the female germ cell, each germ cell contributes one of the pair of genes to the other, thus forming one new pair of genes. The separation occurs by chance. That is, if your father has brown eyes, he may carry a pair of genes for brown eyes or he may have a pair of mixed genes, one-half of the pair producing brown eyes (which, for him, are dominant) and one-half of the pair capable of producing blue eyes. Your mother, on the other hand, may have blue eyes, in which case she carries only blue-eyed genes. Now in the union of germ cells that produced you, if the male cell carried your father's gene for brown eyes to your mother's gene for blue eyes, you will have brown eyes. But you will be a mixed brown, having a pair of genes, one of which produces brown eyes, the other of which produces blue. Thus, when you produce children, you might produce a blue-eyed baby.

If, on the other hand, your father were mixed brown and passed the blue-eyed gene to your mother, you would be blue-eyed, meaning that the pair of genes you possess for eye color carry only blue-eyedness. If you, in turn, married a blue-eyed person, your children would probably have blue eyes. If you married a person with brown eyes, you might have either blue-eyed or brown-eyed children.

The chance nature of genetic selection is best seen perhaps in the determination of sex. Each human being possesses what is called the *sex chromosome*. The female produces X chromosomes (two in number) but the male produces both an X chromosome and a Y chromosome. The male germ cell, then, carries either an X or a Y chromosome, but not both, when it unites with the female germ cell. If the male X is carried to the female (X), a female child (XX) results. If the male germ cell carries a Y chromosome to the female, a male child (XY) is formed. Since thousands of male germ cells are present each time the sex act is performed, but only one female egg (and then only at certain times), the random or chance nature of fertilization and heredity is obvious, for only one of the germ cells from the male can unite with the germ cell of the female. Remember, too, that each germ cell (whether male or female) carries one-half of a pair of characteristics that unite to form one complete pair of characteristics in the new cell.

Physical and motor growth and development

Physical educators should be familiar with the various physical characteristics, in addition to those already presented, that are present in human beings from infancy to adulthood. A thorough knowledge of these factors will enable a physical educator to plan a program of activity that will meet the needs and interests of each individual with whom he works. Such a knowledge would include the following:

1. Various ages by which individuals are classified
2. Various aspects of physical and motor growth during infancy, preschool years, the elementary school period, and adolescence
3. Physiological differences between males and females
4. General rules that should be followed in respect to physical and motor growth and development

AGES OF DEVELOPMENT. Individuals are classified in various ways according to age. The most common are estimations of chronological, anatomical, physiological, and mental age. These may all be helpful to the teacher of physical education.

Chronological age represents the age of an individual in calendar years and months. *Anatomical* age is usually related to the ossification of bones. Quite frequently the small bones in the wrist are used for this purpose. An x-ray examination is needed to determine anatomical age. Sometimes the

stage of dentition is also used to determine this type of age. *Physiological* age is related to puberty. It may be determined in some cases by the quality and texture of the pubic hair in boys and by menstruation in girls. The last classification is *mental* age, which is arrived at by determining, through tests, the degree to which an individual has adjusted to his environment and is able to solve certain problems.

Although the physical educator will be interested in all the age classifications of the individuals with whom he works, he should have special interest in the physiological age. It seems that this, more than any other age classification, is a determining factor in arranging a program of activities adapted to the needs and interests of any one person.

PHYSICAL AND MOTOR GROWTH AT VARIOUS LEVELS. The characteristics of physical and motor growth in the child during infancy, the preschool years, elementary school, and adolescence are very interesting for the physical educator. From a study of these characteristics, one can see that the child, a dynamic individual, craves activity. The type of program provided should depend to a great degree upon child growth and development characteristics, such as the maturation level of the child.

Infancy. During prenatal life the fetus grows very rapidly. For example, there is an increase in height to an average of 20½ inches. After birth, growth continues to be rapid for a period of 2 years and then begins to slow down. At birth and for about 18 months thereafter, the head is big in proportion to the rest of the body.

Development occurs from the head downward or in the *cephalocaudal* direction. The fact that the arms develop faster than the legs is an indication of this. During prenatal life the arm buds develop before the leg buds. Development also is from the axes of the body to the extremities or in the *proximodistal* direction. For example, the ability to use the hand develops in the palm of the hand before the fingers. This may be seen by watching a baby manipulate a block. He pushes it around with the palm of his hand for some time before he is able to pick it up with his fingers.

In discussing the cephalocaudal and proximodistal directions of development, it seems wise to bring out information as to whether educational programs for young children should be concerned mainly with big-muscle activity or with the fine-muscle activity that is associated with the use of the fingers, eyes, and the like. Many educators claim that the child's main concern during the growing years should be big-muscle activity. This is based on the premise that fine-muscle coordinations develop after the large-muscle coordinations in the child. Many times such fine-muscle skills as reading, writing, and the like are utilized in the educational process too early in life and thus prevent the child from engaging in activities that more rightfully belong on the earlier levels. Jersild, on the other hand, points out that there is some basis for this argument but that it is not entirely true. He points out that a child can pick up objects with his thumb and forefinger and perform many manual manipulations, thus utilizing the fine muscles, before he is able to walk and run, activities that utilize the large muscles. According to Jersild the choice of play materials should not be based only on whether they involve large-muscle or small-muscle activity but should provide for both types of activity. On the basis of physiological facts it would seem that big-muscle activity plays an important part in normal growth and development and that during the growing years the child should have ample opportunity for such activity in order to become a well-developed, healthy human being.

Other implications for physical educators include a knowledge of the infant's skeleton. The skeleton is largely made up of cartilage and fibrous tissues, and as a result the bones are soft. Proper care must be given to avoid deformities and postural difficulties. The spine of a child is very flexible, and for proper development it should receive proper physical activity. This will minimize the possibility of increased lumbar curve.

Preschool years. During the preschool years the child develops many physical skills. He develops skills in running, climbing, and skipping. These not only aid in his physical development but also provide a basis for social relationship. He associates with other children and finds out how they react to their environment. During this period the child gains great pleasure from his physical activity. This affects his emotional life. As he gains ability in certain physical acts, he gains self-confidence. He has better use of his arms and legs and utilizes more and more skills. This motor development makes possible more avenues of learning as he begins to explore his environment.

Certain maturation levels should be recognized in children. If allowed to develop independently to a certain point, a child will do things as a part of the natural course of growth. Jersild lists several examples of this. He explains how 2-year-old children were prompted to button their own clothes. However, at the end of several

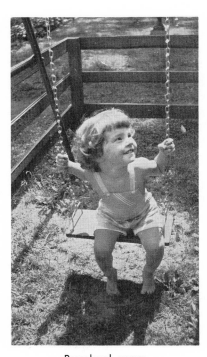

Preschool years.

weeks of practice they did not do any better than another group of children of the same age who had not practiced. He shows how this also applies in the learning of such skills as skipping and tricycling. The motor skills that are provided for children should definitely be related to their readiness to utilize and perform them. Jersild points out that we need more research into the skills that children should have at various ages. More should be known about skills that are of value in themselves, as distinguished from skills that develop a child socially and intellectually, and skills useful for a limited period of time, as contrasted with skills that are developed for future use.

Motor learning has been recognized as an essential for all children and important to the social and emotional life of a child. It helps him to become independent. It plays a part in his intellectual development. Through motor skills the child acquires concepts as to size and weight and finds out about such things as gravity and balance. Emotionally they help him to solve problems that would otherwise enrage and stump him. Newell Kephart, former head of the Achievement Center at Purdue University, has conducted much research that supports the relation of motor skills to the mental as well as physical development of the child.

Elementary school years. During his elementary school years the child acquires fundamental skills that affect his present existence and that he will use throughout life. According to a study of men 20 years old and older, it was found that many of their hobbies and adult leisure-time interests were based on their childhood experiences. The physical educator should recognize this as having implication for his work. If adults are to have physical skill in various activities, their foundation should be laid during the early years of life.

During the elementary school years the child develops socially. He makes contacts through motor activities. He is accepted by the group if he can participate with some degree of skill. He gains independence by learning to do things by himself. He increases his knowledge in respect to his environment. In all this development, motor skills play an important part. Through them he develops his "whole" organism.

Physical educators need to know what skills children possess at certain age levels, those skills possessed by most children and those possessed by just a few, the importance of skills in the lives of children, and the environmental factors contributing to or thwarting skill development. These are essential facts if physical education is to contribute further in the development of the child.

Adolescence. During adolescent years the body reaches maximum powers in the use of its musculature. This also applies to its capacity to learn motor skills.

During the elementary years boys are superior to girls in many activities, such as running, jumping, and throwing. This is even more pronounced in adolescent years. This can be explained by the fact that boys have more opportunities than girls to participate in these activities and also because of certain anatomical differences. A girl has a wider pelvis, and the angle of attachment of the femur to the thigh is different in girls than in boys. Boys are also stronger than girls. Girls are generally larger than boys from about 10 to 14 years of age, but after the age of 14 or 15, boys become larger and much stronger. Despite the fact that girls are larger than boys from the ages of 10 to 14, they do not have the same degree of skill proficiency that boys have. After the age of 14 or 15 boys and girls should probably not participate together in the more strenuous types of physical activity because of the fact that boys are achieving their greatest development in growth and strength while girls are not.

In the middle and later adolescent years activity decreases in most individuals. In a large part, this decrease results from interest in an occupation, decrease in the number of different activities in which one can engage, and social and other interests that appear to be stronger. Available evidence shows that there are more excuses from physical education classes in high school than elementary and junior high school. This falling off of activity continues into adult life and produces one of the problems with which physical educators should be concerned. The public should be better informed as to the value of adapted activity throughout life.

Postadolescent years. At this age physiological maturity has been reached. Boys are still developing muscularly. Improved motor coordination becomes evident in those youths who are active in many different types of physical activity. These are years when endurance increases, emotional balance is better, there is an interest in physical attractiveness, and recreational activities become popular. It is a time when people have an increased interest in their body conformation and sometimes use various techniques such as exercises and diet pills in an attempt to change their body size. It is also a time when strong convictions and ideals are being developed, prejudices and antagonisms become intensified, there is a desire for deeper friendships, and much thought is given to the future. There is a need during these postadolescent years for periodic health examinations, for information about proper weight control, for opportunities to participate in coeducational and recreational activities, for experiences in helping others in the development of skills and playing of games, for practice in planning for many social activities, for opportunities to gain increased skill and competence in activity areas of their choice, and for practice in critical thinking and problem solving.

DIFFERENCES IN BOYS AND GIRLS. The physical educator should be cognizant of certain differences in the physical makeup of boys and girls. The pelvic girdle of the female is much broader than that of the male and does not completely develop until in the twenties. This means that activities that would result in any pull on this region should be guarded against. Boys are stronger than girls, especially in the shoulder

girdle region. The thigh bones of girls join the pelvis at a more oblique angle than that of boys. The center of gravity is lower in girls. In respect to body weight the muscular strength of girls is lower than in boys.

In respect to strength, research has indicated that the female is less responsive to training than the male. It has been found that the body temperature of the female rises 2° to 3° C. higher than the males before the sweating and cooling off process begins. Such a factor must be taken into consideration in dealing with vigorous physical activities, such as swimming in hot weather. Other differences include a more stable knee joint in girls than in boys, greater length of bones in boys than girls, and, on the average, greater height and weight in boys than girls. The skeletal structure of the female makes her more susceptible to athletic injuries than the male. Injuries involving overstraining, such as in foot deficiencies and tendon inflammations, have been found to be more common in the female.

Activities that are provided for girls and women should be selected in light of psychological as well as physiological considerations. Those that emphasize feminine qualities such as grace and rhythm and involve a minimum of body contact should receive priority. Furthermore, regularity in engaging in physical activity should be stressed, even during the menstrual period, if there are no harmful results.

Implications of growth and development characteristics for athletics for junior high school students

One of the most controversial areas in athletic programs is the one concerned with junior high school boys.

Biologically, children in grades seven to nine are composed of preadolescents and young adolescents. In grade seven, among 11-, 12-, and 13-year-old children, preadolescents predominate—approximately two-thirds are boys and one-third girls. In grade 8, among 12-, 13-, and 14-year-olds, young adolescents increase in number. In grade 9,

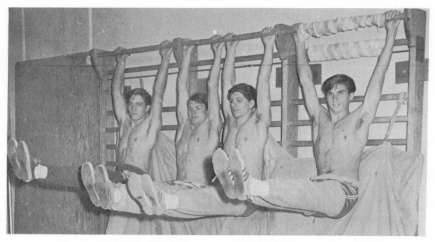

The La Sierra, California, high school physical fitness program.

among 13-, 14-, and 15-year-olds, young adolescents predominate.

Preadolescents are children who belong to later childhood. They have not yet experienced the growth spurt. Instead, growth is usually slow. Young adolescents are characterized by fast-growing arms and legs, changing facial features, broadening hips and shoulders, and changing voices. They resemble men and women more than they do children.

The growth spurt, experienced by junior high school students, is a very rapid and spectacular one both from its outward expression in the form of height, weight, and size and also in respect to sensitive biochemical activity resulting in internal physical changes.

Girls normally have their growth spurt between the ages of 8½ and 11½ years, reaching a peak at about 12½ years and leveling off at 15 to 16 years of age. Boys begin later than girls, with their growth spurt normally occurring between the ages of 10½ and 14½ and with the peak being reached at about 14½. Following this there is a gradual decline, the rate of growth usually being complete between the ages of 17 and 20.

Biologically, an adapted program of activities is needed to meet the changing physical makeup of the junior high school student. The period of growth and development through which the student is passing requires a program adapted to his needs. There is a special need for team-type activities that will satisfy the "gang" urge. There is a need for competition. There is a need for a wide variety of activities that will help in the development of body control, enable each student to experience success, provide consideration for energy output and fatigue, and protect the sensitive individual. There is a need for activities that will offer a channel of release for tensions rather than increase the amount of tension. Furthermore, in selecting activities, the danger of injury to the skeletal framework, as well as dangers in regard to students overextending themselves to the point of exhaustion through competitive activity, must be kept in mind. There is a need to keep accurate records of growth and achievement, to have a program of health supervision and medical services, and to make provision for work in body mechanics.

Because of the uneven way in which growth takes place, it is difficult to know how old a child is during the early adolescent period. "Old" in this frame of reference does not refer to years but to other kinds of age—age of his skeleton, mental age, physiological maturity, and emotional maturity. This raises the question as to how students can be properly grouped for forms of athletic activity that in many instances should rightfully be limited to the "older" youngsters.

Implications of growth and development characteristics for girls' and women's athletics

The question of athletics for girls is a highly controversial matter. The questions of how much, how little, and what is a happy medium are frequently raised with enthusiastic supporters on all sides of the issue. There seems to be a general consensus that athletics can render a valuable service to girls. The question arises as to what type of program can best render this service. Girls can develop a better state of total fitness, skills for worthy use of leisure time, and other desirable qualities and attributes, just as boys and men can. However, it must be recognized that girls and women are not boys and men. There are many biological, sociological, and other differences that must be taken into consideration. It is impossible to take the boys' program and duplicate it for the girls without any changes.

Critics of athletic competition for girls have frequently declared that such competition can interfere with the female's menstrual cycle and cause problems associated with the reproductive system. Much of this criticism, however, has not been fully substantiated. On the other hand, physical activity for girls has been found to improve the development of abdominal and spinal muscles, which in turn may prove beneficial in the progress of pregnancy. Dr. Evelyn Gendel* has stated that those girls who have had little physical activity may have increased postpartum problems of back pain. Physical activities that strengthen the abdominal muscles can alleviate this discomfort.

It is important that the women in charge

of the girls' program and those who do the officiating be qualified. There is need for training programs that will aid women in their preparation as teachers, coaches, and officials. There is need for the nation's women sports leaders to unite their efforts and organize the type of program that will most benefit the girl athlete. The Division of Girls' and Women's Sports of the American Association for Health, Physical Education, and Recreation has established guidelines for girl athletes. These guidelines should be reviewed and followed wherever such programs exist.

In the next few years there will be an increasing demand for more athletic competition for girls. The current women's liberation movement has been instrumental in emphasizing the point that women should be emancipated politically, socially, economically, and sexually. Women are now desiring to be emancipated athletically. For example, the women jockey is becoming a more frequent sight at many race tracks. Athletic competition for girls is a concern for physical educators and one that needs further research.

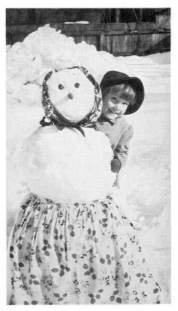

The normal child needs from 2 to 6 hours of activity a day.

---

*Gendel, Evelyn S.: Women and the medical aspects of sports, Journal of School Health **37:** 427-431, 1967.

General rules pertinent to physical and motor growth and development

Certain general principles may be stated in respect to physical and motor growth and development. The physical educator should continually be conscious of these principles in planning and directing a physical education program for children:

1. The normal child needs from 2 to 6 hours of activity a day. Since all of his activity cannot take place during school hours, the time spent in activity in school should be devoted to providing instruction that may be utilized in after-school hours.
2. Aside from heredity and the nutritive environment, the organic systems of the body can be developed only through muscular activity.
3. Because of the softness of a young child's bones, particular attention should be given to the prevention of postural abnormalities.
4. A child's physiological age is an important consideration in determining the type of physical education program best fitted to his growth and development.
5. Large-muscle activity is an essential for the proper growth and development of normal children.
6. The various parts of a child's body grow at different rates of speed.
7. A child's intellectual, social, and emotional growth and development are greatly increased through motor activity.
8. A "skills" program should take into consideration the maturation levels of children.
9. Disease, malnutrition, and insufficient exercise are causes of growth disturbances in children.
10. Skills utilized in adult leisure hours are frequently acquired during childhood.
11. The acquisition of skills aids the awkward, adolescent child to obtain satisfaction and enjoyment through participation.
12. Adolescent boys and girls should participate in physical education programs that are adapted to their needs and physiological make-up.
13. The values of physical activity to everyone, regardless of age and regardless of sex, should be brought to the attention of all.

Body types

Psychologists often classify individuals on the basis of "body types" or physique. This is based on the body structure of an individual. Through such a classification, it has been thought possible to distinguish certain physiological and personality traits that might be associated with each type.

One method of classification is that promulgated by Kretschmer, who classified the human body into four groupings based upon physical features. Types distinguished are the *asthenic,* a word which has a Greek derivation and means "without strength," referring to those individuals who are lean, slim, shallow chested, and tall in proportion to their weight; the *athletic,* from Greek meaning "a contender for a prize"— the muscular individual, the fellow with broad shoulders and well-developed chest, robust and strong; the *pyknic,* from the Greek meaning "thick" and referring to the individual who has a broad, rounded figure, large head, heavy neck, and ruddy face; and the *dysplastic,* in the Greek meaning "badly formed" and designating individuals who have abnormal bodies and have builds that are abnormal and not found in the asthenic, athletic, and pyknic types.

Within certain limits body types may be used as an indication of athletic ability. For example, the pyknic type usually will be interested in a sport such as football, soccer, or hockey, whereas the asthenic type will choose running or tennis. Classifications based on body types, however, are not always reliable, and physical educators should be careful as to how much they rely on them as a basis for classifying groups for physical education activities. Age, physiological maturity, interests, skill, size, strength, physical fitness, and other similar criteria should be used with the various body-type classification in making such judgments.

Another classification that has been used divides body types into *endomorph,* which is similar to Kretschmer's "pyknic" type; *mesomorph,* similar to the "athletic" type, and *ectomorph,* similar to the "asthenic" type. Sheldon uses these classifications and has developed a system of somatotyping whereby an individual's body classification can be more accurately analyzed by giving it a number classification showing relationship to endomorph, mesomorph, or ectomorph. This is based on the premise that there are no clear-cut or absolute "endomorphs," "mesomorphs," or "ectomorphs." Instead, body build represents a variation of all three. Sheldon then goes on to give a detailed description of the various somatotypes that he has found in his research.

Willgoose relates body types and physical fitness. Table 15-1 shows that within certain groups of somatotypes there are different interests and abilities in athletics. Willgoose points out there is some overlapping in this structure but that it might be useful in considering athletic performance.

Body mechanics

The attitudes about good posture have changed from that of a rigid, static, upright, unnatural position to one of efficient, graceful, yet somewhat relaxed body movement. Physical educators are concerned with dynamic posture in sitting, standing, walking, running, and other body positions. The aim is to have each individual develop a body carriage suited to his own body build. The best posture will be characterized by balance and proper alignment of body segments to give one maximum support and movement with the least strain.

Good posture is valuable for appearance since it influences the concept others have of the individual. One's posture may even influence self-concepts and attitude of mind. Good posture makes for efficiency of movement since poor posture causes additional muscular effort, fatigue, and undue strain. In some cases the strain may be enough to alter structure, resulting in limited use of body parts. In extreme cases chronic strain may lead to arthritic conditions.

Poor posture may be the result of several causes including weak musculature, faulty diet, fatigue, disease, arthritis, vision and hearing defects, overweight and obesity, skeletal defects, faulty postural habits, and injuries such as back strain. Even negative attitudes toward exercise and desirable posture can be basic causes of poor body carriage.

Physical educators must be aware of the various deviations in body mechanics. Devi-

Table 15-1. Body types and physical fitness*

Mesomorphic endomorphs	Endomorphic mesomorphs	Extreme mesomorphs	Ectomorphic mesomorphs	Mesomorphic ectomorphs
(S-types: 631, 532, 541, 542, 543)†	**(S-types: 452, 361, 462, 451, 453)**	**(S-types: 171, 162, 262, 172, 252)**	**(S-types: 253, 254, 163, 164, 265)**	**(S-types: 235, 126, 136, 145, 146)**
Table tennis	Baseball	Sprints	Lightweight wrestling	Bicycling
Floating (swimming)	Football (lineman)	Basketball	Long-distance running	Cross-country
Croquet	Heavyweight boxing	Middleweight boxing	Tennis	Table tennis
Fly and bait casting	Heavyweight wrestling	Middleweight wrestling	Gymnastics	Basketball center (short periods)
Bowling	Swimming	Quarterbacks	Weight lifting	Archery
	Soccer (backs)	Football (backs)	Javelin	(Also many athletic games, except those requiring weight and sheer strength)
	Ice hockey (backs)	Divers	Pole vault	
	Weight tossing	Tumbling	High jump	
		Lacrosse	Fencing	
		Soccer (forwards)	Badminton	
		Ice hockey (forwards)	Skiing	
		Handball	Jockey	

*Willgoose, Carl E.: Journal of Health, Physical Education, and Recreation **27:**26, 1956.
†S-types in the table refer to those body types given in Sheldon, William H.: Atlas of men, New York, 1954, Harper and Row, Publishers.

ations in body mechanics can either be *functional* or *structural*. Functional deviations can be corrected. They are primarily associated with muscles and ligaments and exercises can help alleviate the problem. Structural deviations are those that have not been corrected in time and have become permanent. Physical educators must be especially concerned with the functional deviations since students can, in many cases, be aided by proper exercise programs.

QUESTIONS AND EXERCISES

1. Why is it necessary for the physical educator to be able to interpret physical education from the biological point of view?
2. What is the status of America's health? What are the implications for physical education?
3. What is the extent of preventable health defects and diseases in the United States?
4. Trace the role of physical education in the evolution of man.
5. What are the biological defects of man in light of his structure? What are the implications for physical education?
6. Why is it essential for physical educators to understand the makeup of each of the following parts of the human body: skeleton, musculature, circulatory system, respiratory system, nervous system, digestive system, excretory system, endocrine system, integumentary system, and reproductive system?
7. Select one of your classes and categorize members into endomorphs, mesomorphs, or ectomorphs.
8. Identify each of the following: chronological age, anatomical age, physiological age, mental age, asthenic body build, Sheldon, maturation, cephalocaudal development, proximodistal development, and Jersild.
9. Describe what you would believe to be an ideal education for a child from birth until 10 years of age.
10. Construct a chart depicting the physical and motor growth of a child during infancy, the preschool years, elementary school years, adolescence, and postadolescence.
11. Develop an outline of a physical education program for each of the following age ranges based on information provided in this chapter concerned with child growth and development, characteristics, and needs: 1 to 5 years, 5 to 7 years, 8 to 10 years, 11 to 13 years, and 14 to 16 years of age.
12. What part does heredity play in physical differentiation?
13. Discuss several additional factors that affect man's growth and relate these factors to their implications for physical education.

Reading assignment
Bucher, Charles A., and Goldman, Myra: Dimensions of physical education, St. Louis, 1969, The C. V. Mosby Co., Reading selections 37, 41, and 43.

SELECTED REFERENCES

American Association for Health, Physical Education, and Recreation: Children and fitness, 1964; The growing years—adolescence, 1962; Washington, D. C., The Association.

The Athletic Institute in cooperation with the American College of Sports Medicine: Health and fitness in the modern world, a collection of papers presented at the Institute of Normal Human Anatomy, Viala Regina Elena, 289, and the Ministry of Foreign Affairs, Rome, Italy, 1961, The Athletic Institute.

Bartley, F. H., and Chute, E.: Fatigue and impairment in man, New York, 1947, McGraw-Hill Book Co.

Bucher, Charles A.: Administrative dimensions of health and physical education, including athletics, St. Louis, 1971, The C. V. Mosby Co.

Bucher, Charles A.: Interscholastic athletics at the junior high school level, Albany, New York, 1965, The University of the State of New York.

Bucher, Charles A., and Reade, Evelyn M.: Physical education and health in the elementary school, New York, 1971, The Macmillan Co.

Bucher, Charles A., Olsen, Einar A., and Willgoose, Carl E.: The foundations of health, New York, 1967, Appleton-Century-Crofts.

California Association for Health, Physical Education, and Recreation: Values inherent in the daily program of physical education, Journal of California Association of Health, Physical Education, and Recreation, special issue, March, 1965.

Competitive athletics for children of elementary school age, Pediatrics **42**:703, 1968.

Department of Classroom Teachers, American Education Research Association of the National Education Association: What research says to the teacher. In Hunsicker, Paul: Physical fitness, 1963, The National Education Association.

Gendel, Evelyn S.: Women and the medical aspects of sports, Journal of School Health **37**:427-431, 1967.

Jennings, Herbert: The biological basis of human nature, New York, 1930, W. W. Norton & Co., Inc.

Johnson, Warren R., editor: Science and medicine of exercise and sports, 1960, New York, Harper and Row, Publishers.

Kretschmer, E.: Physique and character (translated by W. J. H. Sprott), London, 1925, Kegan Paul, Trench, Trubner.

Mitchem, John: Isometric exercise—an evaluation, The Physical Educator **20**:28, 1963.

National Association for Physical Education of College Women and National College Physical Education Association for Men: Science and physical education, Quest, Winter Issue, Monograph III, December, 1964.

Ryan, Allan J.: Medical care of the athlete, New York, 1962, McGraw-Hill Book Co.

Selye, Hans: The stress of life, New York, 1956, McGraw-Hill Book Co.

Sheldon, W. H.: The varieties of human physique, New York, 1940, Harper and Row, Publishers.

Steinhaus, Arthur H.: How to keep fit and like it, Chicago, 1957, The Dartnell Corp.

Still, Joseph W.: Man's potential—and his performance, New York Times Magazine, November 24, 1957.

Time, Inc.: The healthy life, Time-Life Books Special Report, New York, 1966, Time, Inc.

16/Biological fitness

The health of the people is the foundation upon which all their happiness and all their powers as a state depend.

DISRAELI

EDUCATION FOR FITNESS

Since many youths and adults do not fully understand and appreciate the importance of health and fitness, a heavy responsibility rests upon the shoulders of educators. If a nation is to remain strong physically, mentally, spiritually, and socially, there must be *education* for *fitness*. Furthermore, this education must take place largely through the formal processes of physical education, health education, and recreation programs in our schools and colleges. Knowledge about the human body must be imparted, desirable health attitudes inculcated, and proper health practices instilled. The responsibility for accomplishing this herculean task must be assumed mainly by physical educators, health educators, and recreation educators. They must continually strive for sound school and community programs in their special fields. They must interpret articulately the need for educational institutions to educate not only in science and mathematics but also in those essentials that comprise other aspects of total fitness. This is a major challenge that faces society in the days and years ahead. If educators can accomplish this goal, they will not only render a valuable contribution to their country but to the health and happiness of millions of human beings as well.

WHAT DOES "PHYSICAL FITNESS" MEAN TO CHILDREN AND YOUNG PEOPLE?

In order to discover what the term *physical fitness* means to elementary, high school, and college students, 10,000 children and young people were surveyed throughout the United States. The answers given were then analyzed to determine the most common concepts held by students in regard to their understanding of the term *physical fitness*.

The survey showed that a uniform meaning of the term *physical fitness* has not been communicated to students in our schools and colleges. The variations in the answers obtained in the survey may mean that there is a lack of uniformity in the understanding of the term by teachers in the field, that there is very little, if any, teaching being done as to the meaning of this term, that students are formulating their own definitions, and/or that the home and community are influencing the student's understanding of this term.

Elementary school

At the elementary school level the most common answer given by all students, and also by the majority of the girls surveyed at this level, was that physical fitness means "to be healthy." Among the boys, the most prevalent answer given was that it means "to keep the body in shape." The other most frequently mentioned answers by both boys and girls were that it means "exercise," "to be good in sports," and "to have good body coordination."

Boys and girls in elementary school are passing through a very formative period. It would seem important that meaningful basic concepts regarding the meaning of physical fitness be communicated to them at their level of understanding. Since the home has a great influence on the child's thinking, it also implies that parents should be informed in regard to the meaning of physical fitness and its place in a physical education program.

Junior high school

Among the girls at the junior high school level, the term *physical fitness* takes on a different meaning from the girls' elementary school interpretation. Identification of the term *exercise* with physical fitness has now become the number one answer, while the concept "to be healthy" has moved to second place. This may indicate that girls are now being introduced to formal exercise in physical education classes and that teachers are stressing the importance of exercise as a means of becoming physically fit.

The second most prevalent answer among the girls was that physical fitness means "to be healthy." This answer may possibly indicate that the home and community continue to influence the student's thinking. Health is frequently stressed in the home and among neighbors and other members of the community.

Junior high school boys gave the same answer as to the primary meaning of the term *physical fitness* as did the elementary school boys. They both placed the greatest emphasis on "keeping the body in shape." The survey seemed to indicate that from the elementary school to the junior high school level there is no significant change in the meaning of the term *physical fitness* among the boys. The fact that this answer has been constant may indicate that teachers and parents have accepted this interpretation of physical fitness and are continuing to emphasize this point of view. The general thinking of a significant segment of our

society stresses the importance and desirability of boys "keeping their bodies in shape."

"To be healthy" was the third most prevalent answer among the junior high school boys, the second most common answer offered by junior high school girls, and was first on the list for elementary school girls, as expressing their understanding of the term *physical fitness*. The second most prevalent answer among the junior high school boys was that physical fitness and "exercise" are synonymous. This was the third most prevalent answer offered by the elementary school boys. As with the girls, this may indicate that boys are also being influenced by the introduction of formal exercise into their physical education classes. The emphasis given by boys to the definition "to keep their bodies in shape" may also be a reflection of the feeling in our society that this is what the term *physical fitness* means.

At the junior high school level we find the introduction of two new terms used by the students to define physical fitness. One of the new answers was that physical fitness means "conditioning your body." Possibly the students who gave this answer were merely using a more sophisticated terminology for "keeping the body in shape." The introduction of this new statement may have no significance except to show that students at this age level are able to express themselves in a more articulate manner. The other new term that was introduced was that physical fitness means "good body coordination." This answer may be a reflection of the teachings taking place in physical education classes. It may also imply that teachers are attempting to give these students a more meaningful understanding of the term.

High school

The most prevalent answer given by boys on the high school level in regard to the meaning of physical fitness was that it means "to keep the body in shape." The second most common answer offered by the high school boys was one that was rarely mentioned at the lower educational levels, namely, that physical fitness means "to be good in sports." Since boys are exposed to a greater emphasis on sports in high school and engage in both team and individual sports, this may provide the answer as to why this sport is stressed by high school boys.

The data for the high school level also show, for the first time in the survey, that the answer "endurance" is given. This may indicate that in some schools physical educators are attempting to increase the scope of the concept that they are teaching. It may also be an indication of the influence of factors outside the school such as television, magazines, and general public opinion.

The second most frequent answer given by junior high school girls in regard to the meaning of the term *physical fitness* was that it means "to be healthy." High school girls placed this answer first. This may indicate that students are receiving more health instruction at the high school level and that there is more emphasis being placed on the relation of health and physical fitness.

The next answer in order of frequency given by high school girls was that physical fitness means "to keep the body in shape." This is an age when girls are maturing physically, interested in boys, and conscious of good health practices. Consequently, girls are interested in doing all those things that will help them to be most attractive to the boys.

High school girls are less apt to define the term *physical fitness* as meaning "sports" or "exercise" than are junior high school girls.

College

When asked to define the term *physical fitness,* most college boys felt it meant "to be strong and healthy." The concept of strength, along with health, was introduced at the college level. College men students also introduced a new dimension in regard to physical fitness: "coordination of mind and body." Evidently some students had grasped the concept of the "unity of man."

The largest percentage of college women still interpreted physical fitness as meaning "to be healthy." A concept of physical fitness also given by college girls involved a consideration of physical fitness as meaning the "ability to do everyday tasks." It was the first time that this answer appeared and might indicate a better understanding of the functional aspects of physical fitness in day-to-day living.

Some implications that might be drawn from the survey

The implications of this survey as to what children and young people regard as the meaning of the term *physical fitness* include the following:

1. As an objective of physical education, students do not clearly understand the meaning of physical fitness and its place in educational programs.
2. There is a need for communicating the meaning of the term *physical fitness* to students at all educational levels and to the public in general.
3. Physical educators should assume the responsibility for communicating key concepts to students in regard to terms such as *physical fitness.* This responsibility should be part of the subject matter and the theory underlying their field of endeavor.
4. There should be better communication between professional leaders in physical education and those practitioners functioning in schools, colleges, and various agencies at the "grass roots" level.
5. Physical education cannot be limited to activity alone. There must also be provision for getting at basic concepts underlying the field of physical education and making sure these basic concepts are understood by all persons concerned.

This chapter is designed to define and analyze the terms *fitness* and *physical fitness* and to discuss the implications these terms have for the profession of physical education.

FITNESS AND HEALTH*

According to the Greek poet Homer, one setting for the adventurous wanderings of

---

*Parts of this discussion have been adapted from Bucher, Charles A.: Health and fitness, Educational Leadership **20**:356, 1963.

Odysseus was on the island of the Phaeacians. There, King Alcinous arranged to have the best of his athletes perform for his guest. After a superb and spectacular display of sports feats, Odysseus was asked if he too wished to demonstrate his skill. Seizing a discus larger than had been used by any of his counterparts and dashing on the field with a heavy cloak restricting his movements, he opened wide the eyes of his competitors by showing his superior strength and fitness in hurling the missile farther than all the rest.

History is replete with illustrations of peoples throughout the world who considered physical prowess and strong, healthy bodies the vital ingredients for survival and power. The desire for physical excellence and well-being has its roots deeply embedded in historical tradition. For early man the ability to survive was dependent to a large degree upon his accuracy with the bow and arrow, swiftness of foot, strength of muscle, and ability to withstand trying physical ordeals. Nature literally kicked him into activity, as one historian relates.

As man became more and more civilized, the concept of "survival of the fittest" was augmented by other catalytic agents that propelled him into action. Statements from two of the world's great thinkers illustrate these motivating factors. Aristotle said: "The body is the temple of the soul and to reach harmony of body, mind and spirit, the body must be physically fit." John Locke wrote: "A sound mind in a sound body is a short but full description of a happy state in this world; he that has these two has little more to wish for."

As motives for well-being have changed, so have the preventive and medical procedures for achieving and maintaining fitness and health. Herb medicines, witch doctors, healing chants, and bloodletting remedies have given way to wonder drugs, immunizations, and vitamins. Today there is much scientific knowledge to direct human beings assuredly along the path to good health. And according to the health experts, the way each human being lives will be a major determining factor for the

health and fitness of that individual. Although heredity plays a part, to a large degree health and fitness are acquired characteristics. The food that is eaten, amount of rest obtained, physical activity engaged in, and other health practices that are followed play important roles in determining human welfare. In other words, it is important to follow a good health regimen if one is to be healthy and fit. This is especially important today in an automated society where advertising lures, medical quackery, fake shortcuts to health, and other temptations embrace human beings on all sides.

In order to help people follow a healthful regimen, *education* is essential. It is important to educate students about English so that they can communicate articulately with their fellow human beings, about mathematics so that they can add their grocery bills accurately, and about the fine arts so that they can appreciate and enjoy Picasso and Beethoven. It is also important to educate people about their physical selves so that they can function most efficiently as human beings and accomplish all they are capable of achieving. And to attain this objective they need to know scientific facts essential to good health, possess desirable health attitudes, develop skills to make activity exciting and enjoyable, and be physically active. The end result will be productive, vigorous, and rewarding lives. And as Will Durant advises, health is mostly within each person's will. "In many cases, sickness is a crime," this philosopher states. "We have done something physiologically foolish, and nature is being hard put to it to repair our mistakes. The pain we endure is the tuition we pay for our instruction in living."

Much of this education should take place early in life when the organic foundations are being laid, skills are more easily learned, and attitudes are formed. Unfortunately, too many people do not recognize the need for this education until cholesterol deposits have closed their arteries, ulcers have penetrated their duodenum, or cancer has started its insidious attack upon their lungs. As one wise man has said, "We never appreciate health so much as when we lose it." Although it may be difficult to change the health habits of adults, schools and colleges *can* and *should* educate young people about their health and fitness. This is not only essential from the individual's point of view but also in view of this country's national posture. The late President Kennedy stated: "The strength of our democracy is no greater than the collective well-being of our people. The vigor of our country is no stronger than the vitality and will of our countrymen. The level of physical, mental, moral, and spiritual fitness of every American citizen must be our constant concern."

The fact that 10 million out of 40 million school children could not pass a screening test of minimum physical fitness and that many more had undesirable health practices offers some evidence that our educational programs have been inadequate in this regard.

Sound school physical education and health programs are needed. In order to have outstanding programs, educators must have a clear understanding of the philosophy of physical education and health and their worth in education. The following definition of terms and concepts will be of help in setting the stage for education for fitness of young and old people alike.

1. *Fitness implies more than physical fitness.* Fitness is the ability of a person to live a full and balanced existence. The totally fit person possesses physical well-being but also such qualities as good human relations, maturity, and high ethical standards. He also satisfies such basic needs as love, affection, security, and self-respect. School health and physical education programs are vitally concerned with physical fitness but also strive to contribute to total health and fitness.

2. *Physical fitness includes more than muscular strength.* The term *physical fitness* implies soundness of such body organs as the heart and lungs, a human mechanism that performs efficiently under exer-

Physical fitness includes more than muscular strength.

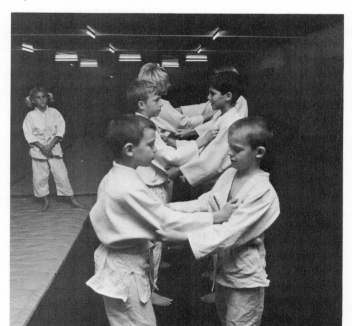

FROM MICHELSON, MIKE: JUDO: NOW IT'S A SAFE FAMILY SPORT,
TODAY'S HEALTH, FEBRUARY, 1969.

cise or work conditions (such as having sufficient stamina and strength to engage in vigorous physical activity), and a reasonable measure of skill in the performance of selected physical activities. Physical fitness is related to the tasks the person must perform, his potential for physical effort, and the relationship of his physical fitness to his total self. The same degree of physical fitness is not necessary for everyone. It should be sufficient to meet the requirements of the job plus a little extra as a reserve for emergencies. The student who plays football needs a different type of physical fitness from the student who plays in the school orchestra. The question "fitness for what?" must always be asked. Furthermore, determining the physical fitness of a person must be done in relationship to his own human resources and not those of others. It depends on his potentialities in the light of his own physical makeup. Finally, physical fitness cannot be considered by itself but, instead, as it is affected by mental, emotional, and social factors as well. Human beings function as a whole and not as segmented parts.

3. *Physical education is not the same as health education.* Although closely allied, health and physical education are separate fields of specialization. Whereas physical education is concerned primarily with education of and through the physical, the school health program is concerned with teaching for health (for example, imparting facts about good nutrition), living healthfully at school (for example, providing healthful physical and emotional environment), and providing services for health improvement (for example, instituting measures for communicable disease control).

4. *Both health and physical education contribute to physical fitness.* The student needs to engage in regular physical activity but, in addition, needs to understand the impact this activity has on his organism. The student needs to have activities fitted to his individual requirements but also to have these activities conducted in a safe and healthful environment. The student should develop skill in various sports but also should develop skill in first aid and home nursing. These are only a few examples of how the health and physical education programs complement and supplement each other in the achievement of the objective of physical fitness.

5. *Health education and physical education must be integral parts of the educational program in order to most effectively achieve the goal of physical fitness.* These subjects are not frills or appendages of the school's curriculum, nor are they a means for entertaining students. They should be vital parts of every educational program in this country. Only as they are so recognized will it be possible to achieve the goal of fitness and health for all young people. Furthermore, such recognition cannot be merely in the form of lip service but must be repeatedly injected into programming, scheduling, and other practices that reflect the true educational philosophy of each school.

6. *Good leadership is the key to good health and physical education.* The good health or physical education teacher is not someone who merely looks healthy, can produce a string of sports victories, or give a good speech before the Rotary Club. Leadership is basic to the health and physical education professions, and this means men and women who know their subject, the boys and girls they are teaching, and the best methods and techniques for teaching.

7. *Physical fitness is not synonymous with physical education.* Physical fitness is *one* objective of physical education. It is important to have physically fit boys and girls. However, as long as the word *education* is a part of the term *physical education,* there are other responsibilities. Developing physical skills, imparting knowledge about the human organism, and using the body as a vehicle for achieving desirable social traits also represent desirable goals. Any program or curriculum aimed merely at building strength and muscle is failing in its educational mission.

8. *Interschool athletics represent only one part of the total physical education program that contributes to physical fitness.* The school physical education program includes the class program for all students, the adapted program that fits the activities to handicapped or atypical individuals, the intramural and extramural program that provides a laboratory experience for the skills and knowledge imparted in the class program, and the interscholastic athletic program for those students with exceptional physical skill. All four of these aspects of the physical education program must function in a manner that affords balance and harmony and allows for the achievement of physical fitness and other objectives for *all* students.

9. *The development of physical skills is a major contribution to long-term physical fitness of students.* Obstacle courses and calisthenics represent forms of "canned" activities that yield organic benefits to the student, but a major contribution of any physical education program is to teach boys and girls a wide variety of physical skills. Skills are the motivating agents that will accelerate a boy and girl to engage in activities and promote physical fitness, not only in the present but throughout a lifetime as well.

10. *Administrative support and understanding are needed to achieve physical fitness.* The quality of school health and physical education programs will be largely determined by the administrative leadership of the school and community. Boards of education, superintendents of schools, principals, and other administrative officials will decide the prestige these programs have in the eyes of the students, whether credit is given to the subjects when calculating the requirements for graduation, how much money is provided in the budget for their development, the attention given to girls as well as to boys, the degree of emphasis on physically underdeveloped students as compared to gifted athletes, and the answers to other administrative matters that affect the physical fitness of students.

PATHS TO PHYSICAL FITNESS

Physical fitness?*

You know the model of your car,
You know just what its powers are,
You treat it with a deal of care,
Nor tax it more than it will bear.

But as to Self—that's different;
Your mechanism may be bent,
Your carburetor gone to grass,
Your engine just a rusty mass.

Your wheels may wobble and your cogs
Be handed over to the dogs
And then you skip and skid and slide
Without a thought of things inside.

What fools, indeed, we mortals are,
To lavish care upon a car,
And ne'er a bit of time to see
About our own machinery.

JOHN KENDRICK HANGS

The American Medical Association has outlined seven paths that lead to physical fitness. The physical educator should recognize the many-faceted approach to physical fitness and thereby understand that this quality cannot be achieved solely through physical activity.

1. *Proper medical care*—To be physically fit requires regular medical examinations, immunizations against communicable diseases, emergency care, and prompt treatment by qualified medical personnel when such care is warranted.

2. *Nutrition*—"You are what you eat" has much meaning in regard to physical fitness. The right kind of food should be eaten in the right amounts.

3. *Dental services*—Good oral hygiene is essential to physical fitness. This means regular visits to the dentist, treatment of dental caries, and proper mastication.

4. *Exercise*—Exercise is important, but to have a salutary effect there must be a proper selection of activities adapted to the age, condition, and other needs of the individual, together with proper exposure to these activities in terms of time and intensity of workout.

5. *Satisfying work*—Work that is adapted to one's interests and abilities and performed in a satisfying working climate is essential to physical fitness. There should be good mental attitude, recognition, and a sense of achievement and belonging.

*Quoted in Sportscope, October 15, 1962, Chicago, The Athletic Institute, Inc.

6. *Healthy play and recreation*—To achieve physical fitness requires play and recreation in an atmosphere that has as its by-products fun, enjoyable companionship, and happy thoughts.

7. *Rest and relaxation*—Adequate sleep, rest, and relaxation are essential to good health and physical fitness.

COMPONENTS OF PHYSICAL FITNESS

Larson and Yocom* surveyed physiological research and listed the following ten factors as the components of physical fitness. These have implications for the physical education profession. They are presented here in adapted form.

---

*Larson, Leonard A., and Yocom, Rachael Dunaven: Measurement and evaluation in physical health, recreation, and education, St. Louis, 1951, The C. V. Mosby Co., pp. 158-162.

1. *Resistance to disease.* Heredity and environment both help to determine the ability of the individual to resist disease. Among the important environmental factors are diet, exercise and recreation, rest habits, and proper personal hygiene.

2. *Muscular strength and muscular endurance.* A person who has sufficient strength and endurance can sustain vigorous activity and perform strenuous work over an extended period. For an individual to be physically fit, he must have strong and efficient muscles. He must have a balanced proportion of good muscle fibers, the ability to bring the needed number of muscle fibers into play when there is work to be done by the muscles, efficient body levers, a working rhythm, and good coordination.

3. *Cardiovascular–respiratory endurance.* When a person contracts a series of muscle groups over a period of time long enough to put a strain on his circulatory and respiratory systems, but without causing a stoppage of the work, that individual has cardiovascular-respiratory endurance. These

The milking machine.

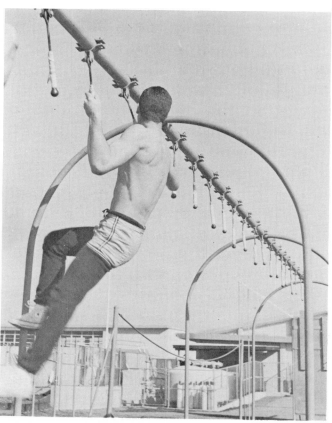

LA SIERRA HIGH SCHOOL, LA SIERRA, CALIF.

two systems are important to fitness because they work together to supply the muscles with fuel and oxygen, both of which are needed for muscular contractions. The more efficient the cardiovascular and respiratory systems of the individual, the longer he will be able to sustain work, since his muscles will be well supplied with their fuel and oxygen. The individual who has a high degree of this kind of endurance has improved his physical fitness, since his muscles receive large supplies of fuel and oxygen; he has a slower pulse rate and lower blood pressure; his lungs have a larger surface area, allowing for the absorption of more oxygen by his blood; he has a larger supply of red corpuscles, which also aid in increasing the oxygen supply; and he is less prone to fatigue.

4. *Muscular power.* Muscular power is explosive power such as that needed for putting the shot, high jumping, and sprinting. A person who has muscular power also has two of the components of muscular power: strength and speed. The powerful individual is able to use his speed and strength in an efficient, coordinated, and skillful manner.

5. *Flexibility.* Total body flexibility depends on the flexibility of the individual body joints and their supporting structures. Flexibility infers that the body is capable of making a wide range of movements, such as those needed for swimming, diving, and tumbling. The more flexible a person is, the less energy he spends in accomplishing a skill.

6. *Speed.* A person who possesses speed is able to make a series of similar movements in a short span of time. Speed in swimming relates to the number of arm and leg strokes a swimmer takes in a given period of time. Muscular strength and the aspect of speed are highly related.

7. *Agility.* The agile individual can change the position of his body in space efficiently and easily. Agility, strength, and endurance are important factors in agility. Agility is particularly important to the hurdler in track, lacrosse player, and diver.

8. *Coordination.* The coordinated individual is able to put together a series of movements into a flowing and rhythmical pattern. Different kinds of activities and bodily movements require different kinds of coordination. Agility, balance, and speed are important components of coordination.

9. *Balance.* Balance is the maintenance of equilibrium through neuromuscular control. Many of the skills of physical education, such as tumbling, trampolining, and skiing, require good balance. Coordination is a factor in balance and, for some skills, agility also plays a part.

10. *Accuracy.* The accurate individual can control the movement of one object toward another, such as pitching in baseball, throwing for a goal in lacrosse, or casting a fishing fly. Although there is some relationship between accuracy and balance, they are not related closely enough to have a strong dependency on each other.

EXERCISE AND PHYSICAL FITNESS*

Scientists attending a 1967 session of the Federation of American Societies for Experimental Biology heard about an experiment at Howard University where three dozen roosters ran a mile a day on a treadmill five times a week for a period of almost 6 months. The birds were fed on a diet high in cholesterol, a fatty substance that clings to the insides of the arteries—often closing them as rust clogs a pipe. When the arteries of the roosters were examined after the 6 months of exercise, little if any deposits of cholesterol were found. However, in sedentary birds that were also used in the experiment, fat stuck to the arteries. The fats even invaded the coronary arteries, the small blood vessels that feed blood to the heart muscle itself and that if clogged bring on a coronary heart attack by starving the heart of oxygen.

This is not an isolated piece of evidence. Dr. Menard Gertler, of New York University, has demonstrated that the physical activity of the U. S. Marines' basic training keeps the fat content of the blood down, even though the men were eating large amounts of calories each day consisting of animal fats—just the type that is supposed to increase fat and cholesterol in the blood.

A Harvard group of researchers investigated the farmers of a 2-mile-high Swiss village in the Alps. Each day the men climbed 3,000 feet to farm a plateau. Although they ate a high-animal-fat diet, the blood cholesterol levels were down.

Other experiments have shown that exercise decreases the tendency of the blood to clot and increases the capacity of the blood to dissolve clots already formed.

In general, exercise lowers blood pressure and slows heart rate, two important considerations in heart conditions.

Being active is not a sometimes thing but

---

*Parts of this discussion have been quoted and parts adapted from Bucher, Charles A.: Today's Health (published by the American Medical Association) **34:**24, 1956.

A stiff but reliable test of fitness.

		EIGHTEEN TESTS OF FITNESS	NORMAL MEN (% PASSED)	NORMAL WOMEN (% PASSED)	YOU
BALANCE	1	Assume a diver's stance, arms outstretched, standing on your toes with your eyes closed. Hold this stance—and your balance—for 20 seconds.	95%	56%	
	2	Squat with your palms on the floor. Tip forward, resting your legs on your elbows, toes off the ground in a squat handstand, and hold for 10 seconds.	25%	14%	
	3	With your finger touching the floor, walk in a circle around it 10 times in 30 seconds. Then walk a straight 10-foot line within five seconds.	1%	36%	
AGILITY	4	Keeping your legs together and knees straight, bend at the waist and touch the floor with your finger tips. Women should touch palms of their hands.	75%	86%	
	5	Slowly bend from a sitting position, knees flat, until your forehead is eight inches, or two fists, one atop the other, from the floor.	67%	73%	
	6	Lying on your stomach with your feet pinned to the floor and your fingers laced behind your neck, raise your chin until it is 18 inches from the floor.	35%	25%	
POWER	7	Kneel with your insteps flat on the floor. Using just your back and arms, spring erect, both feet together, and hold your balance for three seconds.	65%	25%	
	8	From a standing position, jack-spring from the floor, touching your toes at waist height without bending your legs. Repeat five times quickly.	38%	13%	
	9	Repeat six times: (1) squat; (2) kick legs backward; (3) kick legs forward between arms; (4) turn over; (5) squat; (6) stand.	10%	14%	
FLEXIBILITY	10	With a partner who is lying down (and who is within 10 pounds of your weight), lift and carry him fireman-style—all in 10 seconds from floor to carry.	94%	54%	
	11	With your hands on your hips and the back of your head on a partner's knee or the edge of a chair or sofa, hold your body rigid for 30 seconds.	78%	66%	
	12	Lying prone, with arms outstretched, lift your midsection four inches in an extended press-up using just hands and toes. Women may use forearms.	1%	60%	
STRENGTH	13	Do a standing broad jump the length of your height. If you are under 25, the distance should be the same as your height plus one foot.	71%	8%	
	14	Do 15 full-length push-ups with your hands positioned beneath your shoulders. Women should do 30 push-ups, keeping their knees on the floor.	65%	34%	
	15	Chin yourself, or, on your back, straddled by a partner, grasp his hands and pull up until your chest strikes his legs. Men repeat 20 times, women 10.	79%	73%	
ENDURANCE	16	Sit on the floor with your knees stiff. With hands on hips, lean back so your legs come off the floor in a V-sit, and hold 60 seconds.	68%	40%	
	17	Run in place for two minutes at double time, or 180 steps per minute. Then take three breaths and hold your breath for 30 seconds.	15%	12%	
	18	Do 200 two-foot hops, 200 straddle hops, 200 scissor, or alternate stride, hops, 50 hops on each foot and 50 squat jumps.	9%	6%	
		TOTAL PASSING SCORES	10	7	

a continuing must for good health. Exercise is needed all year long. The benefits of physical activity cannot be "canned up" when the temperature is hovering in the 80's and "dished out" as it drops into the 20's any more than the body can be put in cold storage on Labor Day and thawed on the Fourth of July. For proper functioning, the human organism needs this essential ingredient on a regular basis, just as it demands nutritious food every day.

Many busy men and women limit their sports and activity to the summer months. There are others who even deplore the thought of getting into action at any time of the year. Those who hate exercise love to soothe their guilty consciences and flabby muscles by talking about the animal kingdom. The lazy tortoise avoids exercise and lives 200 years or more. The clumsy elephant saves his strength and reaches the ripe old age of 100 years. Flies that buzz around the fastest die the soonest. Businessmen sag lower into their living room chairs and mothers playing bridge settle deeper into their corsets, saying "Why exercise?"

Dr. Edward C. Schneider, a famous physiologist, after a lifetime study of the effects of exercise, came to the conclusion that: "Frequently repeated exercise, extending over months and years . . . is necessary for healthy existence; it is a physiologic need of a primitive kind which cannot safely be eliminated by civilization. It is difficult to find men who have been injured by muscular exercise but easy to find many who have failed of normal development and been ruined by the lack of it."

The "don'ts" of exercise are well known. Don't exercise after 40 years of age. Don't exercise when you're tired, when it's cold, or after eating. Don't exercise—it will injure your heart and you will die sooner. More should be said about the "do's." You do need exercise to get the most out of life. You do need exercise to keep in the best of health. Exercise is good for the normal heart. Exercise contributes to good mental health.

Dr. George W. Calver, former physician for the Supreme Court and Congress, outlined ten commandments for keeping these men fit. Two of these were "exercise rationally" and "play enthusiastically." As Dr. Calver counseled: "Give 5% of your time to keeping well and you won't have to give 100% getting over being sick."

The worth of exercise rests upon a basic principle, the law of use. Hippocrates called attention to this many hundreds of years ago, when he said: "That which is used develops and that which is not used wastes away." Modern medical practice recognizes the law of use.

Although there are many claims for exercise that are not true, many accusations against it are also false. Two of these are that exercise will shorten life and that it is harmful to the heart. Sir Alan Rook, former Senior Health Officer of Cambridge University, compared the longevity of 834 sportsmen from his university with a group of "intellectuals" and men chosen at random. Sir Alan concluded: "No evidence could be adduced from the information available that cardiovascular causes of death were more prominent in the sportsmen or occurred at an earlier age." Other research studies have come to the same conclusion.

Medical authorities state that proper exercise cannot harm the heart. Dr. E. Cowles Andrus, former president of the American Heart Association, advises: ". . . it is clear that strenuous exercise, properly supervised, does not cause disease in the normal heart." Dr. Paul Dudley White, world-renowned authority on heart disease, reasons this way: Men who slow down at 40 years of age may have a heart attack sooner. For some reason that cannot be explained at the present time, such a slowdown seems to increase the possibility of hardening of the arteries. He capped his reasoning with this remark: "The general warning to stop vigorous exercise at 40 seems to me ridiculous." Dr. White cites five benefits from exercise:

1. Maintains muscle tone
2. Relieves nervous tensions and provides relaxation

3. Aids digestion
4. Helps to control obesity
5. Improves functioning of the lungs by deepening of respiration

In addition to Dr. White's benefits, other advantages of exercise cited by experts include:

1. Added strength and endurance help in performing daily tasks with less fatigue
2. Better movement accrues for the human body
3. Exercise helps to maintain health of the heart and blood vessels
4. Exercise helps in the building of a desirable self-concept
5. Exercise helps in the prevention of accidents

Other fitness myths that have been cited include: middle age begins at 40 years of age—chronologically it starts at about 26 years of age; hardening of the arteries is a natural part of getting old—not necessarily, blood vessels are dependent partially on regular exercise to keep in shape; rest or sleep is the best way to eliminate fatigue —not always, physical activity can act as an antidote to some kinds of fatigue; youngsters will be harmed through sustained exercise—it depends, if they are fit, their physical endurance is great and the exercise will be conducive to good health; and there are shortcuts to fitness—no, the truth rests in a continuing program of activity, good nutrition, rest, sleep, relaxation, and adequate health care.

The values of exercise are not limited to the body; they also contribute to sound mental health. Exercise makes a person feel better. I spoke with at least 1,000 people on this subject. In addition, my students have surveyed at least 10,000 more. Comments follow a pattern; "I feel more alive when I exercise"; "I have more energy"; "I don't feel as tired in the evening"; "I can do a lot more work." Those who exercise regularly never fail to mention that exercise makes them feel better. If a person feels better, his attitude toward others will probably be friendlier. He is happier, makes wiser decisions, and his world in general looks better.

The benefits to sound mental health are especially great when a person engages in games and sports. He finds release from tensions, relaxes, forgets his troubles, and loses himself in the game. Dr. William Menninger, the famous psychiatrist, points out that physical activity provides an outlet for instinctive aggressive drives by enabling an individual to "blow off steam," provides relaxation, and is a supplement for daily work. He stresses the fact that "recreation, which is literally re-creating relaxation from regular activity, is a morale builder. It is not a luxury, a waste of time or a sin."

Socialization is also provided in many games and sports. Psychologists say every human being has the desire to belong to a club, gang, or association. This is an essential human need. Games and sports offer opportunity for recognition and a feeling that one belongs to a group. Like the ex-con said who was recently caught in an Eastern city: "I'm glad to go back to jail. Here I'm nothing, but up there I'm first baseman on the baseball team."

Although exercise has many physical, mental, and social benefits, this does not mean a person should rush out and buy himself a tennis racket and schedule three sets of tennis for Saturday afternoon. In order to secure these benefits, exercise must be used with discretion. Following are some suggestions that reflect the opinion of medical experts and provide good advice for physical educators:

1. Encourage a thorough medical examination at regular intervals to determine the type of exercise most beneficial to the individual.
2. Encourage people to select, if possible, a sport or an activity around the house, such as gardening, in preference to calisthenics. The mental and social values are greater.
3. After 40 years of age, encourage people to cut down on the "explosive" sports requiring fast starts, quick stops, and prolonged activity without rest. Examples are badminton, tennis, handball singles, and basketball.
4. If a person is out of training in a sport, advise him to return to action gradually. A little today and a little more tomorrow is a good prescription.

5. Encourage persons to exercise out-of-doors if possible.
6. Encourage persons to select activities that are adapted to them.
7. Encourage people to give their full attention to the activity and leave their worries at the office.
8. Encourage individuals engaging in sports that involve body contact or other hazards to use essential protective equipment, especially for head, neck, eyes, and teeth.
9. Encourage individuals to play in areas where safety precautions have been taken to avoid the danger of injuries.
10. Encourage individuals to participate with others of the approximate same degree of skill, training, and size when these factors are pertinent to the competition.
11. The way a person recuperates after exercise should be a guide in its wise use. Breathing and heart rate should not be excessively fast 10 minutes after stopping exercise. Extreme fatigue should not persist

2 hours after stopping. The activity should not cause broken sleep at night or a tired feeling the next day. If any of these symptoms occur, the activity should be cut down. If they continue, the person should see his doctor. Exercise is good, but it must be adapted to the individual's needs.

Exercise and general health

Exercise and training have important implications for the general health of a person. Studies of 5,000 patients at the Columbia Presbyterian Medical Center in New York City and the Institute of Physical Medicine and Rehabilitation, New York University, indicated that approximately 80% of the patients with low back pain experienced this difficulty because of muscle weakness or stiffness. Follow-up studies showed that pain symptoms decreased as

Physical fitness testing in a high school in Tainan, Taiwan. This was part of the test program carried out in Southeast Asia to compare results to those of the performance of American children.

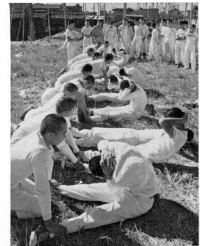
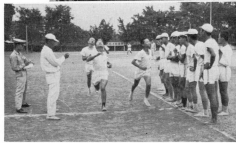
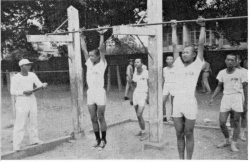

COURTESY DR. GUNSUN HOH, REPUBLIC OF CHINA.

muscle strength and flexibility increased. If exercise was stopped, the ailments came back again. Other studies in recent years have added to a gradually accumulating volume of evidence that exercise has a salutary impact on degenerative diseases, on slowing the aging process, on the ability of an individual to meet emergencies, and on the prevention of vascular degeneration.

Steinhaus took twenty-five popular sports and rated each in respect to various components of physical fitness. The participant can use Table 16-1 as a checklist to determine what activities will best meet his fitness needs.

Isotonic and isometric exercises*

Muscles function by contracting in such a manner that the muscle shortens and the ends are brought together (concentric), or the muscle lengthens and the ends go away from the center as in the beginning of a pull-up when one lowers himself into a hanging position (eccentric) (isotonic). Or, a muscle contracts when the muscle builds up tension and holds without any shortening or lengthening (static or isometric is derived from the words *iso,* meaning same, and *metric,* meaning length).

Isometric exercises have become very popular. Athletes are using them to become better baseball, football, and basketball players. Some patients convalescing in hospitals are finding them helpful in restoring the strength lost while being sick. Handicapped individuals offer testimonials that they have therapeutic value. The weak, physically underdeveloped person is often amazed at their results.

The worth of isometric exercises to the athletic world has been expounded through the sports news channels. Several years ago the chief trainer of the champion Louisiana State University Tiger football team and the Olympic team used isometrics to win fame for the athletes under his care. World

*This discussion is based on Bucher, Charles A., and Nagel, John: Isometrics: new method for new muscles, unpublished.

record holders in the 100-yard dash adopted them to improve their performance. Professional basketball players have claimed they improved their basketball ability. Athletes in high schools across the country have been helped by isometric exercises. Weight lifters, high jumpers, as well as many players from the San Francisco 49'ers, Pittsburgh Pirates, and a host of other notables and teams, are converts to isometrics. Current champions in many athletic events use isometric exercise in their training programs.

If these claims of isometrics are true, the value of this system of physical activity is not limited in use to star high school, college, and professional athletes. It can be used by anyone who has the desire to improve his strength. If a person is a little on the weak side, isometrics may be better suited to him than to the superhealthy, physically fit fellow because his improvement will be more rapid and pronounced. This fact was demonstrated as far back as 1958 when isometrics proved their value to some average high school boys. In a study conducted by Rarick and Larsen, the students performed a daily, single, 6-second workout. After only 6 weeks the boys, regardless of whether they were tall, short, or skinny, improved their strength. This experiment, together with other studies, impressed many professional physical educators with the worth of isometrics for students.

WHAT IS ISOMETRIC EXERCISE AS COMPARED TO ISOTONIC EXERCISE? Since physical educators are interested in building strength, a first concern is to know what strength is. A professor at the University of California defines it as the ability to work against resistance. In everyday terms it is known as possessing that physical quality that enables a person to lift a 50-pound bag of cement, climb a rope in the gymnasium, or lift a girl in his arms.

Strength, when combined with other physical elements, yields additional qualities important to any person who wants to get the most out of his body. For example, strength combined with speed gives power. Power is that quality that permits Wilt Chamberlain to jump high and snare rebounds off the board, Willie Mays to throw a baseball with rifle-shot precision to home plate from center field, and Jim Ryun to sprint like a deer down the cinder path.

The traditional way of building strength is to get muscles into action by increasing the resistance offered them. Terms commonly used for this form of exercise are *isotonic* and *dynamic*. The classical story is of the man who started lifting a small animal weighing about 25 pounds and continued to lift the animal each day until it became full grown, weighing over 200 pounds. The man's muscles gained strength as the workload was progressively increased from day to day. The people who lift weights in the school gymnasium or YMCA are trying to do the same thing—build strength by following what is called the principle of overload. They gradually increase the amount of weight they lift.

In isotonic or dynamic contraction, the muscle shortens and the resistance, such as that offered when a stack of books is lifted from a school desk, is overcome. Physical work is accomplished by utilizing movement and resistance in the exercise. Isometric contractions, on the other hand, are static types of contractions since there is no joint or muscle movement. Instead, the muscle is put in a state of tension. All the energy that is expended in contracting the muscle isometrically is converted into heat. The resistance, whether it be a radiator, desk, office file, wall, or anything immovable, cannot be overcome. In other words, a force is exerted against an immovable object in which neither muscle nor object moves but in which the pressure or exertion is applied to create a tension within the contracting muscle.

Here is a simple example. Place yourself between two walls. Put your back against one wall and your hands against the other wall. Now push with all your strength against the wall. Even though you grunt and groan and give it all you have

as you contract your muscles maximally, it is impossible to move the resistance, in this case the wall. This is the way strength is developed in isometric exercise. As you can see, it is a very simple procedure. There are still several points that need to be known before starting to exercise, such as how much force to apply and how long to apply it, as well as what to do after a desirable level of strength has been achieved.

WHERE DID IT ALL START? When did isometric exercise start? What is its history? Briefly, the principles underlying isometric contractions have been public domain for years. One physiologist relates how scientists shortly after World War I used frogs in their experiments. When they tied down one of the frog's legs but not the other, they were surprised to find that the leg that could not move still gained considerable strength. The muscles in the immobilized leg were in a state of static tension and thus strength was developed. These researchers had the basic knowledge about isometrics but for some reason dropped their laboratory work and did not apply the idea to building strength in human beings. Some 40 years ago research in this field was conducted at a college famous for training physical educators, Springfield College in Massachusetts. However, the results were not conclusive and the experiments were discontinued. Not much was heard about isometrics for the next 20 years. Then, in 1953 two German physiologists, Dr. T. Hettinger and Dr. E. A. Muller, did considerable research and published their findings in a German magazine. This article attracted considerable attention and created anew throughout the world an interest in isometric exercises. In America such men as Steinhaus, Karpovich, Drury, McCloy, Rasch, Morehouse, and Bender, realizing the significance of the Germans' study, started conducting their own experiments. Many of their findings confirmed the work done in Europe—isometric exercises are of real value in building strength in human beings.

In the last 15 years an increased interest in applying this method of exercise to patients and in the treatment of injuries was developed.

Probably the greatest boost was given when it was found that isometric contractions had value for athletic performance. When school and college personnel and the coaches, trainers, and owners of professional teams heard the news they were very much interested. Today, although some physiologists have reservations about all the claims made for isometrics, there is general agreement that they can play an important role in developing body strength.

WHAT RESULTS CAN BE EXPECTED? How much strength can one expect to develop in his body through this form of exercise? How long will it take to do the

A series of exercises recommended by the American Medical Association.

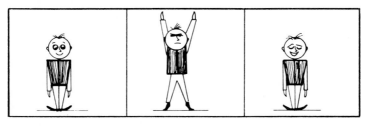

1. THE STRETCHER (Minimum 4; Maximum 10)
(1) Stand erect; (2) Spread feet apart, reach high with hands, rise on toes; (3) Return to starting position.

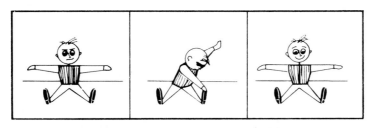

2. THE TWISTER (Minimum 6; Maximum 15)
(1) Sit erect with legs straight, feet apart, hands out wide; (2) Touch right hand to left toe, keeping left arm back and horizontal; (3) Return and exercise opposites.

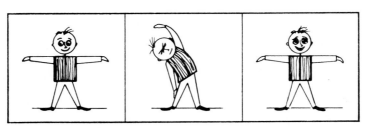

3. THE SIDE BENDER (Minimum 6; Maximum 15)
(1) Stand erect, feet apart, hands out wide; (2) Raise left arm straight over head, slide right arm down leg; (3) Return and exercise opposites.

Continued.

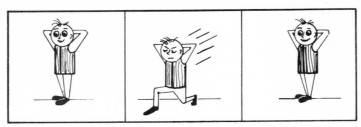

4. THE STRIDE SQUAT (Minimum 6; Maximum 15)
(1) Stand erect, hands behind head; (2) Stride forward deeply with right leg, keep left toe in place, keep bent left knee off floor; (3) Return and exercise opposites.

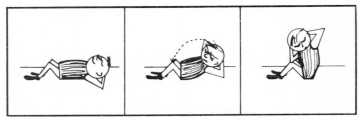

5. THE CURL (Minimum 6; Maximum 15)
(1) Lie on back, knees bent, hands behind head; (2) Tuck chin, "curl" as far forward as possible, aiming right elbow to left knee; (3) Return and exercise opposites.

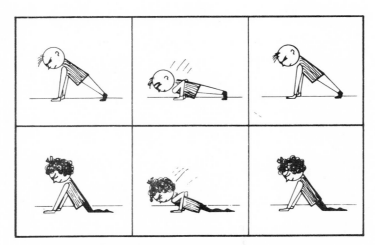

6. THE PUSH-UP (Minimum 6; Maximum 15)
(1) For men: On hands and toes; For women: On hands and lower legs; For both: Keep trunk and neck straight, fingers forward; (2) Lower trunk to two inches from floor; (3) Return.

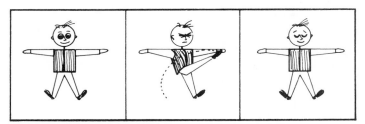

7. THE COMPRESSOR (Minimum 6; Maximum 15)
(1) Lie on back, hands out wide, feet apart; (2) Roll onto left hip, keep legs straight and right arm on floor, touch right toe to left hand; (3) Return and exercise opposites.

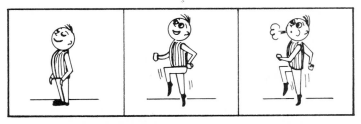

8. THE HIGH-STEPPER (Minimum 10 Steps; Maximum 20 Steps)
(1) Stand erect, elbows bent, fists clenched; (2) Run in place, pump knees and arms vigorously.

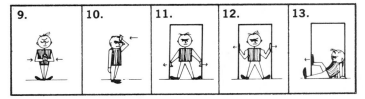

ISOMETRIC EXERCISES — which involve muscular contractions without movement — follow. Hold each contraction forcefully for six seconds. Repeating is not necessary.

9. THE ORGAN GRINDER Push hand against hand, then pull hand against hand.

10. THE THINKER Push forehead against palm; then push back of head against palm(s).

11. THE BIRD Push back of hand against door jambs; then push palms in same manner.

12. THE SAMSON Push palms against door jambs; then straighten arms high against jambs and push again.

13. THE SIESTA Sitting with back against one door jamb, push foot against other side; then push other foot in same manner.

FROM PHYSICAL FITNESS, CHICAGO, 1964, AMERICAN MEDICAL ASSOCIATION.

job? Muller and Hettinger found that one short isometric contraction of a muscle involving less than maximum force (they suggest two-thirds effort) and performed daily for 6 seconds over a period of 5 or 6 weeks would increase strength at the rate of 5% a week. This estimate is believed to be too generous by most American researchers, who believe 2% a week is a better estimate. Simple arithmetic will show that less than 1 minute would be required to exercise a muscle group per week. An entire exercise program involving the major muscle groups, such as those of the arms, abdomen, shoulders, and back, will take about 5 minutes per day, including rest periods. On the other hand, if a person is lifting a barbell, he might have used up this much time in merely chalking his hands, to say nothing of the 1 to 2 hours a day, three times a week, required to do lifts. One estimate has been made that 10 seconds of isometric contractions can be equal to 100 or more isotonic contractions. If this is true, it would be possible to elicit many more strength gains in 10 minutes of isometric work than in 1 hour of isotonic exercise.

Isometric contractions get results, according to many researchers. McCloy, one of America's pioneers in this area, concluded as a result of his experiments that when these exercises are engaged in regularly for a period of 1 year a normal person's muscles can be strengthened as much as 100% and those of a physically underdeveloped individual as much as 150%.

After a person has gained the necessary strength he must still continue to exercise. The benefits cannot be "canned up" and forgotten. But one encouraging note—a person does not need to spend as much time to maintain the desired strength level. Muller felt that one isometric contraction per day at one-fifth maximal effort was sufficient. McCloy suggested that for the first year strength can be maintained by a workout once a week and after 12 months by a session once every 30 days. Other researchers are more conservative in their estimates.

A person should not abandon all the dynamic exercise done in weight training.

Isometrics are not the complete answer to strength and fitness. Probably the biggest drawback is their inability to develop stamina and endurance, those qualities that permit a person to engage in vigorous activity for extended periods of time without becoming exhausted. But as part of a total fitness program they should help because strength is essential to good physical performance, whether it is pole vaulting, lifting a ladder to paint the house, or hiking through the woods. Isometric exercise will help to build this needed strength. And in order to make up for some of those qualities that cannot be developed, a person might engage in some running, swimming, or similar type of activity. Or else isometric contractions can be supplementary to regular workouts in sports. Of course, if a person is not following any exercise program at the present time, isometrics should prove helpful.

SOME RESEARCH FINDINGS ON ISOMETRIC AND ISOTONIC EXERCISES. Physical educators should be acquainted with the research in respect to isometric and isotonic exercises and use these studies as a guide to their utilization of these techniques. Selected research studies* indicate the following:

1. Both forms of exercise, isotonic and isometric, build muscular strength. However, the evidence to date shows little if any difference in the effectiveness of the two forms of achieving strength increase—results of over a dozen studies indicated this conclusion.
2. Isometrics can be carried on in many different locations, including one's office or while waiting for a train.
3. The motivation factor is usually not as great in the case of isometrics as with isotonics.
4. Studies have not shown a strength gain of 5% per week (claimed by some persons) for 10 weeks (50% for the entire period) when a single 6-second contraction was used against resistance equal to two-thirds of the muscle's strength. Most studies support a strength gain, but it has not been as great. Many of them show only 2% or 3% a week.

---

*Clarke, H. Harrison: Physical fitness newsletter, Research Review, No. 3, May, 1965. For other references, see end of chapter.

5. Rarick and Larsen found that strength that was retained after the exercise programs were followed over a period of time was greater in the case of isotonic than isometric exercises.
6. Bender, Kaplan, and Johnson found that isometric contractions were often harmful when exercises of a gross nature, such as pressing the whole body upward against a bar, were used. Many times the wrong muscles are developed.
7. Bender and Kaplan found that isometric contractions must be executed at various angles throughout the range of motion if benefits are to accrue, rather than at one point in the range of motion of a joint.
8. Royce found there is a greater interference in circulation to an exercising muscle in isometric than in isotonic contractions.
9. Clarke found that oxygen debt is 40% greater in isometric exercises.
10. Thompson found that the effects of isometric and isotonic work have different effects on blood pressure.
11. Berger found that isotonic exercises will improve jumping ability better than will isometrics.
12. The evidence from existing research seems to favor isotonic exercise rather than isometric exercise as a means of conditioning a muscle.

Exercise and the daily program of physical education in the schools

A few years ago the daily period of physical education was challenged by some California legislators. In order to show the need for the daily program, the CAHPER published a special issue of its journal,* which contained a wealth of statements and research findings supporting the daily period of physical education. Statements and scientific evidence were listed from cardiologists, American Medical Association, California Heart Association, physiologists and psychologists, nutritionists, educators, school administrators' associations, defense authorities, Parent-Teacher Associations, students, and the President's Council on Physical Fitness and Sports. Some of the arguments set forth for a daily program were: (1) it is essential to the physical fitness of the students, (2) it provides a badly

*Values inherent in the daily program of physical education, Journal of the California Association for Health, Physical Education, and Recreation, March, 1965, Special Issue.

needed break from intellectual demands, (3) it is needed for the optimal functioning of the brain, (4) it is a preventive measure against heart disease, (5) it helps to prevent obesity, (6) it develops necessary strength and endurance, (7) it enables individuals to meet emergencies more effectively, (8) it is conducive to good mental health, (9) it reduces tension, (10) it develops muscle tone, (11) it contributes to emotional fitness, (12) it helps to ensure a healthy populace, and (13) it contributes to scholastic achievement.

TRAINING AND PHYSICAL FITNESS

There are many aspects of training that are pertinent to a high state of physical fitness.

Principles of training

Some principles of training have been compiled by Forbes Carlile.* These will be helpful to the reader who is interested in helping his students achieve peak performance in sports or other forms of physical activity. They are presented in adapted form.

1. The training load should follow the principles of frequency and intensity. The load must be severe and frequently applied so that the body can adapt maximally to a particular activity.
2. Training is an individual problem. As such, factors like age, work and study load, physical makeup, time available for sleep and rest, and training facilities available are important considerations in arranging a training schedule for any person.
3. Physical and emotional stresses, in addition to the training exercise routine, must be taken into consideration for each individual. For example, such conditions as manual labor performed, daily traveling, and emotional pressures from home, school, and other sources are important considerations.
4. Excessive stress on the individual will lower the performance level and therefore attention should be constantly given for manifestations of stress.
5. Periods of rest and physical and mental

*Carlile, Forbes: Ten principles of training, Track Techniques **1**:23, 1960.

relaxation must be interwoven with doses of exercise in order to get the best results. This is true during a single training session as well as week by week.

6. Training for a particular sport and many times for different events within a sport (such as sprinters and distance runners in track) is specific and geared to the particular sport or event. Therefore, training procedures for one sport or activity are not necessarily helpful for other sports or activities.
7. Flexibility and strength are two components that are essential to free-flowing movements and efficiency in sports performance. There should be provision for exercises that develop these qualities especially during the off-season. Such exercises should be carefully designed and directed at specific groups of muscles and joints. Scientifically designed weight-training exercises plus stretching exercises are especially good.
8. Interval training has been found to be one of the best procedures for a modern training schedule. This consists of rhythmically carrying out an activity from 30 seconds to 1 minute at fairly intense effort (but not all out). Each period of exercise is followed by 10 seconds to 2 minutes of slow recuperative activity.
9. Nutrition is an important consideration in any training schedule. Therefore, the person in training should adhere to a good diet that contains the essential food groups.
10. Three popular conditioning and training techniques today are as follows:
    A. *Circuit training*—this represents a series of exercises, usually ten, that are performed in a circuit and in a progressive manner, doing a prescribed allocation of work at each station, and then checking the progress against the clock. As the performer becomes stronger, the number of repetitions and the quality of the exercise are increased. Activities should be selected with care.
    B. *Fartlek* (Swedish for speed play)—this is free-relaxed running. The course usually consists of a soft surface and considerable uphill and downhill running. The following schedule is recommended: (a) easy running for 5 to 10 minutes, (b) steady, fast running, (c) easy running with wind sprints for 50 to 60 yards, (d) rapid walking for 5 minutes, (e) uphill running, and (f) maintaining a fast pace for about 1 minute.
    C. *Interval training*—this has been briefly mentioned above. Four factors that are important in using this technique are: (a) distance (to build endurance)—should be long enough to create a stress

in the performer, (b) speed—runner increases speed over a designated distance that is possible to repeat allowing rest between each run, (c) number of repetitions—depends upon its value or purpose, and (d) rest or recovery period —the recovery interval is gradually reduced as training progresses.
11. The most important fact in a program of training is to achieve the goals of physical readiness and psychological readiness when your schedule indicates it is important.

Effects of training

The results derived from regular periods of muscular work or exercise are many and varied. The individual who participates regularly in exercise adapted to his needs and thereby attains a state of physical fitness may be called "trained." The individual who allows his muscles to get soft and flabby and is in a poor physical condition may be referred to as "untrained."

Space does not permit listing all the advantages of the "trained" state. Therefore, certain advantages that seem to stand out as being important to the vital organs of one's body will be mentioned here.

EFFECTS OF TRAINING ON GENERAL HEALTH OF HEART MUSCLE. There is evidence available to show that the heart muscle increases in size through use. With greater demands placed upon the heart through physical activity, a hypertrophic condition exists. This is a healthy condition. The term *athletic heart* has often been used to connote a heart that has pathological or diseased indications because of participation in physical activity. Physiologists maintain this is incorrect. Instead, they indicate that an "athletic heart" is a normal condition that follows the law of use. The law of use may be stated in these terms: "that which is used develops and that which is not used atrophies." This applies to all of the muscles of the body. Since the heart is a muscle, this condition indicates a stronger and better developed heart.

There is considerable controversy over whether a heart may be impaired through extreme muscular effort. There is general agreement that a child with a normal heart cannot damage this vital organ through ex-

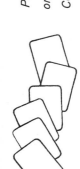

CIRCUIT TRAINING

a dynamic tool
for improving
the fitness of
**AMERICA'S
YOUTH**
at the time of
greatest need—
TODAY!

*Prepared for the President's Council
on Physical Fitness and Sports by the
Courtesy of Sears, Roebuck and Company.*

Sears
SPORTS CENTER
Where the new ideas are

ercise. The controversy concerns individuals 35 or 40 years of age. The proponents of the theory that a sound and normal heart cannot be impaired through activity are many. Others feel that sudden, explosive exertions may cause heart strain. A report published by the American Association for Health, Physical Education, and Recreation, prepared after considerable research by eminent medical doctors, physiologists, and health and physical educators, points out that the normal heart and circulatory system become stronger through use. However, the report continues, strenuous competitive physical activity should not be engaged in by older persons *unless* they have done this regularly and have kept themselves physically fit.

EFFECTS OF TRAINING ON STROKE VOLUME OF HEART. As a result of research on such men as DeMar, the great marathon runner, Olympic athletes, and others, it is generally agreed that there is a greater volume of blood per heartbeat pumped through the body of the trained person than the untrained person. The research on DeMar showed that his heart pumped 22 liters of blood as contrasted with 10.2 liters in an untrained individual.

EFFECTS OF TRAINING ON PULSE RATE. As a result of evidence gathered from tests performed on Olympic athletes and others, there appears to be evidence that the trained individual has a lower pulse rate than the untrained person. One estimate has been made that the heart of a person beats from six to eight beats slower when he is in training as compared to when he is out of training. In many athletes, pulse rates are ten, twenty, and as much as thirty beats lower than in those individuals who follow sedentary pursuits.

Before exercise the trained individual's heart has a lower rate than an untrained person's heart, but under exercise both increase about the same proportion.

Individuals convalescing from an illness show by their pulse rates the effects of training. As their condition improves and they become more physically fit, their pulse rate decreases. If the pulse rate does not go down, it is interpreted as a lack of improvement in their physical fitness.

The pulse rate of the trained individual returns to normal much more quickly after exercise than does the pulse rate of the untrained individual. Many cardiovascular tests have been patterned on this premise.

EFFECTS OF TRAINING ON BLOOD. The rate of lactic acid formation is lower in the trained individual, resulting in a lower blood lactate concentration. This allows for greater work output on the part of the trained individual. Lactic acid is the substance that is transferred from glucose when a muscle contracts. The more lactic acid, the more fatigued an individual will become. Lactic acid begins to appear in the blood when the oxygen supply gets low and is inadequate. It escapes from the muscles and goes into the blood. Some of it is buffered. The liver transforms some of it into glycogen, and then it is sent back to the muscles as needed in the form of blood sugar. Some is eliminated through the kidneys.

In addition to the lower rate of lactic acid formation, another effect of training on the blood is the reduction in the osmotic resistance of red corpuscles. It is thought that this may result from the rise in body temperature during muscular work.

EFFECTS OF TRAINING ON ARTERIAL BLOOD PRESSURES. Schneider and Karpovich point out that experiments on DeMar showed that the increase in blood pressure is less in the trained individual than in the untrained individual. They further point out that under exercise DeMar's systolic blood pressure increase was 50 mm. Hg, whereas the increase in an untrained man, who was used as a means of comparison, was 125 mm. Hg.

Karpovich, in a later work, refers to additional studies in which this condition has also held true.

The relation of blood pressure to muscular work depends on duration of the exercise, intensity, and rate of performance.

EFFECTS OF TRAINING ON RED CORPUSCLES. There is considerable disagreement as to the effect of training on the red corpuscle count. However, there appears to be agreement that, as a result of training, the bone marrow becomes redder, indicating an increased rate of blood manufacture. As a result of this agreement, it seems reasonable to conclude that there is an increase in the number of red corpuscles in the trained individual.

The person who follows a sedentary or inactive existence and then pursues strenuous work destroys a considerable number of red corpuscles, which it takes several days to restore. A period of anemia results, and the individual is not fit to follow strenuous muscular effort for a period of several days. However, the trained individual has developed the red marrow in his bones. Any ordinary destruction of red corpuscles, for any given time, does not affect the individual because the loss is quickly made up. In the trained individual there is a better balance between the destruction and manufacture of red corpuscles.

EFFECTS OF TRAINING ON WHITE BLOOD CELLS. More knowledge is needed concerning the effects of training on the white blood cells. However, it seems clear that the white blood cells or leukocytes increase in number in the blood after a period of muscular work, whether it be mild or severe. The increase in the white blood cells seems to vary in proportion to the degree of intensity of muscular work. It is thought by many that the increase can be credited to a redistribution of the cells in the vascular system.

EFFECTS OF TRAINING ON RESPIRATION. Evidence is available to show that there are several effects of training on the respiratory system. Some of these are as follows:

1. There is greater expansion of the chest. This is true during the early years but not especially during adulthood.
2. There is a slower rate of breathing. Some evidence shows that the trained person takes as little as six to eight breaths a minute, as compared to eighteen to twenty by the untrained person.
3. The depth of the chest is increased.
4. The blood is exposed to oxygen over a greater area. This is not true of sedentary or inactive individuals because a greater portion of their lungs becomes closed off to air that is inhaled.

5. There is deep diaphragmatic breathing. In the untrained person, the diaphragm moves very little.
6. In performing similar work, a trained individual takes in smaller amounts of air and absorbs oxygen from the air in greater amounts than does an individual not in training. It is believed that the increased number of capillaries in the lungs caused by greater amounts of blood being exposed to the air at any given time is responsible for this economy in respiration.

EFFECTS OF TRAINING ON THE MUSCULAR SYSTEM. Evidence is available to show that there are several beneficial effects of training on the muscular system. Some of these are as follows:

1. The sarcolemma of the muscle fibers (the part that surrounds each fiber by a connective tissue sheath) becomes thicker and stronger.
2. The amount of connective tissue within the muscle thickens.
3. The size of the muscle increases. It is believed that muscle fibers increase in size but do not increase in number.
4. The muscle has greater strength. It is necessary to exercise a muscle in order to increase its strength. It is reputed that Milo of Crotona, a 17-year-old boy weighing 149 pounds, lifted a bull daily. The bull weighed 75 pounds to start and finally weighed 290 pounds. The boy's muscles increased in strength through use as the bull increased in size.
5. The muscle gains in endurance. An experiment is reported on an ergograph being attached to the flexor muscles of a finger and the number of contractions recorded. The increase was from 273 contractions to 918.
6. There is a chemical change in the muscle. There is an increase in phosphocreatine content, glycogen, nonnitrogenous substances, and hemoglobin. All of these aid the muscles in working more efficiently.
7. The nerve impulse travels more readily across the motor end plate in the muscle fiber.
8. There is a greater number of capillaries. This results in better circulation of blood to muscles.

EFFECTS OF TRAINING ON THE DIGESTIVE AND EXCRETORY SYSTEMS. Exercise helps to keep the digestive and excretory organs in good condition. The nerves and muscles of the stomach and intestines become well toned and better able to function in an efficient manner. Also, exercise usually makes a person hungry, and, in general, hunger can improve digestion.

EFFECTS OF TRAINING ON THE NERVOUS SYSTEM. The nerves and muscle work together because the muscles are controlled by the nerves. Messages are relayed by the nerves to the muscles, which react in the way the individual wishes, whether by running, playing a musical instrument, or hitting a tennis ball. Consequently, any kind of muscular exercise enhances nerve-muscle coordination. Furthermore, nervous fatigue may be lessened by pleasant physical activity because the nervous fatigue that has accumulated through anxiety or mental work is offset through muscular activity.

EFFECTS OF TRAINING ON THE ENDOCRINE SYSTEM. There is some evidence that the hormones produced by the adrenal medulla (adrenaline and noradrenaline) are affected by training. The plasma level of noradrenaline has been found to increase considerably during exercise while that of adrenaline is only slightly increased. Increased amounts of noradrenaline are responsible for vasoconstriction of the heart, while increased amounts of adrenaline are responsible for the increased metabolic rate of the body. Adrenaline and noradrenaline prepare the organism for action by increasing the blood pressure and heart rate of the individual. These hormones are also responsible for the release of more energy by the organism, thus aiding the individual in his strenuous activities.

EFFECTS OF TRAINING ON BODY TEMPERATURE. Increased muscular activity generates more body heat. In demanding activities such as long-distance running, the deep muscle temperature of the body has been known to rise to over 100° F. Such increases in muscle temperature also produce a rise in body temperature. The heat that has been generated by such an activity must be dissipated. Sweating is the prime body mechanism for the dissipation of heat. Research has shown that during training, the composition of sweat differs from one person to another. The larger, heavier man is likely to produce more sweat than the smaller man. The skin temperature of the organism is related to the environment more so than the body temperature is. Exercising in a cold environment may result in the skin temperature dropping down to 80° F., while the body temperature, because of the muscular activity that is taking place, still remains over 100° F.

EFFECTS OF TRAINING ON THE FEMALE. There has been concern in recent years that training can interfere with the sexual and reproductive functions of the female. Research by Klaus[*] has indicated that women are more susceptible to athletic injuries than men. There is considerable evidence to support the claim that females should not engage in training during pregnancy because of the greater demands placed on the heart. However, observation of female athletes has shown that there is no disturbance on the onset of menarche. It had been thought that athletic women would have difficulty in delivery because of the development of the abdominal walls. Research by Dr. Evelyn Gendel[†] has indicated that athletic women have quick and easy deliveries. Gendel points out that females should participate in training programs that increase their abdominal strength and circulation because of the beneficial effects this can have on their reproductive ability.

DIFFERENCES BETWEEN TRAINED AND UNTRAINED INDIVIDUALS. A trained individual is in a better state of physical fitness than the individual who follows a sedentary, inactive life. When two individuals, one trained and one untrained, of approximately the same build are performing the same amount of moderate muscular work, there is evidence to indicate that the trained individual has a lower oxygen consumption, lower pulse rate, larger stroke volume per

[*]Klaus, E. J.: The athletic status of woman. In Jokl, E., and Simon, E., editors: International research in sport and physical education, Springfield, Illinois, 1964, Charles C Thomas, Publisher.

[†]Gendel, Evelyn S.: Women and the medical aspects of sports, Journal of School Health **37:** 427-431, 1967.

heartbeat, less rise in blood pressure, greater red and white corpuscle counts, slower rate of breathing, lower rate of lactic acid formation, and a faster return to normal of blood pressure and heart rate. The heart becomes more efficient and is able to circulate more blood while beating less frequently. Furthermore, in work of a very strenuous nature that cannot be performed for any great period of time, the trained individual has greater endurance, a capacity for higher oxygen consumption, and a faster return to normal of heart rate and blood pressure. Training results in a more efficient organism. Since a greater efficiency of heart action enables a larger flow of blood to reach the muscles and thus ensure an increased supply of fuel and oxygen, more work is performed at less cost; improvements are brought about in respect to strength, power, neuromuscular coordination, and endurance; there is a better coordination and timing of movements; and an improved state of physical fitness results.

Oxygen and training and fitness

One of the most controversial questions in athletics concerns the use of oxygen as an aid to performance. It might seem logical to some persons that oxygen would increase fitness by producing a greater capacity for exertion and recovery. However, because oxygen cannot be stored, this is not the case. Research by Miller* has shown that inhalation of oxygen before an event does not affect performance or rate of recovery. Miller, in a study of performers using the treadmill, indicated that the greatest benefit to the performer that oxygen may have is psychological. Most coaches agree that athletes should not be conditioned to the use of oxygen because of the psychological effect it may have if the athlete is deprived of its use at an important event.

*Miller, A. T., Jr.: Influence of oxygen administration on cardiovascular function during exercise and recovery, Journal of Applied Physiology **5:**165-168, 1952.

Environment and training and fitness

It is important to have an understanding of the effects of the environment on physiological state. The environment characterized by pollution will definitely decrease participation in activities. Smog has been known to lower the motivation of runners because of chest discomforts and increasing eye irritations caused by this type of pollution. An understanding of the influence of the environment on activities is important. This discussion is concerned with activities that take place in a cold environment, a hot environment, and high altitudes.

In a cold environment, such as on the ski slopes, athletes must realize the importance of proper dress. The greatest danger to an athlete exercising in a cold environment is the sudden changes in temperature. Temperatures may drop 30° to 40° during a day of skiing. The participant's dress should be comfortable and protective at any time during the changes in temperatures. Many athletes perspire a great deal even in a cold environment. It is not rare to see a football player walking off the field in Green Bay, Wisconsin, in the middle of winter with sweat running down his face. Metabolic rates increase when engaging in vigorous activities regardless of cold or warm weather environments, and the body must dissipate the heat that accumulates by sweating.

Research has indicated that athletes who compete in cold weather environments and perform vigorous activities should wear light clothing that allows sweating. Not all people react to a cold environment in the same manner. Physique is an important factor in determining who can exercise in a cold environment with the least body discomfort. Research has indicated that the heavier man, because of greater fat tissue, will be better able to withstand exercising in a cold environment. Fat tissue is an insulator and preserves heat.

An individual who exercises in a hot environment usually faces more problems than one who exercises in a cold environment. For example, in a hot, humid environment such as in Nevada, the air is both hot and extremely humid. Sweating will be difficult in such an environment because of the deficiency in the volume of air available. The human body is limited as to the amount of heat it can tolerate. Too much exposure can lead to heat cramps, heat exhaustion, and heat stroke.

Heat cramps are caused primarily by a deficiency in salt. During strenuous exercising in a hot environment there is a great deal of salt loss. Heat exhaustion occurs when there is too great a stress on the circulatory system of the body and the body's heat controlling system fails. The individual will normally feel cold and dizzy, there is an immediate increase in body temperature, and medical treatment is necessary. Heat stroke, a state of exhaustion usually accompanied by fever caused by exposure to extensive heat over an extended period of time, has been a leading cause of death for many young football players who engage in this vigorous activity during the summer. Coaches must take adequate precautions with their players to avoid overexertion under such climatic conditions. The National Federation of State High School Athletic Associations and the Committee on the Medical Aspects of Sports of the American Medical Association* have indicated that frequent rest breaks, ample supplies of drinking water, and increased salt intake will help to decrease the possibilities of heat disorders during vigorous workouts in extremely high temperatures.

The 1968 Olympic Games held in Mexico City raised questions as to the ability of athletes to participate in activities at high altitudes. Could athletes who set records at sea level retain their titles at an altitude 7,349 feet above sea level or lose them to athletes who participated in activities at high altitudes for many years? For the most part, the majority of champion athletes left Mexico City with their titles. However, others succumbed to the altitude and lost their competitive edge. What effect does the altitude have on the body while exercising? High altitudes decrease the availability of oxygen to the tissues because the partial pressure of oxygen is lower at high altitudes than at sea level. Events most affected by high altitudes are such events as running and swimming lasting longer than 2 minutes, because performance in prolonged events depends largely on inspired air. Before engaging in exercises at high altitudes, it is important to acclimate to this environment. Dr. Merrit H. Stiles,* the Chairman of the Medical and Training Services Committee of the United States Olympic Committee, stated that vigorous workouts speed up acclimatization and improve performance at high altitudes. Dr. Stiles indicated that 2 to 3 weeks of training at high altitudes will adapt a person to this environment. The adaptive changes the organism undergoes increase the cardiac output and maximum oxygen uptake of the performer.

Warm-up and training and fitness

A major discussion today concerns the use of some type of warm-up procedure before engaging in physical activity. The physical educator and coach should be familiar with the available evidence before determining whether or not to use the warm-up or how to use it most effectively.

Neuberger,† in an analysis of the research on warm-up appearing in the *Research Quarterly* of the American Association of Health, Physical Education, and Recreation over a 13-year period, indicated that 95% of the studies demonstrated that to achieve peak physical performance the individual should warm up. Warm-ups have been found to increase speed, strength, muscular endurance, and power. The re-

---

*Tips on Athletic Training XII, American Medical Association, Committee on the Medical Aspects of Sports, 1970, p. 8.

*Olympic planners discount fear of Mexican altitudes, Medicine in Sports, vol. 8, no. I, January, 1968.

†Neuberger, Tom: What the *Research Quarterly* says about warm-up, Journal of Health, Physical Education, and Recreation **40:**75-77, 1969.

search indicates that vigorous, long warm-ups are better than less moderate ones. Related warm-ups (those similar to the activity to be engaged in) are preferable to unrelated ones because of the practice effect that also results. Attitudes toward warm-up are also related to efficiency in performance. An individual with a positive attitude toward warm-up appears to benefit more from such an experience than one who has a negative attitude. It has been determined that combinations of intensity and duration contribute to the desired effects of a warm-up. Insufficient warm-up does not achieve the high level of muscle strength and temperature desired, and excessive warm-up can lead to fatigue and thus decrease the performance level.

Warm-ups have been found to be important in preventing injury and muscle soreness. It appears that muscle injury can result when vigorous exercises are not preceded by a related warm-up. An effective quick warm-up can also be an effective

motivator. Students who get satisfaction from an effective warm-up usually have a stronger desire to participate in the activity. By contrast, a poor warm-up can lead to fatigue and boredom, limiting the students' attention and ultimately resulting in a poor program.

Jogging and training and fitness

In recent years jogging, which is basicly a combination of walking and running, has become popular as an aid to keeping physically fit. It has received wide approval from many groups because it is a sustained type of exercise that is noncompetitive. An individual does not have to possess any particular skill in order to jog, and the majority of joggers range in age from 35 to 65. Advocates of jogging feel that men and women up to the age of 65 can learn to jog at a good pace. It is extremely important for an individual to have a medical examination and to discover the limits of his heart's endurance, however, before be-

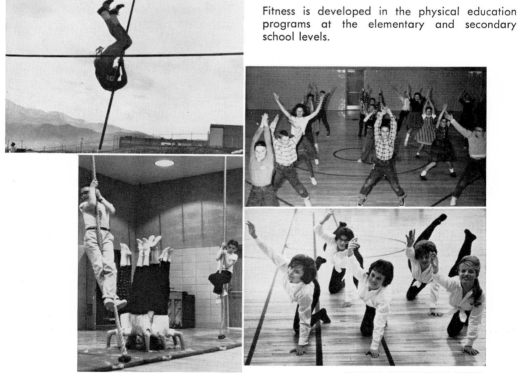

Fitness is developed in the physical education programs at the elementary and secondary school levels.

COLORADO SPRINGS PUBLIC SCHOOL,
COLORADO SPRINGS, COLO.

ginning to jog. Jogging has been found beneficial to some heart-attack victims because it increases the flow of blood to the damaged heart, and it may also help some heart-attack victims to rebuild the endurance in their heart and lungs. Dr. Kenneth H. Cooper,* author of the much publicized book entitled *Aerobics,* has stated that exercises such as jogging force the body to become conditioned to an increased need for oxygen. When the body reaches the level of fitness that meets this need, the cardiopulmonary and oxygen transport systems become more efficient. Among other benefits, jogging also helps the healthy individual who wants to lose weight.

DETERRENTS TO FITNESS

There are several deterrents to a high state of fitness. Some of the more important of these are tobacco, alcohol, and drugs.

Tobacco and fitness

Smoking speeds up the pulse rate, raises the blood pressure, constricts the blood vessels, and may cause other physical damage. In recent investigations there has been some evidence that cigarette smoking interferes with the ability of red blood cells to release oxygen to body tissue. Although the evidence is not fully conclusive, there is some indication that blood from heavy smokers should be rejected for donation purposes because of this deficiency. Smoking has also been linked to many diseases. For example, the correlation between cancer and smoking has been established. There is considerable evidence to indicate that smoking is detrimental to the maintenance of physical fitness. There is no evidence to indicate that it contributes to a higher level of physical performance.

Studies have been conducted in respect to smoking and physical performance. One study of 2,000 runners was conducted over several track seasons. It showed that the nonsmokers took more first places in

competition than did those runners who smoked. Another study showed that students who do not smoke grow more in height, weight, and lung capacity than do those who smoke. The increase in the chest development among the nonsmokers was also greater. Tests of physical steadiness have shown that nonsmokers are far steadier than smokers.

Coaches and physical educators are almost unanimous in feeling that athletic performance and muscular power are lessened through smoking. They feel that fatigue begins earlier among the smokers. Very few coaches of high school and college teams knowingly permit their athletes to smoke. Knute Rockne, a former famous coach at Notre Dame, said: "Tobacco slows the reflexes and any advertising that says it helps an athlete is falsehood and fraud."

Alcohol and fitness

Alcohol depresses the central nervous system. It acts on the higher brain centers that affect decisions, judgment, and memory. The control of the lower brain centers are lost, reaction time is slowed, and physical and emotional pain are reacted to more slowly.

Coaches, almost universally, will not permit their athletes to drink during the seasons of play or at any time during the school year. As in smoking, although there is considerable evidence to show that alcohol hinders physical performance, there is no evidence to show that it improves performance in any way. A great number of automobile accidents can be attributed to loss of control through drinking.

Although drinking has become a popular social custom in our society, the young man or woman who is striving to achieve or maintain a high level of fitness should objectively examine the evidence that shows the result of such a habit.

Drugs and fitness

Marijuana, heroin, LSD (lysergic acid diethylamide), and similar drugs detach a person from reality. They make him oblivious to danger. They induce a sense of well-

*Cooper, Kenneth H.: The role of exercise in our contemporary society, Journal of Health, Physical Education and Recreation **40:**24, 1968.

being by postponing feelings of fatigue. And they start a habit of use that is very difficult to stop.

The use of such drugs as amphetamine (found in pep pills), marijuana, cocaine, heroin, and LSD has become popular among a few of this nation's young people. Amphetamines have been found to produce toxic side effects and cause a person to become dependent on them. Research has indicated that amphetamines do not improve an individual's performance but, rather, they give the individual an illusory feeling that he has improved his performance.

Some drugs have also been used in sports where a high level of energy is required, as in long-distance cycling races. Such a practice is denounced by physical educators, coaches, and sports medicine associations. Athletes at the present time are utilizing drugs known as anabolic steroids. Many athletes, such as weight lifters, have been known to receive large doses of the male sex hormone known as testosterone. Such drugs can have serious side effects on the user. Large doses can cause atrophy of the tubules and also interfere with the functioning of the prostate gland.

The use of drugs such as marijuana, heroin, and LSD is against the law. The continued use of drugs brings about a permanent physical deterioration.

Caffeine, which can be found in coffee, tea, and cola, is a stimulant. Moderate doses of caffeine can increase motor activity. Large doses, however, can decrease the pulse rate, blood pressure, and respiratory rate and produce nervousness. Caffeine has also been found to interfere with carbohydrate and protein metabolism, which is necessary for the production of energy. Most researchers agree that large amounts of caffeine should not be a part of the athlete's daily diet.

WEIGHT CONTROL

There is no easy path to weight reduction. There are no reliable gimmicks or shortcuts. And too many persons are overweight. Weight control involves watching one's diet and following a healthful regime, including regular amounts of physical activity. If a person is careful about his caloric intake and engages regularly in physical activity, there will be a gradual weight reduction. However, in some cases, persons step up their exercise and similarly step up their appetite, resulting in an excessive food intake.

Some research has indicated that exercise does not necessarily increase appetite and thereby make it more difficult to lose weight. The research by Mayer* and his colleagues has shown that, contrary to popular belief, exercise does not necessarily result in greater food intake. An important factor is whether the individual was active to start with. If sedentary in his pursuits there can be a step-up of activity without increase in appetite. Conversely, if activity is decreased below a certain point, depending upon the individual, appetite does not decrease correspondingly. In some cases it may, in fact, increase.

In a few cases obesity may be the result of disease. If a person suspects some disturbance, the first step should be to go to a physician for advice. There is great danger in following any highly commercialized solution involving gadgets and appetite depressant pills. To follow the advice of any person other than a qualified physician is risky and may not only result in a loss of hundreds of dollars but be harmful to one's health.

As far as "spot reducing" goes, medical opinion says "No."† This is an erroneous belief. Weight reduction in such special areas of the body as the hips, thighs, and buttocks is not possible. There is no physiological basis for such claims. Only through a general weight reduction program can a person hope to affect the areas mentioned.

---

*Mayer, J.: Exercise and weight control. In Exercise and fitness, Athletic Institute, 1960.
Mayer, J.: Exercise and weight control. In Johnson, Warren, editor: Science and medicine of exercise and sport, New York, 1960, Harper and Row, Publishers, chap. 16.
†Journal of the American Medical Association, May 14, 1955.

Balancing calorie intake and outgo.

TYPE OF FOOD	NUMBER OF CALORIES PER SERVING	SLEEPING	READING	TYPING
RAW CARROT	42	36	23	18
BOILED EGG	77	66	43	33
BREAD AND BUTTER	78	67	43	34
TWO STRIPS OF BACON	96	82	53	41
LARGE APPLE	101	87	56	44
FRIED EGG	110	94	61	47
ONE GLASS OF BEER	114	98	63	49
GELATIN WITH CREAM	117	100	65	50
ONE GLASS OF ORANGE JUICE	120	103	67	52
PANCAKE WITH SYRUP	124	106	69	53
ONE GLASS OF MILK	166	142	92	71
CHEESE PIZZA	180	154	100	77
DRY CEREAL WITH MILK AND SUGAR	200	171	111	86
HALF A BREAST OF FRIED CHICKEN	232	199	129	100
T-BONE STEAK	235	201	131	101
ICE-CREAM SODA	255	219	142	110
TUNA-FISH SALAD SANDWICH	278	238	154	119
HAMBURGER	350	300	194	150
ONE-SIXTH APPLE PIE	377	323	209	162
SPAGHETTI	396	339	220	170
STRAWBERRY SHORTCAKE	400	343	222	172

Numbers in activity columns are minutes

BOWLING	GOLF	ROWING	WALKING	TENNIS	BICYCLING	STAIR-CLIMBING	SWIMMING	RUNNING
10	8	8	8	6	5	4	4	2
17	15	15	15	11	9	8	7	4
18	16	16	15	11	10	8	7	4
22	19	19	18	14	12	10	9	5
23	20	20	19	14	12	10	9	5
25	22	22	21	15	13	11	10	6
26	23	23	22	16	14	12	10	6
27	23	23	23	16	14	12	10	6
27	24	24	23	17	15	12	11	6
28	25	25	24	17	15	13	11	6
38	33	33	32	23	20	17	15	9
41	36	36	35	25	22	18	16	9
45	40	40	38	28	24	20	18	10
53	46	46	45	33	28	24	21	12
53	47	47	45	33	29	24	21	12
58	51	51	49	36	31	26	23	13
63	56	56	53	39	34	28	25	14
80	70	70	67	49	43	36	31	18
86	75	75	73	53	46	38	34	19
90	79	79	76	56	48	40	35	20
91	80	80	77	56	49	41	36	21

Claims made for massage and shaking devices are also ineffective, according to authoritative opinion. Dr. Peter V. Karpovich, a respected expert in the field of physiology and associated with Springfield College in Massachusetts, says that the claims of self-massage and shaking devices for loss or redistribution of fat deposits are based on misrepresentation of facts. They are useless as a means of weight loss.

STRESS

Stress, according to Dr. Hans Selye,* is essentially the rate of all the wear and tear caused by life. Each person experiences some degree of stress during each moment of existence. Stress can be caused by an injury, but it can also be caused by a happy occasion. Stress can be good, and it can also be bad for a person.

The important thing is that the body must be prepared to meet stress. The formula for enjoying life is learning how to make adjustments in a world that is constantly changing and in which events do not always run smoothly. These adjustments can be more readily made by the person who understands his body and the ways and means of meeting stress. It is felt that to some extent disorders involving such things as nervous disturbances, high blood pressure, and ulcers are caused by lack of understanding in knowing how to adapt.

Selye points out that stress has three phases. The first is the alarm that is sounded by the endocrine, circulatory, or nervous systems. If the stressor persists, the body offers a resistance in an attempt to combat the stressor agents. Finally, if the battle is not waged successfully, the body enters a stage of exhaustion that can have very severe consequences.

Ernest Michael,† in reviewing several research studies concerned with the endocrine and autonomic nervous systems, has in-

dicated that regular exercises may increase the sensitivity of the adrenal glands. Such an increase in sensitivity may result in a greater response to stress. The important thing for the physical educator to recognize is that physical activity, it is believed, can help to break the chain of harmful stress and thus have a beneficial impact upon the body. Therefore, in order to maintain a proper body balance, activity is essential and should be encouraged as an antidote to those harmful stressful experiences that appear in every person's life.

FATIGUE

Fatigue is a phenomenon that all individuals experience. It is a temporary inability of the muscular system to perform efficiently. It is felt at the end of a hard day's work, after strong muscular effort, when one has time on his hands with nothing to do, after one has passed through an exciting experience, and after periods of intense emotional strain. It results in a decrease in the ability to do work and a feeling of uneasiness. It is a phenomenon that may be aided by sleep, recreation, and physical activity.

There are different types of fatigue. First, there is a *physical* fatigue which a person experiences after a hard day's work, after extreme muscular work, after playing tennis all day, or after pitching hay for 8 hours. The cure for physical fatigue is a good sleep. Second, there is *mental* fatigue. This is the type of fatigue a person experiences after cramming 5 hours for an examination, after working on his income tax a whole evening, or after finishing the monthly report to the boss. Mental fatigue may also be the result of nothing to do or boredom. When a person sits around without anything to occupy the mind, yawns start to appear and a state of mental fatigue ensues. Finally, mental fatigue may be the result of a trying emotional experience, such as attending the funeral of a close friend, getting angry at your next-door neighbor, or worrying about where the next meal is coming from. In many cases the cure for

---

*Selye, Hans: The stress of life, New York, 1956, McGraw-Hill Book Co.

†Michael, Ernest D.: Stress adaption through exercise, Research Quarterly **28:**50-54, 1957.

mental fatigue is participation in some form of recreational activity. When a person is engaged in painting a beautiful picture, weaving a rug, trying to catch a bass, or getting par on the golf course, he forgets about his mental problems, boredom, and emotional upsets and enjoys living. Fatigue disappears and the individual is ready to conquer new worlds.

Karpovich lists six places where fatigue may be located. There are three possible seats of fatigue apart from the central nervous system. These are in the fiber of the muscle, at the points of union between the muscle fiber and its nerve or motor end plate, and in the motor nerve fiber. The other three possible seats of fatigue are located within the central nervous system. These are at the synapse, where impulses pass from one neuron to another and where fatigue causes the transmitting of impulses to be slowed, in the nerve cell body, and in the secondary end organs.

Teacher fatigue*

Fatigue, as related to our energy and performance, can be both harmful and beneficial. Constructively, it can induce us to refreshing sleep or sound the warning signal that exhaustion is not far off. Destructively, it can destroy initiative or transform us from exuberant, active human beings into tired, lifeless creatures oblivious of our responsibilities.

Teaching is one of the most fatiguing of all the professions. Students sap the teacher's energy; papers to be graded or extracurricular activities drain vitality; evening meetings or other after-school responsibilities interrupt rest.

Teacher fatigue can be alleviated by action proceeding from an analysis of the factors causing it and an understanding of how they can be minimized.

Environmental factors may contribute to fatigue. A teacher's bank account of energy

---

*This discussion is based on an article by Bucher, Charles A.: National Education Association Journal, December, 1959.

may be depleted in schools that are located next door to noisy factories or that have poor systems of ventilation, dim lighting, or overheated classrooms.

Type of work can also affect the degree of fatigue. Too much work or unsatisfying or monotonous work can result in mental fatigue. Too much physical labor can cause muscular weariness.

The attitude of a teacher toward his work may be a source of trouble. Whether he regards the position as challenging or boring makes a difference. The poor physical condition of the instructor or a lack of cultural, recreational, or community interests may be the culprit. Emotions such as hate, frustration, and anxiety are notable troublemakers. The teacher's daily habits with regard to diet, exercise, relaxation, rest, and play can also contribute to or help alleviate fatigue.

Cutting down on fatigue requires the help of the teacher and the school. Some things the teacher can do to deal with the problem are as follows:

1. Be inwardly motivated and propelled toward accomplishing school tasks. If a teacher does not recognize the importance of teaching and does not derive satisfaction from his job, the fatigue is probably from boredom.
2. Try to cut down on emotional turmoil by planning, by facing problems realistically, and by setting attainable standards. Work to develop self-control and try not to become involved in feelings of anger, fear, hate, and frustration.
3. Eliminate monotony by varying tasks. Throw out the class plan that has been used over and over again. Vary the daily schedule. Get a "new look."
4. Live a balanced life that involves participating in some vigorous activity, following a nutritious diet, getting ample rest and relaxation, and spending a few moments each day in self-evaluation. All work and no play also makes dull teachers.
5. Try to cut down on routine chores.
6. Practice some techniques for relaxation. Gardening is better than television, and making a set of bookends is often more refreshing than stretching out on the sofa.
7. Remember fatigue is cumulative; rest before it builds up.

Some universities and colleges have es-

Table 16-1. Physical fitness ratings of popular sports in the United States*

Sport	Endurance	Agility	Strength			Age range recommended
			Leg	Abdomen	Arm and shoulders	
Archery	L	L	L	M	H	All ages
Badminton	H-M	H	H	M	M	Singles to 50
Basketball	H	H	H	L	L	Under 30
Baseball	M	H	H	M	M	Under 45
Bicycling	M	L	H	L	L	All ages
Bowling	L	L	M	L	M	All ages
Boating	M	L	M	M	H	All ages
Field hockey	H	H	H	M	M	Under 30
Football	H	H	H	H	H	Under 30
Golf	L	L	M	L	L	All ages
Handball	H-M	H	H	M	H	Singles to 45
Heavy apparatus Tumbling	L	H	H-M	H	H	Under 45
Hiking	M	L	H	L	L	All ages
Horseshoes	L	L	L	L	M	All ages
Judo	H	H	H	H	H	Under 30
Lifesaving	H	M	H	H	H	Under 45
Skating Speed	H	M	H	M	L	Under 45
Figure	M	H	H	L	L	All ages
Skiing	H	H	H	M	M	Under 45
Soccer	H	H	H	M	L	Under 45
Swimming Recreational	M	L	M	L	M	All ages
Competitive	H	M	H	M	H	Under 30
Table tennis	L	M	M	L	L	All ages
Tennis	H-M	H	H	M	M	Singles to 45
Track Distance	H	L	H	M	M	Under 45
Sprints	M	M	H	M	M	Under 45
Volleyball	L	M	M	L	M	All ages
Wrestling	H	H	H	H	H	Under 30

Key to abbreviations: H, high; M, medium; L, low (fitness values).

*Steinhaus, Arthur H.: How to keep fit and like it, Chicago, 1957, The Dartnell Corp., p. 70; copyrighted by George Williams College.

tablished Faculty Fitness Programs. At the University of Arizona* the school's Department of Health, Physical Education, and Recreation created an exercise program that was aimed at making vigorous exercise a regular part of the daily routine of faculty members who led a sedentary existence. The daily exercise program consisted of 20 minutes of light calisthenics, flexibility, and muscular endurance exercises and 20 min-

---

*Munroe, Richard A.: Faculty fitness program at the University of Arizona, Physical Fitness News Letter, series XV, no. 3, November, 1968, pp. 2-4.

utes of sustained movement, such as running and jogging. Faculty members participating in the program not only felt better but also lost weight and improved their oxygen intake.

RELAXATION AND RECREATION

Relaxation contributes to one's health and may actually be in the form of physical activity. Relaxation is essentially a mental phenomenon concerned with the reduction of tensions that could originate from muscular activity but that are more likely to result from pressures of contemporary living. Today's way of life has created high-tension living. Mounting pressures have resulted in an increase of certain mental and physical ailments. Ulcers, heart attacks, and nervous and psychiatric disorders may be related to states of tension.

A technique for achieving relaxation or nervous reeducation has been developed by Jacobson.* It has two basic steps.

In the first step the individual learns to recognize muscle tension in subtle as well as in gross forms. Gross tension is easily identified. With fists tightly clenched, he holds his arms outstretched to the side at shoulder height for 1 minute. He observes the feeling of exertion and discomfort in the forearms and shoulders. The arms are dropped to the side and the muscles of the arms and hands relaxed completely. The effortless relaxation which Dr. Jacobson calls the "negative of exertion" can be noted. Subtle tension, involving less muscle effort than that just illustrated, is sometimes difficult to detect. It takes concentration and practice to learn to recognize minor tension in the trunk, neck, face, throat, and other body parts.

In the second step the individual learns to relax completely. First, the large muscle groups—arms, legs, trunk, and neck—are relaxed. Then the forehead, eyes, face, and even the throat have tension eased through a program of passive relaxation. Carried out in the proper fashion, the program teaches the subject to relax his whole body to the point of negative exertion. The result is a release of tension, an antidote to fatigue, and also an inducement to sleep.

Leisure-time activities such as games and sports, hobbies and avocations, and intellectual and artistic endeavors like painting and sculpturing are considered to be excellent means for eliminating boredom and tension. These recreational activities provide a means of relaxation. Long abused as simply childish diversion or amusement,

---

*Jacobson, Edmund: Anxiety and tension control, a physiological approach, Philadelphia, 1964, J. B. Lippincott Co.

recreation is being suggested as an antidote for some of the tensions each person experiences in his daily life.

FITNESS STATE OF THE UNION— A PROFESSIONAL CHALLENGE

A positive or a negative picture can be painted for the state of the Union's fitness. On the positive side it can be shown that there are fewer deaths today per 1,000 population than existed five decades ago and that the average life expectancy has increased since 1900.

Deaths per 1,000 population for the 1-year to 24-year age group:
    1910—5.6 deaths
    1960—0.8 death
Deaths per 1,000 population for the 25-year to 44-year age group:
    1910—7.6 deaths
    1960—2.3 deaths
Average length of life:
    The average length of life for babies born in 1969 is 70.5 years as compared with 47.3 years for babies born in 1900.
Persons who were 45 years of age in 1959:
    These persons could on the average expect to live another 29.3 years as compared to 24.8 years for those persons who reached 45 years of age in 1900.

These health statistics are encouraging and to a large degree are a tribute to better hospital and medical care in the United States. But it is not sufficient to make a judgment on the nation's fitness by looking only at this bright side of the coin. The other side must also be considered—the negative side. The fitness state of the union cannot be judged solely by deaths per 1,000 persons or length of life. It is important also to be cognizant of such factors as the vigor, strength, emotional stability, and the muscular state of the union—factors basic to the full development and use of each person's inherent capacities. Educators must be concerned not only with whether people are alive or dead but also with such factors as how vigorous a life they are living, how healthy they are, how emotionally fit they are, and how well they have developed all the facets of their total makeup. When educators take a look in this direction, the outlook is not as favorable and there is still much work to be done.

1. On validated physical fitness tests American youths lag far behind their counterparts in England, Austria, Italy, Switzerland, Denmark, Japan, and other countries around the world.
2. During recent years nearly one-half of Americans called up for the armed services were turned down for moral or physical deficiencies.
3. Approximately one-half of all hospital beds are occupied by patients suffering from some form of mental illness.
4. The rate of failure has risen steadily on the fitness examinations of college freshmen in some institutions of higher learning.
5. An estimated 60% of the nation's schoolchildren do not participate in a daily program of vigorous physical activity.
6. In a recent year schools in five states, working in cooperation with the President's Council on Physical Fitness and Sports, gave standardized physical tests to more than 200,000 students. Nearly one-half of the youngsters failed to meet minimum standards of strength, agility, and flexibility. Fewer than one in ten passed more comprehensive tests of physical achievement.
7. Only an estimated 28% of the schools in this country have adequate health and physical education programs.

PRESIDENT'S COUNCIL ON PHYSICAL FITNESS AND SPORTS

As a result of the Kraus-Weber studies of the physical fitness status of American and European youth, President Eisenhower created the President's Council on Youth Fitness, the name being changed to the President's Council on Physical Fitness by President Kennedy. During President Lyndon Johnson's administration the name was changed to the President's Council on Physical Fitness and Sports.

Under Eisenhower's administration a nationwide program was established that emphasized cooperation with state, city, and town officials to raise the nation's fitness level. When President Kennedy came into office, he appointed Charles B. Wilkinson, football coach of the University of Oklahoma, his special presidential consultant and placed the Council under his direction. The Council developed and organized, with the cooperation and help of nineteen lead-

ing school and medical organizations (the American Association for Health, Physical Education, and Recreation played a most active role), a suggested program of physical fitness for the nation's schools. President Nixon also reorganized the President's Council on Physical Fitness and Sports and directed the Council to study the status of school physical education, physical fitness programs, and the physical fitness of America's adults and to revise the literature in regard to youth and adult physical fitness.

The President's Council on Physical Fitness and Sports has devoted much time to promoting a school-centered program for physical fitness. In addition, it has accomplished special working relationships with institutions of higher learning, community groups, voluntary agencies, and other key organizations. It has mobilized mass media to communicate to the general public the need to be fit. It has utilized television, movies, radio, and articles in national magazines very effectively in this promotional campaign.

The President's Council on Physical Fitness and Sports in recent years has been responsible for the conduct of various regional physical fitness clinics that have featured some of the nation's physical fitness leaders and also the Council staff. Statewide councils or commissions have been established in many states by either the governor of the state or other agency or organization. State superintendents of education have indicated their active support of the physical fitness movement in approximately one-half of the states. Statewide conferences on fitness have been held in a majority of the states in the country. Several fitness films have been produced. Publications have been printed for all segments of the population, including boys, girls, and adults. Materials have been prepared for release to television stations, radio stations, and other communication media. Millions of dollars worth of free advertising has been made available to the Council. Presidential Fitness Awards have been established and demonstration centers have been developed.

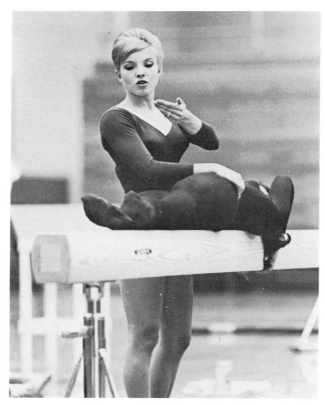

Representatives of the President's Council on Physical Fitness and Sports participating in demonstrations for the Council.

The demonstration centers merit further discussion. For example, in California, schools were selected as state and national physical education demonstration centers. The purpose of these centers is to focus attention upon outstanding school programs of health and physical education that contribute to the development of a physically fit youth. The centers in California have attracted much attention with school administrators and other interested persons visiting them.

The President's Council on Physical Fitness and Sports is also concerned with summer programs in physical education. In conjunction with the National Collegiate Athletic Association, it has established the National Summer Youth Sports Program (NSYSP).* This program provides disad-

*Newsletter, President's Council on Physical Fitness and Sports, pp. 1-2.

vantaged youth of cities the opportunity to participate in planned physical activities. Children and young people receive physical examinations, daily meals, and sports instruction and have the opportunity to participate in competitive events. The staff of the NSYSP is largely composed of physical educators, coaches, and athletes, with many of the latter coming from city ghetto areas.

The President's Council on Physical Fitness and Sports believes the following elements are basic to instruction in physical education and health:

1. Full recognition by physical educators, health educators, parents, citizens, and school administrators that the attainment and maintenance of physical fitness is a basic responsibility of physical education and health education.

2. A daily class period allotted to physical education, grades K through twelve.

3. During this period, every girl and boy

participates in sufficient vigorous activity to insure the benefits which result from exercise. This is the unique function of physical education.

4. Every physical education class should be conducted to provide proper warm-up, sequence of activities, progressive development of strength, endurance, and other physical attributes.

5. Teachers must, themselves, project the image of fitness. They always should endeavor to be examples through personal appearance, enthusiasm, and participation.

6. In addition to the period allotted for physical education, sufficient curriculum time should be provided to adequately teach healthful and safe living, which includes an understanding of the effects of inactivity and the role of exercise in the development and maintenance of good health.

In order of priority, the Council's objectives include:

1. To encourage all elementary and secondary schools to provide a physical education program which includes the four basic concepts . . . :

   (a) Every child should have a medical examination, with proper follow-through, upon entrance to school, and periodically thereafter at least three additional times in his school career.

   (b) Use of a screening test to identify the physically underdeveloped child, and provision of a developmental program to meet individual needs.

   (c) A daily physical education period which conforms to items 2 and 3 above.

   (d) Use of a comprehensive testing program to evaluate pupil progress and to motivate improvement.

2. To encourage elementary and secondary schools to work toward quality programs, encompassing the administrative standards set forth in the "Blue Book."

3. To develop basic recommendations for health education . . . and to work for the implementation of the recommendations.

4. To establish suggested guide lines for health education and physical education at various grade levels to encourage progressively developmental programs in school systems throughout the country. (Because of the increasing mobility and urbanization of the American population, such guide lines are recommended to encourage equalized opportunities for all our children and youth.)

5. To develop basic recommendations to insure the physical fitness of college students.*

The U. S. Office of Education surveyed the nation's schools to find the impact on

---

*President's Council on Physical Fitness: Policy statement on school health and physical education (mimeographed).

physical education of the President's Council and found that 56% of the 108,000 public schools improved their programs during one school year. Improvement meant they added a screening test to identify physically underdeveloped pupils, and/or a comprehensive test of physical achievement, and/or more vigorous physical activity during the class period.

John F. Sweeney, Director of Guidance and Counseling for the Springfield, Missouri, public schools, conducted a special study for the President's Council that attempted to determine some relationships between academic performance and physical fitness. Sweeney was interested in finding out how students who maintain a high level of physical fitness performed in their academic work and also what their attitude was toward school and their studies. The research rated students in four areas: (1) grade average, (2) attendance, (3) participation in extracurricular activities, and (4) attitude. There were two student groups, one a very select group of 442 freshmen and juniors who had passed a comprehensive test of physical achievement and ranked in the upper 40% of their classes on the basis of physical performance. The other group was composed of 200 juniors and freshmen whose records were taken at random from the school files. Equal numbers of boys and girls were in both groups. The select group's collective grade average was better, they participated in 50% more extracurricular activities, missed fewer days of school, and had a more enthusiastic attitude toward their schoolwork.

PROGRESS BEING MADE TO IMPROVE PHYSICAL FITNESS OF NATION'S CHILDREN AND YOUTH

Data indicate that progress is being made in improving the physical fitness of American youth. According to information released by the President's Council on Physical Fitness and Sports, the 1960's witnessed improvement in physical achievement standards among the nation's youth. For example, 9.2 million children are participating in school physical education programs; four out of every five pupils now successfully pass standardized physical fitness tests (only two out of three passed in 1961); 68% of all schools have strengthened their physical activity programs; the number of parochial schools providing physical education instruction has doubled; and seventeen states have raised their school physical education requirements. Rhode Island and West Virginia have established state supervisory positions in health, physical education, and recreation.

A survey conducted by Hunsicker and Reiff* and supported by the Cooperative Research Program of the U. S. Office of Education shows the progress made in grades five through twelve when the AAHPER Youth Fitness Test was used as the instrument of measurement. There was an increase in the physical fitness level of public school children during the 7-year period. Initially the test was given to approximately 8,000 pupils in order to develop national norms for the seven-item test. Seven years later a similar group of pupils was given the same test and fared much better than their counterparts did several years earlier. A comparison on two items of the text, for example, shows that when the tests were first given, a 15-year-old boy ran 600 yards in 2 minutes, 19 seconds and did 45 sit-ups, while a 15-year-old girl ran 600 yards in 3 minutes, 19 seconds and did 18 sit-ups. Seven years later, on the other hand, the 15-year-old boy ran 600 yards in 2 minutes and did 73 sit-ups, while the 15-year-old girl ran 600 yards in 2 minutes and did 28 sit-ups.

A survey conducted by the Division of Health, Physical Education, and Recreation in New York State during a 2-year span shows the improvement in the physical fitness of students in one of the nation's most populous states.* Initially 25% of those students in grades four to twelve were physically underdeveloped as indicated by the New York State Physical Fitness Screening Test, whereas 2 years later only 12% were classified as underdeveloped. The lowest physical fitness levels were found at the elementary school level and the highest at the high school level. Throughout the school years boys were slightly above the girls in their physical fitness achievement levels. At all grade levels public school pupils were significantly higher in their physical achievement levels than private school pupils.

Reasons given for the progress made by New York State students in achieving higher physical fitness levels in recent years include the increased national, state, and local emphasis upon physical fitness, the recognition by pupils of the importance of physical fitness in their own lives, and the increased skill development by pupils in the "lifetime" sports.

Still room for improvement

There is still much progress to be made in improving the nation's level of physical fitness. For example, an estimated 14% of the children in school today do not participate in any physical activity program, and an additional 27% participate only 1 or 2 days per week; only about four schools in ten provide physical education programs 5 days per week; and approximately 23% of the schools have administered the American Association for Health, Physical Education, and Recreation seven-item physical achievement test, but on this test only 57% of the boys and 51% of the girls were reported to have scored "satisfactory" on all items.

Tests also show that American boys and girls in their physical development are weak in such areas as the shoulder girdle. They are also lacking in endurance and flexibility.

---

*Hunsicker, Paul A., and Reiff, Guy G.: A survey and comparison of youth fitness, 1958–1965, Ann Arbor, 1965, University of Michigan Press.

*Straub, William: State survey shows 130,040 pupils physically unfit, New York State Journal of Health, Physical Education, and Recreation **19:**22 (fall issue), 1967.

Statistics show that approximately one-half of the draftees being disqualified from the armed services are failing because of physical reasons. Furthermore, records show that one out of every four Americans is overweight.

PROGRESS BEING MADE IN ADULT FITNESS

The children and youth of America are not the only members of the nation's population becoming physical fitness minded. Adults are conscious of the state of their physical fitness. The President's Council on Physical Fitness and Sports has contributed much to this movement by publishing a pamphlet entitled *Adult Physical Fitness,* which provides a home exercise program for men and women, and also by distributing information on exercise, aging, and other pertinent subjects. The Young Men's Christian Association has provided special

Comparison of test results.

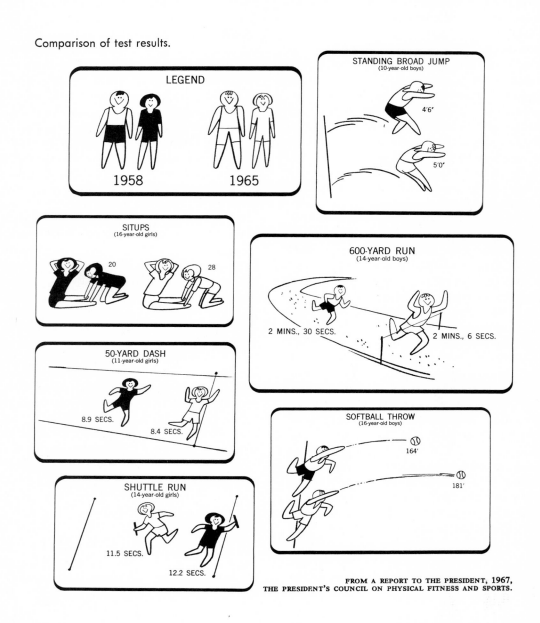

FROM A REPORT TO THE PRESIDENT, 1967, THE PRESIDENT'S COUNCIL ON PHYSICAL FITNESS AND SPORTS.

clinics, programs, and pilot studies on physical fitness for adults, including business executives. Industrial concerns have developed fitness and recreation programs for their personnel on a large scale throughout the country. The armed forces have shown increased interest in how they can better physically train the men in uniform. Also, such organizations as the American Medical Association, parent-teacher associations, adult education organizations, athletic clubs, and gymnastic organizations have given emphasis to the adult fitness movement.

The need for adult physical fitness is a result of several conditions. Some of the more pertinent factors are the increased leisure, the changing nature of man's work involving less and less activity, the pressures and speed of modern existence, the prevalence of heart disease and other ailments where exercise is thought to be a preventive factor, and the desire for greater productivity.

Industrial organizations have expanded their fitness programs in recent years. Physical activities are very popular, including such sports as softball, bowling, basketball, golf, tennis, volleyball, judo, aquatics, badminton, and handball. These activities are offered under conditions where individuals, couples, and families can participate and where industrial leagues provide activity for the more competitively minded persons.

In addition to a broad program of activities for the rank and file of the working population, executives are also being provided programs. Exercise routines, massage, weight-control programs, sports competition, and many other activities are being offered. The Gates Rubber Company in Colorado has created a gymnasium in their plant in order to give their workers an opportunity to exercise. Industrial concerns feel that the large investment they have in their key men must be protected, and so physical fitness programs are coming into vogue to help increase the productivity of the executive class and also increase their service in number of years to the company. Industrial companies are also involved in

research in the area of physical fitness.*

In 1966 an experimental facility and program was implemented by the National Aeronautics and Space Administration's Division of Occupational Medicine. In conjunction with the President's Council on Physical Fitness and Sports and Bio-Dynamics, Inc., this facility serves as a research laboratory where studies are made on the health of industrial executives. The facility is known as the physical stress laboratory because its prime concern is determining the effects of stress on the health of executives. The program is also aimed at increasing the executive's motivation for physical activity and reducing the deterrents to exercise that exist.

The Central YMCA of greater New York in recent years has conducted several Executive Fitness Weekends. At these sessions various physical fitness tests are administered to executives and recommendations are made in regard to exercise programs.

Communities† are also becoming more involved in improving the fitness level of their adult citizens. Recently the Eugene, Oregon, *Register-Guard* newspaper established an Adult Fitness School. The School's purposes are primarily concerned with educating the area's adults in the importance of physical fitness for good health and teaching principles of exercise, diet, and rest applicable in one's day-to-day activities. The school also gives each adult an experience in a physical activity, helps each adult plan a program of physical fitness, and orients him as to community facilities available.

PROGRESS BEING MADE IN PHYSICAL FITNESS FOR THE ATYPICAL INDIVIDUAL

In recent years it has been recognized that physical fitness programs can benefit

---

*Duggar, Benjamin C., and Swengros, Glenn V.: The design of physical activity programs for industry, Journal of Occupational Medicine 11(6): 322-329, 1969.

†Register-Guard and Gary Winen team up, Physical Fitness Newsletter, series XVII, no. 2, October, 1970, pp. 5-6.

those individuals who suffer from mental and emotional problems. Today, in the United States, it is estimated there are over 5.4 million emotionally disturbed children between the ages of 5 to 17 and over 2.7 million mentally retarded persons under the age of 21. Professionals who work with delinquent youngsters point out that many such persons are not physically fit, and many suffer from severe emotional and physical problems. The Physical Education Department at the Youth Development Center in New Castle, Pennsylvania,* has stated that most delinquents are healthy and physically able; however, their physical ability has not been properly developed. Authorities at the Center point out that delinquent youths have not received the proper education as to how to use their physical abilities for something other than self-protection and violence. Their program stresses physical fitness and swimming activities. Their officers indicate that students become motivated to participate in the program when they realize that they can develop more self-respect by becoming physically fit.

It has also been found that physical activities can be beneficial in aiding the psychiatric patient. Marusak† studied the effects of exercise on the psychiatric patient, and on the basis of his observations it was found that physical exercises were of value in channeling aggression, increasing socialization, and improving the fitness level of these people.

All children need the opportunity to achieve success. The educable mentally retarded boy, for example, has improved his physical fitness through participation in planned physical education experiences. Amiel Solomon and Roy Pangle,‡ in a

---

*Libicer, Stephen J., Jr.: The name of the game is fitness, Outlook 1(2):1, 4, 1969.

†Marusak, F. M.: The use of corrective therapy in a psychiatric treatment program, Journal of the Association of Physical and Mental Rehabilitation 5:9-11, 1952.

‡Solomon, Amiel, and Pangle, Roy: Demonstrating physical fitness improvement in the EMR, Exceptional Children, November, 1967, pp. 177-181.

study of educable mentally retarded boys, administered the AAHPER Youth Physical Fitness Test to a group of forty-two youngsters. After an 8-week period of planned activities, the group that received the training increased their level of fitness.

FITNESS SUCCESS FORMULA

Newspaper and magazine articles and television and radio commercials are sounding the need for a tougher, stronger, and more physically fit youth. Schools and communities are building spacious gymnasiums, playgrounds, and athletic facilities. Taxpayers are pumping thousands of hard-earned dollars into exercise and sports programs.

But is the answer to physical fitness as simple as this? Will providing the facilities, the leagues, the equipment, and the opportunities for youth to be participants be enough to yield the desired results?

The answer is NO. A physically fit population cannot be achieved solely through exercise programs for a captive youth in the schools and dazzling athletic programs in the communities of the nation. There are many physically fit adults who never exercised in a school gymnasium or played in an organized community recreation program, but they had something that many young people do not have—respect for their bodies and a determination to stay in "top" shape. They wanted to be physically fit because they knew it was good for them, and so they provided time and their own means to achieve this goal.

Today's American boys and girls have better food, medical care, and housing than any generation preceding them. They weigh more, are taller, have less disease, and possess firmer foundations for a strong, healthy body than most youngsters around the world. It is paradoxical, therefore, to find that tests of physical fitness picture them as soft, flabby, and weak. These muscular yardsticks show America's young people cannot run without puffing, perform sit-ups without groaning, or lift without grunting. And when they were compared with their counterparts abroad, they came out second best. Why?

The explanation being clarioned to the local communities is that our youngsters do not exercise enough. To correct this situation these remedies are cited: "Get them into sports." "Build more gymnasiums and swimming pools." "Put them on bicycles." "Make them walk to school." "Turn off the television set." "Give them calisthenics."

Educators and public-spirited citizens listen to this advice and conclude that the answer to physically inept young people is to provide a daily program of exercise in the schools and a wide variety of sports programs in the community. Simply by providing opportunities for physical activity, they feel our youth will become strong and tough. BUT WILL THEY?

What school personnel and the public in general must recognize is that to get the desired results, boys and girls must also be inwardly motivated to want to be physically fit. The reason children and youth are soft is not only that they do not have the opportunity to achieve physical fitness but also that they do not fully appreciate and know why physical fitness is important to themselves and to their country. They do not see the relationship between their fitness and their personal success, health, and productivity. They do not know simple physiological facts that would help them to understand what happens to their bodies when they exercise regularly. They do not possess skill to motivate them into activity. There is nothing inside that propels them into action.

Also, young people do not seem to fully appreciate the stake they have in the future of this country and how they can most contribute. They do not seem to understand that to be physically fit is fundamental to the preservation of the democratic way of life and the accomplishment of national purposes. Democracy is not a spectator sport. It is a game where all Americans are participants, and today's life-and-death struggle demands all-out effort on the part of each person. This requires total fitness, including intellectual, physical, and emotional fitness.

I invited five teen-agers with high IQ's into a graduate-school education class at New York University. These boys and girls represented outstanding high schools in New York, Pennsylvania, and New Jersey. Each of these schools had broad physical education and athletic programs. In a frank exchange of opinion, these youngsters showed they were devoid of information as to what physical fitness is and the physiological benefits accruing from exercise. They possessed few physical skills and felt the main purpose of the physical education and athletic program is to have some fun and improve school morale.

I spent a sabbatical traveling 6,500 miles and visiting many high schools and colleges throughout the United States. It was very disturbing to find that many young people think it is smart to cheat on their health. They feel it is high fashion, sophisticated, or romantic to smoke two packs of cigarettes a day, drink a coke and eat a candy bar for lunch, and go to bed at 2 A.M. They think they will get by without any bad effects.

I traveled around the world observing education programs in many parts of the globe. One thing that impressed me in Japan, where comparative tests have shown their young people to be much more physically fit than in the United States, is that textbooks, lectures, and discussions are a part of many physical education programs. The schools and colleges attempt to get at the "why" of the activity as well as the activity itself. Many higher education institutions, for example, follow this type of program.

The United States has a very intelligent crop of young people, and they are not going to sweat or puff unless given a good reason. And if they are to be physically fit, they are going to have to understand and know that the time spent in the pursuit of this goal has its rewards.

The importance of educating young people in health matters is shown by a study conducted by the American Cancer Society among 22,000 high school students in Portland, Oregon. The research team set out to determine what type of approach was best in influencing smoking among students. Of the five different approaches that were used, the most effective was that of providing the facts about smoking and then allowing the student to decide whether or not to smoke on the basis of this knowledge. Previous to the study, each successive school grade had a higher percentage of smokers than the preceding grade. For example, 14.5% of the freshmen boys smoked, whereas 35.4% of the senior boys smoked. But after a year's study of basic facts, the student body as a whole showed that the number of new students who took up smoking dropped from 13% to 7.7% among the boys and 6.4% to 2.1% among the girls. The researchers projecting these figures over a 4-year period estimated that about 20% of the high school students who would ordinarily be smoking regularly by graduation time would not do so.

When young people become educated about desirable health practices, it helps to ensure an intelligent choice because they KNOW it is the wise thing to do. Boys and girls need to be *physically educated* to understand why they should have such essentials as regular physical activity, good nutrition, and proper rest and sleep. This approach will get results.

What are the essential ingredients for a physically educated youth? The answer is written into this formula:

**Knowledge + Attitude + Skill + Activity =
Physical fitness**

Knowledge

Today's boys and girls need to know the facts about physical fitness. First of all, young people should recognize that physical fitness is the basis for excellent performance whether as a student, scientist, teacher, mechanic, or leisure-time sports enthusiast. As President Kennedy pointed out: "The foundation of intellectual fitness

is physical fitness." Well-being is a means to an end, the end being a more productive, vigorous, interesting, and rewarding life.

Boys and girls need to know that physical fitness is more than just having enough strength to chin themselves and carry out their daily duties. It also means having a sound, healthy heart, lungs, and musculature and other aspects of medical fitness; and the best time to get good organic development is before 20 years of age. It means having the necessary stamina, speed, agility, endurance, and coordination to use bodily equipment in an efficient manner; and it means possessing physical skills that will enable a person to engage in sports successfully.

Young people need simple physiological knowledge, such as this: Exercise makes the blood circulate faster to meet the need for more oxygen and food; as a result the cells of the body benefit; the blood manufactures more red cells and hemoglobin; and the cells are better nourished and grow larger so that the muscles gain in strength and flexibility.

Boys and girls should know that the values of exercise rest upon the application of three scientifically based principles.

1. *Frequency.* The benefits cannot be stored; they are only gained through regular participation.
2. *Duration.* A sufficient length of time is needed to give the body a good workout.
3. *Intensity.* The activity must be vigorous enough to place a load on the circulatory and respiratory systems.

Young people need to know that, although the path to physical fitness is the result of heredity and the absence of strains and drains on the human system, the most important consideration for them is *the way they live*—kind of food they eat, exercise they get, hours they sleep, and other health habits they follow.

Fallacies need to be exploded, such as the one that exercise is the best means of weight reduction. Although it plays a part, the best means of weight reduction is through caloric reduction. To burn up 1 pound of fat, one scientist has estimated that a 155-pound man must walk 144 miles at the rate of 2 miles an hour or do 5,714 push-ups.

Attitude

Facts and knowledge are not enough to ensure physical fitness, however. Examples of men, women, and young people who possess the knowledge but do not act accordingly are replete in every community. The woman who knows that a lump in her breast requires medical attention but fails to see her physician, the man who knows the value of seat belts in his car but does not take the time to have them installed, and the boy who knows milk is good for him but reaches for soda pop are illustrative evidence to support this premise.

Attitude is important to physical fitness. The interest in and desire for well-being is the catalyst that sparks the boy and girl to want to apply the knowledge they know to be true. Mothers and fathers play an important role in the development of proper attitudes among youth. If a father remarks that he had rather have a soggy body than a soggy mind (as though it were an "either-or" proposition), his children are likely to react the same way and try to avoid physical activity. The development of an interest in health and being healthy, a determination to be physically active, and desire to develop all of one's potentials are important attitudes to develop.

Skill

The need for motor skills is also an important part of becoming physically educated. As a boy develops skill in skating, his interest in the activity increases and he spends much of his leisure time in perfecting this skill. The girl who develops skill in swimming does the same thing. In addition to physical fitness, skill kindles within a person the desire for action and competition. Skill provides such essential human needs as recognition, belonging, and the joy of accomplishment. Many tired business-men get up at 7 A.M. on Saturday and Sunday mornings because they have developed the skill of hitting a small, white ball 250 yards down the fairway, and they are more physically fit for doing so.

One of the main contributions a school or community can make to their boys and girls is to develop a wide variety of physical activity skills for each season of the year: archery, handball, squash, volleyball, skiing, field hockey, dance, and many more activities. These skills will contribute to year-round and life-long physical fitness, since the youngster will not only enjoy participating during school hours but also will be active on his own after school, on holidays, during vacation periods, and throughout life. One criterion of a good education program is what the boy and girl do when they are away from the teacher and the school, and skills will help to ensure that such time is spent in a constructive manner.

The ability of youth to develop skills accents the need for more instruction during this golden age of skill learning in activities than can be engaged in throughout a lifetime. Only about one out of 1,000 students will probably engage in baseball when they leave school, but the number increases sharply in tennis, golf, and badminton.

Each boy and girl should develop skills in such fundamental movements as running, throwing, and jumping and in such basic activities as swimming, as well as in various sports for each season of the year.

Activity

With scientifically based knowledge, wholesome health attitudes, and a wide variety of physical skills, activity becomes meaningful. Young people will engage in healthful physical exercise regularly because they know it is just as essential to their body as good food and because they want to be fit so that they can become all they are capable of becoming. Furthermore, with this knowledge, attitude, and skill, activity will be a part of their personal regimen throughout life.

Long-term physical fitness is not going to be accomplished by calisthenics and sports programs carried out in a vacuum. Long-term physical fitness for each of our young people will only become a reality when every boy and girl clearly understands the need for such activity, has the desire to be physically fit, and possesses the skills to make activity exciting and enjoyable. When children and young people have acquired these essentials, they can be called *physically educated,* recognizing that this is what will make coming generations healthy and the nation physically strong. The development of physically educated youth requires opportunities for participation in healthful physical activity. But even more important is the need for teachers and youth leaders who are dedicated to the task of helping all boys and girls and who recognize the importance of exercising the brain as well as the muscle cells in developing physically fit youth.

ROLE OF SCHOOL AND COMMUNITY IN FITNESS

One of the chief avenues for reaching the youth of America is the schools. Here are a few reasons why the schools are an important part of the fitness picture:

1. They are the only agency through which nearly 60 million children and youth can be reached directly.
2. They have teachers trained for instilling youngsters with the desire to be fit and for carrying out conditioning programs.
3. It has been estimated that 80% of all the physical activity skills acquired during a lifetime are learned by children between the ages of 7 and 17 years.

Education in its broadest sense means preparation for life. It should help each individual to become all he is capable of being. Therefore it is inexorably tied in with fitness. Education must be concerned with developing in each individual optimum organic health, vitality, emotional stability, social consciousness, knowledge, wholesome attitudes, and spiritual and moral qualities. Only as it accomplishes this task will it achieve its destiny in the American way of life.

Schools have the responsibility for providing many opportunities for understanding and developing fitness. The schools should be "fitness conscious." Programs must be constituted so that experiences and services contribute to fitness. This means that health knowledge, attitudes, and practices are stressed; protective health services are provided; physical activities are available to and engaged in by all, not just the few who are skilled; necessary facilities are provided; the environment is conducive to proper growth and development; experiences in every area stress proper social and ethical behavior.

Leadership exemplifies fitness, and fitness is the responsibility of all disciplines in the school and all teachers and staff. It should permeate the entire program and all persons connected with it. It is not the responsibility of only one area and just a few people.

Schools should provide community leadership in this area. The schools, however, represent only one force for developing a fit populace. The home, the church, recreational agencies, volunteer groups, and other organizations also have major contributions to make. Schools should work closely with and play a leading role in mobilizing the entire resources of each community to do the job.

Children and youth should want to be fit. Unless this desire is resident in each child, the way of life that results in fitness will not be achieved. By the time children leave school behind and enter into adult life, the importance of fitness in achieving personal ambitions and desires, in feeling well and happy, in living most and serving best, and in contributing to a strong nation must be inculcated in every boy and girl.

This is a responsible role for our professions to pursue and a very necessary one. It is a challenge we must meet if we are not to become "a nation of softies." Physical education can make a significant contribution to fitness for living. If it achieves its four main objectives of organic development, skill development, mental development, and social development, it will contribute not only to the physical but also to the total fitness of the individual.

The President's Council on Physical Fitness and Sports raises questions that should be asked in respect to each person's school, child, community, and personal fitness program. They are presented here in adapted form.*

Your school's physical education and health program

Does it emphasize vigorous activity?
Is each boy and girl involved?
Does it have evaluation procedures to identify physically underdeveloped pupils?
Is there outstanding professional leadership?
Are the physical education facilities adequate?
Is provision made for health instruction and services?

Your child

Is he overweight?
Is he underdeveloped?
Has he developed skill in several sports and games?
Have health defects been corrected?
Does he have proper health care?
How does he spend his free time?
How are his energy and stamina?

Your community

Does it provide a recreation program for all persons?
Have fitness centers and clubs been established?
Is instruction provided?
Are the facilities adequate and used year-round?
Has a community recreation committee representative of the entire community been established?

You

When was your last medical checkup?
Do you engage in some form of vigorous physical activity each day?
Are you providing for your health needs?

---

*President's Council on Physical Fitness and Sports, Physical fitness facts, Washington, D. C., 1964.

QUESTIONS AND EXERCISES

1. Trace the history of the current fitness movement and discuss its implications for the professions of physical education, health, and recreation.
2. Why is it important that boys and girls fully understand the meaning of the term *physical fitness?* How can physical fitness educators help to educate for fitness?
3. What is the relationship of exercise to physical fitness?
4. Formulate a physical fitness program for an average school system. Justify your program completely.
5. To what degree should physical education confine itself solely to the development of physical fitness?
6. Discuss and compare the value of isometric and isotonic exercises.
7. How does the "trained" person differ from the "untrained" person?
8. Who are five leaders in the profession who have played important roles in bringing the importance of physical education to the public?
9. What relationship is there between physical education and a commercial "trim-line" club?
10. What are some of the characteristics of the physically fit individual?

Reading assignment

Bucher, Charles A., and Goldman, Myra: Dimensions of physical education, St. Louis, 1969, The C. V. Mosby Co., Reading selections 39 to 42.

SELECTED REFERENCES

American Association for Health, Physical Education, and Recreation: Journal of Health, Physical Education, and Recreation, vol. 29, September, 1958.

Bender, Jay A. and Kaplan, Harold M.: The multiple angle testing method for the evaluation of muscle strength, Journal of Bone and Joint Surgery 45A:135, 1963.

Bender, Jay A., Kaplan, Harold, M., and Johnson, Alex J.: Isometrics: a critique of faddism versus facts, Journal of Health, Physical Education, and Recreation 34:22, 1963.

Berger, Richard A.: Effects of dynamic and static training on vertical jump ability, Research Quarterly, 34:419, 1963.

Bucher, Charles A.: Administration of health and physical education programs including athletics, St. Louis, 1971, The C. V. Mosby Co.

Bucher, Charles A.: Fitness and health (editorial), Educational Leadership 20:356, 1963.

Bucher, Charles A., Koening, Constance, and Barnhard, Milton: Methods and materials for secondary school physical education, St. Louis, 1970, The C. V. Mosby Co.

Bucher, Charles A., Olsen, Einar A., and Willgoose, Carl E.: The foundations of health, New York, 1967, Appleton-Century-Crofts.

Bucher, Charles A., and Reade, Evelyn M.: Physical education and health in the elementary school, New York, 1971, The Macmillan Co.

Clarke, David H.: The energy cost of isometric exercise, Research Quarterly 31:3, 1960.

College Physical Education Association: Fit for college, Washington, D. C., 1959, American Association for Health, Physical Education, and Recreation.

Cooper, Kenneth H.: The role of exercise in our contemporary society, Journal of Health, Physical Education, and Recreation 40:24, 1969.

de Vries, Hebert A.: Physiology of exercise for physical education and athletics, Dubuque, Iowa, 1969, Wm. C. Brown Company.

Duggar, Benjamin C., and Swengros, Glenn V.: The design of physical activity programs for industry, Journal of Occupational Medicine 11(6):322-329, 1969.

Gendel, Evelyn S.: Women and the medical aspects of sports, Journal of School Health 37:427-431, 1967.

Home visitations continued; Physical Fitness Newsletter, series XVI, no. 6, February, 1970, pp. 5-6.

Hunsicker, Paul: What research says to the teacher, Physical Fitness, Washington, D. C., 1963, The National Education Association.

Journal of Sports Medicine and Physical Fitness, official journal of the Fédération Internationale de Medicine Sportive, published by Edizioni Minerva Medica (Torino, Italy). See all issues.

Klaus, E. J.: The athletic status of women. In Jokl, E., and Simon, E., editors: International research and sport and physical education, Springfield, Illinois, 1964, Charles C Thomas, Publisher.

Libicer, Stephen J., Jr.: The name of the game is fitness, Outlook 1(2):1, 4, 1969.

Marusak, F. M.: The use of corrective therapy in a psychiatric treatment program, Journal of the Association of Physical and Mental Rehabilitation 5:9-11, 1952.

Michael, Ernest D.: Stress adaption through exercise, Research Quarterly 28:50-54, 1957.

Miller, A. T., Jr.: Influence of oxygen administration on cardiovascular function during exercise and recovery, Journal of Applied Physiology 5:165-168, 1952.

Munroe, Richard A.: Faculty fitness program at the University of Arizona, Physical Fitness Newsletter, series XV, no. 3, November, 1968, pp. 2-4.

Neuberger, Tom: What the Research Quarterly says about warm-ups, Journal of Health, Physical Education, and Recreation 40:75-77, 1969.

Newsletter, President's Council on Physical Fitness and Sports, pp. 1-2.

Olympic planners discount fear of Mexican altitudes, Medicine in Sports, vol. 8, No. 1, January, 1968.

Rarick, Lawrence G., and Larsen, Gene L.: Observations on frequency and intensity of isometric muscular effort in developing static strength in pre-pubescent males, Research Quarterly 29:476, 1954.

Register-Guard and Gary Winen team up, Physical Fitness Newsletter, series XVII, no. 2, October, 1970, pp. 5-6.

Royce, Joseph: Isometric fatigue curves in human muscle with normal and occluded circulation, Research Quarterly 29:333, 1958.

Selye, Hans: The stress of life, New York, 1956, McGraw-Hill Book Co.

Solomon, Amiel, and Pangle, Roy: Demonstrating physical fitness improvement in the EMR, Exceptional Children, November, 1967, pp. 177-181.

Thompson, Clem W.: Some physiological effects of isometric and isotonic work in man, Research Quarterly 25:476, 1954.

Tips on Athletic Training XII, American Medical Association, Committee on the Medical Aspects of Sports, 1970, p. 8.

YMCA, Journal of Physical Education, vol. 64, November-December, 1966, Special Fitness Issue.

Your child's health and fitness, insert in National Education Association Journal 51:33, 1962.

Additional materials on the subject of fitness may be secured from the President's Council on Physical Fitness and Sports, Washington, D. C., and the American Association for Health, Physical Education, and Recreation, 1201 Sixteenth Street N. W., Washington, D. C. 20036.

17/Psychological interpretations of physical education

Psychology is a science that studies the individual (also the group—social psychology) and his activities from the time he is conceived until the time he dies. It studies his behavior, his ways of reacting, and how he learns. It is concerned with the many traits, feelings, and actions that make up the mind. It compares the normal to the abnormal person and the criminal to the law-abiding citizen.

The word *psychology* comes from the Greek words *psyche,* meaning mind or soul, and *logos,* meaning science. Therefore, from these Greek words it can be seen that psychology is the science of the mind and the soul. The psychologist studies human nature scientifically and, rather than formulate conclusions from casual observations, he sorts out and checks and rechecks human characteristics under reliable conditions. In this manner and through the use of acceptable scientific evaluation, it is possible for him to determine the condition under which certain human characteristics will operate. The data derived through the psychologist's work should theoretically be objective and free from prejudice and bias and focus attention on an impartial and realistic examination of all the evidence.

ELEMENTS OF LEARNING

Learning implies a change in a person—a change in his method of both practicing and performing a skill or changing an attitude toward a particular thing. Learning implies a progressive change of behavior in an individual, although some changes are rapid, such as when insight into a problem is perceived. It implies a change that occurs as a result of experience or practice. It results in the modification of behavior as a result of training or environment. It involves such aspects as obtaining knowledge, improving one's skill in an activity, solving a problem, or making an adjustment to a new situation. It implies that knowledge or skill has been acquired through instruction received in school or some other setting or through a person's own initiative in personal study. Learning goes on all through life. It starts as a result of a felt need. When old forms of behavior are no longer capable of meeting new situations, a felt need results. When a person finds that his present equipment or methods of response are inadequate to solve a need, he may become aware that some change is necessary either in the environment, himself, or both. For example, when a skill is not performed proficiently enough to receive commendation and approval from others, there may be a felt need to improve this skill, or he may have internalized his own standards and not need the group as his judge.

In order to have an effective learning situation, there are certain basic forces of which education must be cognizant. These basic forces serve as the frame of reference for the conduct of learning and teaching in the school environment. Some of the most important forces influencing learning are motivation, individual differences, and intelligence. The role of maturation is also considered.

Motivation and learning

Motivation is a basic factor to effective learning. The term *motive* refers to a condition within the individual that initiates activity directed toward a goal. Needs and drives form the basic framework for motivation. When the individual senses an unfulfilled need, he is moved to do something about it. The desire within a human being prompts him to seek a solution to his recognized need through an appropriate line of action. From the phenomenological point of view, certain needs can arise from the environment. These forces are from the outside. A comprehensive theory of motivation should take these forces into account.

This line of action may require practice, effort, mastery of knowledge, or other behavior in order to be successful. For example, if an individual is hungry he becomes motivated to seek food, while, at a higher level, the individual who desires to pass an examination so he will be permitted to practice law will be desirous of acquiring the necessary knowledge.

A. H. Maslow* has developed a theory of motivation arranged in order from the most immature to the most mature needs.

1. *Physiological needs.* At the lowest level are the physiological needs. Here the individual is concerned with survival, and the need for food is seen as basic to the protection of the physiological being.
2. *Safety needs.* At this level the individual seeks to discover ways of avoiding danger. The individual prefers the known to the unknown and finds that he must establish feelings of security before he is free to do other things.
3. *Love and belonging needs.* The need for affection, love, and friendship fall in this group. The individual desires to be accepted by others, and having their approval enhances his feeling of adequacy and worth.
4. *Esteem needs.* The need to be respected by others appears at this level. The desire to be recognized as important is dominant, and the individual engages in activities that he hopes will lead him to situations where he can win the respect of his peers.
5. *Self-actualization.* This is the highest level

---

*Maslow, A. H.: A theory of human motivation, Psychological Review **50**:370-396, 1943.

of maturity. Here the individual is truly himself. At this level the individual develops to his full potential and becomes all that he is capable of becoming.

Maslow's theory of motivation is important to educators. Each individual in our school system needs the opportunity to develop to his full potential. In a classroom situation, to a large extent, the child's needs for affection, belonging, approval, esteem, and self-actualization are dependent upon the teacher. If the child is given the opportunity to participate in activities important to him and is given the chance to succeed, his needs are satisfied. Accordingly, teachers should organize their programs so that each individual is given the opportunity to satisfy his needs. Physical education teachers are in an excellent position to provide the individual student with the opportunity to participate in activities that will lead to the satisfaction of his basic needs. In physical education, the student is given the opportunity to satisfy his need for belonging, for example, by being given the opportunity to play on a team. Here the individual gains the affection, friendship, approval, and respect of his fellow classmates.

It is important to also recognize that the child's parents or parent substitutes play a vital role in the development and satisfaction of these needs.

Maturation and learning

Maturation is concerned with determining whether or not an individual has reached a certain stage in his development that will enable him to perform a desired task. Psychologists have long adovcated the principle that learning should be adjusted to the level of maturation of the individual and have viewed learning as an adjustment to the environment. At the same time it should be understood that the learner is not always merely adjusting to the environment. He has to restructure it in order to meet the requirements of the task or situation. Sometimes this restructuring takes place within the individual and sometimes within the environment. Sometimes both the individual and the environment are in dynamic inter-action. Psychologist Jean Piaget* has been chiefly concerned with the individual child's adjustment to the environment in which he lives and has attempted to determine the optimum time for presenting learning experiences to the individual. Piaget sees four major stages of the individual's growth.

1. *Sensory-motor stage.* This stage lasts from birth to about 2 years of age. At this stage the child becomes aware of his muscles and various senses and discovers mechanisms for dealing with objects and events. The beginning of language development also takes place during this stage of development.
2. *Preoperational stage.* This stage begins about 2 years of age and continues to about age 6. Language development is the dominating factor during this stage. Through his new-found use of words, the child expresses his feelings about the environment he inhabits. The child at this stage depends on trial and error and intuition to solve the various problems with which he is presented. It should be noted that the trial and error

is not one that is blindly done. Insight is involved at this stage. Motor skill development begins to take form during this stage.
3. *Concrete operation stage.* This stage begins at age 7 and lasts until the child is 11 years old. At this stage the child understands the relationships among various concrete operational groupings. The child develops the ability to solve physical problems and becomes aware of the concept of reversibility (that for any operation there is an opposite operation that cancels it). Improved motor skill development also takes place at this stage, with the child developing greater movement patterns.
4. *Formal operations stage.* This stage begins at about age 11 and sets the foundation for the individual's adult thinking. At this stage the individual acquires the capacity for abstract thought. Logical reasoning and problem solving are dominant during this stage.

Through his four developmental stages, Piaget has described the physical and intellectual growth of an individual. His greatest contribution to psychology lies in his finding that learning proceeds most rapidly when experiences presented to the individual are geared to his physical and intellectual abil-

---

*Jennings, Frank G.: Jean Piaget: notes on learning, Saturday Review, May 20, 1967, pp. 81-83.

Modern dancers in outdoor concert.

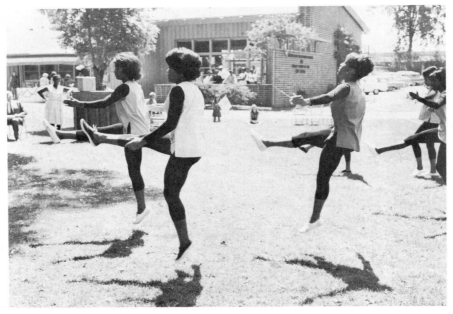

ity. For example, according to Piaget, a child should not be presented with problems to solve that require abstract thought until he reaches the formal operations stage of his development.

All teachers must have a clear understanding of the concept of maturation. A program of research is necessary to help determine the intricate relationship between maturation and learning. When physical education teachers present motor skills to their students, it is essential that they discover whether the child has reached a certain level of development that will enable him to perform successfully. For example, if a boy is to learn a skill such as the shot put, he must be physically mature to make such an activity possible. If the teacher attempts to develop this skill before the student reaches the level of maturity necessary, he will waste his time and may decrease the student's motivation for learning the skill. The student may also harm himself.

Individual differences and learning

In any classroom situation the teacher must provide for the individual differences found among the students. In a typical physical education class, for example, the teacher is faced with a group of boys or girls who differ in physical qualities; some are big while others are small, and some possess greater motor ability than others. There are social and economic differences; some students come from middle-class families, while others are members of the lower class or products of broken homes. There are personality differences among the students; some students are outgoing while others are very shy and withdrawn. Teachers must be aware of the differences found among their students. The teacher who is instructing a class of ghetto* youths, for example, must be aware of the fact that he must be a strong model for these students. Students who come from broken homes need the guidance and support of the teach-

er if they are to develop to their full potential. The teacher who recognizes the need to give some students, such as the shy and withdrawn boy, a little more motivation than others will play a strong role in the child's development.

Intelligence and learning

In addition to physical, social, economic, and personality differences, there are also differences in intelligence that must be recognized. In consulting the literature, one is made aware of the fact that there are many different theories as to what constitutes intelligence. The question of whether we have one intelligence or several different intelligences has been well documented. Spearman* espoused the theory of general and specific intelligence. His theory emphasizes that all mental activities have in common a general factor of intelligence, designated g, and a specific factor of intelligence, designated s, that is related only to particular activities.

Thurstone† believed general intelligence is made up of several "primary mental abilities." The primary mental abilities named were numbers (such as the ability to do arithmetic problems), verbal meaning, spatial perception, word fluency, reasoning, memory, and perceptual speed. Thurstone attempted to prove that these primary mental abilities are independent of one another. However, in testing, those who scored high on one ability such as reasoning also scored high on other abilities, thus indicating that these primary abilities may really be an expression of one general ability.

Recent attempts to define intelligence have estimated that there may be well over 100 individual components of intelligence.

It is apparent that teachers must have an understanding of the principle of intelligence and some means for measuring the

---

*The concept of ghetto as originally developed in Europe is different from the concept in America.

*Spearman, Charles: The abilities of man, New York, 1927, The Macmillan Co.

†Thurstone, L. L.: Primary mental abilities, Psychometric Monograph No. I, Chicago University Press, 1938, p. 9.

intelligence level of their students* if they are to present meaningful learning experiences. Both the general factor and multifactor theories of intelligence have produced a great number of tests to measure intelligence. Tests such as the Stanford-Binet and the Wechsler Intelligence Scale for Children are individual tests of intelligence based on a general theory of intelligence and are concentrated heavily on measuring verbal and numerical abilities. Differential aptitude tests are tests that measure the multifactor theory of intelligence. They measure verbal reasoning, numerical abilities, mechanical reasoning, clerical speed, spelling, language usage, and accuracy. The scores that an individual receives on an intelligence test such as the Stanford-Binet are known as IQ. *IQ* refers to intelligence quotient and is a ratio of the student's mental age to chronological age multiplied by 100 ($\frac{ma}{ca} \times 100$). An IQ in the low 70's indicates an intellectual deficiency, while a score over 130 indicates a high intelligence level. Within a class scores on an intelligence test may range from the low 80's and even lower to well over 130.

Educators must be cognizant of these scores. For those children who score above 130, the question may be asked: Does the class atmosphere satisfy the intellectual needs of these students? The physical educator must be aware of those students in his class who may feel the activities in which they are participating are not stimulating enough. On the other hand, those children who are identified as academically weak may need extra help in discovering the solution to various tasks they are required to solve. Physical educators must have a good assessment of their students, which means that individual differences are discovered in order to provide students with the activities that will meet their needs.

*In New York City schools, it should be noted, group IQ tests are not given. Reading scores are now used by grade advisers to aid in teaching students.

THEORIES OF LEARNING

Psychologists have attempted to explain the phenomenon of learning and to answer such questions as how it best takes place and what are the laws under which it operates. The basic theories of learning, for purposes of discussion, may be said to be divided into two broad categories. The first category may be called the connectionist theories. These theories state that learning consists of a bond or connection between a stimulus and a response or responses. The second category may be called cognitive theories. Those psychologists that support these theories feel that the various perceptions, beliefs, or attitudes (cognitions or mental images) that a human being has concerning his environment determine what type of behavior the human being will have. The manner in which these "cognitions" are modified by the experience that the human being has indicates the learning that takes place. The basic principles underlying the cognitive theories were developed by the Gestalt psychologists.

Thorndike's laws of learning

E. L. Thorndike, a psychologist whose theories of learning have had a great impact on educators and education, believed in a stimulus—response theory, or S–R bond theory. His laws of readiness, exercise, and effect have influenced educational programs.

Thorndike developed these laws that set forth the conditions under which learning best takes place. Because psychology is a relatively new science and because there are many contradictory views as to various psychological principles, laws of learning should not be regarded as the final word. However, they are working principles and, as such, deserve the attention of all physical educators who desire to seek the most efficient and effective ways of teaching.

LAW OF READINESS. The law of readiness means that an individual will learn much more effectively and rapidly if he is "ready" —if he has matured to that point and if there is a felt need. Learning will be satisfying if materials are presented when an individual meets these standards. This law also works in reverse. It will be annoying and dissatisfying to do something when the individual is not ready. The closer an individual is to reaching the point of readiness, the more satisfying the act.

In physical education activities the teacher should determine whether the child is ready in respect to various sensory and kinesthetic mechanisms and in respect to strength in some cases. The teacher should ask such questions as: Does the child have the capacity, at this time, for certain skills? Does he have the proper background of experience? Is the material being presented timely? Should it be postponed until some future time, or is now the time to present it? Most physical educators agree, for example, that athletic competition on an interscholastic basis should not be part of the program for elementary school children. The child is not mentally, emotionally, and physically ready for such an experience. There is also considerable agreement that fine-muscle activity should not play too pronounced a part in the program for young children. Instead, their program should largely consist of activities that involve the large muscles.

The law of readiness also has implications for the learning of skills. An adult has difficulty hitting a baseball, riding a bicycle, throwing a football, and performing other physical activities if he has not developed some skill in these activities during his youth. During youth, on the other hand, individuals can perform reasonably well in these skills without too much difficulty. They are at the proper maturation level for the learning of such skills, and their neuromuscular equipment has developed to a point where skills are learned more economically and effectively. They do not mind passing through an awkward trial-and-error period. Physical educators should bear this in mind and set as their goal the development in youth of many interesting and varied skills. In this way children will have the foundational equipment when they reach

adulthood to engage in a variety of physical education activities that will provide many enjoyable hours of wholesome recreation.

LAW OF EXERCISE. The law of exercise, in respect to the development of skills in physical education, means that practice makes for better coordination, more rhythmical movement, less expenditure of energy, more skill, and better performance. As a result of practice, the pathway between stimulus and response becomes more pronounced and permanent.

In many ways this law of learning is similar to the law of use and disuse. As a result of continual practice, strength is gained, but as a result of disuse, weakness ensues.

Learning in education is acquired by doing. In order to master the skill of bowling, swimming, or handball a person must practice. However, it should be restated that practice does not necessarily ensure perfection of the skill. Mere repetition does not mean greater skill. Practice must be meaningful, with proper attention being given to all phases of the learning process. The learner, through repetition and a clear conception of what is to be done, steadily makes progress toward the goal he is attempting to attain. Repetition, however, should not be blind. It is during the process of "repetition" that learning takes place.

LAW OF EFFECT. The law of effect maintains that an individual will be more likely to repeat experiences that are satisfying to him than those experiences that are annoying. If experiences are annoying, the learner will shift to other, satisfying responses.

This law of learning, as applied to physical education, means that every attempt should be made to provide situations in which individuals experience success and have a satisfying and enjoyable experience. Leadership is an important factor. Under certain types of leadership undesirable experiences would be satisfying. One coach might approve of hitting an opponent and make this an enjoyable experience. Under other coaches such an act would be an annoying experience because it would be condemned and would not be tolerated. Leadership is the key to good teaching.

Guthrie's contiguity theory

Edwin R. Guthrie* developed the contiguity theory of learning, which emphasizes the stimulus-response association. Contiguity means that a response that is evoked by a stimulus will be repeated whenever that same stimulus reoccurs. The strengthening of the connection between the stimulus and the response takes place in a single trial. Guthrie believed that since associations can occur with one trial and last forever, there is no need for anything like rewards or motivation to explain learning. However, although Guthrie holds that the

---

*Guthrie, E. P.: The psychology of learning (revised edition), New York, 1952, Harper and Row, Publishers.

full connection is established in one trial, it usually appears to take place gradually. This means that all stimuli cues are not always presented in the same manner, and for this reason many stimulus-response associations must be made. In every learning situation, for example, there are various combinations of stimuli that are presented and the correct responses need to be established for each situation. Guthrie holds that repetition and practice are essential in learning in order for the individual to become aware of the stimuli that will evoke the correct response.

In physical education we can apply Guthrie's theory to the learning of a skill such as the high jump. If a youngster desires to be proficient in this skill, he must make sure that his bodily movements are always the same each time he approaches the bar. The individual must be aware of all the surrounding stimuli such as the runway and position of the bar. The proficient

Physical education skills should be taught in the most effective way possible. Tennis instruction using stroke developer.

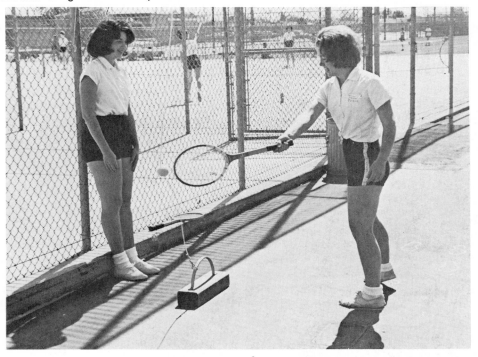

high jumper will be one who has established a successful pattern for his movements and does not deviate from it. Even the slightest change in stimuli can evoke an incorrect response. The youngster who becomes distracted by the noise of the spectators finds it difficult to clear the bar if he has been used to practicing in complete silence. According to Guthrie's theory, this youngster should practice under conditions that he faces during actual competition, for in order to achieve his best performance he must be aware of all the stimuli that are present at the time of competition.

Hull's reinforcement theory

Clark L. Hull* sees learning as a direct influence of reinforcement. He has established his theory on the influence of need and its reduction as the prime elements in learning. In his theory Hull emphasizes that learning occurs when the individual adapts himself to his environment and that such adaptation is necessary for survival. When needs arise the individual's survival is threatened, and the individual must act in a certain manner to reduce the need. The responses that the individual makes that lead to the reduction of the need are reinforced, resulting in habits or learning. According to Hull's theory, a stimulus causes a response that results in a need. The need evokes a response on the part of the individual, which reduces the need. The response that resulted in the reduction of the need is then reinforced, which develops habits or learning. Hull employed drive and primary reinforcement in his early work. Later he used ideas such as drive stimulus reduction and secondary reinforcement.

Hull's theory emphasizes that habits or learning result from reactions set into motion by needs. In physical education the teacher plays an important part in satisfying the needs of the student. Teachers who explain the psychological and sociological bases for participating in an activity may stimulate students to a larger degree than those who present the activity without any rationale. To elicit correct responses from students, the teacher presents material that is meaningful, and therefore lesson plans consist of material important to the learner.

In Hull's theory the child learns by doing—drive reduction is a doing phenomenon. In physical education the child arrives at the solution to many problems through his own efforts. For example, the student practices the "kip" on the low bar and after many attempts becomes aware that he is not achieving success because of the position of his arms or other weakness. Upon discovering the correct position, the student repeats it over and over to reinforce it. The result is the correct movement on the low bar. The habit is learned. Further repetition of the activity with the correct response leads to a feeling of satisfaction on the part of the student, for the need is no longer a problem.

One of the major implications of Hull's theory to physical education is his finding that practice periods that are extremely long or lacking in reinforcement inhibit learning. An example of this is the pole vaulter who practices hour after hour. After a long period of practice without any reinforcement, he finds it difficult to clear his usual height. However, Hull states that the inhibitions decrease after rest periods, and the next day the vaulter can again clear his accustomed height. Thus practice periods play an important role in determining the performance of an individual.

Skinner's operant conditioning theory

The main feature of B. F. Skinner's* operant conditioning theory is the fact that the stimulus that reinforces the responses does not precede it but rather follows it. In operant conditioning, behavior is elicited by the individual rather than the stimuli. In this theory of learning the individual organism first makes the desired response

---

*Hull, Clark L.: Principles of behavior, New York, 1943, Appleton-Century-Crofts.

*Skinner, B. F.: The behavior of organisms, New York, 1938, Appleton-Century-Crofts.

and then is rewarded. Reinforcement is contingent on the desired response. Skinner's main emphasis is that the individual repeats at a future time the behavior that has been previously reinforced. Behaviors that are not reinforced are not usually repeated. When the individual is rewarded, he elicits that behavior again. Extinction occurs when the behavior is no longer reinforced.

Skinner makes the point that since teachers cannot always wait for behavior to manifest itself, they must sometimes shape the behavior of the individual. In teaching any physical skill it is recognized that reinforcement is extremely valuable. For example, if the teacher desires a student to learn how to take the jump shot, he encourages the student to learn the proper form. When the student is shooting at the peak of his jump, in the correct manner, the teacher indicates approval to the student. The student becomes aware of the proper form and continues to use it, because he knows the skill is being properly performed according to the teacher's standard.

Skinner has placed great emphasis on the use of audiovisual aids and teaching machines because of their reinforcement value. Since the teacher cannot reinforce the behavior of all children in a class, such machines may be useful, although some psychologists believe that they may interfere with the organization of materials into structural wholes. Through the use of such new innovations as the videotape replay, the student sees himself in action and discovers his deficiencies. Such devices prove beneficial in reinforcing learning in large classes where the teacher cannot cope with all the individual problems that arise.

Gestalt theory

The Gestalt psychologists such as Max Wertheimer, Kurt Koffka, Wolfgang Kohler, and Kurt Lewin are greatly concerned with form and shapes. Gestalt theory is more concerned with perception than learning. One of the most important Gestalt prin-

ciples having implications for physical education is the whole method theory. This theory is based on the premise that a person reacts as a whole to any situation. The whole individual attempts to achieve a goal. Furthermore, the greater the insight or understanding an individual has concerning the goal he wishes to attain, such as paddling a canoe or guiding a bowling ball to a strike, the greater will be his degree of skill in that activity. An individual reacts differently each time he performs a physical act. Therefore it is not just a question of practice, as it would be if he performed it the same way each time. Instead, the more insight he has of the complete act, the greater his skill. The individual performs the whole act and does it until he gains an insight into the situation or until he gets the "feel" or the "hang" of it. Since insight is so important, dependent conditions such as a person's capacity, previous experience, and experimental setup are necessary considerations.

Psychoanalytic theory of learning

Psychoanalysis is a genetic as well as a dynamic theory. Learning is related to the psychosocial stages of development and must take into account that it may be affected by unconscious forces and in certain cases leads to repression, fixation, and regression. All of these unconscious forces are involved in the psychoanalytic theory of learning. Freud's theory stressed the importance of cognitive control in the development of a rational ego.

MOTOR LEARNING

Learning has previously been described as a progressive change in behavior resulting from experience or practice. As we have seen, many theories have attempted to explain how such a process occurs. Physical educators are primarily concerned with the learning of motor skills. Basically speaking, motor learning is learning involving the neuromuscular system of the body. As with learning theories in general, attempts

As a general rule, learning is more effective when skills are taught as whole skills and not in parts.

COURTESY NATIONAL BROADCASTING CO.

have been made to explain how the process of learning a motor skill occurs.

Factors and conditions that promote the learning of motor skills

At this point it is necessary to consider some of the major factors and conditions that promote the learning of motor skills.

1. *Perception is one of the most important concepts in motor learning.* Perception refers to the process of receiving and distinguishing among the available stimuli presented in any situation. It is apparent that organizing information about one's environment and interpreting it correctly are important to learning. One prime determinant in a student's attempt to acquire a motor skill is his ability to perceive the world around him. It is essential in motor skill learning for an individual to perceive speed, distances, and shapes of objects. Deficiencies in any of these areas makes the learning of motor skills more difficult. For example, the student who has visual perception problems finds it difficult to play baseball because he is unable to follow the flight of the ball.

One of the major attempts at explaining the relationship of perception and motor learning has been made by Bryant J. Cratty.* Cratty established a "three level theory of perceptual-motor behavior." This theory makes the assumption that the factors involved in the three levels influence the individual's learning and performance. *At the first level* are general factors in performance, including aspiration level, arousal, and task analysis. The attributes at this level influence cognition, verbalization, and several perceptual-motor abilities, such as figure-ground perception and perception of muscular tensions. *At the second level* are the main perceptual motor ability traits such as arm-leg speed, finger-wrist speed, ballistic strength, static strength, trunk strength, and wrist-arm accuracy. *At the third and highest level* are factors specific

to the task and situation, such as motivation, past experiences, practice conditions, the characteristics of the situation in which the task is performed, and the movement patterns involved.

Cratty advises the physical educator and coach to become familiar with all three levels of influence upon perceptual-motor performance. He emphasizes the point that attention should be focused toward their mutual influence in the learning process because there are both general and specific factors involved in the learning of motor skills. For example, the lower level of the theory is associated with the alertness and arousal of the performer, which is in turn influenced by the higher level, because at this level the individual is given an assessment of his performance that will determine his further alertness and arousal. Poor visual feedback, for example, will interfere with one's alertness and decrease his level of performance.

Cratty's theory and others that have attempted to explain the relationship between perception and motor learning have been instrumental in providing the direction needed in this important area. However, more research is necessary before any definite conclusions can be reached as to the influence of perception in the learning of motor skills.

2. *The student should have an understanding of the nervous system because of its possible assistance in the development of a motor skill.*

The complicated mechanism of the nervous system controls and regulates an individual's behavior and is the key to the development of neuromuscular skill. The process by which this is performed is very interesting.

Neuromuscular skill is developed as a result of an impulse traveling through a reflex arc. The reflex arc is the path from a sense organ through a nerve center to a muscle. It is composed of three neurons, a neuron being a nerve cell including all of its various branches. The impulse enters through a nerve fiber, commonly known as

---

*Cratty, Bryant J.: A three level theory of perceptual-motor behavior, Quest (Monograph VI), May, 1966, pp. 3-10.

the receptor or sensory nerve, goes through a connector, and passes on to the effector or motor nerve.

The receptor or sensory nerve reacts to certain stimuli in the environment. These nerves may be found in such parts of the human body as the eyes, ears, tongue, nose, skin, muscles, and joints. These specialized sensory nerves, however, react to only certain types of stimuli. For example, the ears will not react to smell or the eyes to sound. They are the media through which the individual responds to the various conditions of his environment. The connector nerve is that part of the reflex arc that connects the receptor or sensory nerve with the effector or motor nerve. The spinal cord is a connecting center in the simplest type of reflex arc, whereas the brain, as well as the spinal cord, is used in complex reflex arcs. The effector or motor nerves are the response mechanisms. As a result of impulses traveling through the reflex arc, muscular contraction and glandular activity take place. The sensory nerves carry impulses to the nerve center; the connectors relay them to the response organs; and the motor nerves carry impulses away from the nerve center to the muscles. In many ways this resembles a telephone exchange; there are many wires carrying messages to and from the central office. The receptor or sensory cells, the connector cells, and the effector or motor cells are numerous. For example, it is estimated that there are millions in the receptor organs of the eyes alone.

To have neuromuscular activity, there must be a path or connection between the effectors and the receptors. The lines that carry the messages or impulses from the receptors to the effectors are the nerves. There are nerves throughout the body. The nerves in the muscles lead to and from the brain and the spinal column. The message comes in on a sensory nerve to the spinal cord or the brain. There it is transmitted to a motor neuron, which in turn carries it to a group of muscle fibers and makes them contract. Many authorities believe the nerve impulse to be an electrochemical wave transmitted over nerve fibers. As one practices an activity and as learning takes place, it is believed there is a neural growth—dendrites and axons at the synapses develop and grow. The "all-or-none" principle applies to nerves and muscles. A nerve fiber or a muscle fiber discharges all of its available energy when it is stimulated. Neuromuscular skill is developed when a pattern is laid between the sense organs and the muscles. Continuous practice in the performance of physical acts conditions the nervous and muscular systems to a point where habits and skills are performed with increasing degrees of coordination in activity.

3. *Effective motor learning is based on certain prerequisite factors.* According to McCloy,* there are prerequisites to effective motor learning. These are muscular strength, dynamic energy, ability to change direction, flexibility, agility, peripheral vision, visual acuity, concentration, an understanding of the mechanics of the activity, and an absence of inhibitory factors.

4. *Skills should not be offered to students unless they have reached a level of development commensurate with the degree of difficulty of the skill.* This principle refers to the concept of maturation previously discussed. Maturation is growth that takes place without any special training, stimulus, or practice—it just happens. It is closely associated with the physiological development of all individuals. Therefore, the material must be adapted to individual maturation levels. Tennis should not be part of the primary grade physical education curriculum because the student is not ready for the activity at this time. Teachers of motor skills must determine the optimum time at which the individual is ready to learn a skill and should provide the atmosphere most beneficial for its learning. Muscular development, strength, endurance, emotional stability, and other factors are criteria that should be taken into considera-

---

*McCloy, Charles H.: Research Quarterly **17:** 28, 1946.

tion in determining the maturation levels for various physical education activities.

5. *Each individual is different from every other individual.* The concept of individual differences has previously been discussed. However, it is necessary to make the point once again that teachers must be aware of the fact that individuals are different from one another and that these differences must be recognized if learning is to occur.

6. *The physical educator should be familiar with the learning curve as it applies to individuals.* Learning curves are not always constant, and they are different for each individual. The learning curve depends on the person, the material being learned, and the conditions surrounding the learning. Learning may start out with an initial spurt and then be followed by a period in which progress is not so rapid, or there may be no progress at all.

The initial spurt in learning may have been caused as a result of such factors as the enthusiasm for a new activity, mastering the easier parts of the task first, or the utilization of old habits in the first stages of practicing the new activity. All of these factors may be present from time to time in the teaching of soccer, badminton, handball, and other physical education activities.

Many learning curves also show that progress slows down as practice continues. This would seem to be true of many physical education activities wherein the easier acts are acquired first; as the activity becomes increasingly difficult, the learning rate is not so rapid as during the early stages. The physical education instructor should take such conditions into consideration instead of immediately coming to the conclusion that perhaps this instruction is inadequate or that the individuals in his class are not quick to learn.

A period in which there is a leveling off of learning is known as a plateau. It may be the result of a variety of reasons, such as loss of interest, failure to grasp a clear concept of the goal to be attained, preparation for a shift from a lower to a higher level in the learning process, or poor learning conditions. Physical educators should be cognizant of plateaus and the conditions causing little or no apparent progress in the activity. They should be especially careful not to introduce certain concepts or skills too rapidly, without allowing sufficient time for their mastery. They should also be on the lookout for certain physical handicaps to learning progress, such as fatigue, eye trouble, or lack of strength. Certain individuals cannot go beyond a given point because of physiological limits in respect to such things as speed, endurance, or some other physical characteristic. Physiological limits are absolute and cannot be surmounted and should be so recognized by physical education instructors. However, problems caused by physiological limits are rare, and in most cases it is the psychological limit that has to be overcome. By utilizing techniques to motivate the interest and enthusiasm of the learner, this goal can be accomplished.

7. *Learning takes place most effectively when the student has a motive for wanting to learn.* The role of motivation in the learning process has previously been stated (see p. 478). In motor skill learning its role is most important to the physical educator.

Motivation is an inducement to action. Usually, the greater the motivation, the more rapid is the learning. Motives should be of the intrinsic rather than the extraneous type. Rewards, awards, and marks should not be a means of motivating activity. The worth of the activity in itself should be the motive. In physical education activities, such motives as the desire to develop one's body, the desire to develop skill in an activity so that leisure hours may be spent in an enjoyable manner, the desire to become a member of a group, and the desire to maintain one's health are worthwhile motives. When these are present, the stage is set for learning to take place.

8. *Learning takes place much more effectively when the student intends to learn.* If the student makes up his mind that he intends to learn a certain skill, if he arrives

at the point where he sees a need for the skill, the learning situation is much more wholesome. Meaningful learning experiences presented by the teacher influence the student's intent to learn. Physical educators should stress the need of physical activity for enriched living. As the need is recognized, the intent to learn becomes greater and learning takes place more effectively.

9. *Education is a doing phenomenon—a person learns by doing.* A person learns through his own responses, meaning practice or a repetition of the act. During this repetition or practice, errors should be avoided as much as possible, and the ones that are made should be corrected. (See p. 482 for further discussion of this topic.)

10. *The student should know the goals toward which he is working.* Learning progresses much faster when goals are clear. Mental practice or thinking through the movement desired should be utilized more extensively in skill learning than it is. The student should have a clear picture of what constitutes a successful performance. For example, if high jumping is being taught, the proper form and technique should be clearly demonstrated and discussed. This can be done by the instructor discussing, demonstrating, and/or utilizing the many filmstrips and other visual aids that are available to show what is involved in the execution of the skill. In this way, after practicing for a time, the student can compare his performance with the successful performance and can change his responses accordingly. As he approaches the standard that has been set, the goal toward which he is working becomes increasingly clear. A knowledge of the goal enables the individual to see the problem as a whole and so see it in a coherent pattern. The physical education teacher must make sure that the goal is within the reach of the student. Unrealistic goals result in problems for the teacher and the student. When students realize that they cannot reach the goals that have been set for them, tensions arise and frustrations result, decreasing the motivation for learning.

11. *The student should receive feedback that indicates the progress that he is making.* There are basically two kinds of feedback available to the student during the performance of a motor skill. Internal feedback is related to the concept of *kinesthesis,* while external feedback is related to the concept known as *knowledge of results.* Kinesthesis is associated with the feeling of the movement and has been recognized as being a conscious muscle sense. This conscious muscle sense is extremely important to the student during the performance of a motor skill. For example, during the shot put the teacher may tell the student to feel the movement of his body as he releases the metal ball. The feel of the movement during and after completion of this skill gives an indication to the student of his performance. If he feels an awkward rather than a smooth fluid motion, it indicates that he is not performing correctly. Students need to develop a feeling for the correct way to run, jump, or throw. Physical education teachers should help their students to improve their "kinesthetic sense." When teachers discover their students performing the correct movements in a particular skill, they might inform the student of their findings and ask the student questions about the movement. For example, after a student successfully throws a curve ball, the teacher might ask the student: "Did you feel the ball break off your fingers?" In such a manner the teacher alerts the student to the feel of the movement and, if performed correctly, hopefully it will be repeated.

External feedback or knowledge of results is also extremely valuable to the student during and after the completion of a motor skill. Knowledge that one is progressing toward a set goal is encouraging and promotes a better learning situation. Research shows that when students are aware of the progress they are making (through charts or other media), the learning process is stepped up and the learner enjoys his work to a much greater degree. Knowledge of results should give an analytical self-evaluation in order to be important to the student during the learning of a motor skill. Although students view themselves on video-tape replay, for example, if they have been inadequately prepared to analyze movements, viewing will be ineffective. Physical education teachers should make students aware of the elements that constitute a correct movement as opposed to an incorrect one.

12. *Progress will be much more rapid when the learner gains satisfaction from the learning situation.* Satisfaction is associated with success. As the learner is successful in mastering a particular physical skill, his desire to learn increases so that he can experience additional success. On the contrary, if he does not experience satisfaction, the situation often becomes distasteful, and the learner turns to areas in which he may experience this satisfaction. Many individuals become dissatisfied with physical education because they do not have a satisfactory experience. The physical education instructor

may give his attention to the individuals who are most skillful and overlook the "dub" and the less skilled member of the class. The instructor should attempt to make sure that all members of a physical education class gain satisfaction from the activities in which they engage. Praise or other forms of rewards, to be most effective, should follow as soon as possible after the desired behavior is attained, and the best type of reward is that which gives a person a sense of achievement.

13. *The length and distribution of practice periods are important considerations for effective learning. Massed practice* refers to long and continuous practice periods, while *distributed practice* refers to practice periods interrupted by rest intervals. Questions of whether to emphasize massed or distributed practice in the learning of motor skills have perplexed physical educators for many years. There are no

Cartridge loop projector used in high school golf instruction program.

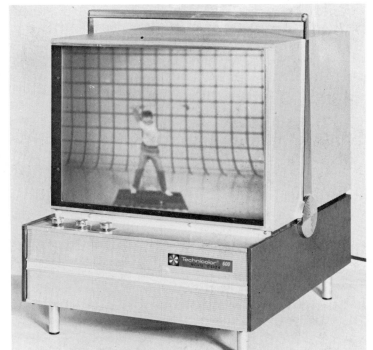

definite conclusions as to which method more easily facilitates the learning of motor skills since research in this area is very contradictory. However, there is some agreement that practice periods are most profitable when they are short and spaced over a period of time. The number of repetitions, such as shots at the basket or serves in tennis, should be considered as the unit of practice rather than the total number of minutes spent in the practice session. Forgetting proceeds rapidly at first and then more and more slowly in the learning situation. Furthermore, fatigue works adversely on the rate of learning and also on the accuracy of learning.

According to some psychologists, when subject matter is very interesting and meaningful to the learner, practice periods may be made longer. Therefore, it seems the length and spacing of periods should be adjusted to the class and material being learned. For example, if the physical educator has a class in volleyball that is very much interested and enthusiastic about this activity, the length of the instruction period could be longer, and the time between practice periods could be less than when he is working with a class that is indifferent and uninterested and that cannot see the need for developing skill in such an activity. New innovations in teaching such as flexible scheduling of class periods gives the physical education teacher a greater opportunity to utilize the principles of massed and distributed practice.

14. *As a general rule, learning is more effective when skills are taught as whole skills and not in parts.* In physical education it seems that the whole method should be followed when the material to be taught is a functional and integrated whole. This means that in swimming, which is a functional whole, the total act of swimming is taught. You learn to swim by using your arms and legs, and this can be taught as a whole. However, the research indicates that complex skills should be broken down into their basic parts. In a complex sport such as football the game consists of blocking,

broken-field running, tackling, passing, punting, and the like. In such a complex sport each of these skills represents a part of the whole that is football. However, they represent a functional and integrated whole by themselves and, as such, should be taught separately.

15. *Overlearning has value in the acquisition of motor skills.* The initial practice in the learning of a motor skill is important in determining how long the skill remains in possession of the learner. A partially learned skill does not remain in possession of the learner as long as one that is overlearned, that is, practiced until it establishes a pattern in the nervous system. If a skill is mastered and there is continual practice of the accomplishment, considerable time elapses before such a skill is lost to the learner.

A good example of this is the ability to swim. Once the skill has been mastered an individual can still swim even after long lapses without practice in this activity. This applies to many other physical education activities. If a student wants to remember a skill, he should overlearn it through continued practice. However, it should be pointed out that overlearning when overdone results in diminishing returns.

16. *Speed rather than accuracy should be emphasized in the initial stages of motor skill learning.* Physical educators are often required to make a judgment as to whether speed or accuracy should be emphasized in the initial stages of skill learning. Although some psychologists maintain that speed may lead in some cases to blindness in thinking, other researchers emphasize the speed factor. It would be desirable to be able to emphasize both speed and accuracy; however, this is not always possible. In physical education many skills are carried on primarily by momentum, and according to some research, speed should be emphasized in the initial stages of such learning. At this stage an emphasis on accuracy interferes with the dvelopment of momentum needed to carry on the movement. In teaching golf and tennis skills that require momentum in order to be

performed successfully, it is important to emphasize speed in the early stages of learning. For example, if the student attempts to develop accuracy while learning to drive the golf ball, he is forced to use a less desirous level of speed. Research indicates that such a student does not develop the level of speed needed to perform the skill successfully. Physical education teachers should make students cognizant of the fact that by practicing the skill at speeds they will utilize when actually performing the skill, accuracy will also tend to improve.

17. *Transfer of training can facilitate the learning of motor skills.* Transfer of training is based on the premise that a skill learned in one situation can be used in another situation. For example, the student who knows how to play tennis takes readily to badminton because both skills require similar strokes and the use of a racquet. Most psychologists agree that positive transfer most likely occurs when two tasks have similar part-whole relations involved. Again, to use the example of racquet games, since many racquet games such as platform tennis, squash, tennis, and badminton have similar part-wholes involved, considerable transfer takes place. Transfer, however, is not automatic. The more meaningful and purposeful an experience, the more likelihood of transfer. Transfer of training occurs to a greater degree with more intelligent participants, in situations that are similar, when there is an attitude and an effort on the part of the learner to effect transfer, when there is an understanding of the principles or procedures that are foundational to the initial task, and in situations where one teaches for transfer.

Physical educators must also be aware of the concept known as *negative transfer*. Negative transfer occurs when one task interferes with the learning of a second task. For example, a young man being introduced to the game of golf for the first time experiences difficulty in swinging the club because of his previous experience in another skill such as baseball. Perhaps you have heard the expression: "You're swinging the golf club like a baseball bat."

Recently physical educators and coaches have become interested in transferring skills learned in practice sessions to game-like situations and have attempted to make their drills as game-like as possible. For example, during practice sessions before a basketball game, coaches have their substitutes initiate the actions of their next opponents so that when the varsity takes the floor on the night of the game, they are familiar with the opponents' style of play.

18. *Mental practice can enhance the learning of motor skills.* Mental practice is the symbolic rehearsal of a skill with the absence of gross muscular movements. The physical educator should be concerned with the role of mental practice in skill learning. Research seems to indicate that although physical practice is superior to mental practice, mental practice is better than no practice at all. A combination of physical and mental practice is best. For example, since all students cannot practice a physical skill at the same time, they can practice mentally while waiting their turn to perform. While one student is performing on the high bar, for example, another student can mentally review the essential elements that must be mastered. Of course, mental practice can also take place at other times. Research shows mental practice is a valuable procedure when combined with overt practice in the motor activity. Through encouraging mental practice the physical education teacher may be able to increase the student's level of performance in motor skills. Questions concerning the most effective means of directing mental practice and the optimum time for utilizing mental practice must be more fully researched before definite conclusions can be reached as to the true worth of mental practice in the learning of motor skills.

19. *A knowledge of mechanical principles increases the student's total understanding of the activity in which he is participating.* A knowledge of mechanical principles that involve levers, laws of motion,

gravity, and other factors are closely related to skill performance. Physical educators should be able to give their students sound rationale for the skills they are performing based upon a knowledge of basic mechanical principles. For example, the bones of your body are levers. Their action resembles the action of levers found outside the body. A lever is an inflexible bar that rotates around a fixed point called a *fulcrum*. In order for a lever to rotate, some force must move the lever. Your bones are the inflexible bars that form the levers in your body. Your joints are the fulcrums, and your muscles supply the force to move the bones. Your body levers act each time you move. They help you to balance, cover distance, apply force, and develop speed.

You use your head as a lever when you hit a soccer ball with it. You contact the ball with your forehead, the fulcrum being at the base of your skull, the muscles of your body and neck supplying the power. You use your forearm as a lever when you spike a volleyball. The fulcrum is in your elbow. The muscles of your upper arm supply the power and your hand does the hitting.

Principles of gravity offer another example. Gravity acts on every object, including your body. Gravity pulls downward. The pull of gravity affects the energy your muscles release. At times your muscles must work extra hard to help you execute a movement because of the pull of gravity.

20. *Implementation of the principle of reinforcement will enhance learning.* One of the most fundamental laws of learning is reinforcement. In essence it means that the behavior most likely to emerge in any given situation is one that is reinforced or found successful in a previous similar situation. Therefore, the best-planned learning situation will provide for an accumulation of successes. The reinforcement (reward) should follow the desired behavior almost immediately and should be associated with the behavior in order to be most effective. (See p. 484 for more complete discussion of reinforcement.)

21. *Errors should be eliminated early in the learning period.* As one of our popular magazines states: "It's easier to start a habit than to stop one." When instructing in such skills as field hockey and softball, the physical education teacher should attempt to eliminate incorrect performance as early as possible so that errors do not become a fixed part of the participant's performance. Inefficient methods, once learned, are difficult to correct.

22. *The learning situation should be such that optimum conditions are present for efficient learning.* This means that distracting elements have been eliminated from the setting, the proper mental set has been established in the mind of the student, the proper equipment and facilities are available, the learner has the proper background to understand and appreciate the material that is to be presented, and the conditions are such that a challenging teaching situation is present.

23. *A learning situation is greatly improved if the student diagnoses his own movements and arrives at definite conclusions as to what errors he is committing.* Self-criticism is much more conducive to good learning than teacher criticism. If the student discovers his own mistakes, they are corrected much more readily than if discovered by someone else. A masterful teacher will develop teaching situations in which the student is led to self-criticism. This is a sign of good teaching. In physical education activities the student should be encouraged to analyze his own performance so that he may determine for himself where improvement can be made. This, in turn, will result in a more meaningful experience.

24. *The leadership provided determines to a great degree how much learning will take place.* As far as a child is concerned, a leader does not usually have to motivate the desire to engage in physical activity. It is a part of the child's makeup. However, the leader should set up certain situations to achieve other values. The physical educator should make sure that the

student has a clear picture of the goal to be accomplished. The instructor should be continually alert to detect correct and incorrect responses in the activities comprising the physical education program. He should encourage correct performance. This is a stimulus to more success. The physical educator should be able to present material on the pupil's level of understanding, should recognize individual differences, and should utilize his personality to further the teaching situation.

25. *The student should become less and less dependent upon the physical education instructor for help and guidance.* During the early periods of instruction when the basic techniques of the skill are being learned, instruction and help are needed frequently. However, as the fundamentals are mastered, the student should rely less upon the teacher's help and more upon his own resources. Excessive direction by the teacher may result in apathy, defiance, escape, or scapegoating.

26. *Physical education teachers must be concerned with more than just the teaching of motor skills.* When an individual is engaged in a skill or activity, he learns more than just the details of that one skill or activity. In tennis, for example, he learns such skills as serving and volleying. At the same time, however, he learns about tennis racquets and how they are constructed. He learns about tennis shoes, about the various types of composition for surfaces of tennis courts, and about the construction of tennis balls. He also learns about the other participants with whom he is associating, about his instructor, about rules of sportsmanship, about tolerance, about respect for the individual, about competition, and about respect for opponents. These are the concomitants of learning. The concomitants in a learning situation should be recognized as being just as important as the technical aspects of the skill that the teacher is attempting to present. One of the principal differences between an excellent and a mediocre teacher is that the mediocre teacher is concerned only with the teaching

of the mechanical aspects of a certain skill to the students, whereas the excellent teacher is concerned with the entire learning situation and how the learner reacts to the "whole" situation. A physical educator should not only be concerned with the neuromuscular or physical development of the individual; he should also be concerned with his mental, emotional, and social development.

OTHER PSYCHOLOGICAL BASES FOR PHYSICAL EDUCATION

In addition to helping physical educators teach their subject matter in a more meaningful manner, psychology is related in other ways to their field of endeavor.

Physical education and psychological development

Psychology is concerned with human behavior, and physical activity can affect behavior in many ways. Scott lists seven ways in which physical activity contributes to psychological development.*

1. *Attitudes are changed.* Physical education can contribute to the development of wholesome attitudes toward such factors as exercise, learning of motor skills, fitness, and use of leisure hours. The desire for and interest in physical activity will play a very important role in determining the support the profession of physical education obtains in trying to achieve its goals of a fit population.

2. *Social efficiency is improved.* Physical education has the potential, it is believed, to contribute to proper group adjustments, to the development of such desirable social traits as honesty, sportsmanship, and reliability, and to the development of a socially desirable personality. Social efficiency is discussed in Chapter 18.

3. *Improved sensory perception and responses accrue.* Although the research is inconclusive, there is some feeling that physical education can help to make a person

---

*Scott, M. Gladys: The contributions of physical activity to psychological development, Research Quarterly **31:**307, 1960.

more sensitive and responsive to his environment through the development of such characteristics as speed, visual perception, reaction time, depth perception, and kinesthetic awareness.

4. *Improved sense of well-being exists.* Physical education, it is believed, contributes to good mental health. Through play and various forms of physical activity, an opportunity is afforded for emotional release and having fun, and it provides a supplement for daily work. Being physically active contributes to the development of a healthy personality. As William Menninger, a famous psychiatrist, stated in a speech: "Good mental health is directly related to the capacity and willingness of an individual to play. Regardless of his objections, resistances, or past practice, any individual will make a wise investment for himself if he does plan time for his play and takes it seriously."

5. *Better relaxation is promoted.* Physical education has some support to show it can help to release muscular tension, together with affording an efficient motor response. Through selected forms of physical activity, there is some evidence that some forms of stress can be alleviated and thereby relaxation promoted in the individual.

6. *Relief is provided on psychosomatic problems.* More research should be conducted to determine the contributions of physical education to certain physical states such as chronic fatigue, dysmenorrhea, and phobias. Scott points out there is more objective evidence on the effects of exercise on dysmenorrhea than on the other aspects.

7. *Skills are acquired.* One of physical education's greatest contributions is through the development of physical skills in its programs.

The science of psychology plays an important part in the teaching of physical education activities. Members of the physical education profession are interested in learning the best ways to teach skills, which should be taught in the most efficient and economical way possible. Therefore, the purpose of this chapter is to give the student a brief introduction to psychology as a foundation for the learning process in physical education.

Motives for participation in physical education activities

Teachers must have an understanding of the behavioral characteristics of their students. In physical education it is necessary for the teacher to be aware of the reasons why students participate in physical activities. Cogan* lists several motives.

1. *Health and fitness.* This is an extremely important motive for participation in physical education. Associated with this motive is the student's desire to develop physical endurance and strength. Because society has placed a high value on the need for a good physique, students participate in physical education in order to improve their general appearance and thus win the admiration of members of the opposite sex and their peers.

2. *Social approval.* Students participate in physical education because of their desire to win social approval. The youth from the ghetto often participates in physical activities because this is one area where he can succeed and not face discrimination. Students who cannot obtain academic recognition may look to physical activities as a vehicle to win the respect and admiration of others. Students who are shy and withdrawn may participate in physical education to develop the relationship with others that they are lacking. Cogan also indicates that students participate in physical education because of a desire to gain understanding of other people that leads to the development of more positive relationships. Dancing, as an example given by Cogan, gives the student the opportunity for socially accepted body contact with members of the opposite sex.

3. *Competition, self-evaluation, and social control.* Through physical education activities the student can compete with others and assess his own liabilities and limitations. Students have a desire to compete in physical education activities because through them they can develop self-control and learn such ethical qualities as honesty and good sportsmanship.

4. *Self-esteem.* Students participate in physical education because of the desire to master particular skills and thus improve self-esteem. The boy or girl who achieves success and gains skill in such sports as tennis or bowling feels a sense of

*Cogan, Max: Motives for participation in physical education, National College Physical Education Association for Men, Proceedings of Annual Meetings, January 10-13, 1968, pp. 56-63.

accomplishment, which in turn raises his self-esteem.

5. *Creative experience.* Students participate in physical education because they desire a creative experience. Cogan indicates that the qualities of spontaneity, imagination, love of adventure, and new situations are often associated with physical education activities and satisfy the needs of students looking for creative activities. Creativity is expressed in many activities such as athletic contests, where teams develop new plays in order to out-think opponents, and through dance, where students express feelings and emotions without using spoken language.

6. *Integration of personality.* Students participate in physical education activities to relieve their tensions and frustrations. Physical education is an important outlet for aggressive behavior because it provides a setting where the student can reduce his tensions and frustrations in a socially accepted manner. Students realize that psychological problems can result if too much time is spent working with no time for relaxation; thus, they participate in physical education activities as an escape from daily work routine.

7. *Development of specific skills.* Students are motivated to participate in physical education activities in order to improve their performance in a particular sport or activity in which they have particular interest. For example, some students participate in physical education activities in order to improve their ability for self-defense.

The psychologist is interested in people's attitudes toward physical activity and also the various phenomena associated with skill learning. Cratty* lists some reasons why physical educators as well as psychologists should be interested in such relationships.

1. The social psychologist is interested in determining the attitude of young people and adults toward physical activity.
2. The physiological psychologist is interested in the relationship of such things as stress and tension to vigorous physical activity.
3. The clinical psychologist and psychiatrist are interested in such things as body image and self-concepts in the formation of a healthy personality. Some of them have also advanced the thesis that to improve such things as cognition, visual perception, speech and hearing, perceptual-motor characteristics must be taken into consideration.
4. Many psychological variables relate to phys-

ical activity directly involving the teaching-learning situation, the way human beings behave, and the impact of physical practice in behavioral change.
5. Many psychological parameters relate to sports that concern themselves with such factors as mental preparation of the athlete, problems of motivation, nature of movement perception, personality development of athletes, and the therapeutic values of competition.
6. Professional preparation institutions have introduced courses in recent years concerned with motor learning and psychology of motor activity.
7. Many questions need to be answered by our profession such as: What is the nature of kinesthesis? How often should physical education be taught each week? What are the causes of muscular tension? What are the conditions for the retention of a skill? The answers to these and other questions involving psychological factors will result in a superior program of physical education.

Personality development and athletics

The role of athletics in personality development is extremely important to the physical educator. Although an individual's personality is formed early in life, it can be modified by later experiences. Psychologists recognize that participation in athletics can contribute to personality development. In some cases competitive athletics satisfy such basic needs as recognition, belonging, self-respect, and feelings of achievement, as well as provide a wholesome outlet for the drive for physical activity and creativity. These are desirable psychological effects that aid in molding socially acceptable personalities. At the same time, however, competitive athletics can produce harmful effects. If they are conducted in light of adult interests, community pressures, and as ends in themselves, rather than as a means of fuller psychological development of students, such competition can result in undesirable social and emotional effects.

Since participation in athletics may affect an individual's personality in either a positive or negative manner, it is important for physical educators to understand why students prefer to participate in one sport or activity rather than another. Students select

*Cratty, Bryant J.: Psychological bases of physical activity, Journal of Health, Physical Education, and Recreation **36**:71, 1965.

a particular activity because of their personality. Thune,* in a comparison of weight lifters and non–weight lifters, found weight lifters to be shy, withdrawn, and often lacking confidence, and he concluded that people with this type of personality prefer this sport as opposed to others. Many students who are introverted and shy prefer the individual sports such as golf or tennis, while the extroverted student prefers the team sports such as baseball or football.

Singer,† in collecting data on student preferences in physical education, found that college students selected bowling as their first choice as opposed to the team sports. Singer concluded that the choice was made because students at this age want to demonstrate personal skill in activities satisfying to them. Recreation and coeducational activities were found to be popular among college students because they are associated with adulthood. Young children, however, since they are not as interested in coeducational activities, would be more apt to choose team sports and body contact activities.

Much research has been done in the area of personality and athletics. Studies have attempted mainly to determine the personality characteristics of the performer. In a study on the personality of the male athlete, Ogilvie‡ found that those athletes who achieved a high degree of success in sports were mainly extroverted. Top athletes were found to have a need to achieve success, had a need for an outlet for aggression, had the desire to dominate others, were confident, and were found to be extremely independent.

Most of the research in this area is inconclusive because ineffective measuring devices and techniques were used. Hopefully there will be improved techniques in the future that will provide valid information about the personality of the athlete. This will help physical educators and coaches to create programs that best meet the needs of their students.

Self-attitudes

Physical education teachers must be concerned with improving self-attitudes of their students. Research indicates that physical education can be an important vehicle in the improvement of one's self-image. Recent investigations disclose that athletic success is associated with personal and social adjustments that improve the student's feeling of worth and esteem. Physical fitness development improves an individual's mental health, and motor skill learning improves an individual's inner feelings of worth.

Body image is an important concern to students. In a day and age where society places great importance on a good physique, individuals should develop healthy attitudes toward their body. The attitudes and feelings of a person toward his body affects his personality development. Sheldon and Stevens* have indicated that a person with a particular type of physique may have a definite stereotyped behavior. For example, he may view his body as something ugly, lack confidence in its performance, or believe that it is something that is well developed and can meet the challenge of any physical situation. Such feelings will affect his relations with other people and also his role in a physical education experience.

Body image is particularly important during the adolescent period. For example, some research has shown that when a boy's physique is small, not well developed, and weak over an extended period of time, his behavior is affected. He will become overly shy or assertive and will reflect internal discord. The person who matures late may find his relations with classmates affected when he is kept out of games because his classmates

---

*Thune, John B.: Personality of weightlifters, Research Quarterly **20:**296-306, 1949.

†Singer, Robert N.: Motor learning and human performance, New York, 1968, The Macmillan Co., p. 319.

‡Ogilvie, Bruce C.: The personality of the male athlete, The American Academy of Physical Education **1:**45-51, 1968.

*Sheldon, W. H., and Stevens, S. S.: The varieties of temperament, New York, 1942, Harper & Row, Publishers.

desire to be successful in their game experience. He may consequently develop an unfavorable attitude toward physical activity. On the other hand, the person who matures early may find that although he was always the star during his early game experiences in adolescence, as other persons matured he lost this status and the adjustment presented some difficulties. Other personality problems have been found in such individuals as boys with feminine characteristics, students with narcissistic characteristics, and boys and girls who possess certain types of body mechanics and posture.

As physical educators understand the role of body image, they will be better able to understand why various students have certain attitudes and feelings toward physical activity and the contributions that physical education can make to these persons.

PHYSICAL EDUCATION AND ACADEMIC ACHIEVEMENT*

Although 9-year-old Susan has normal intelligence, she could not master the fundamentals of arithmetic, social studies, English, and writing, regardless of how hard she tried. Her academic difficulties were compounded by a partial paralysis of the right side of her body. After her parents and teachers had tried unsuccessfully to help her, she was referred to the Achievement Center for Children at Purdue University, where much research has been done on children with academic difficulties.

At the Center, Susan spent 2½ years in a specially designed program of motor activity under skilled leadership. As a result, her academic and physical improvement was termed "miraculous" by her mother, the principal, and her classroom teacher. Her report card jumped two letter grades in every school subject, and for the first time she was able to participate in a full schedule of classroom activities.

---

*This section is adapted from an article by Bucher, Charles A.: Health and physical education and academic achievement, NEA Journal **54:**38-40, 1965.

Susan is just one of numerous children, most of whom do not have a physical handicap like hers, who have been helped to improve academically at the Center by taking part in a program of motor activities used as an integral part of a perceptual-motor training program.

More research is needed to establish and define the exact relationship of physical activity, motor skills, and health to academic achievement, but the evidence to date firmly establishes the fact that a close affinity exists. Indeed, the kind of physical education program that leads to improved physical and social fitness and health are vital to the education and academic achievement of every boy and girl.

This fact has been recognized throughout history by some of the world's most profound thinkers. For example, Socrates stressed that poor health can contribute to grave mistakes in thinking. Comenius noted: "Intellectual progress is conditioned at every step by bodily vigor. To attain the best results, physical exercise must accompany and condition mental training." Rousseau observed that "an enfeebled body enervated the mind" and included a rich program of physical activities for *Emile.*

More recently, such authorities as Arnold Gesell, Arthur T. Jersild, and the Swiss psychologist Jean Piaget found that a child's earliest learnings are motor in nature (involving neuromuscular systems and resulting in movement such as running, jumping, reaching, and the like) and form the foundation for subsequent learnings.

As D. H. Radler and Newell C. Kephart wrote in their authoritative book *Success Through Play:* "Motor activity of some kind underlies all behavior including higher thought processes. In fact behavior . . . can function no better than do the basic motor abilities upon which it is based."

Academic achievement refers to the progress a child makes in school as measured by his scores on achievement tests, his grade-point averages, his promotion from grade to grade, and the development of proper attitudes. As any experienced teacher knows, academic achievement requires more than intellectual capacity. Non-intellectual factors, such as the will to achieve, health, and self-concept, are almost certain to play an important part in a student's ability to achieve academically.

Physical education is related to academic achievement in at least four ways: (1) through emphasis on the development of motor skills, (2) by promoting physical fitness, (3) by imparting knowledge and modifying behavior in regard to good health practices, and (4) by aiding in the process of social and emotional development, which leads to a more positive self-concept.

Typical of the research studies confirming the relationship between motor skills and academic achievement is that of G. L. Rarick and Robert McKee, who studied twenty third graders grouped according to their motor proficiency. The study showed that the group with high motor proficiency had a greater number who achieved "excellent" or "good" ratings in reading, writing, and comprehension than the group with low motor efficiency.

In another study, Jack Keogh and David Benson experimented with the motor characteristics of forty-three under-achieving boys, ages 10 to 14, enrolled in the Psy-

Relationship of academic performance to physical fitness.

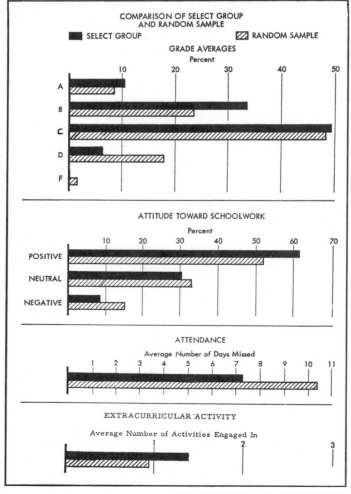

FROM WILKINSON, C. B.: REPORT TO THE
PRESIDENT, DECEMBER 10, 1962.

chology Clinic School at UCLA. They found that, as individuals, half of the boys from 10 to 12 years old exhibited poor motor performance.

James H. Humphrey* found that motor activities are beneficial in developing skills and concepts in reading, mathematics, and science. Humphrey indicates that if an academic skill or concept is practiced during a physical education activity, that skill or concept is learned faster. For example, children can be taught the science concept of the "complete circuit" by participating in a simple activity such as the straddle ball relay. In this activity the children standing in line one behind the other, legs outstretched, roll a ball between their legs, the ball is considered the electric current, while the children are the circuit. When the ball goes outside one of the student's legs, the teacher can impose upon the students the fact that the circuit is broken. Students can get a fuller insight into the meaning of the concept being taught. Humphrey further indicates that many advanced academic skills and concepts can be introduced to children at an early age through the use of motor activities as a vehicle for learning.

A. H. Ismail, N. Kephart, and C. C. Cowell, utilizing motor aptitude tests, found that IQ and academic success could be predicted from these tests, with balance and coordination items the best predictors for estimating achievement.

Other studies indicate that the child's first learnings accrue from an interaction with his physical and social environment. Physical action provides the experience to clarify and make meaningful concepts of size, shape, direction, and other characteristics. In addition, through physical activities he experiences sensations, he has new feelings, and he develops new interests as well as satisfies old curiosities.

The importance of physical fitness was stressed by Lewis Terman more than 25

*Humphrey, James H.: Academic skill and concept development through motor activity, The American Academy of Physical Education 1:29-35, 1968.

years ago. After working with gifted children he stated: "Results of physical measurements and medical examinations provide a striking contrast to the popular stereotype of the child prodigy, so commonly depicted as a pathetic creature, an overserious, undersized, sickly, bespectacled child." He went on to say that physical weakness was found nearly 30% fewer times in children of higher intelligence than in those of lower intelligence.

Many research studies since Terman have supported the contention that physical fitness is related to academic achievement.

H. H. Clarke and Boyd O. Jarman, in a study of boys of ages 9, 12, and 15, found a consistent tendency for the high groups on various strength and growth measures to have higher means on both academic achievement tests and grade-point averages than low groups. Studies conducted at the universities of Oregon and Iowa and at Syracuse and West Point have shown a significant relationship between physical fitness and academic success and between physical fitness and leadership qualities. David Brace, F. R. Rogers, Clayton Shay, Marcia Hart, and others have done extensive research showing relationships between scholastic and academic success and physical fitness.

Through the development of desirable attitudes and the application of health knowledge, the student achieves his maximum strength, energy, endurance, recuperative power, and sensory acuity. Furthermore, the effective physical education program helps boys and girls to understand and appreciate the value of good health as a means of achieving their greatest productivity, effectiveness, and happiness as individuals.

Some research has shown a relationship between scholastic success and the degree to which a student is accepted by his peer group. Similarly, the boy or girl who is well grounded in motor skills usually possesses social status among his or her peers.

For example, J. B. Merriman found that

such qualities as poise, ascendency, and self-assurance were significantly more developed in students of high motor ability than in those with low motor ability.

Other research shows that popularity in adolescent boys is more closely associated with physical and athletic ability than with intelligence; that leadership qualities are most prevalent among school boys (and West Point cadets) who score high on physical fitness tests; and that well-adjusted students tend to participate in sports to a greater extent than poorly adjusted students.

Physical education not only affects social development but emotional development as well. Games provide release from tension after long periods of study; furthermore, achievement in physical activities gives students a sense of pride that pays dividends in emotional satisfaction and well-being.

In this sense, the value of physical education may be greater for educationally subnormal students than for average boys and girls. James N. Oliver, lecturer in education at the University of Birmingham, England, has done much research on educationally subnormal boys and has found that systematic and progressive physical conditioning yields marked mental and physical improvement. He believes such improvement resulted from the boys' feelings of achievement and of consequent improved adjustment.

The value of physical education will depend largely upon whether or not they meet the following criteria:

The physical education program includes a variety of daily movement experiences and instruction in many basic motor activities, aimed not at making the student a superior performer in one or two but stressing a modest performance in all, consistent with his developmental level. It also helps each student to achieve physically according to desirable standards.

The physical education program provides boys and girls with accurate and significant health knowledge related to their individual needs and interests. There is also concern for health services and a healthful physical and emotional environment.

The physical education program is accorded educational respectability so that students and parents will more readily appreciate its value and seek the benefits it offers.

By providing these essentials, the school will help to ensure a high standard of academic achievement on the part of all boys and girls.

GETTING AT THE "WHY" OF THE ACTIVITY

There is the beginning of a trend in physical education to get at the "why" of the activity as well as the activity itself. This is evidenced by the publication of high school textbooks; assignments given to students to investigate various physiological, psychological, and sociological factors related to the role of physical activity and human development; findings of some research studies that indicate that mental practice is effective in skill learning; the provision for classroom activity in state syllabuses, and the emphasis upon conceptualized teaching with a realization that the most effective way to help students form general concepts is to present the concepts in many different and varied situations. Watson* indicates this and points out, in addition, that the formation of concepts can be furthered by providing many different experiences, some of which will be contrasting— some that include and some that do not include the desired concept—and then to encourage the formulation of the general concept and its application to specific situations that are different from those in which the concept was learned.

For many years physical educators have been primarily activity oriented. Programs have been centered around calisthenics, games, sports, obstacle courses, dance, and other physical activities. There has been little classroom activity where assignments are given, discussions held, laboratory experiences conducted, questions answered, scientific principles of physical activity pre-

---

*Watson, Goodwin: What do we know about learning? NEA Journal **52**:20, 1963.

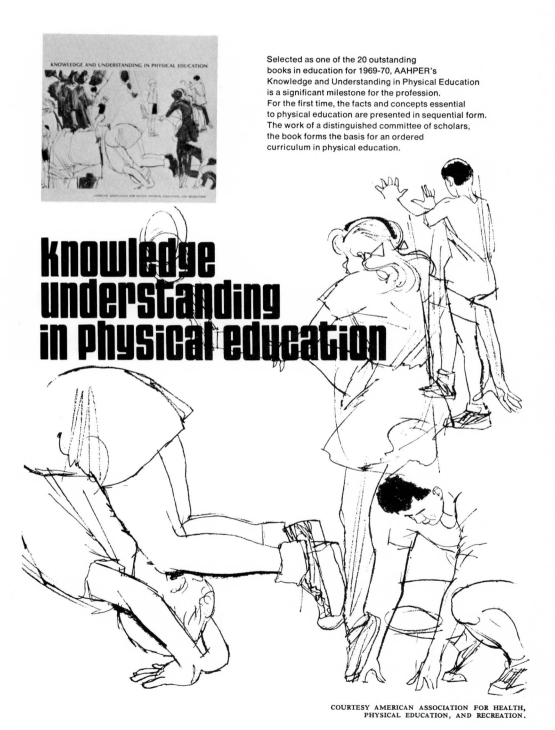

Selected as one of the 20 outstanding
books in education for 1969-70, AAHPER's
Knowledge and Understanding in Physical Education
is a significant milestone for the profession.
For the first time, the facts and concepts essential
to physical education are presented in sequential form.
The work of a distinguished committee of scholars,
the book forms the basis for an ordered
curriculum in physical education.

COURTESY AMERICAN ASSOCIATION FOR HEALTH,
PHYSICAL EDUCATION, AND RECREATION.

sented and interpreted, history of sports revealed, as well as rules, strategies, and other subject matter related to physical education presented. Some physical educators have discussed with high school students the subject of physical education in order to determine what knowledge, for example, they had regarding the physiological basis for physical activity. Unfortunately, most of these students did not know why physical education is important to them as individuals and the contributions it makes to their physiological, psychological, and sociological betterment. They did not know why exercise is important on a regular basis in planning their week-to-week schedules. Some students felt that physical activity is desirable to provide a break between classes and a means of having fun. Girls found it difficult to see the relationship between beauty and physical activity. Most students did not understand why physical education should be a requirement in our schools and colleges. Most of our students have not been physically educated in this sense. It is the feeling of more and more persons in the profession that all students who graduate from our schools and colleges should understand and appreciate the scientific values that accrue to the person who includes physical activity as part of his routine throughout life. It is the feeling of this group that the carryover values of school and college physical education programs will be much greater if such subject matter is presented. These persons would hasten to explain, however, that they would continue to stress activity, but at the same time provision would be made periodically for classroom experiences and for reading and mental problem-solving experiences.

Physical educators must attempt to carry out this new approach to the teaching of physical education. By concentrating on the why of the activity, students will more fully understand the importance of physical education in their total development, and the profession of physical education will be taking an important step in establishing itself as an integral part of the educational process.

DEVELOPMENTS AFFECTING THE LEARNING PROCESS

There are several developments on the educational scene that portend to influence the learning process. These include programmed instruction, team teaching, flexible scheduling, creativity, sensitivity training, educational television, ability grouping, and class reorganization. Because of the impact these trends may have on physical education, a short discussion is devoted to each.

Programmed instruction

Programmed learning is available in many forms, but the advent of teaching machines is the best known of the various kinds of mechanical devices that utilize programmed materials. The first person believed to have experimented with teaching machines was Sidney L. Pressey at Ohio State University in the 1920's. B. F. Skinner, a psychologist at Harvard University, has given great impetus to this method of teaching, which is being used in several subject-matter areas and in some schools across the country. It has implications for physical education, especially in the area of getting across knowledge, understanding, and appreciation associated with such factors as physiological facts, rules of games, techniques, and health materials.

The basic psychological principles that seem to make the teaching machine a valuable auxiliary aid to the teacher are:

1. *Learning appears to progress best when acquired in small steps.* Programmed learning is based on the principle that subject matter should be broken down into small doses and that the student should be led from the simple to the complex in the learning process. However, it should be pointed out that where the steps are broken into pieces, not parts, this can interfere with the learning process.

2. *The learning process encourages the student to actively participate.* Each stu-

dent participates by answering questions, analyzing his progress, and progressing as he achieves. He cannot be a passive spectator. He becomes actively involved in the learning process.

3. *Rewards reinforce learning.* The student is immediately informed if his answer is correct, if he is making progress, and if he can go on to more difficult material. This reward usually proves to be a satisfying experience and enhances the learning process.

4. *The student sets his own pace.* Programmed learning is tailored to either the fast or the slow learner. The individual proceeds at his own rate, but in either case he learns.

5. *The student learns when he is ready.* Programmed instruction is adjusted to the concept of readiness. It only presents the student with learning experiences that he is capable of mastering.

6. *The student is given the opportunity to achieve success.* Because of the way teaching machines are constructed and through their technique of prompting the learner, programmed instruction helps the student discover the correct answer to the problem.

Teaching machines usually function by asking questions of the student through the medium of an item, a sentence that appears in a small window, or some other method of presentation. If a space is left for a missing word, for example, the student would answer the item and then by manipulating a lever determine the right answer. The student knows immediately if his answer is correct. He then moves on to the next question. Some machines repeat questions at the end of the lesson.

The results from programmed learning have been encouraging and augur well as an effective means of instruction. In some cases a programmed text is used rather than the teaching machine. Subject matter fields such as psychology, logic, music, and foreign language have been utilized with some degree of success. In physical education the benefits of programmed instruction have

not yet been fully realized. It is extremely difficult, if not impossible, to program motor skills. However, programmed instruction can be beneficial in teaching a sport like basketball. Many basic principles, rules, and strategies of the game can be programmed. Programmed learning will never eliminate or replace teachers, but it can free them from routine drills and other forms of robot learning.

Team teaching

In its barest essentials, team teaching takes place whenever more than one teacher has responsibility for the same group of children at a given time. In its more highly organized existence, team teaching involves an instructional team of teachers who are specialists in certain areas, together with some who are nonprofessional. The team usually varies from three to six teachers responsible for 150 children or more. The students instructed by the team may all be in the same grade or in different grades and the classes in one subject or groups of subjects. The teaching team is responsible for the planning, teaching, and evaluation of the educational program for the group of children with whom they are working. One of the teachers is named the team leader and is responsible for program coordination.

Hundreds of communities throughout the United States are engaged in or planning some form of team teaching. It has been utilized in the field of physical education with success.

The Dade County, Florida, public schools* have utilized team teaching programs. Officials concerned with the program have stated that the primary advantages of the program are:

1. Instructor-pupil ratio may be varied with the type of activity, ability level, or facilities available.
2. The department is able to utilize the talents

*Reams, David, and Bleier, T. J.: Developing team teaching in physical education, Journal of Health, Physical Education, and Recreation **39:**50, 1968.

and interests of individual staff members to the best advantage.

3. The pupil has the benefit of the talents of several instructors rather than being limited to one person during an entire year.
4. Adaptation to abilities can become a reality rather than a desire. Each level should have specific lesson plans based on the general abilities of that group. This enables the pupils to better establish goals for their progression through the physical education program.

Evergreen Park High School in Evergreen Park, Illinois, utilizes team teaching in physical education.* In this community large-group instruction is utilized in such areas as warm-up drills, special programs and tournaments, and health instruction. These large groups are broken down into smaller groups for discussion of certain health instruction and matters that can be handled effectively in this manner. It has been found that team teaching in this community has resulted in greater flexibility. Changes can be made as the need arises; each teacher in the department plays a part in each class; outside resources, such as teachers from

---

*Clein, Marvin I.: A new approach to the physical education schedule, Journal of Health, Physical Education, and Recreation **33**:34, 1962.

other departments, and the community, are utilized more frequently; the needs of students are better met; the planning period provides for better teaching and evaluation; more benefits accrue for the intramural program; members of the department can better exploit their own specialties; better teacher-pupil ratio exists; and there is more effective supervision and control of classes.

Flexible scheduling

Flexible scheduling, sometimes called modular scheduling because of the time units involved—most frequently about 20 minutes each—is a term used to describe a school schedule in which classes do not meet for the same length of time each day. Flexible scheduling uses blocks of time to build periods of different length. For example, one module might be 20 minutes in length, a double module would be 40 minutes, a triple module would be 60 minutes, and a quadruple module would be 80 minutes. Time is left between each module for organization of classes.

One advantage of flexible scheduling over the traditional pattern of fixed scheduling, or the same allotment of time

Team teaching at Evergreen Park High School, Evergreen Park, Ill. Physical education instructors meet daily in a common planning period.

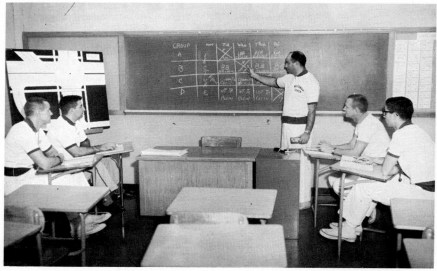

per day to a subject, is that flexible scheduling enables subjects to have varying times for instruction. For example, teachers say that usually more time is necessary in a science laboratory than for instruction in a foreign language newly introduced to students. It has been pointed out that a foreign language can be most effectively taught in shorter time periods at more frequent intervals. Flexible scheduling also provides more instructional time, more opportunity for small group instruction, and less time in study halls where learning time is not always put to the best use. With flexible scheduling it is possible to have subject matter and courses presented under more optimum conditions, on an individual basis, and in smaller or larger groups, as best meets the needs of the subject and teacher.

With flexible scheduling it is also possible to increase the length of the school day, giving students the opportunity to do more of their school work at school, where there is greater instructional assistance available. Flexible scheduling also allows programs to be expanded not only for the academically gifted but also for the below average student. Flexible scheduling allows the teacher more time for preparation, planning, and instruction.

Team teaching at Evergreen Park High School, Evergreen Park, Ill. The large group (center) and its breakdown into small groups. Team members are utilized in areas of their best abilities.

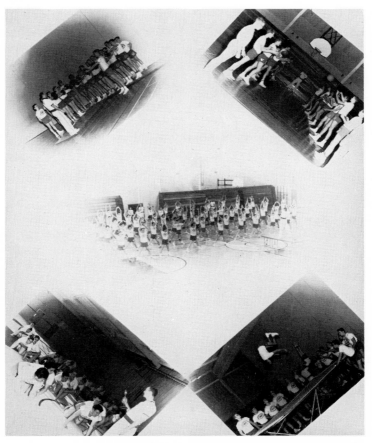

FROM CLEIN, MARVIN I.: JOURNAL OF HEALTH, PHYSICAL EDUCATION, AND RECREATION **33**:34, 1962.

Creativity

There is increased interest and stress in education on promoting creativity in the teaching process and in helping to release the creative talents of students. Creativity, as used here, is the process of giving birth to an idea. It involves thinking, exploring, and examining and a reconstruction of experiences and formation into new patterns.

Creativity can be injected into teaching. Following are some basic principles involved in creative teaching that have been reiterated by Henry, as a result of a lecture he heard.*

1. Creativity is not absolute; there are different levels.
2. Creativity arises from a love of children and helping them to learn.
3. Self-realization is a cardinal principle of creative teaching.
4. Meaningful and aesthetic learning is the outcome of creative teaching.
5. The climate of the classroom must be conducive to creative learning.
6. Problem situations give rise to creativity.
7. A creative teacher is not restricted to a textbook or course of study.
8. A creative teacher helps to direct the creative abilities of children into the right channels.

Certain characteristics contribute to creativity. Strang identifies these qualities as follows†:

1. The creative child *possesses imagination*. All kinds of new ideas and problems cross the child's mind, perhaps not new to adults but original with the child.
2. The creative child *has a purpose*. There is method and an objective in the young person's mind, and creativity stems from this purpose.
3. The creative child *desires experience*. He is curious and wants to explore, and this motivating force should be nourished.
4. The creative child *is puzzled*. The answers to many things in the environment and

events that occur are not readily apparent and there is a desire to know.

5. The creative child *exploits the present*. He is not concerned with the past or the future; it is the job at hand that commands his attention—a requisite for creativity.
6. The creative child *enjoys spontaneous play*. There is a desire to toy with different ideas, to see new relationships, and to have fun doing it.

Strang goes on to point out that a child's creativeness is enhanced by the teacher's questions and comments if they encourage him to participate, choose, and have fun. However, if the reaction is negative, if there are too many "don'ts" or if there is too much criticism, this tends to suppress creative tendencies.

Physical educators can be more creative in their own teaching by developing new ideas of presenting material, utilizing facilities, scheduling classes, and evaluating and carrying out other responsibilities. They can also open up the creative reservoirs of their students by encouraging new ideas and new movement concepts and by involving pupils more in the planning of educational experiences.

Sensitivity training or human awareness

A recent innovation in some educational programs, both at the school and college level, is sensitivity training, or, as it is sometimes called, human awareness. It has been the subject of sufficient discussion to warrant its inclusion in this section of the text.

In sensitivity training participants work together in a small group situation in an attempt to better understand themselves and other people. The training group is typically called a T group. The person who leads the group is referred to as the trainer. His role is to help the group learn from its experiences.

The purpose of sensitivity training is to learn through an analysis of our own and other people's experiences. Most groups meet for a total of 10 to 45 hours. Some of these periods are usually marathon sessions that go on for several hours and

*Henry, Charles D.: Developing hints in promoting creativity in the classroom, The Physical Educator **15:**58, 1958. (Taken from notes from a lecture by Dr. H. L. Richards of Grambling College, Grambling, La.)

†Strang, Ruth: The creative child, National Parent-Teacher **54:**14, 1960.

where fatigue plays a part in helping members of the group to reveal their true feelings, reactions, perceptions, and behavior. The group does not have a fixed agenda or a definite structure in its meetings. Instead, the trainer initially points out that the participants themselves will be the forces that determine how individual behavior is influenced and that the data for learning will be the behavior of the members of the group.

Assumptions underlying T group sensitivity training is that each member of the group is responsible for his own learning, the trainer facilitates the learning experience, and the experiences of the group are examined in sufficient detail so that valid generalizations may be drawn. Furthermore, assumptions include that a member of the group will be most likely to learn when honest relationships are established with other people. Sensitivity sessions, it is claimed, enable persons to be open, honest, and direct with each other. Finally, an assumption is made that human relations skills will be developed as a person examines and understands the values underlying his own behavior and is able to practice new behavior patterns and to see the reactions achieved.

There is little valid research to date to support the worth of sensitivity training. However, some generalizations that appear to have support from the work done thus far are that persons who have been exposed to such training are more likely to improve their managerial skills with the persons with whom they work on the job, that every person who pursues such training does not profit equally from the experience, that personal testimonials support the beneficial impact that it has on their lives, and that such hazards as serious stress and mental disturbance during training occur in not more than 1% of the participants.

IMPLICATIONS OF SENSITIVITY TRAINING FOR PHYSICAL EDUCATION

Some educators feel that what is purported to be sensitivity training is best furthered in a setting in which people are actively interacting with one another. The teacher or trainer, as he is called, is the most important single factor in establishing a good program. The teacher creates a climate where the student feels free to express his feelings about himself, his friends, his teachers, or school in general. In this atmosphere where students can freely express themselves, individuals can improve their social development, relationships with other members of the class, and in some cases their performance in the subject matter. In this context physical education can play an important role. Physical education provides a laboratory for improving human relationships because in the gymnasium and out on the playing fields students are interacting with one another. Within certain limits physical education teachers should encourage students to express their feelings about themselves, their classmates, and the program in which they are participating.

Ability grouping

Ability grouping is being utilized more and more in the school systems of the United States. Students are being classified according to their intelligence, achievement, and other factors that impinge on their school record. Ability grouping has its advocates and also those who oppose such methods.

Ability grouping, according to some leaders in the field, has potential for grouping physical education classes into meaningful units for instructional purposes. For example, having students with low physical fitness ratings in one group facilitates meeting their needs in this area; having boys and girls of the same skill ability together makes it easier to teach effectively. In other words, a homogeneous grouping rather than a heterogeneous one makes it possible to concentrate on special activities and techniques readily adapted to the needs of the group in question.

Effective ability grouping depends upon staff, facilities, and valid methods of identifying pupils' abilities. If it is to do the job that is needed, providing better learning experiences for children and youth with a variety of skills, intelligence, physical traits, and mental abilities, then, according to Essex, the following items should be kept in mind*:

1. The foremost purpose of the American school should be kept in mind—all children should have some of their school experiences in a typical classroom situation.
2. Ability grouping will be more successful if parents understand individual differences. Mothers and fathers as well as teachers must understand that each child is different from the others.
3. Parents need to understand that ability grouping is aimed at helping all children and not just a few. The aim of ability grouping is to help each child experience challenges that he can meet successfully and not fail.
4. The program should provide for a continuous and comprehensive identification of children's abilities. Children change; therefore, changes in grouping will be necessary from time to time if the child's best interests are to be met.
5. There should be conferences between teachers and parents. Through home and school meetings a better understanding can be created.
6. Patterns of ability groupings will vary from community to community; therefore, the type of ability grouping in any one school system should be developed on the basis of the needs within that educational program.

Class reorganization

Trump has utilized a report on secondary education in general to forecast a future secondary school health, physical education, and recreation program. Among the new approaches he indicates will take place are the following†:

1. Class size will vary with the purpose and content of instruction. There will be large, small, and medium-sized classes. There will be large groups of students for lectures and demonstrations and small groups for discussions and for work in the laboratories.
2. A student in the future physical education program will spend once a week as a mem-

ber of a large group, once a week as a member of a class of fifteen students, and 120 minutes twice a week in the laboratory.
3. Six kinds of staff members will be in charge of the program. These six are professional teachers, instruction assistants, general aides to help with technical services, clerks, community consultants, and professional consultants.
4. Teachers will have more time to plan and evaluate their instruction.
5. The quality of teachers will be improved.

EDUCATIONAL INSTRUCTIONAL MEDIA

Audiovisual aids are being utilized to a greater degree in educational institutions than ever before. Educators have come to realize that the sensory experiences provided by audiovisual aids can make learning much more effective. Research in the use of audiovisual aids has found that aids contribute to a greater understanding of learning experiences. For example, the teacher may discuss the butterfly stroke in swimming; however, this concept may not be clear to the student because he cannot visualize the actual movements. By providing a film or picture of the stroke, the student gets a clearer picture of its component parts. Audiovisual aids also increase student interest and motivation for learning. When teachers break from their traditional verbal-centered approach and utilize such aids as television or films, students are freed from the boredom that frequently takes place in many learning experiences. The innovation of new techniques such as the videotape lets students see themselves in action, thus increasing their desire to perform.

Some of the most important visual aids having implications for physical education are (1) educational television, (2) the overhead projector, (3) videotapes, and (4) single concept loop films.

Educational television

Physical education is a subject for which television has great potential. Some of the advantages include the following:

1. Physical education can be interpreted in its correct light to the public. Today, many people do not understand the true meaning of physical education; consequently, there

*Essex, Martin: How good is ability grouping? National Parent-Teacher **54:**16, 1959.
†Trump, J. Lloyd, and Baynham, Dorsey: Focus on change—guide to better schools, Chicago, 1961, Rand McNally & Co.

is a great need for better ways of reaching the general public.

2. Physical education can utilize master teachers. By utilizing the very best instruction, an excellent job can be accomplished in presenting physical education to the public.

3. Physical education can reach a larger audience. Television reaches into classrooms, play centers, and homes that would never be exposed under ordinary circumstances.

4. Physical education classes in an entire city system or in many systems can benefit from closed-circuit television. New methods can be utilized, new materials demonstrated, new activities introduced, and many other innovations can be accomplished through educational television. New ideas that would not ordinarily be available to many schools, teachers, and people can be disseminated.

5. Physical education can exploit close-up television techniques to advantage. The zoom lens and other techniques make it possible to provide excellent instruction in how to perform skills and other physical activities correctly.

The potential of educational television for physical education is great. Physical edu-

New techniques for teaching.

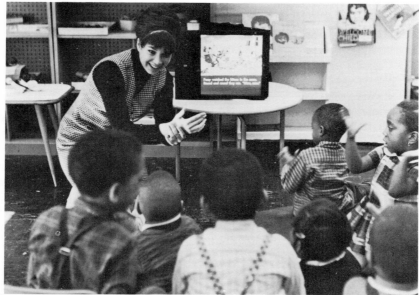

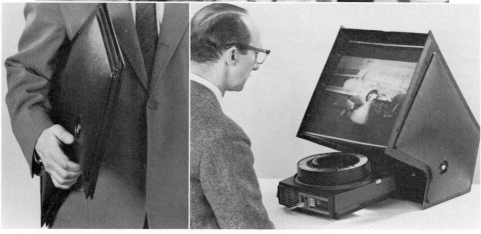

cators should acquaint themselves with the techniques, opportunities, and ways and means by which television can be utilized in their field.

Overhead projector

The overhead projector is a compact, lightweight machine that is easily operable. The material projected is in the form of a transparency made of film. There are various ways to make a transparency. Some transparencies such as a diagram or play are reproduced from the original document by a copying machine. Companies such as 3M have been instrumental in providing research in this area.

Botwin* lists several features of the overhead projector applicable in physical education.

1. It enables a brilliant image in black and white or color to be projected in a lighted room or gymnasium.
2. It enables teachers to face their students because of the normal front room position the overhead assumes.
3. It permits the teacher to present various concepts, ideas, and skill development to small, average, or large classes.
4. It enables a pen or pencil pointer to be used with the projection, thus directing the attention of the class to various details on the screen.
5. It enables teachers to use a grease pencil and thus write over the transparency.
6. It allows teachers to control the rate at which information is presented.
7. It permits the use of overlays so that the teacher can superimpose additional materials. In the teaching of skill progression this method reduces complex skills or difficult movements to their simplest design.
8. It enables the simulation of motion on the transparency through the use of a polarizing spinner.
9. It permits the teacher through the use of copying machines to duplicate the materials presented on the transparencies. Each student can be given a duplicate copy that will serve as an excellent follow-up for skill teaching.

---

*Botwin, Louis: The media approach, a happening in physical education, The Physical Educator **25:**119, 1968.

Videotapes

Videotapes are an asset in many physical education programs. The videotape records a student participating in learning a motor skill and provides instant review. After each attempt at a skill is recorded, the student can visualize and analyze his performance. The insight the student gains from seeing himself in action can be extremely beneficial in improving his understanding of the skill and thus increase his level of performance. For example, the student sees himself throwing a baseball and discovers that he is not following through in his delivery. The videotape, with its slow motion and stop action techniques, is instrumental in discovering deficient performance.

Loop films

Loop films are also beneficial in physical education programs. The 8-mm. single concept film cartridge system requires no threading or rewinding. The teacher simply inserts the cartridge in the slot in the loop projector and the machine is turned on. Each film loop deals with a specific topic and is very concise. Loop films are used to teach various skills such as in gymnastics. For example, a student experiencing difficulty in mastering a particular piece of apparatus such as the trampoline selects a loop film on the trampoline and analyzes the performance. The student can stop the film at any time and study the specific phase causing him difficulty. Loop films can be an important contribution to learning because as a student views a single concept film he can proceed at his own rate of understanding and interest.

Other aids such as charts, pictures, and recordings also are used in physical education.

The audiovisual aids mentioned are extremely important in physical education. Their importance is as an aid that supplements rather than replaces the teaching of the qualified physical education instructor. A major abuse of audiovisual aids is that some teachers use them as substitutes. This is wrong since learning is most beneficial when there is a face-to-face exchange of ideas between the teacher and the student. Audiovisual aids play an important role in the learning process, but their role must remain secondary to personal instruction.

ADMINISTRATIVE DEVELOPMENTS AFFECTING THE LEARNING PROCESS

Until the nineteenth century, most public education in the United States was conducted in the "little red schoolhouse," a structure containing one classroom and one teacher, or, at the most, two classrooms and two teachers. These rooms were filled with pupils of varying ages studying on many different levels. During the latter half of the nineteenth century student enrollment greatly multiplied, thus increasing the need for more teachers, more classrooms, and more schools. At this time, the first graded schools in the United States emerged, and units of knowledge were established and given grade labels.

School enrollments again showed a large increase in the early part of the twentieth century, almost doubling in every decade, with the bulk of the increase in the high school age groups. In 1918, the Commission on Reorganization of Secondary Education investigated high school curriculums in an attempt to make this phase of education conform more closely to practical aims. This evaluation resulted in the formulation of the Cardinal Principles of Education and brought, at least in theory, general education closer to the needs of the masses. However, the standard curriculums were little changed as a result of the report, and all pupils, regardless of ability, were exposed to the same courses and were taught by the same methods.

As the twentieth century progressed, the needs of each individual, rather than the masses, began to dominate educational thought. Researchers pointed out the variations in creativity, ability, need, and interest, and education began to emphasize individual inquiry while placing less stress on the learning of rigid, formalized bodies of knowledge.

Only recently have our schools, and the secondary schools in particular, come under criticism from both educators and parents. Only minor changes in curriculums took place until the start of the space age. Previous to this time, the status quo was almost unequivocally accepted.

Currently, both the federal government and private industry, among other groups, are influencing educational thought through research, experimentation, and the application of technological discoveries and innovations. This influence is having an effect on curriculums in education by placing an increased emphasis on content, creativity, and school organization.

Some of the most widely applied and discussed innovations of recent years are briefly detailed in the following paragraphs. Each educator needs to be aware of not only the newest trends in his own field but also of those of education in general. Each new trend has an implication, and possibly an application, for every educational field.

The nongraded school

One of the first attempts at organizing a nongraded elementary school took place in St. Louis, Missouri, in 1868. During the late 1800's communities in New York and Colorado were experimenting with nongraded schools and were giving specialized help for both slow and fast learners. In 1957–1958, nongraded schools were in operation in forty-four communities in twenty-one states, and in 1961 there were nongraded schools in more than 500 communities. Currently, many geographically scattered school systems are experimenting with nongrading, particularly on the elementary school level.

Nongrading is simply the removal of grade labels from some, or all, of the classes in a school or school system, allowing the learner to proceed at his own pace. Appleton, Wisconsin, offers a good example of this kind of educational organization. Under the Appleton Continuous Progress Plan report cards, promotion, and grade retention are eliminated. Each individual is encouraged to work up to the limits of his own capacity and thus advances at his own most comfortable and practical rate.

The teacher in the nongraded school serves as a motivator to instill in his students the desire to learn. He is also a guidance counselor and discovers the hidden problems that may be interfering with the student's learning process. Serving as a guide for each student, the teacher selects material suitable to the needs, interests, and abilities of each individual student and then provides appropriately more difficult material as success is achieved.

The student in the nongraded school realizes that he plays an extremely important role in deciding how and what he learns. The student in such an educational setting works on his own and determines for himself the material that best fits his own individual needs, abilities, and interests.

The basic premise of the nongraded school is the recognition of individual differences between learners, and within the learner himself, and the need to teach through, rather than around, these differences.

The nongraded school evolved mainly through discontent with existent school organization and curriculums. Other reasons for nongrading have been:

1. To allow for greater flexibility in pupil placement and for uninterrupted pupil progress
2. To find, and put into use, better educational procedures
3. To provide for irregular pupil progression
4. To remove the stigma of nonpromotion and relieve the tensions created by skipping
5. To provide for more continuous upward progress of all pupils, regardless of their individual rates of learning
6. To provide a more workable educational framework centered around the pupil

The middle school

The question as to what is the most desirable pattern of grade organization is the topic of many discussions among school administrators, teachers, and the lay public. One survey of 366 unified school systems with pupil enrollment of 12,000 or more, conducted by the Educational Research Service, showed that 71% of these school systems were organized on the 6-3-3 plan, 10% on the 8-4 organization, and 6% on a 6-2-4 pattern. Other patterns include 7-5, 6-6, 5-3-4, and 7-2-3.

The pattern of organization being considered by many school systems today is the middle school concept.

The NEA* has suggested that certain features be part of the middle school.

1. There should be a span of at least three grades between five and eight to permit a gradual transition from elementary school to high school.
2. There should be an emerging departmental structure in each higher grade to provide for a gradual transition from the self-contained classroom in the elementary school to the departmentalized high school.
3. There should be a variety of flexible approaches to instruction such as team teaching, flexible scheduling, individualized instruction, independent study, and tutorial programs as means of motivating children to discover how to learn.
4. There should be courses taught that involve an interdisciplinary or multidisciplinary approach.
5. There should be a well-organized guidance program to provide for the special needs of this age group.
6. There should be some faculty members who have both elementary and secondary certification or teachers with each type of training until special preparation and certification are available for this level.
7. There should be limited attention to interschool sports and social activities.

The last feature is important to physical educators. One of the main aims of the middle school is to hold back social pressures that face students entering high school. Most research indicates that youngsters in grades five through eight should not participate in interscholastic athletics, citing mainly the emotional and social pressures

*Middle schools in theory and fact, NEA Research Bulletin **48:**49, 1969.

involved. The middle school places emphasis on athletics that take place within the boundaries of the school. Regular physical education programs and intramural athletics are highly valued for children at this age.

Some of the reasons for the middle school concept are as follows:

1. There is an opportunity for more departmentalization than found in the elementary schools but less than found in the high schools, especially in such fields as science, mathematics, art, and music.
2. There is an opportunity for greater stimulation of students and better facilities and equipment, such as laboratories and shops.
3. There is an opportunity for special teachers and special programs essential for children passing through the early adolescent period.
4. Students today have subjects that were taught much later in the school program years ago. For example, in terms of the required curriculum, the fourth grader today is in advance of the sixth grader years ago. Therefore, the middle school concept is applicable to the present educational era.
5. There is a better opportunity for student grouping and meeting individual differences.
6. There is a better opportunity for guidance services to be extended into the lower grades.
7. There is a better opportunity for a more personalized approach than is possible under other types of organization.
8. The ninth-grade youngsters are more mature and can fit into the high school program, permitting them to take advanced courses.
9. There is better opportunity for a gradual change from self-sustained classroom to complete departmentalization.

Some of the reasons against the middle school are as follows:

1. There is lack of evidence to support its value because of its relative newness.
2. There are social adjustment problems in placing ninth graders with twelfth graders.
3. Youngsters in the middle school will be pushed too hard academically and socially.
4. Administrative techniques and procedures would need to be altered.

Year-round school

The need for a year-round school program is increasingly heard whenever educational topics are discussed. Such developments as the child's becoming an economic liability in our modern industrial society, the great technological advance that has resulted in a raising of the minimal requirements for vocational adequacy, the knowledge explosion, and the taking over of many functions of the home by other agencies and institutions have resulted in many people asking the question: Why not have the children in school for a longer period of time?

The year-round school also makes sense to some educators because the school plant is idle during the summer months, although costs for administration, insurance, and capital outlay remain constant. Also, many school-age children do not have constructive programs for the summer months, and teachers would be available in many cases.

Research indicates that year-round attendance does not cause fatigue as some persons suggested it would. There is also evidence that shows the year-round school helps the slow learning pupil to do better in the classroom and the emotionally disturbed child to improve his self-control under such a program. The additional time added to the school year allows for more individual study by the students and provides teachers more opportunity to plan and develop the material they will use in the classroom.

Some of the plans suggested for extending the school year include the staggered quarter plan, in which the calendar year is divided into four quarters with pupils attending three of four quarters and having a vacation for the fourth quarter. Teachers could be hired for either three or four quarters.

A second suggestion is the 48-week school year, which would be divided into four 12-week periods, with the remaining 4 weeks being used for vacation purposes. Teachers would be employed on a 12-month basis.

A third suggestion would be the voluntary summer program, which students could attend if they so desired for purposes of remedial work and avocational, recreational, and enrichment type courses.

The fourth suggestion is the summer program for professional personnel plan. Under this arrangement, teachers would be employed on a 12-month basis and would work 48 weeks and have a 4-week vacation. The students would go to school from 36 to 40 weeks. Teachers would spend the other weeks working on curriculum and instructional planning.

The new curriculums

At the present time, our schools are passing through a rapid state of change. Few people, whether educators, parents, or leaders of our society, are satisfied with the curriculums we have. Few are content with the outcomes of these curriculums. This unrest has sparked the formulation of new objectives and has led to new curriculums based on these new objectives.

New curriculums have been devised by Project English of the U. S. Office of Education, by the School Mathematics Study Group, by the American Institute of Biological Sciences Curriculum Study, by the National Council for the Social Studies, by the Physical Science Study Committee, by the National Science Foundation, by the Chemical Education Material Study, and by the High School Geography Project.

The new curriculums are designed not to present new facts in place of the old but to lead today's students toward self-discovery of facts. The new curriculums give incentive to students, beginning in the elementary years, to be inquisitive, to discover knowledge on their own, and to learn through problem solving. The facts of mathematics, for example, do not change. What does change is the teaching approach, the methodology, and the materials used. Rather than memorization, conceptualization is the keynote. The significant concepts of a subject are learned through discovery and thus understood. Drills and memorization are viewed as the antithesis of learning.

The proponents of the new curriculums believe firmly in a basic and comprehensive education suited to individual needs. They have developed the new curriculums to provide both an enriched and a more

significant education. Thus, they have attempted to make the new curriculums as valid as possible. Not only are the effects of these curriculums on learners investigated but also the effects and demands on the teachers. Comparative pupil progress under new and old curriculums is assessed, as are the goals of the new and the old.

The new curriculums in themselves have presented problems to academicians. While the new materials are widely used in many school systems, other schools have as yet been untouched by the new curriculums. Some academic fields have had vast exposure to the new, while progress in other areas, such as physical education, the arts, and the humanities, have been virtually untouched. Where the new materials have been put into use, the total educational structure has often not been strengthened or revised sufficiently to support the use of the new materials, and teachers are occasionally ill prepared to use them. In some fields, the materials have been updated so frequently that assimilation has been difficult.

Other new trends

Many schools are placing additional emphasis on minority studies. Demands are being made for learning experiences and for programs reflecting the needs and attitudes of minority groups, particularly Negroes, Puerto Ricans, and Mexican-Americans. Many school systems have responded to these demands by creating minority study programs. In some schools such minority study programs are integrated in American history and literature courses, and in other schools separate departments have been created. Schools are also placing additional emphasis on special programs for exceptional children and investigating ways in which these children can be aided in becoming useful adults. Some schools participate in distributive education or in sheltered workshop programs so that vocational training, if even of a limited nature, is assured.

The Elementary and Secondary Education Act of 1965, the first major increase in federal spending for education, provided for on-going opportunity for many school systems to experiment with program improvement and enrichment and to develop better facilities.

Recent conferences* on education have recognized the disparity between the traditional curriculums that are offered and the learning needs of large segments of the population. The Educational System for the 70's (ES'70) has attempted to remedy this problem by bridging the gap between the academic and vocational programs so that all high school students can develop the basic learning and job skills and also be able to meet requirements for further study at institutions of higher learning. The purpose of ES'70 is to develop in each of the participating school districts a student-oriented, individually tailored, effective, and efficient secondary education program.

In the realm of facilities, school architecture is being modernized. The newest schools are often imaginatively designed and at times are built in a decentralized form, so that rather than being multistoried, a large school is low and many-winged. Air-conditioning, below-ground construction, the use of movable air bubbles, and park-like settings characterize the most recent school construction.

Physical educators interested in playing a key role in the future will equip themselves to utilize their abilities to greatest advantage in the years ahead.

A CONCLUDING STATEMENT

Good teachers apply psychological principles to their work. They consider several conditions in fulfilling their duties. They try first to establish rapport between themselves and their students. When this is accomplished, they will be better able to understand, accept, and help each pupil. Their objectives, expectations, and disciplinary

methods are clearly stated and understood. Content of material is adjusted to each student's level of learning and made interesting to motivate each pupil. Practice periods are adapted to the subject matter being taught and to the individual's needs and interests. Good teachers recognize and acknowledge achievements made by students and then set new goals for the boys and girls to obtain. They give each child a sense of worth by letting him contribute and also give him a sense of belonging. They recognize that repetition of useful and significant information is necessary for retention of material. They know it is important to emphasize the rudiments of physical education so that the students will remember and use their skills, attitudes, and knowledge in furthering learning experiences.

As teachers, they are firm in their disciplinary approach. They let pupils know what is expected of them. They understand why pupils act in certain ways. They expect courtesy and fair play. They motivate pupils to do their best work and challenge them so they are proud of their achievements. They are sensitive to each pupil's feelings. They are patient, tolerant, and honest.

The physical education instructor should teach the various activities that comprise his profession in accordance with established psychological principles. If the instructor is thoroughly conversant with the best methodology and resources available for skill teaching, physical education skills will be learned better, time will be saved, and the learner will have a more satisfying and all-around better educational experience. The student who is planning to enter this profession should recognize the value of scientific psychological data.

QUESTIONS AND EXERCISES

1. Define the term *psychology* and discuss its implications for the teaching of physical education.
2. Discuss Maslow's theory of motivation in respect to the teaching of physical education activities.
3. Why are the concepts of motivation, matura-

---

*Bushnell, David: ES '70: a systems approach to educational reform, Education **91**(1):61, 1970.

tion, individual differences, and intelligence important to the physical educator?

4. Discuss Thorndike's, Guthrie's, Skinner's, and Hull's laws of learning. Why are they important in the teaching of motor skills? Discuss the Gestalt and psychoanalytical theories of learning.
5. What is meant by the term *motor learning?*
6. Discuss ten factors or conditions that promote the learning of motor skills.
7. Identify whole method, mental practice, kinesthesis, knowledge of results, massed versus distributed practice, learning curve, mechanical principles, and transfer of training.
8. What is the relationship between leadership and learning?
9. Why is it necessary to overlearn a skill such as swimming?
10. What is meant by concomitant learning? What are some of the concomitants learned in each of the following activities: field hockey, football, basketball, softball, badminton, swimming, and horseback riding.
11. How will the psychological principles of learning help you to become a better physical education teacher?
12. Why is personality development important to the physical educator?
13. What are the implications of "sensitivity training" for physical education?
14. Why is motivation sometimes said to be the "heart of the learning process"?
15. Make a list of the things a physical education teacher can do that will act as incentives to pupil learning.
16. Explain how learning takes place, especially relating your discussion to the learning of physical skills.
17. What is the relationship of physical education to academic achievement?
18. How will the new developments in general education, such as educational television, nongrading, and new grading methods affect physical education?
19. How will the physical education curriculums of the future be affected by new curriculums in general education?

Reading assignment

Bucher, Charles A., and Goldman, Myra: Dimensions of physical education, St. Louis, 1969, The C. V. Mosby Co., Reading selections 44 to 50.

SELECTED REFERENCES

American Association for Health, Physical Education, and Recreation: Motor learning and motor performance, Fitness Series No. 4, 1959; The growing years—adolescence, 1962; Washington, D. C., The Association.

Bigge, Morris L.: Learning theories for teachers, New York, 1964, Harper & Row, Publishers.

Botwin, Louis: The media approach, a happening in physical education, Physical Educator **25:** 119, 1968.

Broer, Marion: Efficiency of human movement, Philadelphia, 1965, W. B. Saunders Co.

Bruner, J. S.: The process of education, Cambridge, 1963, Harvard University Press.

Bucher, Charles A.: Health, physical education, and academic achievement, NEA Journal **54:** 38, 1965.

Bucher, Charles A., and Reade, Evelyn M.: Physical education in the modern elementary school, New York, 1971, The Macmillan Co.

Bushnell, David: ES '70: a systems approach to educational reform, Education **91(1):**61, 1970.

Cogan, Max: Motives for participation in physical education, National College Physical Education Association for Men (Proceedings of Annual Meeting), January 10-13, 1968, pp. 56-67.

Cratty, B. J.: A three level theory of perceptual-motor behavior, Quest (Monograph VI), May, 1966, pp. 3-10.

Cratty, Bryant J.: Movement behavior and motor learning, Philadelphia, 1964, Lea & Febiger.

Cratty, Bryant J.: Psychological bases of physical activity, Journal of Health, Physical Education, and Recreation **36:**71, 1965.

Dewey, John: How we think, Boston, 1933, D. C. Heath & Co.

Goldstein, Jacob, and Wiener, Charles: Visual movement and the bending of phenomenal space, Journal of General Psychology **80:**3, 1969.

Goodlad, John I.: Directions of curriculum change, NEA Journal **55:**33, 1966.

Goodlad, John I., and Anderson, Robert H.: The nongraded elementary school, New York, 1963, Harcourt, Brace, & World, Inc.

Guthrie, E. P.: The psychology of learning (rev. ed.), New York, 1952, Harper & Row, Publishers.

Hermann, Don, and Osness, Wayne: A scientific curriculum design for high school physical education, Journal of Health, Physical Education, and Recreation **37:**23, 1966.

Hilgard, E. R.: Learning theory and its application. In Schramm, W., editor: New teaching aids for the American classroom, Stanford, California, 1960, Institute for Communicative Research.

Hull, C. L.: Principles of behavior, New York, 1943, Appleton-Century-Crofts.

Humphrey, James H.: Academic skill and concept development through motor activity, The American Academy of Physical Education **1:** 29-35, 1968.

Jennings, Frank G.: Jean Piaget; notes on learning, Saturday Review, May 20, 1967, pp. 81-83.

Johnson, Perry B.: An academic approach to college health and physical education, Journal of Health, Physical Education, and Recreation **37:** 23, 1966.

Maslow, A. H.: A theory of human motivation, Psychological Review **50:**370-396, 1943.

Middle schools in theory and fact, NEA Research Bulletin **47:**49, 1969.

National Association of Physical Education for College Women and National College Physical Education Association for Men: A symposium on motor learning, Quest (Monograph VI), May, 1966.

National Education Association: Schools for the sixties, New York, 1963, McGraw-Hill Book Co.

National Society for the Study of Education: Forty-first yearbook, Chicago, 1942, Department of Education, University of Chicago, Part II.

Ogilvie, Bruce C.: The personality of the male athlete, The American Academy of Physical Education **1:**45-51, 1968.

Oxendine, Joseph B.: Psychology of motor learning, New York, 1968, Appleton-Century-Crofts.

Reams, Davids, and Blier, T. J.: Developing team teaching in physical education, Journal of Health, Physical Education, and Recreation **39:** 50, 1968.

Sheldon, W. H., and Stevens, S. S.: The varieties of temperament, New York, 1942, Harper & Row, Publishers.

Singer, Robert N.: Motor learning and human performance, New York, 1968, The Macmillan Co.

Skinner, B. F.: The behavior of organisms, New York, 1938, Appleton-Century-Crofts.

Skinner, B. F.: Reinforcement today, The American Psychologist, March, 1958, pp. 94-99.

Spearman, Charles: The abilities of man, New York, 1927, The Macmillan Co.

Thune, John B.: Personality of weightlifters, Research Quarterly **20:**296-306, 1949.

Thurstone, L. L.: Primary mental abilities, Psychometric Monograph No. I, Chicago, 1938, University of Chicago Press.

Trump, J. Lloyd, and Baynham, Dorsey: Focus on change—guide to better schools, Chicago, 1961, Rand McNally & Co.

Wells, Harold C.: To get beyond the words, Educational Leadership **28**(3)**:**241, 1970.

18/Sociological interpretations of physical education

Sociology is concerned with a study of people, of groups of persons, and of human activities in terms of the groups and institutions in society. It is concerned with the origin of society. It is a science interested in such institutions of society as religion, family, government, education, and recreation. It is a science involved in developing a better social order characterized by good, happiness, tolerance, and racial equality.

Persons associated with educational sociology are concerned primarily with three functions: (1) the influence of education upon social institutions and of group life upon the individual, such as how the school affects the personality or behavior of an individual, (2) the human relations that operate in the school involving pupils, parents, and teachers and how they influence personality and behavior of an individual, and (3) the relation of the school to other institutions and elements of society, as, for example, the impact of education upon natural resources.

Physical education can play an important part in the improvement of the democratic way of life. Play is a socializer. It can do much in promoting the brotherhood of man. To illustrate, the primitive tendency was to strike back if angered by an adversary. Physical education, however, teaches human relationships in accordance with set rules. Participants put forth their best efforts to defeat opponents but in a socially acceptable manner.

CULTURAL VALUES

Social scientists have stated that in man's evolution from his ape-like ancestors he has had an advantage over other members of the animal kingdom, because he has had the ability to transmit learned behavior from one generation to another. The learned behavior that is transmitted is recognized as man's culture. It is a way of thinking, believing, and acting. Each culture has its own unique features that distinguish it from other cultures. The culture of the African Bushman is different from the culture that exists in the United States. The development of a culture will be primarily dependent upon the various interactions that take place in man's adjustment to the social environment that has been created. As man recognizes his role in society, he adjusts and adapts to his environment.

The culture that man transmits from one generation to another consists of both material and nonmaterial developments made by man. The material developments of man are his buildings and machines, to name two, while the nonmaterial developments are concerned with such things as the knowledge and technology he uses.

There are also certain values that are recognized as desirable to ensure the permanence and worth of a culture. The Educational Policies Commission* has listed ten values that are moral and spiritual in character and that represent the foundation upon which a strong society is built. They are presented here to help clarify the influence that cultural values have on education and the sociological implications they

*Educational Policies Commission: Moral and spiritual values in the public schools, Washington, D. C., 1951, National Education Association.

520

have for physical education. These values are reflected in human relationships and affect a person's emotions, sentiments, and ways of behaving.

HUMAN PERSONALITY—BASIC VALUE. The individual has worth. This represents the basic value in life. Physical education should help each individual to possess a feeling of worth and importance and to achieve within his abilities.

MORAL RESPONSIBILITY. Each individual must feel responsible for his own behavior. Human beings must exercise rational judgment in making decisions that will not infringe upon the rights of others. They must perform in a manner that is ethical and right according to established codes of conduct. Physical education should try to inculcate this responsibility in those individuals who participate in its programs.

INSTITUTIONS AS SERVANTS OF MEN. Social institutions, whether they are domestic, educational, cultural, or political, must serve people. They should never exist for themselves but, instead, as agencies that help people to realize their goals.

COMMON CONSENT. The popular will must be the key to understanding. Cooperation must exist. Law, justice, and conformance with existing rules and regulations must be a guideline.

DEVOTION TO TRUTH. The truth must always be sought and social direction guided thereby. Deception, coercion, and intellectual dishonesty must not exist. Schools and physical educators within the schools must help young people to determine the way to find the truth and how to be guided by its revelation.

RESPECT FOR EXCELLENCE. There should be a constant search for excellence of mind, character, and creative ability. Education should help young people to determine their abilities, to select leaders who are most able, and to be excellent producers themselves in all their efforts. Physical education can help people to achieve this important quality by stressing the importance of well-being and good health.

MORAL EQUALITY. All individuals are judged by the same moral standards. The golden rule has been written into all the great religions of the world. Education and physical education must recognize this precept and practice rules of fair play, tolerance, sympathy, and brotherhood.

BROTHERHOOD. There must be a feeling of brotherhood for all persons, whether these individuals are ignorant or bright, feeble or strong, experience misfortune or abound in good fortune. This is a moral responsibility of all citizens. Education and physical education must help young people to develop those traits and qualities that will enhance their usefulness to society.

PURSUIT OF HAPPINESS. Opportunity must be provided for each individual to pursue and achieve happiness. Education and physical education must promote those qualities that provide lasting happiness—deep personal resources, respect and affection for others, and opportunities for making a contribution to humanity.

SPIRITUAL ENRICHMENT. The outlook of people is affected by spiritual belief. Their inner feelings and their emotions are tempered by this same belief. Their behavior is also guided by this quality. Education and physical education should encourage and help individuals to have spiritual enrichment, in which beauty and refinment, esthetic appreciation, and creative abilities represent important considerations.

• • •

These moral and spiritual values are important considerations in discussing and considering the sociological interpretations of physical education. The next step is to look at the nature of man to discover what role these values play in his existence and how these values can best be instilled as part of his makeup.

NATURE OF MAN

The study of sociology shows that man becomes a different type of individual from his original nature when he takes on acquired characteristics of human nature. The traits and characteristics that result in antisocial conduct and cause fear, hate, and worry in the world are acquired characteristics. Man is not born an antisocial being. Man is not born with traits that lead to power seeking, aggrandizement, and intolerance. These traits are acquired through man's environment. Through a better understanding of human nature and through a meaningful educational experience, it is possible to build a better social order for all mankind. The physical educator should understand these things so that he can utilize his work in the development of a better social order.

Original nature of man

Man does not start life as a human being. He originates from cells, and cells are not human. The adjective *human* can be applied only after the acquisition of human traits that encompass the sympathies, passions, and failings of men. Such characteristics as jealousy, greed, and insolence are human traits. They are not present in the cells at birth. *Human* is a term that can be applied to an animal species—a name given to a large number of animals. Only in a very limited sense is man born human. He is, in fact, born an animal and becomes a human being. He becomes a human being when he adapts himself to such characteristics of his culture as tools, laws, religions, and words.

The original nature of man is characterized by involuntary or reflex actions, such as crying, sneezing, coughing, blinking an eyelid, sucking, and wiggling. This is animal nature, which under the influence of man's environment becomes human nature.

Original nature is not predestined to take a certain shape or direction. Instead, it can be molded in patterns that permit human beings to live side by side in a peaceful and happy existence. Physical education has the potentialities to contribute much in this molding process.

Human nature

Human nature is characterized by the acquisition of human traits that are a part of the environment in which an individual lives. It is characterized by intelligence and thinking. Man has a thinking mechanism that enables him to make decisions, to control his behavior, and to adapt to various situations.

From birth, man develops as a social being as well as an individual characterized by self-assertiveness and personal interests and desires. Within a few weeks after birth the child shows an inclination to be a social being. His social activities play an important part in his growth. As the maturing process continues, the child exhibits behavior that is characterized by cooperation and a willingness to be friendly. On the other hand, however, he also exhibits characteristics that display his uniqueness as an individual, his desires, and his likes and dislikes. As time elapses he becomes more cooperative, makes friends, becomes conscious of other people's desires, and acquires to some degree a sympathetic attitude toward the desires of others. Eventually he recognizes the impor-

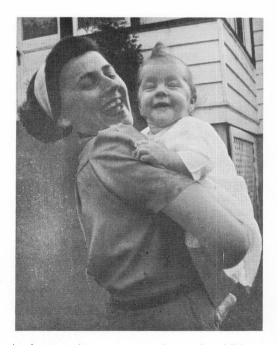

As the maturing process continues, the child exhibits behavior that is characterized by cooperation and a willingness to be friendly.

tance of teamwork, develops convictions and loyalties, and becomes interested in the community in which he lives and in the welfare of the nation as a whole. He also feels a certain responsibility for the welfare of all mankind. At the same time, he has certain vested interests that he aims to protect. He becomes a competitor for recognition, prestige, and material possessions, and he spends most of his time in furthering his own special and personal interests, which seem to be a prime consideration. Thus an individual develops socially. On the one hand, he is interested in the larger world, in other people, and in the welfare of mankind; but conversely, he is interested in the life that revolves around himself and his personal ambitions. Physical education, through the various activities that it offers, has the potentialities for developing social traits that further personal interests and at the same time stress those characteristics that are necessary for group living.

Man's human nature is also characterized by a progressive advance from involuntary action to one of fixed modes of behavior. At birth the individual possesses certain reflexes, such as crying, sneezing, and coughing. Before long he acquires set patterns of reacting to certain experiences, which soon become habits. The baby cries when he wants certain things. The child acquires the habits of wearing clothes, of brushing his teeth, and of saying his prayers before he goes to bed at night. Eventually, as he grows older, he recognizes that the group of people with whom he is associated in a particular environment act in certain ways and have developed certain folkways and mores.

These folkways and mores arise from the needs of the people. People discover in the course of history that certain things give them pleasure and contribute to a more enjoyable existence, whereas other things cause pain and grief. They profit from the experience of previous generations. They find some ways more expedient than others. They adopt certain methods of doing things and turn them into customs, which thus become folkways. Examples of folkways that

have developed among some groups of people are the customs of a man's tipping his hat to a lady, going to town on Saturday afternoon, and eating hot dogs at the ball game.

Most groups of people attempt to improve customs or folkways as they progress. Certain ones are abandoned in light of new developments. Folkways that have been lifted to another or higher plane to better serve the needs and interests and desires of a group of people become mores. They are the folkways that through continued experience have been proved right and true and have the force of law. Examples of mores are such things as having one wife or husband and believing in one God.

Human needs

Another concept that needs the careful consideration of physical educators is what is called "needs" theory. Whenever a person acts he is trying to satisfy a need. Therefore, we should know the needs of our students and of human beings in general and try to satisfy these needs in a constructive manner.

The most obvious human needs are for physical survival and well-being. Others may concern themselves with the physiological, psychological, or sociological makeup of the human being.

The physiological aspects include the needs for oxygen, escape from pain-producing situations, and attention to requirements of thirst, sex, intestinal and bladder elimination, rest, sleep, and hunger. These are important to the individual as a means of survival and comfort. They must be satisfied. This fact is generally recognized by almost everyone.

The psychological needs are less obvious and concern themselves with the mind and emotions. They include love, achievement, affection, belonging, approval, recognition, acceptance, and security. A person needs the feeling of belonging, having status, and becoming something. These are not as easily identified by laymen, but they should be known to educators. Teachers can do much to help satisfy these basic needs of every human being.

The sociological needs are those that pertain to the pattern of how a person fits into society. These needs include cooperation, sharing, gregariousness, and love. They take into account the opinions of others, the desire to influence others, and the security one has within the group. A person's self-esteem is affected by his relations with the group.

Human needs can be realized through work, play, and recreation. If not properly nurtured, they may result in an antisocial action and personal maladjustment. Therefore the professional educator should be cognizant of these human needs and plan definite means of meeting them.

MODES OF SOCIAL LEARNING

According to Havighurst there are three general modes by which children learn from other people.* All three of these methods of social learning operate in a school situation.

REWARD AND PUNISHMENT. A child wants rewards because of the joy and satisfaction they give him. On the other hand, he does not want punishment because of the pain and dissatisfaction that accrue. Rewards and punishments may be material or nonmaterial in nature. For example, the child may receive some money or a word of praise as a reward and a slap on the face or a severe scolding as a punishment.

IMITATION. Imitation of other people is a common mode of learning. Such imitation may be conscious or unconscious. A child may learn early in life that rewards accrue when he does what a father or older brother, teacher, neighbor, scout leader, or movie star wants him to do. Gradually, he takes on patterns of behavior that imitate older persons, particularly ones with whom he feels a close emotional bond. The association results in habits of imitation that are

repeated frequently and, finally, become unconscious in their application.

DIDACTIC TEACHING. When a person with authority or an expert in something tells a child how to perform a particular task or what constitutes desirable behavior under specific situations, learning takes place. Teaching a boy how to bat a ball correctly is an example. This mode of social learning is effective only when accompanied by reward or punishment, or when the teacher, minister, or expert is a model person whom the child desires to imitate. Since this does not always happen, didactic teaching is sometimes a failure. Also, example may have more influence on the child than didactic teaching. For example, if a father smokes he may find it difficult to teach his boy not to smoke.

BUILDING CHARACTER IN YOUTH

Physical education has great potential for building character in children and youth. However, in order to realize this potential, physical educators should be familiar with the stages of character development and the best approaches to achieving this worthy goal.

Havighurst and Peck and associates, with colleagues of the Committee on Human Development at the University of Chicago, studied boys and girls, giving them tests, talking with teachers and parents, and analyzing findings. This study suggests the existence of five stages through which the ordinary person passes in developing character.*

1. *Amoral, impulsive stage.* This is a period during the first year of life or longer when the individual follows his own impulses and has no moral feelings.

2. *Egocentric, expedient stage.* This period is common among children 2 to 4 years of age. It is characterized by some control over impulses in the interest of making good impressions and also self-protec-

*Morris, Van Cleve, and others: Becoming an educator, Boston, 1963, Houghton Mifflin Co., p. 90.

*Peck, Robert F., and others: Psychology of character development, New York, 1960, John Wiley & Sons, Inc.

tion from physical harm. However, there is still the "I" feeling, with focus on individual pleasures and conveniences.

3. *Conforming stage.* From 5 to 10 years of age there exists a period where the individual attempts to conform to the demands of the social group of which he is a part.

4. *Irrational conscience stage.* This is the period when the example and teaching of parents are dominant, normal for children 5 to 10 years of age and older. Some adults continue in this stage. This period is characterized by a strong feeling that the parental code of morality, whether it is right or wrong, is the one that should be followed in a rigid manner.

5. *Rational conscience stage.* This is the highest level of moral conduct. The individual applies reason and experience to his moral code, continually trying to see the various avenues of conduct that are open and the consequences of traveling each avenue. A few adolescents get into this stage; some adults are never able to achieve it.

Some aspects of all or a few of the five stages may be noticeable in the conduct of individuals. Physical educators should recognize these various stages in the boys, girls, and adults with whom they associate and continually strive to develop higher stages of moral conduct. The more the individual can be led to foresee the moral consequences of his own behavior, the higher on the scale he has risen.

In recognition of these five stages, how is character building in youth most effectively realized? Grinnell lists four approaches that have implications for the physical educator. They are as follows*:

1. *Precept.* This method is based on the premise that if young people know what is right they will do it. The church, to a great extent, operates on this principle. There is general agreement that clearly understanding what is right and proper is important knowledge to communicate. However, to be most effective it must be supplemented by

---

*Grinnell, John E.: Character building in youth, Phi Delta Kappan **40**:212, 1959.

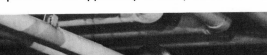

Sports offer an opportunity to satisfy human needs.

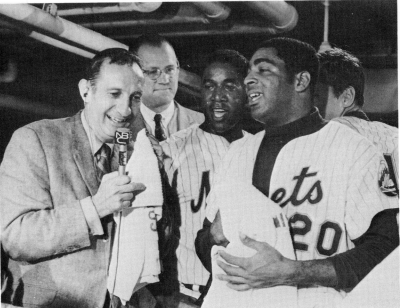

other approaches. In physical education it is very important to have children and youth understand clearly what is considered good moral conduct in a class, in a game, away from parents, and in many other situations. No doubt should be left in their minds as to what is the best conduct under many and varied situations.

2. *Study of lives of men and women.* Young people are impressed with great leaders. The lives of Lincoln, Washington, and Benjamin Franklin, for example, have provided the inspiration for others to achieve high moral goals. This approach can be effective if there is reading and dramatization of important moments of decision that are recaptured from the lives of great people. Such experiences will have an impact upon the conduct of young people. There are many men and women in the history of sport and physical education whose moral conduct and social dedication offer shining examples of the worth of good social conduct and strong character. Branch Rickey, with his belief in and respect for the worth of each individual and the many trying situations he experienced in attempting to achieve what he knew to be right, will always be a cherished part of American sports history and bring inspiration and behavior changes to many boys and girls.

3. *Teacher's example.* The teacher leaves an imprint upon his students, whether it is through his sense of fairness, ability to be a regular person, generosity, or unfailing belief in the truth. Many American presidents have pointed to a teacher as having helped mold their lives. The coach and physical education teacher, because of their close relationship to their pupils, play a unique role in helping to mold good behavior and strong character. Through their examples, much good can be done to realize this objective.

4. *Learning to do by doing.* Grinnell points out that the most effective approach is to influence boys and girls in their moral behavior while they are participating in their school activities. They should be shown what is right and what is wrong and what is just

and unjust. Many teachable moments occur each day in student government activities, sports, and physical education classes in which elements of character can be strengthened. Whether or not proper moral outcomes accrue will dependly largely upon the teacher. Constant supervision, high standards of conduct, strong moral values, and ethical principles will help to make this phase of the educational process a successful venture.

EDUCATING FOR SOCIAL CHANGE

Man's culture, which has been characterized by the formation of groups and the development of social unity, has enabled him to survive. At times, man brings about changes in the culture and social organizations. He makes new technological discoveries, moves from one area to another, organizes new institutions, and establishes new social values. The rate of change in society is dependent upon the culture in which change takes place. New discoveries and inventions influence social change. For example, the invention of the automobile brought about new methods of transportation and other important changes in the American society. Highways had to be built so the automobiles could successfully move about, and new traffic laws had to be written in order to control this new invention. The American people spent more of their leisure hours visiting scenic places, and people from various geographical sections of the country were drawn together as distance and time became less of an obstacle to group interaction.

Social change is also brought about through individual and group motivation. Social movements, for example, have been leading contributors to social change. The common interest that brings people together to form a social movement may be political in nature, such as the antiwar efforts so prevalent among the young people in America today. The common interest may be one of occupation, race, or even age. In the 1930's a social movement was created to help the aged receive retirement benefits.

The government reacted to this movement by enacting the Social Security Act.

Society must also be able to control change because inability to do this can lead to what is called "social disorganization." Society cannot adequately function when it cannot control its change. Entire communities have disappeared because of the inability of its population to adjust to new developments that were taking place. In order to prevent social disorganization, society must plan for change.

It is difficult to find any significant social change or social planning that has occurred in the American society in recent years that has not been influenced by education to some degree. Education not only influences social change, it is also influenced by it. Governments have often turned to education as a means for directing social change. In the United States, at the outbreak of World War II the schools became the training grounds for America's soldiers. Physical fitness programs were expanded in order to make the men of our society more fit for military duty. When peacetime came our educational institutions turned their attention to social planning and attempted to discover ways to improve the health, sanitation, and welfare services in our cities.

Today, society is faced with an environmental crisis. It has been predicted that in the coming decades urban citizens will have to wear gas masks in order to survive the air pollution that will exist. By 1985 it has been estimated that air pollution will reduce the amount of sunlight that reaches the earth by one-half and that increased noise levels caused by our vast technological developments will cause heart disease and impair hearing. The experts say that unless something is done to stop this environmental catastrophe, American society will greatly suffer.

Educators are becoming aware of the fact that our natural resources are being depleted. Ecology has become the catch-word throughout our nation's schools and colleges, and students want to be involved. Some colleges and universities are preparing their physical educators for the role that they are to play in the ecology movement. Queens college* of the City University of New York initiated a program in their department of health and physical education, with the main objective being to provide experiences for familiarizing students with various natural environments, equipping them with the skills that are needed to live in the natural environment, and developing positive attitudes toward the conservation of our natural resources. Recently the American Association of Health, Physical Education, and Recreation's Student Action Council (SAC)† created a program known as Project Life. This program offers an opportunity for every student major in the United States to work either independently or with groups to prevent further destruction of the environment. The Student Action Council is the source of future leaders in the field and can provide a strong catalyst for change. Physical education students should become involved in such activities because of their important social value.

ROLE OF PLAY AS A SOCIALIZING FORCE

Play has the potential for helping man to have better relations with his fellow man and to be a dynamic social force in society. To better understand the social role of play, it is necessary to examine the theories of play and the role of play in man's life.

Theories of play

Sociologists have advanced many theories as to why people play. Some of the more popular of these theories are the surplus-energy or Spencer-Schiller theory, the recreation theory, the relaxation theory, the inheritance or recapitulation theory, the instinct or Groos theory, the social-contact theory, the self-expression theory, the wish-

---

*Loret, John: A happening in the out-of-doors, Journal of Health, Physical Education, and Recreation 40:45-46, 1969.

†American Association for Health, Physical Education, and Recreation: Update, October, 1970, p. 1.

fulfillment theory, the domination theory, and Caillois' theory.

SURPLUS-ENERGY OR SPENCER-SCHILLER THEORY

Friedrich Schiller, a German poet and philosopher (1759-1805), expressed the idea of play as "the aimless expenditure of exuberant energy." This theory points out that human beings have developed many powers that cannot all act at once. As a result of this phenomenon there is an overabundance of time and vigor not utilized in providing for immediate needs. Therefore, many powers are inactive for considerable periods of time. Active, healthy nerve centers accumulate more and more energy during these inactive periods and in time are brought to a point where there must be a letting off of the pressure. Play is an excellent medium of letting off this steam that has developed as a result of the continual bombardment of the organism by a multitude of stimuli. Schiller has also expounded what others have called the "esthetic theory." This theory endorses the concept that man plays as an outlet for his creative imagination and in order to create beauty.

RECREATION THEORY

Guts Muths, the father of physical training in Germany, emphasized the recreative value of play in his book *Games for the Exercise and Recreation of Body and Mind.* This theory has as its premise the idea that the human body needs some form of play as a means of revitalization. Play is a medium of refreshing the body after long hours of work. It aids in the recovery of exhausted energies and is an antidote for tense nerves, mental fatigue, and emotional unrest.

RELAXATION THEORY

In many ways the relaxation theory is similar to the recreation theory. It holds that today's mode of work, which utilizes the small muscles of the eyes and the hands, is hard, tedious, and very fatiguing. This type of work might lead to nervous disorders if the organism does not have some means

whereby it can relax from such an ordeal. Play offers this medium. It helps a person to get out-of-doors and follow such racially old activities as hunting, fishing, hiking, swimming, and camping. These activities relax and rest an individual and leave him refreshed and ready to follow another session of work.

INHERITANCE OR RECAPITULATION THEORY

G. Stanley Hall developed the recapitulation theory. This theory maintains that the past is the key to play. Play has been passed down from generation to generation from earliest times. Play and games are a part of each individual's inheritance. Society repeats the fundamental activities of play that were utilized by earliest man. Such activities as running, throwing, striking, climbing, leaping, carrying, and jumping have been part of our daily life for generations. Today, the sports and games that are played are just variations of these racially old activities.

INSTINCT OR GROOS THEORY

The instinct theory declares that human beings have an instinctive tendency to be active at various stages of their lifetime. A child breathes, laughs, cries, creeps, pulls himself up, stands, walks, runs, and throws at various periods of his development. These are instinctive with him and appear naturally during the course of development. Therefore, play is something that just naturally happens as a matter of growth and development. It is not something that is planned or purposely injected as a means of utilizing time. Instead, it is something that is natural and part of man's makeup.

SOCIAL-CONTACT THEORY

Human beings are born of parents. The parents are members of a certain group, culture, and society. Consequently, to a great extent, the human being takes on activities from his surroundings. An individual will adopt the games of the group of which he is a part. In the United States this might be baseball; in England, cricket; in Spain, bullfighting; and in Norway, skiing.

Self-expression theory

Bernard S. Mason expresses a modern theory of play. He points out that man is an active creature, that his physiological and anatomical structure places limits on his activity, that his degree of physical fitness at any time affects the kind of activity in which he engages, and that psychological inclinations that are the result of physiological needs and learned responses, habits, or attitudes propel him into certain types of play activities.

Wish-fulfillment theory

Man wishes and dreams for many things during his lifetime that can never come true. The young man who wants to be a major league baseball player or football player can, for example, turn to play activities as a means of satisfying these desires. The youngster who plays centerfield on a baseball team and declares "I'm Willie Mays" and the youngster who throws a football pass exclaiming "I'm Joe Namath" are achieving a sense of fulfillment they might not otherwise be able to get.

Domination theory

Associated with man's aggressive behavior is his desire to dominate others. In many aspects of life man wants to outdo his fellow man. Play activities provide man with the opportunity to satisfy this desire. By playing on a team an individual is given the opportunity to rise to a position where he is recognized as the best player. An activity such as track and field provides man with an opportunity to defeat his opponent.

Caillois' theories of play

In his book entitled *Man, Play, and Games,** Roger Caillois, a French sociologist, describes four types of play. He uses the terms *agon, alea, mimicry,* and *ilinx* as the titles of these groups, which may be translated into the categories of *competition, chance, simulation,* and *vertigo.*

*Caillois, Roger: Man, play, and games, New York, 1961, Free Press.

Competition. This type of play may be illustrated by sports and games of individual skill such as tennis, basketball, or chess. The competition may be very simple, such as when children try to see who can hold their arms out to the side the longest.

Chance. This type of play bases the outcome on a decision that is independent of the players such as in dice, lotto, bingo, or perhaps the counting out of nursery rhymes.

Simulation. This type of play involves simulation or imitation when the player assumes another role from his own such as playing cops and robbers or "farmer in the dell."

Vertigo. This type of play results in the deliberate production of dizziness or confusion or an attempt to destroy stability and bring about momentary disorientation. Examples of this would be children whirling around and falling down or an adult engaging in tightrope walking.

The first two types of play are more common among older youth, whereas the last two are more common among preschool children. The activities in the four types of play range, on one hand, between the extreme of uncontrolled fantasy involving an imaginative gaiety and, on the other hand, with activity that is planned and purposefully aimed at a specific result through the application of skill and effort. Caillois states that all four forms of play are universal and necessary to human development. Persons engaging in them find contributions basic to physical growth and personality development.

Table 18-1 outlines Caillois' classifications of play.

Role of play in man's life and education

People in all periods of history have participated in various activities in order to satisfy basic needs. The need for food resulted in man becoming a hunter. The need to transmit social environment from one generation to another resulted in the formation of the family as a means for man to

Table 18-1. Caillois' classification of games*

Agon (Competition)	Alea (Chance)	Mimicry (Simulation)	Ilinx (Vertigo)
Racing, wrestling, etc., athletics } not regulated	Counting-out rhymes, heads or tails	Children's imitations, games of illusion, tag, arms, masks, disguises	Children "whirling," horseback riding, swinging, waltzing
Boxing, billiards, fencing, checkers, football, chess	Betting, roulette		Valador, traveling carnivals, skiing, mountain climbing, tightrope walking
Contests, sports in general	Simple, complex, and continuing lotteries	Theater, spectacles in general	

*Caillois, Roger: Man, play, and games, New York, 1961, Free Press (see his Table 1, p. 36).

perpetuate himself. The need for order and unity in society resulted in the formation of political organizations. The need for man to worship resulted in the formation of religious institutions. When man has satisfied his basic needs he needs opportunities to engage in play activities that are an escape from his daily routines. Play is an important part of a culture and reflects the behavior of the individuals and groups in society. Sociologists who desire an understanding of individual and group relationships study the play activities of the people in a society.

The play activities that a society participates in are determined by several factors, a few of which are discussed. The *geographical location* is a consideration. People who live in California participate in more play activities out-of-doors than people from North Dakota because of their climate. The *natural resources* that characterize an area are a determinant. The snow-capped mountains of Colorado have been instrumental in popularizing the sport of skiing. The youngster in the inner city will engage in many activities that differ from the youngster on the farm. The type of *industrial and technological development* will determine the play activities that people engage in. The rice farmer in China who works a 14- to 16-hour day in the fields is limited in the activities in which he can participate. *Religion* also influences play. The early Puri-

tans of New England with their strict religious beliefs felt play was a sin and a waste of time.

The development of play as an important part of the American society can be attributed in large measure to the rise in industrialization. Industrialization resulted in a shorter work week and increased the number of leisure hours of America's workers. With this increased time on their hands more citizens turned to sports and play activities during their free time. The congestion that has resulted in America's cities has led to the creation of the playgrounds as a means for inhabitants to satisfy their need for play. Also, the great industrial growth of this country with such attendant problems of urban growth, leisure hours, and sedentary work has accented the need for play as an essential to human health and welfare.

All men and women need the opportunity to participate in play activities. This is especially true of children and youth because of the educational value of play. Play activities give the student the opportunity to imitate real-life situations and also permit him the opportunity to be creative and to express himself through his body. Cognitive development theorists such as Jerome Bruner have stated that children should be involved in many activities in order to develop a sensitivity to the world around them. Educators have indicated that games should become more and more a part of the educational curriculum in the schools. Recent educational developments include the "game theory," which stresses that teaching through the use of games is an important educational asset. Giving the child the opportunity to participate in situations he will face outside the classroom provides him with a picture of the various consequences of his actions. In our complex society it is important for students to become aware of the "real world" while they are still in a setting that will hopefully equip them with the tools needed to solve the problems they will face in the future.

By giving the student the opportunity to participate in many play activities, physical education plays an important role in the social development of that person. The social development objective of physical education represents a worthy goal to which all professionals in this field should contribute.

SPORT AS A SOCIALIZING FORCE

Sport is a dynamic social force in the American culture. As such, it is important to examine this phenomenon more closely.

Sociology of sport

Sport has become a very important part of the American culture, as well as of other cultures throughout the world. It captures newspaper headlines, usurps television screens, produces billions of dollars a year for entrepreneurs, is a consideration in international affairs, and has social, political, legal, and educational overtones.

In the United States, sport has become big business. The major radio and television networks compete for the right to broadcast sporting events. The Columbia Broadcasting System, for example, paid over $41 million for a 2-year contract with the National Football League.

The big business of sport has influenced the nature of college and even secondary school sport. The best teams get the opportunity to appear on television. In order to field the best team a school will attempt to attract top athletes to their institutions, ignoring at times their academic ability. Colleges have come to realize the important drawing power a star athlete can have. A college that can convince an Austin Carr

Professional sports have gone "big time."

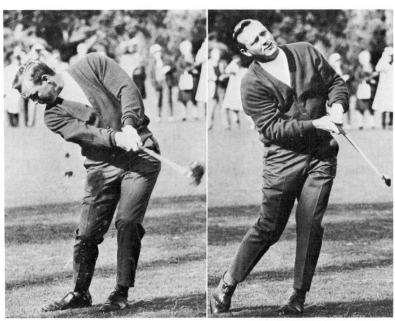

to attend and play on its team will stand a chance of getting on national television and reaping financial and other rewards. Colleges that have excellent academic programs often become better known because of their athletic endeavors.

In order to achieve national recognition, colleges and universities have had to pay great sums of money for their sport programs. According to a survey made by the NCAA, the average amount spent by member schools for athletics in 1 year was $548,000. Schools like Notre Dame and Ohio State average about $1.3 million, with about $670,000 going to football.

Sport is important to society and to physical education. As a medium that permeates nearly every important aspect of life, sport has led some physical educators to believe that it should receive intensive study, particularly as it affects the behavior of human beings and institutions as they form the total social and cultural complex of society. They support their premise by pointing out that, according to some anthropologists and psy-

chologists, games affect social processes and human values. However, these advocates hasten to add that sport sociology should be value free, since such a science would not be used to influence society or individual behavior for or against sport. Instead, the sport sociologist would look at sport in society in an objective manner and report what he finds.

The advocates of a sociology of sport feel that sport sociologists should have a background of psychology, sociology, anthropology, and other behavioral and social sciences. Another requirement would be a background in mathematics and statistics in order to be able to understand the data analysis and other information that form a background for such a science.

Nature and scope of sport

Sport is a highly ambiguous term having many different meanings. Some persons refer to sport when they are speaking of athletic competition, while others refer to sport when they are discussing the organizational

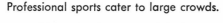

Professional sports cater to large crowds.

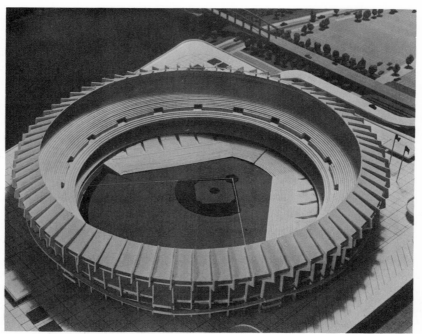

and financial status of a team. John W. Loy, Jr.* has stated that sport should be considered on different planes of discourse in order to understand its nature. He discusses sport as a *game occurrence,* as an *institutionalized game,* as a *social institution,* and as a *social situation.*

SPORT AS A GAME OCCURRENCE

In describing sport as a game, Loy maintains that sport is *playful,* is *competition,* is *physical skill, strategy,* and *chance,* and is *physical prowess.*

Sport as *play* is characterized as being free, separate, uncertain, unproductive, governed by rules, and make-believe. Sport is *free* in the sense that it is voluntary. One chooses the sport in which he wants to participate. The term *separate* means that sport is spatially and temporally limited. The football field, for example, is located within the confines of a stadium and is regulated by rules that control the activities of the players on the field. Sport is *uncertain.* On a third-down situation no one knows for sure what play the quarterback will call. This brings excitement and tension to the event. Sport is *unproductive* in the sense that the only thing produced during any competitive event is the game, and the production of the game is carried out in a fixed setting according to certain rules. Sport is *governed by rules.* The basketball player who receives his fifth personal foul in a college basketball game is automatically disqualified from further play. Sport is *make-believe* in the sense that in a game situation, for example, obstacles are artificially created to be overcome.

Sport as a game occurrence means *competition.* Competition can be between one individual and another, between teams, and between an individual or team and an animate object of nature, such as a bullfight. It can be between an individual or team and an inanimate object of nature, such as in

mountain climbing, and between an individual or team and an "ideal" standard, such as when a team attempts to set a new record.

Sport as a game occurrence means *physical skill, strategy,* and *chance.* Games of physical skill, such as wrestling, are determined by the player's physical ability. Games of strategy, such as checkers, are determined by the player's rational choice among several various possible solutions. Games of chance, such as roulette or a dice game, are determined by guesses.

Sport as a game occurrence means *physical prowess.* The major attribute that distinguishes sport from games is physical prowess. Physical prowess refers to the practice and learning of a skill that must be developed if one is to succeed in sport competition. The physical abilities relevant to success in competition are such qualities as strength, speed, and endurance.

SPORT AS AN INSTITUTIONALIZED GAME

The institutionalization of a game refers to the fact that a game has a past tradition and definite guidelines for future goals. Baseball and football have past traditions and are highly organized, with many plans already in progress for determining the future goals of these sports. Baseball, for example, is in the process of determining what cities are to be given franchises when the next expansion develops. Sport as an institutionalized game is discussed in its *organizational, technological, symbolic,* and *educational* spheres.

The *organizational* aspect of sport is discussed in terms of teams, sponsorship, and government. In a game, team members are usually selected spontaneously, whereas in sport teams are generally selected with care. Once a game is over the team usually disbands, while in sport, once a team is created membership is established and a stable social organization is maintained. In sport there are sponsoring bodies, such as those who sponsor the Little Leagues. On a higher level there are business corporations such as Phillips 66 Oil Company, which sponsors AAU teams. Sport is also governed. There

---

*Loy, John W., Jr.: The nature of sport: a definitional effort, Quest (Monograph X), May, 1968, pp. 1-15.

Cutaway drawing of new Madison Square Garden Sports Entertainment Center, New York City.

NEW 29-STORY OFFICE BUILDING on Seventh Ave. side of site

425-FT.-DIAMETER CLEAR-SPAN ROOF

ROOF IS SUSPENDED BY 48 RADIAL STEEL CABLES OF 3¼ IN. DIAMETER

"COMPRESSION RING" TAKES INWARD PULL OF ROOF-SUPPORTING CABLES

"TENSION RING" ANCHORS CABLES AT CENTER OF ROOF

COLUMNS SUPPORTING COMPRESSION RING BEAR WEIGHT OF ROOF

MADISON SQUARE GARDEN with seating capacity for 20,500 spectators

BOWLING CENTER (48 lanes)

FORUM for games or concerts (5,000 seats)

STREET LEVEL

PENNSYLVANIA STATION (all below street level)

PENNSYLVANIA R. R. AND LONG ISLAND R. R. TRACKS CARRY 650 TRAINS DAILY

EXPRESS ESCALATORS four ft. wide, moving 120 ft. a minute, can evacuate capacity crowd in 22 minutes

EIGHTH AVE. SUBWAY

EIGHTH AVE.

31st St.

33rd St.

ESCALATOR TOWER

TAXI DRIVEWAY

GLASS ENCLOSED PEDESTRIAN MALL CONNECTS OFFICE BUILDING AND SPORTS ARENA

EXTERIOR OF BROWN PRECAST CONCRETE PANELS

L. I. R. R. CONCOURSE

are organizations that control the activities taking place, such as the NCAA at the college level and the AAU at the amateur level.

Sport *technology* denotes the material equipment, physical skills, and body of knowledge necessary for competition. The technological aspects of a sport can be either intrinsic or extrinsic. Intrinsic technological aspects of a sport, like basketball, are the physical skills necessary to play the game effectively. The extrinsic technological aspects are the physical equipment such as the basketball court, the physical skills possessed by the coach, and the knowledge possessed by the coach and spectators.

The *symbolic* aspects of a sport are concerned with the elements of secrecy, display, and ritual. Secrecy occurs when teams hold training sites that are closed to all outsiders. Sport is display in the sense that an

athlete dresses in a uniform. Sport is ritual, such as the shaking of hands between basketball players before the opening jump and the flip of the coin at the 50-yard line prior to the opening kickoff in a football game.

The *educational* sphere of sport is concerned with the transmission of skills and knowledge that is necessary if one is to succeed in sport competition. In sport one needs much skill, knowledge, and expert instruction by coaches to be successful.

SPORT AS A SOCIAL INSTITUTION

When speaking of sport as a social institution, Loy refers to the sport order. The sport order is composed of all social organizations in society that are responsible for organizing, facilitating, and regulating the human actions in sport situations. Four levels of social organizations within the sport order

Sport is a social institution.

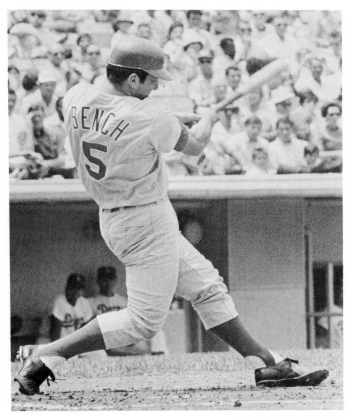

are distinguished: the primary, technical, managerial, and corporate levels. A social organization at the primary level is an informally organized sport team, such as a sandlot baseball team, where there are face-to-face relationships among all members of the team and there is no formal administrative leadership. At the technical level organizations officially designate administrative leadership positions. The college athletic program with its athletic directors and coaches is an example. At the managerial level organizations are too large for each member to know every other member, but they are small enough so that the members know the administrative leadership. The professional sport team is an example of the managerial level. Organizations at the corporate level are very bureaucratic in nature with centralized authority, protocol, and interpersonal relationships. The major governing bodies of professional sport are characteristic of a corporate organization.

SPORT AS A SOCIAL SITUATION

Sport as a social situation or social system, as it is sometimes called, is an important concern for the sport sociologist. The sport sociologist is interested in why man gets involved in sport and what effect his involvement has on other aspects of his life. Involvement in a social system is analyzed in terms of degree and kinds of involvement. Degree of involvement refers to the frequency, duration, and intensity of involvement. Kinds of involvement are expressed in terms of an individual's relationship to the "means of production" of a game. There are producers who are characterized as primary, secondary, and tertiary. The primary producers are the athletes who play the game. The secondary producers do not play the game but have direct technological consequences for the outcome of the game. Secondary producers include club owners, officials, and team doctors. The tertiary producers do not actively engage in the sport and have no direct technological consequences for the outcome of the game. Cheerleaders and bandleaders are examples.

Consumers, like producers, are designated as being primary, secondary, or tertiary. Primary consumers are those who make up the "live" attendance at a sport contest. Secondary consumers are those who become involved in sporting events by viewing them on television or listening to them on the radio. Tertiary consumers become involved in sport through conversations with others and through reading about sport in a newspaper.

Sport is an important part of American culture

From the preceding discussion of the nature of sport it can be seen that sport is not just concerned with two teams meeting each other on the playing field. Sport activities are an important part of the American culture, and sport sociologists face a great challenge in interpreting the role of sport in our way of life. Sport activities in the United States have been found by sociologists to be related to religion, economics, education, and government, to name a few.

Throughout our nation's history, sport has been influenced by the religious beliefs and economic conditions of our nation. As previously expressed, during the early developmental years of our nation sport activities, especially in New England, were severely hampered because of the religious attitude of the Puritan settlers. Today, religious attitudes have changed, and some religious institutions are extremely active in sport. Throughout our nation organizations such as the Catholic Youth Organization and B'nai B'rith provide activities that will give youth the opportunity to participate in sport. Schools and colleges under religious control sponsor sport programs.

Sport and the economic conditions of our nation are closely aligned. When our nation was developing there was little opportunity to participate in sport. However, the rise in industrialization and the resultant increased leisure time has led to an increased awareness of sport. Sport activities have become an important part of the American way of life. Americans by the millions not only take part in sporting events, through active participation, but also spend millions of dollars on sport equipment. They also enjoy sporting events solely as spectators and fans.

In the area of education sport has become a part of the schools and colleges of our nation. Physical education, intramurals, and athletic programs have been created by educational institutions to give the youth of our nation the opportunity to play in these activities. Sport programs in our schools in recent years have been associated with improving the fitness of our youth. The national government under the leadership of President Eisenhower and later Presidents Kennedy, Johnson, and Nixon initiated and is supporting the President's Council on Physical Fitness and Sports, which has been concerned with improving the fitness of our nation's youth.

The *judicial system* has also become involved. The Supreme Court has given indication that sport can no longer be considered just healthy competition; rather, it is now considered big business. Spencer Haywood, professional basketball star, petitioned the Supreme Court in 1971 because he was suspended by the league for having "jumped" the league to play in Seattle. The National Basketball Association, which has a rule against players competing before their twenty-first birthday, declared him ineligible. The Supreme Court ruled in Haywood's favor, declaring that he could not be denied the opportunity to earn a living until his case is finally settled.

At the college and university level the government, through the activities of the Congress, has attempted to resolve the dispute between the NCAA, the governing

One hundred years of football. **A**, Artist Arnold Friberg's painting of the first football game, Princeton at Rutgers, 1869. Bewildered spectators, all 200 to 300 of them, sat on fence rails or in buckboards and watched twenty-five—man teams play soccer-style game. After much "headlong running, wild shouting and frantic kicking," Rutgers won, 6 goals to 4.

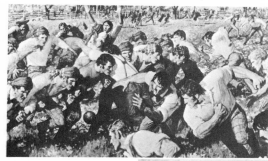
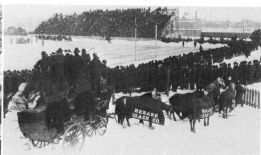
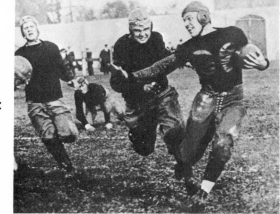

COURTESY UNIVERSITY OF CHICAGO.

body of the nation's colleges athletic programs, and the AAU, the governing body of America's amateur athletes. Each body has attempted to prevent their athletes from participating in events sponsored by the other. In order for America's top athletes to compete against one another, there is need for resolution of this dispute.

The area of sport is extremely vast. Sport sociologists are challenged to help make sport a desirable socializing force in our way of life.

SOME SOCIOLOGICAL IMPLICATIONS OF EDUCATIONAL ATHLETICS

Since athletics play such an important role in the American culture and in physical education programs, it is interesting to examine some of the sociological implications of sports.

Influence of American society on interscholastic athletics

Contemporary America likes athletic competition. This has been evident at the professional level, the college level, the senior high school level, and, in recent years, the junior high school level. Sport has become a part of the American culture. The interest and popularity of athletics have affected educational programs of schools and colleges.

1. *The place of sport in education has been largely determined by society rather than by educators.* Whether or not a sport is popular in schools and colleges depends to a great extent upon the amount of public interest, spectator approval, and newspaper space it generates. This phenomenon has determined in large measure what the "major" and "minor" sports are today. Basketball, track, football, and baseball have rated higher with the American public than other activities. Samuel M. Cooper,* in a doctoral dissertation at Western

Reserve University, indicated that these activities were among the most prominent. This evidence was substantiated further by the National Education Association of Secondary School Principals* in a survey of the interscholastic programs in separately organized junior high schools.

It would appear that what the public supports, educators tend to adopt. Young people grow up in this type of environment and many times are interested in a sport because society has accented its importance, rather than because of the contributions the sport makes to them as individuals.

2. *Athletics many times have become a medium of entertainment rather than serving to fulfill educational objectives.* The popularity of sports in America is frequently related to their value as entertainment rather than their value as education. Thomas Woody, former Professor of Education at the University of Pennsylvania, made direct reference to this development when he stated: "Scholastic contests, despite their best efforts to the contrary, are often spectacles to entertain idle multitudes, rather than to serve educational ends."† Americans thrill to the struggle, competition, and game color that accompany such spectacles. People love competition and are willing to pay to see it. Once the program becomes popular, the school in all too many cases begins to conform to the wishes of the community. The spectators and the entire community want to see a show, and at times the educators either try to please or feel obligated to please.

3. *Community interest in athletics often distorts the program of educational athletics.* In a report on educating children in grades seven and eight, the U. S. Department of Health, Education and Welfare published an article by Gertrude M.

---

*Cooper, Samuel M.: The control of interscholastic athletics, Doctor of Education Dissertation, 1955, Western Reserve University, p. 46.

*National Education Association of Secondary School Principals: A survey of interscholastic junior high athletic programs, November, 1958, pp. 2-3.
†Woody, Thomas: School athletics and social good, Journal of Educational Sociology **28:**246, 1955.

Lewis* on the social and emotional behavior of children at this age. It was reported that society places demands upon children at a very early age. What is demanded, the article pointed out, varies somewhat from one home, one community, or one social economic group to another, but it is considered important that children learn to think and act in the way that most people who live within the community think and act. In regard to junior high athletics, some school administrators and physical education teachers raised a question as to the advisability of interscholastic athletics at the seventh- and eight-grade level, but they refrained from protest since they believed the community, other schools in the region, and the children themselves seem to expect to take part in competitive athletics. The research tended to indicate that the community is indeed a strong motivating force in the shaping of interscholastic athletics.

The interest of the community and the emotional quality and demands of the community in athletics at the high school level were further indicated in a study by Richard Calish† as a master's thesis at the University of Maryland. The purpose of the study was to determine what the problems are among spectators, who causes these problems, in what sports problems exist, at what level of the school population problems prevail, and in what areas the problems exist. The results showed that the community, and not the school, was the group from which stemmed the poor behavior among spectators. Thus the community not only assists to shape the program but to influence how it is conducted during the actual game situation.

4. *Parental interest in schools may increase as a result of athletics.* Athletics may result in an increased interest by the parents in the schools. Mothers and

fathers, through their interest in sports, may become interested in the schools. They may visit the schools, find out about the educational program, and at times attempt to contribute to educational advancement. As a result, better communication may occur between the school and the community.

Many parents desire their children to participate in a successful athletic program. What parents consider a successful program and what educators consider a successful athletic program may be diametrically opposed. Since athletics often place reflected glory upon the parents and relatives of the youngsters, parents frequently want their children to participate and to win.

In a study of the attitudes of parents, teachers, and administrators concerning athletics in grades four through six, conducted by Phebe Martha Scott* of Bradley University, it was found that parents were most favorable as a group to interscholastic competition. The McCue attitude scale was used and distributed to superintendents in cities of 10,000 or more in the Central District of the American Association of Health, Physical Education, and Recreation. They were sent fifty scales to be distributed to parents, teachers, and school officials. This survey found that 78% of the parents were favorable and 22% were unfavorable to athletics in grades four through six. In comparison, administrators were least favorable, with 55% in favor and 45% not in favor of interscholastic competition. The wide range of scores indicated a wide difference of opinion, particularly among teachers and administrators. Parents as a group were more in agreement. Parents sometimes feel that school athletics can improve the social status of their children. Youths at times can increase their social status through athletic achievement more than through intellectual ability.

5. *Pressures on girls' athletics are not as severe.* Society has maintained that

*Lewis, Gertrude M.: Educating children in grades seven and eight, U. S. Department of Health, Education and Welfare Bulletin, 1954, p. 12.
†Calish, Richard: Spectator problems in secondary school athletics, Research Quarterly **25:**261-268, 1954.

*Scott, Phebe Martha: Attitudes toward athletic competition in elementary schools, Research Quarterly **24:**352-359, 1953.

athletic competition for boys is more important than competition for girls; consequently, the community pressures of an athletic program for girls do not exist to the same degree as those pressures so evident on the boys' programs. Girls are exposed to fewer competitive situations than boys, primarily because of the attitude of society. Eleanor Metheny, Professor of Education and Physical Education at the University of Southern California,* published an article concerning the effect of the cultural mores rather than physical consideration upon participation in athletics for girls. She tells of how the women in Russia put the shot and hurl the javelin with a great degree of skill and no evidence of physical damage. "Since there seems to be no differences in physical structure between European and American women, the differences must stem solely from the different concepts of roles appropriate for women in the countries in which they live." She states further that "the resolution of any specific issue relating to girls and athletics is inextricably bound up in these unresolved larger social issues."

Although the pressures are not as great on the girls' programs, this does not mean that they are totally unaffected by the stress placed upon competition for boys. Facilities, leadership, and financial priority for athletics have frequently resulted in a limited program for girls' physical education that places a strain on the class program and the intramural and extramural program. The Educational Policies Commission in *School Athletics*† lists as one of the weaknesses of an interscholastic program the negligence of the girls' programs. Increased concern in this area has resulted in new movements to increase the girls' athletic participation. Some schools have recently decided to allow girls to compete with boys in certain noncontact

sports, and coeducational physical education programs are also being developed.

6. *The current protest movement in society has affected coaches and athletic directors.* Frank B. Jones,* President of the Athletic Institute, has stated that the current protest movement with its riots and student demands has affected the college and secondary school coaches and athletic directors. Jones stated that the coach is being attacked from all sides. Students are turning on him when he has a losing year, faculty and administration turn against him when he asks for more funds, and now even his athletes are turning against him. Racial problems have been a source of great strife for coaches. At Syracuse University in the fall of 1970, eight black football players sat out the season in a racial dispute with the athletic department. At the same time, at the University of Florida, sixty athletes formed a union for a greater voice in programs and policies. The problem of hair length has caused much strife. The athletic director at a high school in California quit his job because his superior, the superintendent of schools, rescinded the grooming policy for athletes after he had suspended several cross-country runners for violating the policy.

Change is characteristic of society; as such, there will be changes in athletics. It is also apparent that some coaches and athletic directors are adjusting to the current situation. Athletic departments in such colleges as Notre Dame, California, and Stanford are making adjustments. Codes of conduct for hair grooming have been relaxed, and there is increased player involvement in policy decisions. In some high schools and colleges students are determining such things as training rules and forms of discipline if these rules are not followed.

7. *The need: proper educational perspective.* Research reveals a need for greater

*Metheny, Eleanor: Relative values in athletics for girls, Journal of Educational Sociology **28:** 268-269, 1955.
†Educational Policies Commission: School athletics, Washington, D. C., 1954, National Educational Association.

*Jones, Frank B.: Intercollegiate and interscholastic athletic program in the 1970's: a report to the Athletic Institute Board of Directors, Sportscope **15**(2):16-17, 1970.

understanding concerning the role of athletics in the school program. Educators, as well as the entire community, need to re-evaluate the relation of society to education as it concern athletics. The manner in which this phase of the school program can best meet the needs of youth should be considered at each educational level.

Beneficial impact athletics can have upon the student

GOOD SPORTSMANSHIP. Competitive athletics, according to some educators and leaders in the field of sports, can teach the art of winning and losing gracefully, the spirit of being fair to others, observance of the spirit as well as the letter of the rules, and the maintenance of a friendly attitude toward all individuals involved in the game situation.

Walter E. Damon* states that competition contributes to team spirit, motivation, and meets the interests of the boys. A boy has the chance to be more than an individual. He can become a part of something. Damon feels that the strain of tough competition, together with the push to win, is not detrimental but is actualy good for all boys and for delinquent or potentially delinquent boys.

COOPERATION. Competitive athletics, some educators feel, provide a social laboratory for the student to learn how to work with others in a cooperative manner, to contribute toward the common purposes of the group, to promote a feeling of social consciousness, and to develop an understanding of the rights and feelings of others. Athletics, they further maintain, may help to further a sense of responsibility for one's own actions and for the entire group. The boys learn to conform to acceptable behavior standards.

James B. Nolan, former Deputy Commissioner of the Police Department in the City of New York, reported that play becomes a way of learning about life—that respect for the rights of others is impressed upon the child through the rules that he is expected to obey and expects his playmates to obey in turn—that he must get along with his own side and guard the rights of the other side, learn about the importance of individual merit, gain a knowledge of fair play and a knowledge of social behavior, the "shall" and the "shall not"—that, in short, there is no bettter arena for democracy.

ACCEPTANCE OF ALL PERSONS REGARDLESS OF RACE, CREED, OR ORIGIN. Competitive athletics may teach the appreciation and acceptance of all persons in terms of their ability, performance, and worth, according to some educators. Individual attitudes are applauded for their achievements regardless of background and team affiliation. Opportunities are afforded for every person to achieve and to be recognized, regardless of economic or social class.

In a study by L. W. McCraw,* of the University of Texas, an investigation was made to determine the relationship between sociometric status and general athletic ability among junior high school boys. The conclusions of this study, on the basis of a statistical analysis of data obtained, revealed that the relationship between sociometric status and athletic ability seemed to be moderately high in almost all of the groups studied. Of the factors included in this study, athletic ability as measured by the athletic index and participation in interscholastic activities and/or intramural athletics were probably the predominant factors in conditioning choices of the "best liked."

TRAITS OF GOOD CITIZENSHIP. It is believed by some educators that competitive athletics help in developing those traits of good citizenship essential to democratic living. These include such qualities as initiative, trustworthiness, dependability, social consciousness, loyalty, and respect for the

---

*Damon, Walter E.: Competitive athletics helps delinquent boys, Journal of Health, Physical Education, and Recreation **29:**14, 1958.

*McCraw, L. W., and Tolbert, J. W.: Sociometric status and athletic ability of junior high school boys, Research Quarterly **24:**72-80, 1953.

individual. Jordan L. Larson,* former president of the American Association of School Administrators, discussed the contributions of athletics to good citizenship. He points out that the ideals of fair play, sportsmanship, and clean living are all part of athletics and are attributes capable of being carried on into adult life. In describing his team in a small school in Iowa many years ago, Mr. Larson states that a great respect was gained for their metropolitan neighbors and that their city neighbors in return began to better understand the boys from the country. From his observations as a coach, athletic official, and school administrator, it was his contention that athletics tended to foster respect for the work of the individual regardless of race, creed, or economic background and that good citizenship qualities could definitely result from competitive play.

LEADERSHIP. Competitive athletics, according to some educators, contribute to qualities of leadership. A study, reviewed in an article by Creighton J. Hale,† was made by Jeanne Doyl Lareau of the University of California. It was reported that girls in grades eight and nine were given the UC Interest Inventory tests to determine the relationship between athletic competition and personal and social adjustment. The results revealed that girls with experience in athletic competition showed better personal and social adjustment, were more popular, and exhibited higher leadership qualities. Thus, it may be that through athletics, opportunities are provided for accepting responsibility, making decisions, influencing others, and developing other qualities important to leadership. As a result, the student may achieve prestige and status in the school and community and this, in turn, may make him a still greater force socially. He may be admired, approved, and appreciated,

all of which may further open the door of possibilities for additional leadership, perhaps in other areas as well as in the field of sports.

FOLLOWERSHIP. Studies by Lareau* and Salz† tend to indicate that competitive athletics develop traits of a successful followership, including such qualities as respect for authority and outstanding leadership, abiding by the rules, cooperation with those is command, a recognition of the rights of others, and a sense of fairness. The student may also learn to take criticism without a feeling of hostility or resentment.

SELF-DISCIPLINE. Athletic competition develops abilities of self-discipline and determination. The rigorous training involved in many athletic events forces an individual to push himself in order to achieve his maximum effort. The athlete must be disciplined to make sacrifices and have the determination to achieve sucess. Winning is not only based on physical skill but also on the will and desire to achieve success.

ADDITIONAL AVENUES FOR SOCIAL ACQUAINTANCES. Competitive athletics, according to some educators, pave the way to new acquaintances, since the athletic appears to be more socially mobile and extroverted than the nonathletic. He has broadened interests, belongs to more organizations, and has many opportunities to meet students from other schools. Some physical educators have stated that interscholastic athletics broadens the social horizon of the child. A wider knowledge of the community may result from the child's contact with children from other schools and neighborhoods.

SOCIAL POISE AND UNDERSTANDING OF SELF. Competitive athletics contribute to social poise, self-composure, and confidence,

*Larson, Jordan L.: Athletics and good citizenship, Journal of Educational Sociology **28**:258-259, 1955.
†Hale, Creighton J.: What research says about athletics for pre-high school age children, Journal of Health, Physical Education, and Recreation **30**: 19, 1959.

*Lareau, Jeanne Doyle: The relationship between athletic competition and personal and social adjustment on junior high school girls, unpublished master's dissertation, University of California, 1950.
†Salz, Art: Comparative study of personalities of little league champions, other players in little league, and non-playing peers, unpublished master's thesis, Pennsylvania State University, 1957.

according to some educators. They also provide man with a socially acceptable outlet for his aggression. Modern man has had to repress his basic aggressive tendencies in order to peacefully exist in society. However, at times, because of the pressure of modern life, there is need for man to "let off steam." The football game or wrestling match is an excellent safety valve for man's aggressive behavior.

Lowell Biddulph,* in a study concerning high school boys, attempted to determine the personal and social adjustment of those boys with high athletic achievement. The results indicated that the superior athletic at the high school level had a higher mean self-adjustment score on the California Test of Personality than other boys. The superior athletes had a significantly higher mean score on the teachers' ratings and sociograms. The athlete also rated considerably higher on the adjustment items as rated by their teachers. The superior athletic group listed more personal friends and were chosen more frequently by others. It was concluded as a result of this study that students ranking high on athletic achievement tests demonstrate significantly a greater degree of personal and social adjustment than those of low athletic achievement.

The athlete may learn to appreciate the uniqueness of each person and more about himself. He is in a position to develop responsibility for his own actions and to acquire a willingness to accept the results of his actions.

SOCIAL CONSCIOUSNESS WITH AN ACCOMPANYING SENSE OF VALUES. According to some physical educators, the athlete develops a concern for his fellow teammates and opponents. He takes increased interest in his school and community. He learns firsthand the importance of sharing with others, adhering to the rules, and the importance of promoting a way of life that fosters morality, ethical behavior, and the concern for individual dignity and worth. He becomes familiar with values concerning what is right and what is wrong, and an adherence to democratic principles and a respect for others is developed.

BETTER RELATIONS WITH THE OPPOSITE SEX. Competitive athletics, it is felt, contribute to a masculine image and, consequently, added appeal to the opposite sex. Also, certain physical urges develop at this stage of growth and development. The child begins to develop an interest in members of the opposite sex. Athletics can help in channeling this urge into the proper perspective without creating sudden social and emotional maladjustments. Athletic participation serves as a healthy outlet through which this problem, induced by the onset of sexual maturation, can be channeled in a healthy direction.

Harmful impact competitive athletics may have upon the student

EGO-CENTERED ATHLETES. There is a great glorification of the star athlete by both the school and the community. These few select youngsters are frequently singled out from the team to receive special publicity and attention. There is a concentration on the few superior players instead of the many. An overemphasis on publicity often results. Consequently, these youngsters may develop inflated ideas about themselves. They begin to assume that they are "special" and should receive extra favors because of their reputations. This desire to be the center of attraction, some educators feel, can very likely grow as they get older and thus continue into adulthood. Samuel Cooper* refers to this glorification of the athlete and indicates that the student is likely to develop false values that he will perpetuate to society.

FALSE VALUES. False values may very likely be developed because of the emphasis placed upon the star athlete or even athletics in general. The team practice session or the

---

*Biddulph, Lowell G.: Athletic achievement and the personal and social adjustment of high school boys, Research Quarterly **25:**1-7, 1954.

*Cooper, Samuel: The control of interscholastic athletics, unpublished Doctor of Education dissertation, Western Reserve University, 1955, p. 46.

actual game may become more important to the youngster than any other out-of-class activity; the youngster may begin to acquire the attitude that he is destined to become an "All-American" and therefore must give his full time to this endeavor. And, as the community becomes more interested in the program, the youngster may become more concerned that the spectator be pleased than he is concerned about his own needs.

Today, according to some newspaper reports, false values are affecting the black athlete. Some black athletes who attend college on athletic scholarships do not graduate because they face enormous pressures on the campus. They may sacrifice educational goals and choose easy courses in order to keep athletic eligibility. Some colleges give scholarships and appear to be interested primarily in the black man's athletic prowess on the playing field rather than his education and ability in the classroom.

HARMFUL PRESSURES. When parents and members of the community develop the kind of interest in interscholastic sports that has as its main objective "winning," pressures that affect the players are very likely to result. A boy may feel the need to win in order to please his public and gain acceptance. Thus, a constant overstimulation of the student progresses as he strives to reach adult goals.

In a study by Elvera Skubic,* of the University of California, concerning little league and middle league baseball, reference was made to the pressures placed upon youngsters in competition. The purpose of this study was to obtain the attitudes of players and their parents toward little league and middle league baseball and elicit suggestions for the improvement of the program. At the close of the season, questionnaires were sent to parents, players, and teachers. Possibly because of the pressures on the players, one-third of the parents responding reported that their sons were too excited after win-

ning or too depressed after losing to eat a normal-sized meal. Also, this excitement, in some cases, interfered with their ability to get to sleep. Of the players responding, about one-third reported that they began to be excited from 30 minutes to over 5 hours before the start of the game; about two-thirds of the boys reported that they did not begin to get excited until shortly before the beginning of the game.

The Joint Committee on Athletic Competition for Children of Elementary and Junior High School Age* made direct reference to the harmful effects of the pressures upon young athletes. In their study, they strongly oppose interscholastics of a "varsity pattern or similarly organized competition under the auspices of other community agencies." This type of competition is "definitely disapproved for children below the ninth grade." The committee listed the type of pressures which they considered to be a direct violation of the above principle. The following involve high-pressure elements of which the committee disapproves:

1. High-pressure practices such as highly organized competition in the form of leagues, publicity, and stress placed upon the individual rather than on the team
2. Tournaments and long seasons
3. Night games
4. Travel beyond the immediate community
5. Partisan spectators
6. "Grooming" of players for the high school
7. Commercial promotions
8. Disproportionate share of facilities and time and attention of staff

LOSS OF IDENTITY. Athletics can lead to a loss of identity on the part of the individual. At a recent symposium† on problems of the black athlete, one of the major problems discussed was the dehumanizing factor of athletics that affects both black

---

*Skubic, Elvera: Studies of little league and middle league baseball, unpublished thesis, University of California, 1953.

*Joint Committee on Athletic Competition for Children of Elementary and Junior High School Age: Desirable athletic competition for children, Washington, D. C., 1952, American Association for Health, Physical Education, and Recreation, pp. 4, 13-24.
†Ruffer, William A.: Symposium on problems of the black athlete, Journal of Health, Physical Education, and Recreation **42**:17, 1971.

and white. Symposium chairman, William Ruffer, emphasized the point that the athlete is not a college student in the generally accepted definition of the term. The college athlete has a special dining arrangement, lives in a separate dormitory, and may take a reduced academic course load. He has a controlled life guided by athletic directors and coaches, who are not always sensitive to his needs. The college athlete has a socially regulated life. He must wear his hair a certain way. He must be careful of his political statements so as not to irritate the athletic department. Although many colleges are reforming their athletic policies, too many are still pursuing strict authoritarian procedures that prevent the athlete from making his own decisions and living his own life.

INEQUITABLE USE OF FACILITIES, LEADERSHIP, AND MONEY. Athletics are only one phase of the total physical education program. Yet the amount of facilities, the number of personnel, and the proportion of money to be spent are often distributed in an unequitable proportion to the interscholastic program. The girls' program, for example, has been known to suffer and be neglected.

DISTORTION OF THE EDUCATIONAL PROGRAM LEADING TO OVERSPECIALIZATION. At times, so great an emphasis is placed upon producing successful athletic teams that the entire educational program may suffer. The academic achievement of both the participants and the nonparticipants may begin to diminish as student interests are captured by the constant excitement and tension of their team and their heroes. The young competitive player may become one-sided in his own interests, with athletics becoming all too large and important in his thinking and purposes. This problem is of concern, especially during the junior high school years. In a bulletin published by the U. S. Department of Health, Education and Welfare,* the preadolescent is described as

having endless interests. He wants to become strong and skillful and to excel in group and team games. But he also wants to explore the many different areas in which his interest falls. This should be an exploratory period for the eighth and ninth grader. Yet athletics may result in an overconcentration in one small area. Referring to the study made by Skubic,* it was found that youngsters spent a disproportionate amount of time playing and practicing baseball; most of the players responding stated that one-half to most of their leisure time during the whole year was spent on baseball.

VIOLENCE. Athletic competition may increase the violent atmosphere that is becoming characteristic of American society. Coaches who place strong emphasis on winning and demand that players win at all costs may find that not only players but spectators also become violent. At athletic events the cry of the crowd to "kill him" and "hit him harder" may be heard. This emotional feeling may carry over after the contest and lead to fights and other forms of violence. The subject of crowd control is a major concern of athletic directors and other educators today. In some cities night contests have been eliminated to help reduce such violence.

LEADERSHIP. Untrained coaches and leaders frequently do not understand the needs of students. Some seem to feel that they are judged by their contribution to the win-loss record rather than by their contribution to the growth and development of the children. The game rather than the child begins to become the center of importance. The coach's concern for the team and the team's record sometimes overshadows the importance of the physical education class for the intramural program.

Conditions under which athletics become valuable sociologically to students

ALL STUDENTS—THE FOCUS OF ATTENTION. There must be equal opportunity

*Lewis, Gertrude M.: Educating children in grades seven and eight, U. S. Department of Health, Education and Welfare Bulletin No. 10, 1954, pp. 4-7.

*Skubic, Elvera: Studies of little league and middle league baseball, unpublished thesis, University of California, 1953.

for all students to participate in the competitive athletic program, with activities included that are individually adapted to the student. Athletics can be valuable when all students are given the opportunity to learn, to practice, and to play and when playing facilities and the coach's time are allocated among all students.

In the study by Biddulph* concerning the relation between personal and social adjustment of high school boys of high athletic achievement and the personal and social adjustment of high school boys of low athletic achievement, his results led him to conclude that athletics should be provided for all boys and not the special few. Since students ranking high in athletic achievement demonstrated a significantly greater degree of personal and social adjustment than those boys with low athletic achievement, Biddulph concluded that it is important for all boys to develop motor ability, with a greater emphasis upon intramural athletic activities rather than upon interscholastic activities, which tend to neglect the majority of boys.

FOCUS ON THE INDIVIDUAL STUDENT. Athletics must be molded and shaped for the student—not the student for athletics. In a study by Katherine Montgomery,† a plan was proposed to determine those principles and procedures in the conduct of competitive athletics for adolescent girls that had been approved by national organizations. Eleven national groups cooperated in this study. Each group recommended individuals qualified by experience and by professional position to serve on a jury of thirty-three to determine the principles. Eighteen states and the District of Columbia were included. It was recommended, as a result of this study, that for athletic competition to be valuable for girls, it should take the form of sports

days where no tournaments are played and a few friendly games with neighboring cities make up the schedule of events. To protect the student from pressures, "championships, athletic records, activities of excessive endurance, strength or speed, travel exceeding two hours, gate receipts, publicity featuring the individual, undue emotional stimulation of players, or any practice not resulting in the welfare of the participants was banned."

In the report by the Joint Committee on Athletic Competition,* the following conditions were revealed as necessary for beneficial effects pertaining to the individual student through participation in competitive athletics: Instruction must be fitted to meet the needs of the players; sports should be included that are appropriate for the age, maturity, skill, stage of growth, and physical makeup of the players; safeguards should be provided for the health and well-being of the participants; the program should be free of undesirable publicity and promotion; and opportunities should be given for a balance of interest and activities on the part of all participants.

OUTGROWTH OF INTRAMURALS AND EXTRAMURALS. The athletic program should represent a natural outgrowth of the intramural and extramural program. The class instructional program and the intramural and extramural programs should be functioning effectively for all students before interschool athletics are considered. Strong physical education classes and intramural programs should form the base of athletic competion in the schools—a base that builds and is finally capped with more highly organized, competitive games of the interscholastic type.

LEADERSHIP. Sound and qualified leadership is essential to the properly functioning athletic program. Elizabeth K. Skin-

---

*Biddulph, Lowell, G.: Athletic achievement and the personal and social adjustment of high school boys, Research Quarterly 25:1-7, 1954.
†Montgomery, Katherine W.: Principles and procedures in the conduct of interscholastic athletics for adolescent girls, Research Quarterly 23:60-67, 1952.

*Joint Committee on Athletic Competition for Children of Elementary and Junior High School Age: Desirable athletic competition for children, Washington, D. C., 1952, American Association for Health, Physical Education, and Recreation, pp. 4, 13-24.

ner* states: "If an activity possesses both desirable and undesirable possibilities, then the problem of leadership becomes of great importance." Leadership plays an important role in setting qualities of fairness, self-control, and honesty. Good coaching, then, together with adequate supervision, must serve to prevent undersirable practices and to eliminate pressures. Leaders must see that the program is always conducted in regard to the best interests of the students.

Implications for the physical education program

The impact that society has had upon athletics in education presents a challenge to educators to (1) properly interpret to the community the role of athletics in education and (2) prevent undersirable pressures and practices that are not educationally sound. When conducted in accordance with desirable standards such as those of leadership and program content, athletics have the potential for accomplishing beneficial effects. However, when not conducted in accordance with desirable standards, athletics can be detrimental and harmful to the student.

YOUTH PROBLEMS IN THE PRESENT DECADE

Adolescent problems are a major concern of parents, schools, churches, other social agencies, and police departments in every section of our country. Physical educators should also be very much concerned. These problems are reflected in part by much of the antisocial behavior that has captured the headlines in the nation's press during the last few years.

On a national scale, J. Edgar Hoover, Director of the Federal Bureau of Investigation, has reported that crime is on the increase and that youths are involved in much of this crime.

The country is concerned with such things

*Skinner, Elizabeth K.: The role of the school in competitive sports for girls, unpublished Doctor of Education dissertation, Teachers College, Columbia University, 1951, p. 107.

as student activism leading to violence, the use of drugs and narcotics, the increase in the number of unwed mothers, and the poor physical condition of youth. Many educators feel that these adolescent problems stem from such basic psychological needs as the necessity for achieving status, gaining economic independence, and being wanted. In order to solve these problems, young people and adults must understand themselves and the culture of which they are a part more fully.

Adolescent problems represent a challenge to every citizen in America. The day and age in which we are living has much to do with youth problems. Today's adolescents have lived during the period of the Vietnam War. They have lived during a period of great internal crisis and have seen major cities such as Detroit and Newark rocked by race riots. Today's youths have seen their fellow classmates shot and killed on our nation's college campuses. These events have left their imprint. A few characteristics of the age in which our youths are living follow.

IT'S AN AGE OF TENSION AND UNCERTAINTY. The world is divided into armed camps. In spite of talks around the peace table, disarmament conferences, United Nations sessions, and other-attempts at friendly relations, there still exists a fear in the minds of most Americans that world war always is a threat as long as power-seeking, hate-inspiring men hold the reins of government in some countries. The Vietnam War has been going on for over a decade. Young men have been concerned that they may be put into uniform at any time and, rather than be exposed to some of the scourges of mankind, some abandoned their homes and moved to more peaceful countries.

There have been confrontations in recent years between adults and youth. The "generation gap" has split families apart. Parents who are unable to communicate with their children often force their offspring to leave home at an earlier age than they normally would.

IT'S AN AGE OF LOW MORALITY. Moral

standards have declined. Movies, television, and literature discuss and depict even the most unnatural and crude aspects of sex. Clothing is designed to reveal everything and conceal nothing. Many college dormitories are coeducational and curfew restrictions nonexistent. Young men and women openly live together and even have children without the formality of a marriage ceremony. Newspapers carry headlines about madmen and their "hippie families" who butcher helpless people. It is an age of extreme drug use that has turned children into muggers and thieves who must commit violent crimes in order to support their habit.

IT'S AN AGE OF PROTEST AND VIOLENCE. The youths on the nation's campuses and in our secondary schools have protested the war and other policies and practices endorsed by our government. The nation's youths have become aware of the pollution problem that is facing our nation and are attempting to voice opinions in this area. In some educational institutions protests have become violent. Colleges have had to shut down temporarily because of student unrest. Confrontations between black and white students have led to disruptions. Shootings, stabbings, and rapes have become a common occurrence in our urban high schools.

IT'S AN AGE OF LEISURE. In 1800 the average work week for Americans was 84 hours; in 1900 it had dropped to 60 hours; in 1925 it was down to 50 hours; and in 1950 it consisted of only 40 hours. Experts predict that with the application of atomic energy to industry it will be reduced to 30 hours a week in the future.

We are living in an age when a tall skyscraper can be clothed with aluminum within one working day. We can board a plane in New York after breakfast and have lunch in Los Angeles. This is an era when, according to Dr. Hurd, former consultant to the Atomic Energy Commission, a completely automatic factory is possible. Machines guided by magnetic tapes running through electronic directors are capable of making many selective motions.

Science is achieving great things for man-

kind by providing more and more leisure hours. But how are these leisure hours being spent? Children are watching television an average of 13 hours a week—adults more. The President of the United States has been concerned over the trend of the youth of America to be spectators rather than participants. More money is spent on comic books than on all the books in elementary and secondary schools—more than four times the budget of all public libraries in the United States.

A CONCLUDING STATEMENT

It has been pointed out that sociology is concerned with a study of people and their institutions and how a better social order may be established. Sociology depends upon education to help in developing happiness, tolerance, and good will in society. Education plays an important part in solving social problems. Its function is to improve society. Physical education, as part of the total educational process, can contribute to this goal. Physical education is a social experience. Through physical activities great strides can be made in achieving social progress and more satisfaction in living. Juvenile delinquency, race prejudice, intolerance, and discrimination perhaps can be alleviated, and progress can be made toward their elimination from our democratic society. Physical education can help to promote a happier and more cohesive and cooperative type of group living. Finally, physical education can help to promote a happier and a more peaceful world by instilling a spirit of fair play in every child, helping in the development of healthy and physically fit individuals, developing an understanding of the worthy use of leisure time, fostering social equality, furthering democratic procedures, promoting the belief in the dignity of man, and developing an appreciation of the simpler things, as against the collection of great possessions and material wealth.

QUESTIONS AND EXERCISES

1. Define the term *sociology*. What implications does this field have for physical education?

2. What challenges are confronting educational sociology in modern-day living?
3. Describe the cultural values characteristic of American society. What are the implications for physical education?
4. How does original nature differ from human nature? What are some of the characteristics of each?
5. Describe how man is interested, on the one hand, in other people and the welfare of mankind and, on the other, is interested in the life that revolves around hmself and his personal ambitions. How can both of these interest categories be realized?
6. What are some of the forces that impel group living?
7. Contrast a hermit's life with your own. What are the advantages and disadvantages of each?
8. What do you feel are possible solutions to present world crises from the standpoint of sociology?
9. What are the essential foundations for successful group living?
10. Describe the social stratification that has taken place in physical education.
11. How can physical educators contribute to social change?
12. What is social learning? How does it relate to physical education?
13. Discuss in detail each of the theories of play. In your own thinking, which theory is the most descriptive of your definition of play? Discuss.
14. Contrast Caillois' theory of play to the seven other theories of play discussed in this chapter.
15. What are the beneficial aspects of competitive athletics? What are the harmful aspects?
16. Discuss the place of sports in education from your own viewpoint.
17. To what extent should physical education activities be provided for the underprivileged youth who inhabit nearly every community in this country? What kind of program should be provided?
18. How can physical education contribute to mental health?
19. Why is it important for physical educators to adapt their program to the older population?
20. What are the social responsibilities of physical educators in the present decade?

Reading assignment

Bucher, Charles A., and Goldman, Myra: Dimensions of physical education, St. Louis, 1969, The C. V. Mosby Co., Reading selections 51 to 56.

SELECTED REFERENCES

Bucher, Charles A.: Administrative dimensions of health and physical education programs, including athletics, St. Louis, 1971, The C. V. Mosby Co.

Bucher, Charles A.: Interscholastic athletics at the junior high school level, Albany, New York, 1965, The University of the State of New York, State Education Department.

Bucher, Charles A., Koening, Constance, and Barnhard, Milton: Methods and materials of secondary school physical education, St. Louis, 1970, The C. V. Mosby Co.

Bucher, Charles A., and Reade, Evelyn M.: Health and physical education in the elementary school, New York, 1971, The Macmillan Co.

Caillois, Roger: Man, play, and games, New York, 1961, The Free Press.

Educational Policies Commission: Moral and spiritual values in the public schools, Washington, D. C., 1951, National Education Association.

Frederickson, Florence Stumpf: Sports and the cultures of man. In Loy, John W., and Kenyon, Gerald S., editors: Sport, culture and society: a reader on the sociology of sport, London, 1969, The Macmillan Co.

Gibson, Dorothy Westby: Social perspectives on education, New York, 1965, John Wiley and Sons, Inc.

Havighurst, Robert S., and Newgarten, Bernice L.: Society on education, Boston, 1957, Allyn & Bacon, Inc.

Jones, Frank B.: Intercollegiate and interscholastic athletic program in the 1970's: a report to the Athletic Institute Board of Directors, Sportscope 15(2):16-17, 1970.

Kallenbach, Warren W., and Hodges, Harold M.: Education and society, Columbus, Ohio, 1963, Charles E. Merrill Books, Inc.

Kenyon, Gerald S., and Loy, John W.: Toward a sociology of sport, Journal of Health, Physical Education, and Recreation 36:24, 1965.

Kraus, Richard: Recreation and leisure in modern society, New York, 1971, Appleton-Century-Crofts.

Loret, John: A happening in the out-of-doors, Journal of Health, Physical Education, and Recreation 40: 45-46, 1969.

Loy, John W.: The nature of sport: a definitional effort, Quest (Monograph X), May, 1968, pp. **1-15.**

Loy, John W., and Kenyon, Gerald S.: Sport, culture and society: a reader on the sociology of sport, London, 1969, The Macmillan Co.

Mercer, Blaine E., and Carr, Edwin R.: Education and the social order, New York, 1960, Holt, Rinehart & Winston.

Morris, Van Cleve, and others: Becoming an educator, Boston, 1963, Houghton Mifflin Co.

Oxendine, Joseph B.: Social development—the forgotten objective? Journal of Health, Physical Education, and Recreation 37:23, 1966.

Parker, Franklin: Sport, play, and physical education in cultural perspective, Journal of Health, Physical Education, and Recreation **36:**29, 1965.

Ruffer, William A.: Symposium on problems of the black athlete, Journal of Health, Physical Education, and Recreation **42:**17, 1971.

Ulrich, Celeste: The social matrix of physical education, Englewood Cliffs, New Jersey, 1968, Prentice-Hall, Inc.

Wilton, W. M.: An early concensus on sportsmanship, The Physical Educator **20:**113, 1963.

Wood, Thomas Denison, and Cassidy, Rosalind Frances: The new physical education, New York, 1931, The Macmillan Co.

PART SIX

Leadership in physical education

19/The teaching profession and physical education
20/Duties of physical education personnel
21/Preparation of the physical education teacher

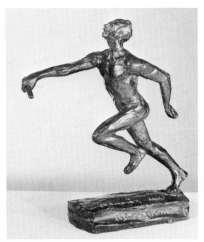

WORK OF R. TAIT
MCKENZIE. COURTESY
JOSEPH BROWN, SCHOOL OF
ARCHITECTURE, PRINCETON
UNIVERSITY.

19/The teaching profession and physical education

Education as a career is attracting outstanding young people to its ranks. The challenge presented by such events and movements as the explosion of knowledge, the poverty program, the pollution of the environment, the civil rights movement, and the developing nations emerging on the world scene has motivated many young men and women to seek educational careers. In turn, they believe that these careers will help them to contribute to the solution of some of the problems that exist in America and throughout the world. Within the field of education, the profession of teaching is attracting the greatest number of our youth.

The teaching profession has more than 2 million men and women employed at the various educational levels. In the elementary and secondary schools combined, about one-third of these teachers are men and two-thirds are women. Contrary to what exists in many fields of endeavor, teachers as a group like their work, as evidenced in a survey conducted by the National Education Assocation that showed that three-fourths of the teachers would choose teaching again if they were starting over in a career. Teachers indicated that the professional relationships with their colleagues, the intellectual stimulation of their work, and the service they rendered to others were some of the factors that marked their enjoyment of teaching. Surveys show that teachers rank higher on social concerns than does the general population. They rank lower in respect to economic concerns, however. In

cognitive abilities, as measured on intelligence tests, students going into teaching rank higher than the general population but lower than those students going into many other professions.

Teaching is one of the favorite choices of a profession for high school and college students today. Surveys consistently show that teaching has great appeal for young people who are trying to decide on a career that holds challenge and satisfactions for the future.

THE TEACHING PROFESSION— WHAT IT OFFERS

Teaching offers many rewards. Probably most important of all is that it offers an opportunity to help shape young people's lives. Other rewards include the privilege of being a member of a profession that is growing in respect and importance in the world as well as in America. It offers an opportunity to mingle with some of the great thinkers and leaders of the academic community. It offers opportunities to travel and to better understand the world. It motivates self-improvement and intellectual growth. It provides increasingly better economic benefits in the form of salaries, retirement benefits, sick leaves, insurance, medical help, and sabbatical leaves. It provides security under the tenure laws that exist in most states.

The rewards that accrue from teaching depend to a large degree upon the individual and what he makes of his opportunities. The inner rewards, plus the financial and other benefits, can be great for the person who

553

applies himself diligently and sincerely to assigned tasks.

THE TEACHING PROFESSION— NEW DEVELOPMENTS

There are many new developments in the teaching profession that should be familiar to each person desiring to become a teacher.

Differentiated staffing

Differentiated staffing means the assignment of personnel to different roles in terms of their training, abilities, career goals, aptitudes, and interests. The primary purpose is to provide for a more individualized program and better service to students, to make greatest use of teacher abilities, and to enable teachers to assume greater responsibilities and receive increases in compensation. Teachers have differentiated levels of responsibility and are paid accordingly.

Some of the rationale and premises upon which differentiated staffing rests include the belief that teachers must have a primary responsibility for teaching and must be relieved of many nonprofessional tasks. Furthermore, teachers should have more responsibility for decision making. In addition, there must be organizational flexibility through the use of flexible scheduling. Also, programs both preservice and in-service in nature must prepare teachers for the roles they play. Finally, teachers should be able to earn salaries comparable to the roles they play, which means that in some cases they would be higher than those of school administrators.

The Kansas City Public School System is an example of a school system that has established a differentiated staffing plan in some of their schools. During the experimental period of this plan they established the following job classifications. The *coordinating instructor* is involved in such tasks as initiating curriculum innovations, selecting and distributing instructional materials, teaching demonstration classes, and developing in-service activities. The *senior instructor* provides leadership in a specific subject-matter area, diagnoses and develops

prescriptions for students, establishes schedules of activities, and supervises the work of student teachers. The *instructor,* a full-time teacher, handles large group instruction in his subject matter specialty and works with students in enriching their learning experiences. The *associate instructor,* a part-time teacher, helps to implement plans developed by the team. The *intern* contributes by participating in teaching and team teaching activities and fulfills the responsibilities provided by the college or university with which he is associated. The *student teacher* is involved in observing and participating in teaching activities as prescribed by the senior instructor and in following the program prescribed by his teacher-training institution. The *paraprofessional* is either a full-time or part-time employee who attends to much clerical work, such as taking attendance, preparing instructional materials, or operating machines.

Since the purpose of differentiated staffing is to utilize teaching resources more effectively, it recognizes the individual differences of teachers and how they can best be used to enhance student learning. There are arguments pro and con for differentiated staffing. More research and experimentation need to take place in order to find the formula that will be most effective for our schools.

In physical education there are many roles that teachers can fulfill. This field should focus its attention on differentiated staffing to determine whether its application will result in a greater learning experience for its students.

Teacher aides

Recently there has been greater and greater utilization of teacher aides. These assistants are sometimes called "auxiliary personnel" or "paraprofessionals." The National Education Association Research Division found that in 1967-1968 there were 29,938 aides reported for 743 school systems. When a similar survey was conducted in 1968-1969, 40,295 teacher aides were being used in 709 school systems with enrollments of 6,000 or more, a distinct gain for the 1-year period. The most recent survey also pointed out that 62.4% of the teacher aides were working in elementary schools and only 12.3% in high schools. Paid teacher aides were used in 84% of the reporting schools.*

Some of the tasks performed by teacher aides include clerical duties such as recording grades, typing, and filing; nonclassroom duties such as helping in lunchroom and playground supervision; assisting with large group instruction such as music and art; grading papers; assisting with small group instruction such as that relating to reading and spelling; helping in the preparation and use of instructional materials such as operating a projector; and performing work connected with the classroom environment such as caring for bulletin boards and monitoring classes.

Student leaders

Another development is the increased use of student leaders in schools and colleges. This is more pronounced at this time primarily because of the stress on student involvement, the need to train leadership for the profession, and the desire to render a greater service to students by providing them more individualized instruction from their better skilled classmates.

Qualifications needed by the student leader include a personality conducive to interaction with other students and faculty, intelligence and sound judgment, interest in other students, love of physical activity, and leadership qualities such as resourcefulness and dependability.

Student leaders are selected in several ways, including a request for volunteers, appointment by the teacher, election by the class, selection based on test results, and selection by the Leader's Club. Student leaders need a period of orientation and training before assuming their responsibilities.

*National Education Association: Use of teacher aids, National Education Association Research Bulletin **47:**62, 1969.

Student leaders may be utilized in several ways, such as class leaders, officials, committee members, supply and equipment managers, program planners, record keepers, office managers, and special events coordinators.

Teaching style

Teaching style is an expression of the educator's individuality in relation to his stated philosophy and program objectives and is being given much attention in today's educational programs. Additionally, an educator's teaching style is reflected in his methodology of teaching and in his class organization and management.

There are two basic kinds of teaching style, teacher centered and student centered. There are many variations and overlappings of these styles that can be applied to educators in general and to physical educators. This discussion will apply to the teaching style utilized by physical educators.

The teacher-centered physical educator is often described as being autocratic. He states his philosophy of physical education in terms of his personal relationship to his profession and his personal conception of the goals of his profession in relation to his own teaching. He will evaluate the basketball unit as a success if he has taught the dribble, the hook shot, and foul shooting to his class so that they can perform to a common standard. The satisfaction to the autocratic physical educator is based not on student success but on teacher accomplishment in terms of teacher-centered objectives. The teacher-centered physical educator is somewhat of a perfectionist and expects all of his students will be able to perform a certain skill in the same way. He does not realize that all students do not have the ability to meet a single standard of performance. His teaching is frequently geared to those students who can measure up to his criteria for success. He is also a rather rigid individual, and his students are motivated more by fear of failure than by an inner desire to succeed. Furthermore, instruction is likely to follow tried-and-tested methodology.

The student-centered physical educator is sometimes thought of as a democratic teacher. His philosophy is stated in terms of the relationship of physical education to general education. His program objectives are stated in terms of student needs and interests, and his evaluation is based upon how well his program has succeeded in meeting these needs and interests. He is especially cognizant of differences in student ability and avoids setting common criteria for skill performance. The student-centered physical educator is usually very flexible and will adapt a lesson if he sees that it is not accomplishing its purpose. He welcomes innovations because he feels that the latest techniques and methodology will better contribute to his students. He also attempts to teach his students to think for themselves, to be creative, to express themselves, and to ask questions.

A teaching style develops gradually and is unique to each educator because of the myriad individual variations and shadings that may be applied to a style. There are various influences that affect the development of an individual's style. Two of the most important are the undergraduate professional preparing program and the student teaching experience. A third influence is the philosophy of the school system.

Teacher accountability

There is increasing stress among educational systems across the country to develop a system of professional accountability for teachers. The aim of such a movement is to develop objective standards as a means of improving school effectiveness. Among other things it is designed to show which teaching and school methods have proved most effective in achieving specific educational goals. It will protect successful teachers against unfair criticisms by providing proof of their effectiveness; for those teachers who are not effective, it will indicate the additional training and help they need to become effective teachers.

It is the belief of some educators and laymen that teachers in the past have not been accountable to a great degree for helping their students achieve a certain standard of performance. Although some teachers have been very dedicated and successful in helping their students to achieve goals far beyond what many students in other school systems achieve, others have been apathetic in regard to their pupil's achievement records. This feeling among some boards of education has led to the negotiation of performance contracts with business establishments whereby certain achievement goals are guaranteed by the business organization making the contract.

There is a need to define the performance objectives of pupils and staff members of every school, assess the school and nonschool factors that influence pupil performance, and develop an administrative structure that can operate effectively on an accountability basis.

At the present time there is considerable discussion concerning how teachers should be evaluated. Questions have been raised as to whether teachers should be rated on the basis of their own performance in the classroom or gymnasium or on the basis of the performance of their pupils and whether their personality should be taken into consideration in the evaluation process.

How teachers are evaluated

Teacher evaluation has become an important consideration in determining promotions, in-service education, tenure, merit salary raises, and, most important, the improvement of teaching. Some general guidelines for the evaluation of teachers include the following.

APPRAISAL SHOULD INVOLVE THE TEACHERS THEMSELVES. Evaluation is a cooperative venture, and teachers should be involved in the development of the criteria for evaluation and should understand the process.

EVALUATION SHOULD BE CENTERED ON PERFORMANCE. The job that is to be accomplished should be the point of focus, with other extraneous factors omitted.

EVALUATION SHOULD BE CONCERNED WITH HELPING THE TEACHER TO GROW ON

Teacher evaluation

TEACHER: Socrates

A. Personal qualifications

	Rating (high to low) 1 2 3 4 5	Comments
1. Personal appearance	☐ ☐ ☐ ☐ ☑	Dresses in an old sheet draped about his body
2. Self-confidence	☐ ☐ ☐ ☐ ☑	Not sure of himself—always asking questions
3. Use of English	☐ ☐ ☐ ☑ ☐	Speaks with a heavy Greek accent
4. Adaptability	☐ ☐ ☐ ☐ ☑	Prone to suicide by poison when under duress

B. Class management

	1 2 3 4 5	Comments
1. Organization	☐ ☐ ☐ ☐ ☑	Does not keep a seating chart
2. Room appearance	☐ ☐ ☐ ☑ ☐	Does not have eye-catching bulletin boards
3. Utilization of supplies	☑ ☐ ☐ ☐ ☐	Does not use supplies

C. Teacher-Pupil relationships

	1 2 3 4 5	Comments
1. Tact and consideration	☐ ☐ ☐ ☐ ☑	Places student in embarrassing situation by asking questions
2. Attitude of class	☐ ☑ ☐ ☐ ☐	Class is friendly

D. Techniques of teaching

	1 2 3 4 5	Comments
1. Daily preparation	☐ ☐ ☐ ☐ ☑	Does not keep daily lesson plans
2. Attention to course of study	☐ ☐ ☑ ☐ ☐	Quite flexible—allows students to wander to different topics
3. Knowledge of subject matter	☐ ☐ ☐ ☐ ☑	Does not know material—has to question pupils to gain knowledge

E. Professional attitude

	1 2 3 4 5	Comments
1. Professional ethics	☐ ☐ ☐ ☐ ☑	Does not belong to professional association or PTA
2. In-service training	☐ ☐ ☐ ☐ ☑	Complete failure here—has not even bothered to attend college
3. Parent relationships	☐ ☐ ☐ ☐ ☑	Needs to improve in this area—parents are trying to get rid of him

RECOMMENDATION: Does not have a place in Education. Should not be rehired.

FROM SATURDAY REVIEW, JULY 21, 1962.

THE JOB. The purpose of evaluation is to help the teacher to evaluate his strengths and weaknesses and to maintain his strengths and reduce his weaknesses.

EVALUATION SHOULD LOOK TO THE FUTURE. It should be concerned with developing a better program and a better school system.

EVALUATION OF TEACHERS SHOULD BE WELL ORGANIZED AND ADMINISTERED. It should be clearly outlined and every teacher should know the step-by-step approach to be followed.

Some of the methods of evaluation of teachers include the following:

OBSERVATION OF TEACHERS IN THE CLASSROOM OR IN THE GYMNASIUM. The National Education Association Research Division, in studying this method, reported that the median length of time for the most recent observation was 22 minutes; about 25% of the teachers were notified 1 day in advance that the observation would take place; and about 50% of the teachers reported that a conference followed the observation period with the teacher's performance being discussed and evaluated. Nearly one-half of the teachers reported that the observation was helpful to them.

STUDENT PROGRESS. With this method, standardized tests are used to determine what progress the student has made as a result of exposure to the teacher.

RATINGS. Ratings vary and may consist of an overall estimate of a teacher's effectiveness or consist of separate evaluations of specific teacher behavior and traits. Self-ratings may also be used. Ratings may be conducted by the teacher's peers, by students, or by administrative personnel and may include judgments based on observation of student progress. Rating scales, in order to be effective, must be based on such criteria as objectivity, reliability, sensitivity, validity, and utility.

At college and university levels the evaluation of teacher performance is sometimes more difficult than at precollege levels because of the unwillingness of the faculty to permit members of the administration, or other persons, to observe them in the class-room, or some other place, for this purpose. Various methods have been devised in institutions of higher learning to rate faculty members, including statements from department heads, ratings by colleagues, ratings by students, and ratings by deans and other administrative personnel.

A question that frequently arises in the development of any system of teacher evaluation is: What constitutes effectiveness as it relates to a teacher in a particular school or college situation? Several studies have been conducted with some interesting findings. For example, there is only a slight correlation between intelligence and the rated success of an instructor. Therefore, the degree of intelligence a teacher has, within reasonable limits, seems to have little value as a criterion. The relationship of knowledge of subject matter to teaching effectiveness appears to be a pertinent factor in particular teaching situations. A teacher's demonstration of good scholarship while a student in college appears to have little positive relationship to good teaching. There is some evidence to show that teachers who have demonstrated high levels of professional knowledge on national teachers' examinations are more effective teachers. However, the evidence here is rather sparse. The relationship of long-term experience to effectiveness also seems to have questionable value. The first 5 years of teaching seems to enhance teacher effectiveness the most. Cultural background, socioeconomic status, sex, and marital status have little value in predicting teacher effectiveness. Finally, there is little evidence to show that any specified aptitude for teaching exists. The studies indicate that more research needs to be done in order to establish what constitutes teacher effectiveness on the job.

Most schools have some system of evaluating teachers, as indicated by a survey conducted by the Research Division of the National Education Association. Some findings from this study include*:

---

*Research Division, National Education Association: Evaluation of teaching, NEA Research Bulletin **47:**67, 1969.

Probationary teachers are evaluated more than those on a permanent status.

In most school systems the principal does the evaluating and in the others he is aided by assistants.

Teachers are usually involved in the evaluation process.

Most teachers feel they should be evaluated.

Teachers dissatisfied with the evaluation may invoke grievance procedures in most school systems.

Most teachers feel the principal should be responsible for the evaluation.

Most teachers feel that the primary purpose of evaluation is to improve teaching competence.

CODE OF ETHICS

The representative assembly of the National Education Association in 1968 adopted a Code of Ethics of the Education Profession. The board of directors of the American Association for Health, Physical Education, and Recreation formally endorsed the code.

The code consists of four principles. *Principle One* outlines the commitment to the *student* and indicates the cooperative, helpful, and professional relationship that exists between the student and teacher. *Principle Two* outlines the commitment to the *public* and spells out the important role of educators in the development of educational programs and policies and their interpretation for the public. *Principle Three* outlines the commitment to the *profession* and indicates the need to raise educational standards, improve the service to people, and develop a worthwhile and respected profession. *Principle Four* outlines the commitment to *professional employment practices* and explains the importance of acting in accordance with high ideals of professional service that embody personal integrity, dignity, and mutual respect.

The code is designed to show the magnitude of the education profession and to judge ourselves and our colleagues in accordance with the provisions of this code.

The National Education Association and affiliate organizations are enforcing the professional code of ethics of the education profession. Examples of such enforcement are the cases of Jim Cherry of Dekalb County, Georgia, and Richard A. White, formerly of Salt Lake City, Utah. Jim Cherry was found guilty on July 28, 1969, of violating the Code of Ethics of the Education Profession, with the result that his expulsion from membership in the NEA was ordered. Richard A. White was suspended from NEA membership for the school year 1969-1970 for violating Principle IV, Section 6 of the Code of Ethics of the Education Profession.*

TEACHER PROBLEMS

As with any professional group, teachers have problems. In attacking these problems, it is necessary to view them in proper perspective, especially in relation to which are the major and which the minor problems throughout the nation. According to a study conducted by the Research Division of the National Education Association,† the five major problems of teachers were identified as: (1) insufficient time for rest and preparation in the school day, (2) large class size, (3) insufficient clerical help, (4) inadequate salary, and (5) inadequate fringe benefits. Less stress was placed upon such problems as lack of public support for schools, ineffective faculty meetings, and poor administration.

QUALIFICATIONS FOR TEACHERS IN GENERAL

Many studies have been made of characteristics of a good teacher and the abilities most useful for a teaching career. Six personal traits are discussed by the Future Teachers of America based on the studies that have been conducted.‡

1. *Do you like to be with people?* If you like group activities, belong to clubs, enjoy serving on committees, know all types of

---

*National Education Association: NEA committee acts on ethics complaint, Today's Education **58:**34, 1969.

†National Education Association: Teacher's problems, NEA Research Bulletin **46:**116, 1968.

‡Future Teachers of America: How's your T.Q. —a check-list to explore your aptitude for teaching, Washington, D. C., National Education Association.

people and are sympathetic to their peculiarities, have a wide circle of friends and are always seeking more, you probably meet this criterion essential to success in teaching.

2. *Are you a good scholar? Do you often lose yourself in a book?* Do you enjoy mastering a subject and read because you want to? Are you in the top one-third of your class, and do you belong to honor societies? Do you recognize that you must learn before you can teach?

3. *Do you have a good sense of humor?* Can you laugh at yourself, not take yourself too seriously, apply a light approach to ease a tense situation, take a happy view of life, shake off the blues quickly, and see the funny side of a situation?

4. *Are you in good physical and mental health?* Since the hours of teaching are long and the work demanding, do you have plenty of pep, energy, and stamina, are you usually poised and emotionally well balanced, do you take criticism without becoming angry or depressed, and do you keep your voice pleasant and calm even when upset?

5. *Do you like to help others?* Do you have the urge to serve others; enjoy working with youngsters; volunteer to help out in church, schools, hospitals, or orphan homes; and offer your services to local charity drives?

6. *Are you often the leader in group activities?* Since a good teacher must have leadership qualities, do you ever organize ac-

Qualities that members of Boys' Clubs believed were needed for leadership.

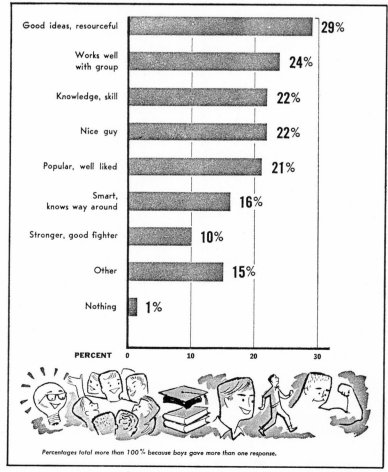

Quality	Percent
Good ideas, resourceful	29%
Works well with group	24%
Knowledge, skill	22%
Nice guy	22%
Popular, well liked	21%
Smart, knows way around	16%
Stronger, good fighter	10%
Other	15%
Nothing	1%

Percentages total more than 100% because boys gave more than one response.

FROM NEEDS AND INTERESTS OF ADOLESCENT BOYS' CLUBS MEMBERS— A NATIONAL SURVEY OF MEMBERS AGED 14 TO 18, NEW YORK, 1960, BOYS' CLUBS OF AMERICA.

A TEACHER'S CREDO

*This I believe**

That when we choose to teach, we choose to serve.

That every child is entitled to the best we have to give, regardless of his personality, his mentality, or his situation.

That our discipline should be firm, consistent, and constructive.

That we should remember that kindness and consideration and trust are not a sign of weakness in a teacher.

That children are hurt by the same things that hurt us—sarcasm and ridicule.

That we should not exact a higher standard of conduct in matters of punctuality, responsibility, and self-control than we ourselves possess.

That we have limitless opportunities to touch lives for good.

That we should treat every child as if he were our very own.

tivities in your circle of friends, have you been elected to office in a club or class, and have you demonstrated leadership ability?

One of the most impressive studies that has been conducted was the one accomplished by Cassel and Johns, of the Fontana Unified School District in California.† The procedure followed was first to analyze more than 1,000 teacher effectiveness reports completed by principals in the Fontana School District. From these reports were listed critical characteristics of effective and ineffective teachers. In addition to extracting the critical characteristics, the "critical incident" technique was used to compile further critical characteristics of effective and ineffective teachers. More than 22,500 critical characteristics were compiled. Positive statement items were paired with negative items and those mentioned most frequently were recorded. They were then arranged into meaningful groupings

*By Mary Livingstone, formerly with Byram Hills Central Schools, Armonk, N. Y.

†Cassel, Russell N., and Johns, W. Lloyd: The critical characteristics of an effective teacher, Bulletin of the National Association of Secondary School Principals **44:**119-124, 1960.

pertinent to outstanding qualifications of teachers. The following list embodies many of these qualifications:

Personal qualities
Integrity
Cooperative
Dynamic personality
Enthusiasm for teaching
Friendly with students and other members of staff
Good mental and physical health
Mature
Sense of humor
Positive in outlook
Approachable
Good intelligence
Creative and imaginative
Dependable and reliable
Ethical in all his activities
Strong sense of moral obligation to youth

Professional preparation
Possesses a general education
Well prepared in subject matter field
Keeps well informed on new trends in education and in special fields
Has special knowledge and competency in understanding of pupils and methodology at educational level where he teaches
Has special knowledge of counseling

Adapts teaching to pupils being taught
Makes every effort to know, understand, and appreciate characteristics and needs of adolescent pupils—knows what they are like, how they feel about themselves, their ideals, behavior patterns, and how they get along with others.
Helps students establish a sound standard of values
Treats each student as a precious and unique personality
Is sympathetic to all students and the problems they face
Helps students evaluate their growth and progress
Takes into consideration the mental, social, emotional, and physical needs of students, regardless of his subject-matter field
Makes learning activity meaningful to student at his stage of growth and development
Insists that what is good for the student is the main criterion for determining what and how a subject is taught
Provides many and varied experiences for students

Professional stature
Active in his profession
Active on school committees
Enjoys teaching
Interested in latest research findings

Participates in community activities
Works well with parents
Interprets professional work to community
Constantly seeks personal and professional improvement

Leadership qualities
Is respected by colleagues and students
Bestows credit on those who have done work
Teaches by example as well as by precept
Gets the most from his students and the students enjoy their studies
Develops an atmosphere of understanding and mutual trust in his classes
Good organizer and planner
Makes sound decisions
Utilizes democratic processes
Interested in all facets of the educational program

Human relations qualities
Observes code of professional ethics at all times
Gets along well with students, administration, and colleagues
Modest in his accomplishments
Keeps educational discussion on professional and not personal basis
Is receptive to constructive criticism
Works for the good of the students

Another study consisted of interviewing several persons as to the qualities and characteristics they thought existed in the best teachers to whom they were exposed. A list of those qualities that were mentioned most frequently are as follows:

1. Teacher knew his subject matter well
2. Teacher took a personal interest in each student
3. Teacher was well respected and respected his students
4. Teacher stimulated his students to think
5. Teacher was interesting and made his subject matter come to life
6. Teacher was an original thinker and creative in his methods
7. Teacher was a fine speaker, presented a neat appearance, and was generally well groomed
8. Teacher had a good sense of humor
9. Teacher was fair and honest in his dealings with his students
10. Teacher was understanding and kind

Another study contrasted effective and ineffective teaching behavior. The information was collected from a survey of supervisors, professors in professional preparation institutions, school principals, student teachers, teachers, and students in education methods courses in professional preparation institutions. Some of the effective behaviors and ineffective behaviors cited were as follows*:

Effective behaviors
1. Alert and enthusiastic
2. Interested in pupils
3. Cheerful
4. Shows self-control
5. Sense of humor
6. Admits own mistakes
7. Fair and impartial
8. Patient
9. Sympathetic with pupils
10. Friendly and courteous
11. Helps pupils with personal problems
12. Offers praise for work well done
13. Encourages pupils to do best
14. Work is planned and well organized
15. Stimulates pupils with interesting material and methods
16. Gives clear directions
17. Discipline is quiet and dignified
18. Gives help willingly
19. Classroom procedure is flexible
20. Tries to foresee difficulties

Ineffective behaviors
1. Appears bored
2. Not interested in pupils
3. Appears unhappy
4. Loses temper
5. Overly serious
6. Does not admit mistakes
7. Has favorites
8. Impatient
9. Uses sarcasm
10. Aloof
11. Appears unaware of personal problems of pupils
12. Is hypercritical
13. No encouragement given
14. Little planning and disorganized
15. Uninteresting materials and methods used
16. Directions are incomplete and vague
17. Ridicules and reprimands at length
18. Does not give help or gives it grudgingly
19. Does not depart from plans—rigid
20. Does not see potential difficulties

QUALIFICATIONS FOR TEACHERS OF PHYSICAL EDUCATION

A young person considering physical education as a career should carefully evaluate his qualifications for this field of work.

*Ryans, David G.: Characteristics of teachers, Washington, D. C., 1960, American Council on Education, Library of Congress.

Need for well-trained teachers in physical education

The physical education profession needs teachers who believe in such credos as the one listed in this chapter; who possess the enthusiasm, culture, and other qualities listed in the employer's letter on p. 564; and who know subject matter, possess skills, are articulate, and command the admiration and respect of their students.

The problem of poor teachers is not foreign to the physical education profession. The great growth in the number of teacher education programs throughout the nation has raised many questions over the years as to the quality of preparation that is being provided. Carl Nordly, former president of the American Association for Health, Physical Education, and Recreation, pointed out that as of February 2, 1948, there were 390 institutions giving professional education in health education, physical education, and recreation—an increase of forty-eight institutions over the previous year. He then emphasized the fact that there was cause for alarm, since many of the prospective teachers being trained in these specialized areas were being poorly prepared for their future responsibilities. William Hughes, former leader in physical education, pointed out that in 1947 more than 300 leaders in the fields of physical education, health education, and recreation listed the education of well-trained leaders as being the most crucial problem with which these professions were faced. The decades of the 1950's and the 1960's have not solved this dilemma. Leadership is still one of the major problems of the profession.

The problem is not only that of preparing teachers in an adequate manner but also one of making sure that only the best students are allowed to become members of the teaching profession. There is little doubt that many young men and women who are capable of becoming superior teachers in our schools never consider the teaching profession as a possible vocation. At the same time, many individuals who are not adequately suited to this profession go through teacher-training institutions. Such a situation must be changed if our educational system is to carry on its work successfully.

General qualifications for physical educators

The physical education profession requires special qualifications for those individuals who wish to be considered as candidates for entrance into this specialized field. Many individuals have entered this profession in the past on the basis of their athletic ability alone, without regard for such qualities as intelligence, scholarship, personality, and technical knowledge. Such a practice must end if the physical education profession is to have prestige in the educational world.

Some of the qualifications that have been mentioned and considered most important by leaders in the field are moral character, leadership, honesty, dependability, adaptability, engaging personality, freedom from organic and functional defects, superior motor capacity, motor skill, high native intelligence, high scholarship, superior social ability, interest in teaching as a profession, desire to help others, competency in oral and written English, and ability to coordinate activities.

The qualification of scholarship is one that is stressed as being especially necessary for our profession. Steinhaus, a former leader in physical education, made this statement years ago, but it is just as true today: "A major obstacle which confronts physical education today in its struggle to become a mighty profession is its shortage in true scholarship . . . primary reason for this is the fact that virtually our only route for recruiting students into our ranks is through the avenue of their interest in sport or some other physical activity."* If prospective candidates for the physical education profession have a high degree of scholarship along with the other important qualifications, the prestige and respect that physical educators will have in the schools, in the community,

---

*Steinhaus, Arthur H.: The next step in teacher training, Journal of Health and Physical Education **10:**141, 1939.

and among the professions will be greatly enhanced.

Specific qualifications for physical educators

The individual desiring to become a member of the physical education profession should be able to meet the following requirements.

HIGH SCHOOL AND COLLEGE

The candidate should be a graduate of an approved high school and an approved college or university preparing teachers for physical education.

INTELLIGENCE AND FOUNDATIONAL SCIENCES

The candidate should possess that degree of intelligence needed to qualify for successful teaching. Furthermore, since the physical education profession is based upon the foundational sciences of anatomy, physiology, biology, kinesiology, sociology, and psychology, the prospective candidate should have some aptitude for these sciences.

ORAL AND WRITTEN ENGLISH

The candidate should meet acceptable standards in oral and written English. The candidate's voice should be audible, pleasant, stimulating, smooth, and unaffected and his choice and organization of words should conform with good English usage. The candidate should be able to write in an acceptable manner with special attention to punctuation, choice of words, sentence structure, and logical organization. The speech of physical educators is under continuous scrutiny, and they are frequently called upon to speak in public. The nature of their positions makes it imperative that they use acceptable English in their speaking and writing.

HEALTH

The candidate should be able to satisfactorily pass health examinations, including an examination of the skin, teeth, eyes, ears, chest, heart, feet, and posture, and show

---

LETTER DESCRIBING TYPE OF PHYSICAL EDUCATION TEACHER AN EMPLOYER DESIRES ON HIS STAFF

Waterloo Public Schools
Waterloo, Iowa

Dear Sir:

Here are some traits that I look for in hiring a teacher of physical education:

I prefer a neat, cultured, enthusiastic person in excellent health with poise and emotional stability.

In checking educational qualifications, I particularly look for the ratings in health, scholarship, discipline and cooperation. It is important that the person is able to cooperate and get along with co-workers. Thus, the individual should be well-adjusted, possess the ability to think practically, and be able to adjust to new situations.

I am interested in a teacher who will be able to have good discipline and at the same time is interested in the welfare of his or her students. It is also important that this person be interested in growing on the job and able to take constructive criticism.

A person with creative ideas who has a wholesome influence on the students as well as his and her fellow teachers is an asset to any faculty.

Once the person is hired and we like his or her work, and he or she is happy in the work, we prefer to have this person stay on the job for a number of years.

Sincerely yours,
Finn B. Ericksen, Director
Health and Physical Education

---

good personal health history, mental health, and emotional stability. The candidate must be free from any physical or mental defects that would prevent successful teaching in physical education. Because of the important part that a teacher plays in shaping a child's life, it is necessary that a candidate with mental disorders, which would adversely affect the child, not be considered for this profession. Furthermore, physical education is a strenuous type of work and therefore demands that members of the profession be in a state of buoyant, robust health in order that they may carry out their duties with efficiency and regularity. They should also remember that they are building healthy bodies; therefore, they should be a good testimonial for their preachments.

PERSONALITY

The candidate should possess a personality suitable for teaching. Such personality traits as enthusiasm, friendliness, cheerfulness, industry, cooperation, firmness and forcefulness in supporting one's convictions, dependability, self-control, integrity, social adaptability, and likableness are factors that can determine in great measure whether an individual will be a success or a failure as a teacher. Whether or not the right social traits are developed in children will depend largely on the personality of the leader. Therefore, it is essential that the teacher of physical education be able to enlist the respect, cooperation, and admiration of the students through his personality, magnetism, and leadership. Frequently one hears teachers described by such phrases as "he has a way with children," or "the children think everything she does is just right." These are the individuals who have personalities that enable them to contribute to a child's development.

INTEREST IN TEACHING

The candidate should have a sincere interest in the teaching of physical education as a profession. Unless an individual has a firm belief in the value of physical education and a desire to help extend the benefits of such an endeavor to others, he should not enter this work. Only if he has a deep conviction that he is rendering a service to mankind will the best job be performed. A person sincerely interested in physical education enjoys teaching individuals to participate in the gamut of activities incorporated in such programs, helping others to realize the happiness and thrilling experiences of participation that he himself enjoys, and helping to develop citizenship traits conducive to democratic living. A person must have a sincere love of the out-of-doors and of all the activities that make up the physical education program, either indoors or out in the open. This means

that anyone interested in being a member of this profession should enjoy such dual and individual sports as tennis, badminton, swimming, golf, and handball and such team sports as field hockey, football, baseball, basketball, and soccer. If an individual does not enjoy these activities, going into this field of endeavor would be similar to a person becoming a sailor who does not like the water or a veterinarian who does not like animals.

MOTOR ABILITY

The candidate should possess an acceptable standard of motor ability. This may be determined through motor ability tests that meet acceptable test criteria. Physical skills are the basis of the entire physical education profession. In order to play tennis, badminton, football, and basketball effectively, it is necessary to have developed some skill in these activities. If the physical educator is to teach various games and activities to others, it is necessary that he have skill in some of them himself. Otherwise, it would be similar to an individual who does not know how to use a saw planning to be a carpenter, a person who cannot drive, a bus driver, or a person who does not know what a spark plug is, an auto mechanic. Physical skills are basic to the physical education profession. Coordination, agility, flexibility, strength, and good reaction time aid greatly in the development of skills. Many of the desirable skills may be developed during the time the prospective teacher of physical education is in college. However, a great amount of time is required in the perfection of skills. Therefore it is important that the individual develop a foundation of skills on the elementary and secondary school levels.

WORKING WITH PEOPLE

The candidate should enjoy working with people. A person is required to associate with human beings when teaching physical education activities. Therefore, a member of the physical education profession should get along well with others, be interested in

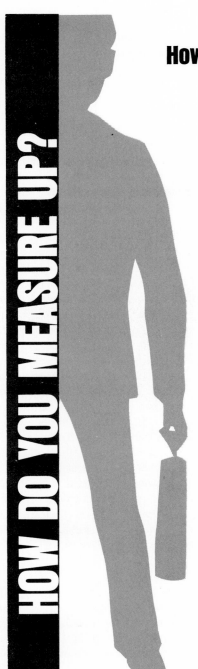

How Do You Measure Up as a Member

- As a first step in determining your professional stature, place a check mark beside the questions you can answer *yes.*

As an individual, do you—

_____Join the united teaching profession—local, state, and national associations—and promote unified professional membership among your colleagues?

_____View your dues as an investment in your profession rather than just another expense?

_____Believe that being a member of the united teaching profession involves more than paying dues—that it includes participating actively, familiarizing yourself with the objectives of your associations, sharing in goal setting, and being a change agent?

_____Identify with your positional organizations (classroom teachers, principals, supervisors, or administrators)?

_____Identify with the associations representing your subject matter area?

_____Keep informed on educational issues through professional journals?

_____Abide by the Code of Ethics of the Education Profession?

_____Participate in political action by discussing issues, campaigning for candidates, and running for offices if you are so inclined?

_____Inform yourself about the economic benefits which may be offered by your local and state organizations?

_____Credit union____Life insurance____Health and accident insurance____Personal liability insurance____Income protection insurance____Tax-deferred annuity program ____Installment financing____Home mortgage loans____ Discount buying.

As a member of your local association, do you—

_____Attend meetings?

_____Volunteer for assignments?

_____Accept committee appointments?

_____Participate in in-service education programs?

_____Lend your efforts in negotiations with the school board by contributing your ideas, serving on the negotiating team, or working on supportive committees?

_____Have a thorough knowledge of grievance procedures so that you can help in referring aggrieved colleagues to the proper persons?

_____Defend teacher rights?

_____Do your part to see to it that classroom teachers, as the largest segment of your association, have an impact commensurate with their number?

_____Work for minority-group involvement in your association program?

_____Reach out to the new teacher, acquaint him with your association's services, encourage him to participate in its activities, and accept him as a member of the team?

_____Support candidates for professional offices who have a record of service to the association; who are committed to the association's goals rather than to their own personal advancement; who speak for the membership?

_____Encourage your association to work with Student NEA chapters in nearby colleges?

_____Promote the Future Teachers of America by supporting

Today's Education • NEA Journal

of the United Teaching Profession?

FTA chapters and by serving as a sponsor?

_____Make sure your association is represented at meetings of your state education association as well as at those of the state classroom teachers association?

_____Make sure that your association uses its full quota of delegates to the Representative Assemblies of the NEA and of its Association of Classroom Teachers?

_____Serve as a delegate to state and national conventions if named?

As a member of the state association, do you—

_____Participate in state and regional meetings?

_____Accept committee assignments?

_____Prepare yourself for office?

_____Read your state association journal and newsletter?

_____Keep abreast of progress in your state association's legislative program?

_____Vote for candidates for public offices who are favorable to the state legislative program?

_____Join your state positional association?

_____Familiarize yourself with its program and services?

As a member of the National Education Association, do you—

_____Make your influence felt in the NEA Representative Assembly by studying NEA resolutions and reports and discussing them with delegates?

_____Attend regional and national conferences?

_____Identify with the Association of Classroom Teachers or your positional association and take advantage of its services?

_____Read ToDAY's EDUCATION and the *NEA Reporter*?

_____Support the NEA DuShane Emergency Fund?

_____Inform yourself and your colleagues about NEA services?

_____Life insurance____Accident insurance____Tax-deferred annuity program____NEA Mutual Fund____Auto leasing ____Research____Publications and other materials____ Field service____Salary and negotiation consultant services ____ Instructional activities ____ Legislative work ____ Travel program____Job referral service____Public relations____Promotion of high standards of teacher preparation, certification, and performance____Protection of professional, civil, and human rights.

Next, write the names of the following in the blanks provided:

Your local association president_____

Your state education association president_____

The president of your state association of classroom teachers or of your positional association_____

Your NEA state director(s)_____

The NEA president_____

The president of NEA's Association of Classroom Teachers or of your positional association_____

The NEA executive secretary_____

The NEA headquarters city_____

See how you measure up as a member of the united teaching profession.

—Jean Heflin, *editorial assistant, Association of Classroom Teachers, NEA.*

March 1969

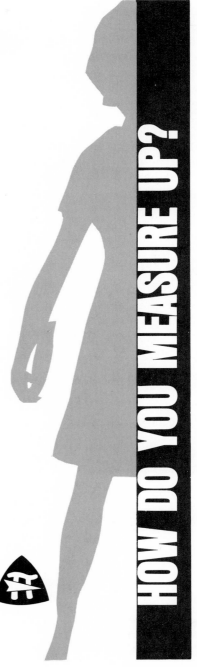

HOW DO YOU MEASURE UP?

people, be able to adapt to various social settings, be able to attain respect, and should enjoy working with children and young people. To satisfy this qualification he should possess such traits as patience, loyalty, tactfulness, sympathetic attitude, sincerity, friendliness, tolerance, reliability, industry, self-control, and good temperament. The effectiveness of the work performed rests upon good human relations. If such relations do not prevail, the objectives for which the profession strives will not be realized.

SENSE OF HUMOR

The candidate should have a sense of humor. The teachers who never crack a smile, tell a joke, or get a "kick" out of life lack an important quality for teaching. Good mental health for both the student and the teacher is dependent upon a sense of humor. The teacher who can see the humor in numerous classroom incidents, a joke told by a colleague, or a remark made by a student possesses a trait that helps him to get along better with others, makes life more interesting for his students and himself, and aids in the dispelling of gloom. Good teachers possess a sense of humor.

The qualifications listed are necessary for all who desire to enter the physical education profession. In establishing such standards it is understood that all individuals are not qualified to be physical educators any more than all are qualified for careers in medicine, law, or social work. A person's future happiness depends upon making the right decision. A poet said it this way:

> Each is given a bag of tools . . .
> A carving block and a book of rules.
> Each must make ere life be done
> A stumbling block or a steppingstone.*

DECIDING WHETHER TO BECOME A TEACHER

Some guidelines that may help the college student or other person in deciding

---

*Quoted from Committee on Vocational Guidance, American Association for Health, Physical Education, and Recreation: Research Quarterly **13:**145, 1942.

whether or not to become a member of the teaching profession include the following:

AN INDIVIDUAL'S INTERESTS AND APTITUDES SHOULD BE CAREFULLY TESTED. The person considering teaching should know that he likes to work with children and young people by actually seeking out experiences in a camp or other situation where he can put himself to the test. Also, there are many tests and other instruments that can be used to objectively analyze a person's aptitude for teaching.

THE PERSON SHOULD MAKE THE DECISION HIMSELF AND NOT PERMIT MOTHER, FATHER, NEIGHBOR, OR CLOSE FRIEND TO MAKE IT FOR HIM. The guidance and advice of others is important and valuable, but the final decision should be made by the individual himself on what is best for him.

AN ANALYSIS OF PERSONALITY IS AN IMPORTANT CONSIDERATION. How well a person can interact with young people, with colleagues on the job, and with the community and other groups of persons should be considered. Furthermore, other aspects of personality such as mental and emotional health, physical health, and prejudices are important considerations.

THE DECISION SHOULD NOT BE RUSHED. A person should be sure that this is the type of work he wants, is best equipped to do, and is where he can make the greatest contribution to society. Such a decision may take time.

THE BEGINNING TEACHER

There is a high turnover rate of first-year teachers. While some teachers change positions after the first year to improve their status, others leave the profession because of dissatisfaction and discouragement and because they have found the job of adjusting to the hard realities of teaching too difficult for them to master. Several research studies have been conducted to determine the reasons teachers give for job satisfaction or dissatisfaction. These include such items as teacher-administrative factors, physical conditions, teacher-community factors, teacher-faculty factors, teacher-student and teacher-parent factors, and salary and security factors.

A survey of fifty teachers indicated the following as some of the problems that beginning teachers face:

1. Difficulties arising as a result of the lack of facilities
2. Large size of classes, making it difficult to teach effectively
3. Teaching assignments in addition to the primary responsibility of teaching physical education
4. Discipline problems with students
5. Conflicting methodology between what beginning teachers were taught in professional preparation institutions and established patterns of experienced teachers
6. Clerical work—difficulty in keeping records up to date
7. Problems encountered in obtaining books and supplies
8. Problems encountered in obtaining cooperative attitude from other teachers
9. Lack of departmental meetings to discuss common problems
10. Failure to find time for personal recreation

Directors of physical education look at problems of beginning teachers

Several directors of physical education in school systems across the nation were contacted to determine what they feel are the most difficult problems faced by beginning teachers. Since these administrators had an opportunity to observe beginning teachers as they embarked on their professional careers, their experiences should be of value in helping new teachers make a good start. The thinking of these administrators may be summarized under the following headings.

ORGANIZATION

Many of the problems of beginning teachers, the directors feel, are caused by poor organization that can easily be corrected. Some of the beginning teachers are not accustomed to moving large groups of students from one place to another and from one formation to another. They are not thoroughly familiar with the various methods of class organization for various activities. Sometimes they do not have proper organi-

zation in respect to caring for uniforms, lockers, towel fees, and many routine duties important in the efficient running of a physical education program.

These problems concerned with organization can be easily remedied if the beginning teacher will study the problems concerned, become familiar with various types of organization, and ask questions and help of experienced teachers.

TEACHING

The beginning teacher is sometimes a very excellent performer himself in various physical education activities and it is hard for him to realize that some students do not know how to throw or jump or perform other basic skills. Also, much time is frequently spent on implementing games rather than in teaching basic fundamentals and skills. The new teacher may not have the ability to organize so as to achieve complete class involvement. Sometimes there is a tendency to teach the units the teacher is interested in and does well and minimize those where he is weak.

The beginning teacher needs to put into effect the tools he has learned during undergraduate training. This includes presenting skills within the ability of the pupil, utilizing appropriate teaching techniques, planning lessons, and finally recognizing his shortcomings in physical education and trying hard to correct the deficiencies through in-service training. Planning is necessary—even the teacher of long experience needs at least a brief written plan. Teaching means to teach an activity or skill and not to "tell" pupils to do something or merely supervise activities in a gymnasium. Rules and regulations should be established and adhered to. Accidents occur at times when rules are not followed. Foreseeability will help to prevent problems from occurring. For example, the climbing ropes should be tied up before class starts rather than having to reprimand students swinging on them after class begins. Finally, the teacher should do self-evaluation each day and faithfully try to eliminate weaknesses and expand strengths.

Teacher-student relationships

Students will frequently test the authority of the new teacher, and sometimes the teacher does not meet the test. Discipline problems may arise and the teacher, instead of facing them directly, refers students to the principal's office. The beginning teacher should recognize that sometimes disciplinary problems are a result of the teacher's lack of planning and class organization. The teacher may expect too much from students. The students may not be adequately motivated. The teacher may show favoritism to certain students, especially athletes.

The beginning teacher needs to establish rapport with pupils, being firm, pleasant, and consistent. He needs to learn to know boys and girls as human beings and not just "numbers" and to establish a friendship with pupils without becoming one of them. Establishing rapport in this manner will require further effort on the part of the new teacher, particularly if he is replacing another teacher who was extremely well liked and respected by the pupils.

Teacher-teacher relationships

Physical education, including sports, tends to isolate teachers of physical education from the rest of the building and often from colleagues in other subject-matter areas. As a result, some beginning teachers fail to realize the importance of participating in general building activities with all teachers, attending faculty meetings regularly, and becoming an integral part of the staff.

From the very beginning the new teacher should become acquainted with other members of the faculty, work cooperatively with them, share committee responsibilities, and try to be respected by all.

Making adjustments

The beginning teacher often finds facilities, staff, equipment, and other conditions on the job far below his expectations and far from ideal. The new teacher should realize that teachers do not always have ideal situations; in fact, very few do. Many of them are faced with poor equipment, limited facilities, changing weather conditions, and other substandard situations.

The new teacher should adjust to the position, the school, other teachers, school policies, procedures, and routines. Regardless of the situation, the conditions that prevail should be accepted as a challenge to see how excellent a teaching job can be accomplished in spite of the limiting factors that exist. The teacher should follow through on the many duties, responsibilities, and "chores" for which he is responsible. There should be an adjustment to existing policy and curriculum, with its inherent demand for skillful budgeting of time. The teacher should recognize his responsibility to the professional principles of physical education and also to the students, faculty, and school of which he is a part.

Teachers can eliminate some problems before assuming the position

The teacher should carefully evaluate the position before accepting its responsibilities. Unfortunately, some teachers accept positions in schools and communities in which they do not fit or belong and, consequently, problems arise. The many complex factors related to proper adjustment on the job are usually associated with the nature of the person, the nature of the environment, and the interaction of the two. It is, therefore, important that the applicant carefully weigh the position that is available and his abilities and personal characteristics for handling this position effectively. If this is done, many of the problems will be foreseen and the qualities and preparation needed to handle them successfully will be evaluated realistically.

Two advance considerations important to the beginning teacher are knowledge of the conditions of employment and pertinent factors about the school and community. Some considerations regarding the conditions of employment include knowledge of classes to be handled, sports to be coached, clubs to be sponsored, homeroom assignments, length of the school day, school obligations, compensation to be received, sick leave, tenure, sabbaticals, health insurance, and other pertinent facts. Only as the beginning teacher has a complete understanding of such responsibilities will he be able to prepare sufficiently, both mentally and physically, for the position. Pertinent factors about the school and community that should be known by the teacher before accepting a position include such items as community traditions, economic status, philosophy of education, political philosophy, projected future growth, and a history of the school and community. These factors will have implications for the type of students to be taught, the parents with whom the teacher will work, the community of which the teacher is to be a part, and the social, political, and educational climate within which the teacher must work.

Induction of beginning teachers

Hunt has discussed a proposal suggested by well-known educator, James B. Conant, which each school system should take into consideration in outlining the duties and responsibilities of the beginning teacher.* They are presented in adapted form. Conant's five recommendations provide that:

Beginning teachers should be given a limited teaching responsibility.

Beginning teachers should be given assistance in gathering instructional materials for their classes.

Beginning teachers should receive the advice of experienced teachers who have their own teaching loads reduced so that they may provide this advice and help.

Beginning teachers should not be assigned students who create problems that are beyond their ability to handle effectively. Instead, these students should be assigned more experienced teachers.

Beginning teachers should be provided an adequate orientation to the community, the neighborhood, and the students that he will have in school.

Beginning teachers would be helped considerably if schools would make such provisions in their respective educational systems.

---

*Hunt, Douglas W.: Induction of beginning teachers, Education Digest **34**:34, 1969.

QUESTIONS AND EXERCISES

1. In approximately 250 words discuss your qualifications for the physical education profession in the light of the standards set forth in this chapter.
2. How would you describe the qualifications for the teaching profession to someone who is considering making teaching a career?
3. To what degree do you feel there is a relationship between the qualifications for a profession and the prestige held by a profession?
4. Why is there a need for well-trained teachers in physical education?
5. What recommendations can be made for the better recruitment and selection of physical educators?
6. Why is scholarship important to physical education work?
7. Prepare a list of standards that could be used as a basis for selecting individuals for training in physical education work.
8. Why is it important for the physical educator to meet acceptable standards in oral and written English?
9. Why is it important for the physical educator to possess an acceptable standard of motor ability?
10. Describe and contrast the various methods of teacher evaluation. Which do you feel might be the most effective and objective? Why?

Reading assignment

Bucher, Charles A., and Goldman, Myra: Dimensions of physical education, St. Louis, 1969, The C. V. Mosby Co., Reading selections 57 to 61.

SELECTED REFERENCES

American Association for Health, Physical Education, and Recreation: Professional preparation in health, physical education and recreation, Washington, D. C., 1962, The Association.

Bain, Helen: We must be reasoning activists, Today's Education **59**:22, 1970.

Bucher, Charles A.: Administration of school health and physical education programs including athletics, St. Louis, 1971, The C. V. Mosby Co.

Bucher, Charles A., Koening, Constance, and Barnhard, Milton: Methods and materials of secondary school physical education, St. Louis, 1970, The C. V. Mosby Co.

Dowell, Linus J.: Action analysis, The Physical Educator **26**:63, 1969.

Filbin, Robert L., and Vogel, Stefan: So you're going to be a teacher, Great Neck, New York, 1962, Barron's Educational Series, Inc.

Goldman, Samuel: The school principal, New York, 1966, The Library of Education, The

Center for Applied Research in Education, Inc., Chapter V.

Harris, Fred R.: The teacher's political role, Today's Education **59:**20, 1970.

National Commission on Teacher Education and Professional Standards: Invitation to teaching, Washington, D. C., 1966, National Education Association.

National Conference on Undergraduate Professional Preparation in Health Education, Physical Education, and Recreation, Jackson's Mill, Weston, West Virginia, May 16-27, 1948: Report, Chicago, 1948, The Athletic Institute.

Skinner, B. F.: The technology of teaching, New York, 1968, Appleton-Century-Crofts.

Stinnett, T. M.: The profession of teaching, New York, 1962, The Library of Education, The Center for Applied Research in Education, Inc.

20/Duties of physical education personnel

The duties performed by physical educators are many and varied and evolve from the responsibilities the physical educator has to students and others concerned with the educational process.

GROUPS TO WHOM PHYSICAL EDUCATORS ARE RESPONSIBLE

The physical education teacher performs duties for the student, the department, the faculty and school, the community, and the profession.

The student

The teacher's first responsibility is to the student. The teacher should know the student physically, mentally, emotionally, and socially. He should know the student's background, his needs, and his characteristics. The teacher should view the student as a growing and maturing human being who can be shaped by the teacher and helped to progress toward worthwhile educational goals. The teacher has the responsibility to help the student develop the skills, master the knowledge, and acquire the attitudes and social qualities that will help him become all that he is capable of becoming.

The department

The teacher is usually one member of a team—the faculty and staff of the department of physical education. The duties that befall the department, such as program planning, grading, testing, counseling, caring for equipment and facilities, and keeping records, must be shared by members of the department. In carrying out these responsibilities, there should be harmonious inter-relationships among members of the department. In addition, ethical standards of conduct should prevail, and there should be mutual support of colleagues. The department will be as strong as its weakest human link, so each member of the staff should strive to be a valuable and important member of the team.

The faculty and school

The teacher must also recognize that he is a member of a school faculty. This position carries with it many responsibilities that are a part of administering a program for students. All teachers must share in this endeavor, which includes obligations in regard to upholding school policies, sharing mutual responsibilities such as supervising student activities, and respecting the total curriculum. Teachers of physical education must see the total educational plan and how all parts of it contribute to the education of young people. Physical education is an important part of the total plan, but at the same time is only one part. Furthermore, since faculty meetings represent an important medium for school planning, discussion of problems, and interpreting to colleagues each area of the curriculum, physical educators have a responsibility to be in attendance at these meetings.

The community

The physical educator has a responsibility to the community. The support a physical education teacher gains for the program of which he is a part depends largely on the program itself and the way in which the citizens of the community view this program. The responsibilities of the physical education staff in developing a close community relationship include presenting a sound program, community-sponsored activities, and supporting worthwhile community endeavors.

The profession

Each physical educator owes some time and effort to the profession of which he is a part. This obligation can be carried out by joining professional organizations, serving on committees and as officers of the associations, and supporting professional endeavors. Physical educators should also be in attendance at professional meetings and be familiar with the literature and developments related to the profession.

RANGE OF DUTIES

The duties performed by physical education personnel include such functions as coaching sports, administering physical fitness tests, teaching games and first aid, monitoring study halls, and performing routine administrative duties. They are not limited to physical education alone. They are also concerned with a wider range of duties essential to the functioning of a school, voluntary agency, camp, church, athletic club, or other organization of which the physical educator is a part.

Although the functions of physical educators are performed in various institutions, they are, nevertheless, very similar in nature. As a general rule, most positions involve some combination of teaching, administrative, community, and other duties that are miscellaneous in nature. Since the majority of students preparing themselves for work in physical education anticipate work in schools and colleges, this area of employment is emphasized.

Physical educators have certain responsibilities that relate to the objectives of their profession, the program of activities, leadership, determining whether objectives are accomplished, and reevaluation of the program in light of results achieved.

GENERAL RESPONSIBILITIES OF THE PHYSICAL EDUCATOR

There are certain responsibilities that each teacher must assume upon accepting a position. These responsibilities are as follows:

Knowing the objectives of the profession of physical education

Planning and administering a physical education program in the light of these objectives

Providing effective leadership in order to achieve these objectives

Scientifically measuring and evaluating the physical education program in order to determine if the objectives are being accomplished

Reevaluating the program of physical education in the light of results obtained through measurement and evaluation techniques

Knowing objectives of profession

In the first place, the physical education person must know and fully understand the objectives of the physical education profession. These objectives include the long-term goals (Chapter 6) as well as the more immediate and specific objectives. By the more immediate and specific objectives are meant those goals that a physical educator attempts to achieve during a lesson, over the course of a week, or during a unit of work. Some examples are the ability to throw with accuracy, to run the 220-yard dash without excessive fatigue, to understand the importance of milk in one's diet, to know the rules of baseball, or to assist a less-skilled player in badminton. These more immediate or specific objectives, along with the long-term goals, should be present in the physical educator's mind, whether he is teaching a class in the public schools, the Young Men's Christian Association, a camp, or a settlement house. They will serve as guides for what he is striving to accomplish today, tomorrow, next year, and ultimately. As a result of a knowledge and understanding of the objectives of physical education, the program will be better planned, the leadership will be better, and the results obtained will be much more fruitful.

Planning a physical education program

The physical educator has the responsibility for planning and administering a program in the light of its objectives. This means that the interests and needs of the individuals whom it will serve, as well as other considerations such as the prevailing philosophy of education, will be taken into consideration. It means that a varied program of activities will be selected that will include movement education experiences, rhythmics and the dance, dual and individual activities, team games, games of low organization, relays, field days, outdoor sports, aquatics, and gymnastics. The percentage of program time devoted to these various activities will depend on the age or grade level concerned. Furthermore, such factors as facilities, personnel, equipment, state legislation, size of class, time allotment, and climatic conditions will be taken into consideration. Provisions will also be made for the physical, social, skill, and intellectual development of the participant. A core and elective program will be utilized at certain age and grade levels.

There has been considerable research on

Today's teachers are expected to . . .

1. Remain alert to significant developments in academic specialty and continue general education in order to avoid obsolescence of knowledge
2. Be a continuing student of the educative process and keep current with respect to innovations in teaching methods and materials
3. Plan with students and fellow teachers
4. Work with curriculum committees
5. Experiment with different content, methods, and materials and keep systematic records of such studies
6. Read and evaluate student work
7. Confer with students and parents regarding pupil progress
8. Counsel and advise students on academic, vocational, and personal concerns
9. Maintain a cumulative file of significant data on each student
10. Develop reading lists, outlines, study guides, drill sheets, and visual materials
11. Prepare tests appropriate to the range of objectives established
12. Type and duplicate tests and other materials for classroom use
13. Arrange for field trips, outside speakers, and other programs relevant to the learning objectives of the class
14. Supervise homeroom, study hall, or lunchroom
15. Supervise playground or recess periods
16. Advise student extracurricular groups, chaperon school functions
17. Keep attendance and academic records
18. Collect money for various drives and sell tickets for school events
19. Order and return films and other visual aids and operate equipment involved
20. Participate in professional-association and learned-society activities
21. Maintain an active interest in civic and community affairs and represent the school in the community effectively
22. Orient and assist beginning teachers
23. Supervise student teachers and cooperate with area colleges in providing opportunities for observation and demonstration.

FROM DENEMARK, GEORGE W.: NEA JOURNAL 55:19, 1966.

Duties assigned to teachers in today's schools.

JOB ANALYSIS FOR AN ELEMENTARY SCHOOL PHYSICAL EDUCATION TEACHER

Mrs. Jacobi of Lafayette Elementary School in Waterloo, Iowa, lists the following as some of her duties:

I teach physical education grades four, five, and six. Many activities are included in the program: games, sports, tumbling, rhythms, rope jumping, ball bouncing, track and field, posture improvement, marching, and exercises for physical fitness. The sports include modified football (football-kickball), soccer (kickball), modified volleyball, modified basketball (captain ball), and softball.

The sixth grade plays several games with other schools each year. An arrangement is made to have members from both schools on the same team. The sixth graders do not compete on a school-against-school basis.

We try to check for physical fitness once a week, i.e., chinning, sit-ups, squat thrusts. The children help check each other in their squads.

After playing a game or after any physical activity we usually discuss what we've done. Suggestions are given for improving our next activity. We discuss what we thought we did well. I stress good sportsmanship and we comment on that. Sometimes I make and give tests over such sports as softball and basketball.

I teach art, literature, and music to grades four, five, and six; and also, fourth grade spelling and social studies.

Some of the things I specifically try to do in my physical education classes are:

1. Offer proper incentives and ideals
2. Help build better citizens—physically, mentally, and morally
3. Develop health habits—posture and exercise
4. Help each child to feel he is needed and has a very important part in everything we do
5. Help each child to work for improvement
6. Help to organize and direct big-muscle activity

the types of programs most suited to various levels of instruction. Years ago a national physical education curriculum was developed based on a committee's research covering a period of 9 years and summarized by LaPorte. This national physical education program was adopted by many elementary and secondary schools and colleges throughout the country. Leaders in physical education too numerous to mention have developed curriculums. Many states have published syllabuses that provide guidance and help in establishing a program for particular geographical regions. The armed forces, voluntary agencies, and various institutions where physical education activities are carried on have developed programs. There is a wealth of material available. The physical education instructor should appraise this material in the light of the objectives of physical education and in terms of his local situation. As a result it will be possible for him to develop a program that meets the needs and interests of the group or groups with whom he is working.

Providing leadership

The physical educator has the responsibility for providing effective leadership in order to achieve the objectives of physical education. Outstanding leadership will be concerned with helping each student to develop to his greatest possible capacity—physically, neuromuscularly, intellectually, and socially.

The program in physical education requires competent leadership. This leadership will be better provided if a person has adequate professional training; understands the problems involved in teaching; and has such essential physical, mental, social, and personality characteristics as vitality, enthusiasm, intelligence, keen powers of observation, respect for the dignity of the individual, sympathy, and patience. A teacher should also be alert to the possibilities in games and other physical education activities as teachable moments for developing desirable human qualities in his students.

The teacher of physical education should also realize that his responsibility extends beyond the immediate group of students with whom he is working to the rest of the school, institution, or agency with which he is associated and out into the community of which he is a part. He should never reach the point where he becomes encased in an ivory tower and feels that he has no responsibility to the community. Every teacher should feel that the wider his associations, the greater his personal enjoyment and happiness and the greater the extension of the benefits of physical education.

The informal and play type of physical education program that sometimes exists today offers an opportunity for the indolent physical educator to conduct a program without providing effective leadership. He can throw out a ball or pass out the equipment and then loaf. In order to provide effective leadership, the physical educator must be alert to every opportunity that arises so that he may aid in developing the individual to his optimum capacity. Effective leadership will not be provided if a ball is thrown out to the physical education class and the instructor goes back to his office to rest or work out a new football play.

Effective leadership also will not be provided by the coach if winning is stressed as the main objective instead of courtesy, sympathy, respect for authority, fairness, and abiding by the rules. Effective leadership will not be provided if physical education classes are neglected and the teacher's entire efforts are put into coaching. Through outstanding leadership the objectives of physical education will be brought nearer to realization.

The teacher's example plays a major role in providing leadership. Whether or not his teachings are effective will depend to a great degree on what example he sets for his students in respect to such things as health habits, sportsmanship qualities, and relationships with people.

Determining whether objectives are being accomplished

The physical educator has the responsibility for utilizing scientifically valid measurement and evaluation techniques in order to determine whether the objectives of physical education are being accomplished.

If the teacher is to evaluate the various types of programs and instruction, if he is to know what he is achieving through these programs and instruction, and if he is to know whether he is meeting the objectives that have been set, it is imperative that he utilize acceptable measurement and evaluation techniques. These will enable him to better determine individual and program weaknesses, quality of instruction, and progress achieved.

Some of the measurement and evaluation techniques used today have failed to be scientifically evaluated or else have fallen below acceptable standards. In view of these conditions, it is necessary to assure oneself that only materials that meet acceptable scientific criteria are used. There are several excellent measurement and evaluation books in physical education that list and discuss scientific instruments and tests that will yield valid results.

JOB ANALYSIS FOR A SECONDARY SCHOOL PHYSICAL EDUCATION TEACHER

Mr. Buck, a secondary school physical education teacher in McKinstry School in Waterloo, Iowa, points out that in his job he performs the following:

1. Teaches physical education classes in such activities as touch football, soccer, rope climbing, rope jumping, handball, dodgeball, crabball, pinball, whiffleball, wrestling, basketball, marching to music, square dancing, softball, track, swimming, and diving

2. Teaches four health classes

3. Gives practical and written tests in physical education activities, physical fitness, attitudes, and lifesaving

4. Coaches football, wrestling, and basketball

5. Conducts intramurals on a homeroom basis

6. Supervises recreation room on days when there are no intramurals

7. Supervises Elks basketball program on Tuesday evenings and swimming on Saturday mornings (programs last about 12 weeks each)

Measurement and evaluation techniques enable a teacher to determine an individual's physical condition, traits, or characteristics in respect to physical, motor, intellectual, and social development. Furthermore, they enable him to evaluate practices concerned with such items as program administration, leadership, facilities, and activities. They may be utilized for purposes of guidance, motivation, diagnosis, pupil classification, prognosis, research, grading, and determining achievement. They should, however, be considered as tools and not as ends in themselves.

Reevaluating program

The physical educator has the responsibility for reevaluating the program in the light of measurement and evaluation results. The results that are compiled, tabulated, and analyzed should aid the teacher in determining whether or not the program being followed and the teaching techniques being used are satisfactory and accomplishing the objectives of physical education. If, through a careful analysis, it appears that progress is not being made, the program and/or the teaching techniques should be reevaluated in light of the findings and the necessary changes made. Such a procedure places physical education on a more scientific basis and enables it to render a greater service to the students in the program. Tests should not be given just for the sake of testing and the results placed in a file and allowed to gather dust. Instead, they should be utilized to further the program and to help the individuals who are participating. Furthermore, they should not take up too much of the time allotted to the program. The activity program should not be sacrificed for a measurement and evaluation program. Instead, it should be aided and strengthened thereby.

CAPACITIES IN WHICH PHYSICAL EDUCATION TEACHERS SERVE

The findings of a national survey that I conducted show that physical educators perform in several capacities.

Teachers of physical education throughout the United States serve in an administrative and/or teaching capacity. The distribution of administrative and teaching positions showed that approximately one-half of both men and women physical educators have a combination of administrative and teaching positions. Many physical educators work in small towns where it is common to find in the public schools one man, the director and teacher of boys' physical education, and one woman, the director and teacher of girls' physical education. This results in the performance of administrative and teaching duties.

Although many physical educators have a combination of administrative positions, others have teaching positions or administrative positions only. The larger the physical education program, the greater the need for personnel whose sole function is teaching and for personnel whose primary responsibility is administration.

Some of the capacities in which physical education teachers served, as revealed by this nationwide survey, are the following:

Positions throughout the country concerned solely with physical education activities, as revealed through this survey, include:

Teacher of physical education
Supervisor and teacher of physical education
Director and teacher of physical education
Supervisor, director, and teacher of physical education
Coach of varsity sports
Director of athletics
Physical educator in the YMCA, YWCA, YMHA, YWHA
Resource physical educator on the elementary level
County supervisor of physical education
Research worker
Supervisor of physical education on the elementary level
Supervisor of physical education on the secondary level
Director of intramurals
Coordinator of physical education
Chairman of the department of physical education

Positions throughout the United States

How high school and elementary school teachers divide the week.

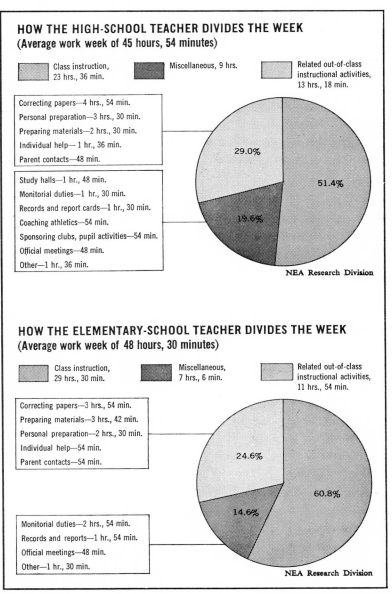

HOW THE HIGH-SCHOOL TEACHER DIVIDES THE WEEK
(Average work week of 45 hours, 54 minutes)

Class instruction,
23 hrs., 36 min.

Miscellaneous, 9 hrs.

Related out-of-class
instructional activities,
13 hrs., 18 min.

Correcting papers—4 hrs., 54 min.
Personal preparation—3 hrs., 30 min.
Preparing materials—2 hrs., 30 min.
Individual help—1 hr., 36 min.
Parent contacts—48 min.

Study halls—1 hr., 48 min.
Monitorial duties—1 hr., 30 min.
Records and report cards—1 hr., 30 min.
Coaching athletics—54 min.
Sponsoring clubs, pupil activities—54 min.
Official meetings—48 min.
Other—1 hr., 36 min.

29.0%

51.4%

19.6%

NEA Research Division

HOW THE ELEMENTARY-SCHOOL TEACHER DIVIDES THE WEEK
(Average work week of 48 hours, 30 minutes)

Class instruction,
29 hrs., 30 min.

Miscellaneous,
7 hrs., 6 min.

Related out-of-class
instructional activities,
11 hrs., 54 min.

Correcting papers—3 hrs., 54 min.
Preparing materials—3 hrs., 42 min.
Personal preparation—2 hrs., 30 min.
Individual help—54 min.
Parent contacts—54 min.

Monitorial duties—2 hrs., 54 min.
Records and reports—1 hr., 54 min.
Official meetings—48 min.
Other—1 hr., 30 min.

24.6%

60.8%

14.6%

NEA Research Division

FROM NEA RESEARCH DIVISION:
NEA JOURNAL, APRIL, 1963.

JOB ANALYSIS FOR A COLLEGE PHYSICAL EDUCATION TEACHER

As a Professor of Education at New York University, I have duties such as the following in the Division of Health, Physical Education, and Recreation:

1. Director of Physical Education involving meetings with staff members, development of curriculums, revision of courses, initiating research projects, answering correspondence from prospective students and active students, and keeping records
2. Supervise research projects
3. Teach four classes per week
4. Attend faculty meetings of School of Education and Division of Health, Physical Education, and Recreation
5. Advise students
6. Attend professional conventions and conferences
7. Serve on All-University, School of Education, and Division committees
8. Teach one off-campus course
9. Prepare brochures and other materials
10. Serve as graduate student organization advisor

concerned with physical education and health duties include:

Supervisor of health and physical education
Director of physical education and health
Supervisor and teacher of health and physical education
Director and teacher of health and physical education
Supervisor, director, and teacher of physical education, and coordinator and teacher of health
Director and teacher of physical education and coordinator and teacher of health
Director and teacher of physical education and teacher of health
Teacher of health and physical education
Director of physical education, health, and recreation

SCHOOL LEVELS OF INSTRUCTION

Teachers of physical education perform duties on all levels of instruction. The high school level has the most teachers of physical education, the junior high school level next, and the elementary level least. Furthermore, there is a marked similarity in the distribution of men and women on the various levels.

Table 20-1. Time allotment in physical education

School systems	High school			Junior high			Elementary		
	Days/ week	Minutes/ period	Total/ week	Days/ week	Minutes/ period	Total/ week	Days/ week	Minutes/ period	Total/ week
No. 1	2½	48	120	2½	48	120	1½	20	30
No. 2	2	53	106	3	65	195	2½	30	75
No. 3	2	45	90	3	45	135	1	45	45
No. 4	2	46	92	2	46	92	2	45	90
No. 5	2½	45	112	2½	45	112	2	30	60
No. 6	5	40	200	5	40	200	2	38	76
No. 7	3	42	126	3	42	126	2	30	60
No. 8	5	48	240	3	45	135	2½	35	88
No. 9	3½	44	154	3	45	135	2	35	70
No. 10	2	45	90	3	45	135	5	30	150
No. 11	5	50	250	5	30	150	5	30	150
No. 12	5	60	300	3	60	180	5	30	150
No. 13	5	52	260	5	52	260	5	40	200
No. 14	2	45	90	2	45	90	2	45	90
No. 15	2	43	86	2	40	80	2	30	60
No. 16	5	55	275	5	55	275	2	45	90
No. 17	2	45	90	2	45	90	5	25	125
No. 18	2	50	100	2	50	100	None	Recess only	
No. 19	3	60	180	3	45	135	5	30	150
No. 20	2	53	106	2	50	100	1	45	45

The majority of teachers have duties on one level of instruction only. However, there are many who have responsibilities on two levels of instruction, and some who have responsibilities on all three levels.

TIME DEVOTED TO PHYSICAL EDUCATION

Table 20-1 shows the results of a national survey of twenty public school systems in respect to number of days per week for physical education, minutes of time usually allocated for physical education per period, and the total time granted to physical education per week. The table provides information on this basis for the elementary, junior high, and senior high schools in each school system surveyed. From a study of this table, the prospective physical education teacher can better understand how much time is devoted to physical education classes in the nation's schools.

TEACHING DUTIES
Physical education activities

Physical educators are called on to teach many and varied forms of physical activity. These include team games, dual and individual sports, rhythms and dancing, formal activities, aquatic activities, outdoor winter sports, gymnastics, and other activities.

The most popular team games on all levels of instruction in the schools (men and women) are baseball, softball, basketball, touch football, volleyball, soccer, and field hockey. The most popular on the elementary level (men and women) are softball, basketball, and volleyball; on the junior high school level, baseball, softball, basketball, soccer, touch football, and volleyball for the men and softball, volleyball, and basketball for the women; on the senior high school level, volleyball, basketball, baseball, softball, football, touch football, and soccer for the men and volleyball, basketball, softball, and field hockey for the women; on the college level, volleyball, baseball, basketball, softball, and touch football for the men and volleyball, basketball, and field hockey for the women.

There is a variety of dual and individual sports offered. Among the ones most frequently included in physical education programs are track, badminton, table tennis, deck tennis, handball, horseshoes, tennis, archery, golf, and shuffleboard. From the widespread use of activities in this category, it seems that greater and greater stress is being placed on this area so as to prepare for many years of enjoyable participation.

There are various types of movement education experiences including rhythms and dancing included in most programs. Social dancing, folk dancing, rhythms, gymnastic dancing, square dancing, tap dancing, and modern dancing are offered. Men as well as women utilize these various types of rhythms and dancing. In the schools, folk dancing, rhythms, social dancing, and square dancing are most popular with both sexes. Only in the area of modern dancing do the men seem to have some hesitancy.

Formal activities are extensively utilized in programs of physical education. Of these activities, calisthenics is the most frequently mentioned, with marching second. Although it is evident that the games type of program is very popular, it still can be seen that many physical educators also utilize some of the more formal activities in their classes.

When facilities make it possible, aquatic activities are a phase of many physical education programs. However, in the public schools the lack of swimming pools makes such an activity impossible for many boys and girls throughout the country. Other agencies, such as the Young Men's Christian Association, frequently have pools as part of their physical plant. The enormous cost involved in including a swimming pool as part of a school plant makes it appear a luxury to many laymen. When aquatic activities are a part of the program, swimming, diving, lifesaving, water games, and sometimes canoeing, sailing, and rowing are offered.

Outdoor winter sports form a group of activities that are included in most programs. Climatic conditions in certain parts of the country and the desire to stay indoors during inclement weather cause many physical educators to omit these sports. When such activities are a part of the program, skating, snow games, ice hockey, skiing, and tobogganing are the most popular.

Gymnastics are included in the majority of physical education programs. Such activities as tumbling, pyramid building, apparatus, rope climbing, and acrobatics are popular.

Some of the other activities offered, which do not seem to fit logically into the previous groupings, are self-testing activities, relays, games of low organization, correctives, and camping. Each of these is very popular throughout the public schools and other agencies of the country that utilize physical education activities in their program.

Health, safety, and driver education

Physical educators may have physical education duties only or they may, in addition, have health education responsibilities. Although health education is making great strides toward having specialized personnel handling the health duties, there is still a lack of adequately trained personnel to take over all of the health duties in the country. Furthermore, many towns are too poor financially to assume the responsibility of having both physical educators and health educators. It is in cases such as these that physical educators are assuming health education responsibilities.

The health education subjects and activities that physical educators are asked to teach and conduct are similar for both men and women. (See Chapter 8 for a fuller discussion of the health education program.)

Besides the teaching of health subjects, the responsibility for holding guidance conferences, administering vision and hearing tests, giving home-bound instruction, and teaching crippled children play an important part in many programs.

Safety education has become an important part of the programs of school systems, and in many cases physical educators are asked to assume duties in this field of endeavor.

Duties include organizing safety patrols, instructing a unit of safety in the health curriculum, cooperating with community agencies interested in promoting a safe community, supervising playgrounds and athletic facilities in a manner that will promote safety, and other responsibilities involving the promotion of safe living in the educational program. In some school systems safety education supervisors are appointed to coordinate the entire safety program. (See also Chapter 8.)

Driver education is becoming a common responsibility of teachers of physical education. The great expansion of this type of education is readily apparent. Studies have shown the effectiveness of driver education in reducing automobile accidents. As a result, some insurance companies offer reduced rates for persons who have pursued this training. Other studies have shown that programs are more effective when offered as a separate course and when the teacher has had special preparation in teaching driver education and traffic safety. (See also Chapter 8.)

Other subjects

In smaller schools especially, administrators frequently hire physical educators who can also teach some other subject. This procedure is followed because of financial limitations, small staffs, and low enrollments.

In determining the duties of physical educators, this national survey found that general science and biology are the subjects most often assigned to physical educators. The second most frequently assigned area is social studies, with such subjects as American history, civics, ancient history, problems of American democracy, and geography on the list. English also ranks high. Such subjects as mathematics, drawing, design, representation, speech correction, industrial arts, lip reading, chemistry, physics, home economics, arts and crafts, agriculture, commercial subjects, and music are also assigned as part of a physical educator's duties in some schools.

MEASUREMENT AND EVALUATION DUTIES

The more popular measurement and evaluation techniques used by physical educators are those that measure the health, physical fitness, knowledge, skill, and adaptability of their students.

The medical examination continues to be the most common procedure for checking on an individual's health status. This is utilized by schools as a routine procedure in examining students periodically and for participation in interscholastic sports and by various agencies and institutions for checking on the advisability of an individual's participating in physical activity. It is conducted by medical doctors.

Other techniques also utilized extensively for determining various physical traits and characteristics are organic, skill, knowledge, and adaptation tests. Organic tests are designed to measure such things as the efficiency and quality of an individual's cardiovascular system, nutritional status, strength, and physical fitness. Skill tests measure such things as an individual's general motor ability, general motor capacity, motor educability, and skill in specific activities. Physical education and health education knowledge tests include such areas as rules, strategies, techniques, health knowledge, and attitudes. Adaptation tests are concerned with measuring certain character and personality traits.

Another evaluation technique that is utilized to some extent has to do with program evaluation. This is concerned with such administrative items in the conduct of a program as leadership, time element, facilities, and participation.

COACHING DUTIES

Both men and women are called upon to coach intramural and interscholastic sports. Such duties are very common in the public schools, increasing progressively from the elementary to the college levels, and are also functions of the individual who works for other agencies.

A study of one state showed that 87.3% of the physical education instructors in the junior high schools and 97.4% of those in the senior high schools of the state had coaching duties. A survey of intramural and/or interscholastic activities that physical educators are called upon to coach showed that an individual preparing to follow this profession should be familiar with many activities. The activities that are most commonly assigned to physical educators as coaching responsibilities are basketball, softball, volleyball, baseball, track, touch football, swimming, tennis, soccer, field hockey (women only), football (men only), speedball, cross country (men only), golf, and bowling. A listing of activities coached by men and women as revealed in this survey is as follows:

Men

Archery	Polo
Baseball	Rifle
Basketball	Skish
Bowling	Soccer
Boxing	Softball
Crew	Speedball
Cross country	Squash racquets
Fencing	Swimming
Flag football	Tennis
Football	Touch football
Golf	Track and field
Gymnastics	Tumbling
Ice hockey	Volleyball
Lacrosse	Wrestling

Women

Archery	Skish
Basketball	Soccer
Baseball	Softball
Bowling	Speedball
Fencing	Swimming
Field hockey	Tennis
Golf	Touch football
Ice hockey	Track and field
Rifle	Volleyball

OTHER DUTIES

Health and physical education teachers are required to perform many duties other than teaching, measuring and evaluating, and coaching. Some of these duties are closely related to their field of endeavor and others are not. The physical educator should realize that they are a part of his job and should endeavor to carry them out just as faithfully as he would his teaching or coaching duties. All are necessary for the efficient operation of a school or other agency. Listed here are some of the duties assigned to physical education teachers.

Administrative duties
  Supervision of plant equipment
  General maintenance and repair of equipment and facilities
  Establishing office regulations and procedures and carrying out departmental policies
  Formulating and administering budget
  Conducting inventories
  Preparing reports on various phases of work
  Maintaining records
  Administering intramural program
  Making arrangements for athletic events
  Securing officials
  Organizing and administering field and play days
  Organizing and administering interschool athletic program
  Preparing attendance reports
  Procuring supplies
  Planning in-service education programs
  Preparing notices and announcements
  Coordinating program with other departments
  Interviewing salesmen
  Developing curriculum materials
  Preparing schedule for classes
  Developing plan for determining pupil marks
  Developing program for evaluation
Special services and activities
  Administering first aid
  Maintaining adequate sanitation
  Speaking at various public gatherings
  Writing for periodicals
  Playground work
  Establishing safety regulations and precautions
  After-school recreation
  Working with athletic association
  Evening recreation
  Working with such organizations as sport clubs, bowling clubs, leaders' clubs, Hi-Y, varsity clubs, booster clubs, and health clubs
  Training cheerleaders
  Organizing assembly programs concerned with health and physical education
  Taking charge of a homeroom
  Taking charge of a study hall
  Directing school plays
  Working with Parent–Teachers Association
  Serving on faculty committees
  Supervising cafeteria
  Supervising noon-hour recreation
  Serving as a school bus driver
  Supervising student and faculty parking of cars

  Chaperoning school affairs
  Planning in-service education programs
  Working with official and voluntary health agencies

TEACHING LOADS

Teaching load varies considerably from school district to school district and from college to college. There is little uniformity, although the National Education Association has suggested that every teacher should have two free periods per day.

Teaching loads should be arranged so that the preparation and planning needed are taken into consideration, as well as the physical and nervous energy expended by a teacher in a class situation. The number of different classes taught per day is a better yardstick in most cases than the number of hours taught per day because of the planning required for each class presentation. The physical educator needs time to consult with teachers, give students additional help, plan the program, and perform the many duties connected with the teaching process.

College and university teaching load is usually computed on a different basis than it is at the elementary and secondary school levels. The normal college load is 12 hours of teaching. However, in some cases the physical education class is not considered on a one-to-one basis. For example, it might take 2 hours in the gymnasium to equal 1 hour in a classroom subject. Of course, the best arrangement is to have teaching in the gymnasium carry the same weight as teaching in the classroom. Also, at the college and university level, other responsibilities such as advisement, research, administration, and some committee assignments may be taken into consideration in figuring load.

SECOND JOBS

According to a National Education Association Research Division survey, about one-fifth of the teachers in this country have second jobs during the school year. This survey covered all teachers and positions and was not limited to those in physical education.

Although second jobs may be necessary in order to support a family when wages are low, this practice is discouraged except in emergency cases. This statement refers to second jobs during the school year and not during vacation periods.

Teaching physical education is a full-time job, not a part-time responsibility. Class preparation, conferences with students and parents, and intramurals and interschool athletic programs will utilize all the time and energy that a teacher has available. A teacher, like any human being, can give his best efforts only so many hours a day. When this limit has been reached, the law of diminishing returns sets in, and inferior services are rendered. The national survey of the National Education Association Research Division showed that all teachers, on the average, work 47.3 hours per week, with an average number of pupils per teacher in elementary school of 29 and in secondary school of 156. Probably physical education teachers exceed the national average in both instances.

COMMUNITY DUTIES

Most physical education teachers throughout the country have community responsibilities. These are usually engaged in voluntarily. However, the special qualifications and skills of a physical education teacher make them a likely target for requests from community groups to assist with youth and other programs. Some of the more common agencies in which all teachers are affiliated are church activities, social or recreational clubs, fraternal or lodge activities, service clubs, civic welfare organizations, and political clubs.

Physical educators should be interested in providing leadership for their communities in programs involving sports, athletics, and recreational activities. By exercising a leadership role they can help to ensure that such programs are organized and administered in the best interests of youths and adults. It also offers an opportunity to interpret physical education to the public in general. In so doing, teachers become respected and important leaders in the community and gain greater support for their school program.

WHAT THE BEGINNING TEACHER OF PHYSICAL EDUCATION SHOULD EXPECT

The beginning teacher of physical education is not going to find an ideal teaching situation when he assumes the first job. Many times the theory that prospective teachers have learned in college is not applicable in a practical situation. The facilities may be limited, the community uninformed, the pupils disinterested, administrators and colleagues uncooperative. These and other obstacles must be hurdled one at a time. However, new teachers should never lose the enthusiasm that prompted them to go into teaching. In time, through hard work and a wholesome attitude, changes will occur and a more desirable teaching situation will develop.

A few factors the beginning teacher should recognize in taking the first job are as follows:

THE WORK DAY AND WORK WEEK WILL BE LONG. The physical education teacher can expect to work 50, 60, or 70 hours weekly. The many duties that need to be performed, students to see, and obligations to render all make for a long day and week. The beginning teacher should expect long hours, but if a good job is done, the rewards will be great.

THE DAILY SCHEDULE WILL BE STRENUOUS. The new teacher may find that he has to work through an entire day with the exception of a small break for lunch. Some schools require teachers of physical education to supervise the parking lot before school, watch the lunch room at the noon hour, see students that need to be disciplined after school, monitor detention halls, and perform 101 tasks. The new teacher should take these extra responsibilities as part of the routine. However, after a period of time has been spent on the job, there should be an attempt to eliminate some of these

Teachers holding extra jobs.

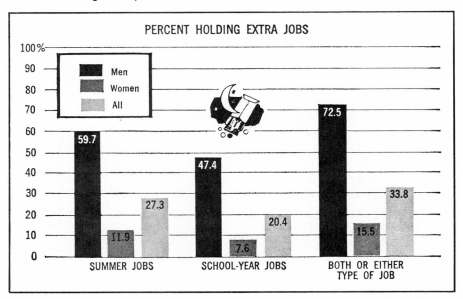

PERCENT HOLDING EXTRA JOBS

Legend: Men, Women, All

- SUMMER JOBS: Men 59.7, Women 11.9, All 27.3
- SCHOOL-YEAR JOBS: Men 47.4, Women 7.6, All 20.4
- BOTH OR EITHER TYPE OF JOB: Men 72.5, Women 15.5, All 33.8

FROM NEA RESEARCH DIVISION:
NEA JOURNAL, APRIL, 1963.

Teachers regularly take part in community activities.

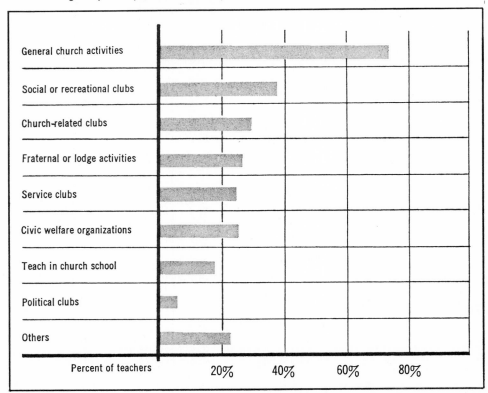

Percent of teachers

- General church activities
- Social or recreational clubs
- Church-related clubs
- Fraternal or lodge activities
- Service clubs
- Civic welfare organizations
- Teach in church school
- Political clubs
- Others

20% 40% 60% 80%

FROM NEA RESEARCH BULLETIN, APRIL, 1959.

undesirable tasks so that more time can be given to the business of teaching.

THE CLERICAL WORK WILL BE HEAVY. The beginning teacher will find himself completing monthly attendance forms, grade slips, requisitions for equipment, and excuses, plus many other records requiring clerical work. All of these take time away from teaching and working with pupils and, as such, cannot be fully justified. However, the teacher should recognize this as part of the job and undertake the responsibility. A new trend called "teacher's aides" may be of help. (See Chapter 19.)

THE MATERIALS AND FACILITIES MAY BE INADEQUATE. Certain materials, in the form of equipment and supplies, as well as adequate facilities in terms of teaching stations for physical education classes, are essential. However, because of the cost, in many communities they are not provided. The beginning teacher should be sympathetic and understanding but, nevertheless, should strive to interpret the need for new materials and facilities so that a better teaching job can be accomplished.

QUESTIONS AND EXERCISES

1. Outline the duties of a teacher of physical education in a school where the enrollment consists of approximately 100 boys and 100 girls.
2. Visit an elementary, junior high, or senior high school and do a job analysis study of one of the physical education positions.
3. Why is it essential that the physical educator be prepared in areas other than physical education?
4. What are the responsibilities of physical educational personnel in respect to each of the following: (a) objectives, (b) program, (c) leadership, and (d) reevaluation?
5. Why is effective leadership essential to the realization of the objectives of physical education?
6. Why is a knowledge of measurement and evaluation techniques essential to the student training for the profession of physical education?
7. For what duties, in areas other than physical education, should the student be trained?
8. Why is a well-rounded, general education background essential to a teacher of physical education in the light of the duties he or she will perform?
9. Write an article of approximately 250 words describing the extent to which your training is preparing you to discharge the duties as outlined in this chapter.

Reading assignment
Bucher, Charles A., and Goldman, Myra: Dimensions of physical education, St. Louis, 1969, The C. V. Mosby Co., Reading selections 60 to 65.

SELECTED REFERENCES

American Association for Health, Physical Education, and Recreation: Careers in physical education for girls: a key to your future, Washington, D. C., 1964, The Association.
American Association for Health, Physical Education, and Recreation: Fit to teach, Washington, D. C., 1957, The Association.
American Association for Health, Physical Education, and Recreation: Physical education and coaching as a career, Washington, D. C., The Association.
Bucher, Charles A.: Administration of school health and physical education programs including athletics, St. Louis, 1971, The C. V. Mosby Co.
Bucher, Charles A.: Administrative dimensions of health and physical education programs, including athletics, St. Louis, 1971, The C. V. Mosby Co.
Bucher, Charles A.: Field days, Journal of Health and Physical Education **19:**22, 1948.
Bucher, Charles A., and Reade, Evelyn M.: Physical education and health in the elementary school, New York, 1971, The Macmillan Co.
Bucher, Charles A., Koening, Constance, and Barnhard, Milton: Methods and materials of secondary school physical education, St. Louis, 1970, The C. V. Mosby Co.
Cassidy, Rosalind: Counseling in the physical education program, New York, 1959, Appleton-Century-Crofts.
LaPorte, William Ralph: A job analysis of the functions of the physical education teacher, Los Angeles, 1951, The University of Southern California Press.
Latchaw, Marjorie, and Brown, Camille: The evaluation process in health education, physical education, and recreation, Englewood Cliffs, New Jersey, 1962, Prentice-Hall, Inc.
Phi Delta Kappa: Teaching as a man's job, Bloomington, Indiana, 1963, Phi Delta Kappa.

21/Preparation of the physical education teacher

Many years ago, Johann Heinrich Pestalozzi, the great Swiss educator, pointed out the responsibility that rests with the teaching profession. The educator, he stressed, must understand the full significance of man himself and human nature. No profession requires greater skill in order to guide human nature properly. What is true of the professional preparation of all teachers is true of the preparation of physical education teachers as well.

The student of physical education, as well as physical education personnel in the field, should be familiar with the role of professional preparation in physical education. Such information will help interested persons to realize what constitutes adequate training for physical education leaders. In turn, they can bring their influence to bear upon teacher-training institutions so that proper preparation will be provided. To a great degree teacher-training institutions have decided—on their own—how physical education teachers should be selected and trained. Many have failed in this responsibility. Good leadership is one of the basic needs in this field today.

OBJECTIVES OF PROFESSIONAL PREPARATION

The goals of professional preparation have been set forth by many professional organizations. These goals include the need to graduate educated men and women who are prepared and committed to teaching, to influence not only the intellectual life of students but also the emotional and ethical aspects of their professional careers, and to acquaint prospective teachers with the rights and responsibilities of professional service.

HISTORY OF PROFESSIONAL PREPARATION

The history of professional preparation programs in physical education dates back more than 100 years. During this time there has been a steady growth in the number and quality of these programs.

Beginnings

Since the first class of teachers was graduated from the Normal Institute of Physical Education in Boston in 1861, the preparation of teachers in physical education has progressed rapidly. The 10 weeks' course at this institution, founded by Dio Lewis, had regular instruction in hygiene, physiology, anatomy, and gymnastics, in addition to an interpretation of and practical work in the "Swedish Movement Cure."

The North American Turnerbund, the second normal school for the training of teachers in physical education, opened its doors in 1866 in New York City, offering a 1-year course. Of the nineteen men who started in attendance, only five received diplomas at the end of the first course. Later the school was moved to Chicago, back to New York, and then to Milwaukee until 1888. In 1889 the school was transferred to Indianapolis for 2 years, was then moved back to Milwaukee, and, finally, in 1907 it was situated permanently in Indianapolis. Gymnastics and gymnastic nomenclature were emphasized, with much concern for medical gymnastics as well as for fencing and swimming.

Dr. Dudley Allen Sargent, one of the early leaders in physical education in America, brought his influence to bear on teacher preparation starting in 1881. The Sargent School, as it was called, trained almost exclusively women who planned to teach physical education. From 1887 to 1919 Dr. Sargent also directed the Harvard University summer courses in physical education.

The Brooklyn Normal School for Physical Education, under the directorship of Dr. William C. Anderson, came into existence in 1886. This school placed principal emphasis upon training the student in the theory and practice of gymnastics. Shortly after the opening of the school in Brooklyn, Dr. Anderson was named to the position of Associate Director of the Yale University Gymnasium in New Haven. With this appointment, the Normal School was moved to New Haven and became the Anderson Normal School of Gymnastics. Dr. Ernst H. Arnold became the director in 1896, and in 1901 the school was named the New Haven Normal School of Gymnastics, eventually to become the Arnold College of Hygiene and Physical Education.*

---

*Now a part of Bridgeport University, Bridgeport, Connecticut.

Goals of professional preparation should include the need to graduate educated men and women.

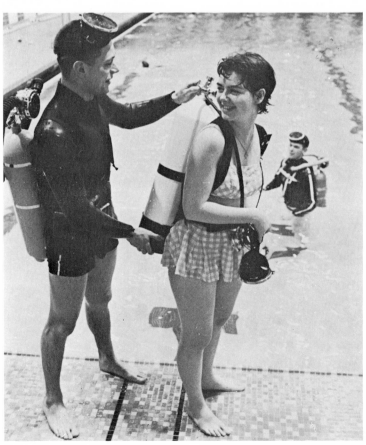

FLINT PUBLIC SCHOOLS, FLINT, MICH.

In the year of 1886 the start of the International Young Men's Christian Association College at Springfield, Massachuetts, was witnessed. This college, better known as Springfield College, offered a professional course for young men who expected to teach physical education in the Young Men's Christian Association. Later the degrees of Bachelor of Physical Education, Master of Physical Education, Bachelor of Science, Master of Education, and Doctor of Physical Education were granted, and many of its graduates accepted positions in public school teaching as well as other related fields. In 1890 a similar training school was opened in Chicago.

In 1889 Mrs. Mary Hemenway established, and later endowed, the Boston Normal School of Gymnastics, which in 1909 became the Department of Hygiene and Physical Education of Wellesley. Baron Posse, a teacher in this Normal School, organized his own gymnasium in 1890, calling it the Posse Normal School of Gymnastics. The school remained under his direction until his death in 1895, at which time Baroness Rose Posse carried on as director. In 1915 Mr. Hartvig Nissen was secured as its president, and the school became known as the Posse-Nissen School of Physical Education.

Prior to World War I, physical educators received their professional preparation primarily in normal schools. A study made by Ruth Elliot in 1927 lists the private normal schools of physical education engaged in training physical education personnel, the date of their establishment, and the length of curricula. This list, shown in Table 21-1, is significant since it indicates the gradual lengthening of curriculums in the training of prospective physical education teachers.

Growth of teacher education programs

The colleges and universities soon followed the normal schools in the preparation of teachers in physical education. The University of Washington, with a professional course in physical education organized in 1896, is usually thought of as the first of

the state universities to offer work in this area. However, in 1894 Bowen, at the State Normal School at Ypsilanti, Michigan, was responsible for the first attempt to train teachers in physical education in a state-controlled institution.

The University of California, Indiana University, and the University of Nebraska initiated courses in this area from 1897 to 1898, placing particular emphasis upon the areas of anthropometry, physical examinations, anatomy, physiology of exercise, hygienic gymnastics, and the history of physical culture.

In the early 1900's privately endowed colleges and universities began to consider training for leadership in physical education. Oberlin College in 1900, Teachers College, Columbia University, in 1903, and Wellesley College in 1909 were among the first of these.

In the early part of the twentieth century, the larger secondary schools began to call for full-time teachers of physical education. State legislation and requirements had much to do with this demand for more emphasis upon teacher training in physical education. Shortly after World War I, approximately thirty-five states passed legislation requiring the teaching of health and physical education in the public schools. Such legislation was a stimulant to teacher preparation in the field of physical education. Until this time, efforts along this line were mainly directed at training gymnastic teachers. The typical curriculum in many of the earlier schools consisted of some theoretical courses, such as anatomy of the bones and muscles, gymnastic nomenclature, and methods in gymnastics and marching. These were included in the program in order to supplement the training received on the gymnasium floor.

A few outstanding leaders in the field of education began to look beyond the mere teaching of gymnastics and subjects related to it and emphasize subjects rich in cultural background, foundation sciences, and courses in the general field of education. In the early 1920's courses in education began to be introduced, as well as courses con-

Table 21-1. Normal schools of physical education*

Name of school	Date estab- lished	Length of present curriculums in years	Degrees granted	Affiliation with college or university
Normal College of the American Gym- nastic Union, Indianapolis, Ind.	1866	1,2,3,4	BPE, MPE	
Sargent School of Physical Education, Cambridge, Mass.	1881	3		
Arnold College of Hygiene and Physical Education (New Haven Normal School of Gymnastics)	1886	2,3	BPE	
International YMCA College, Spring- field, Mass.	1886	2, 4	BPE, MPE	
Chautauqua School of Physical Educa- tion, Chautauqua, N. Y.	1888	1, 3	BS, M Ed	New York University
Formerly Boston Normal School of Gymnastics, Boston, Mass.	1889	2, 5†	MS, AB	1909 became Depart- ment of Hygiene and Physical Education, Wellesley College
School of Physical Education, YMCA College, Chicago, Ill.	1890	4	BPE	
Posse-Nissen School of Physical Educa- tion, Boston, Mass.	1890	1, 3		
Savage School of Physical Education, New York, N. Y.	1898	3		
Chicago Normal School of Physical Education, Chicago, Ill.	1903	1,2,3		
American College of Physical Educa- tion, Chicago, Ill.	1908	2,3,4	BPE	
Battle Creek College, School of Physical Education, Battle Creek, Mich.	1909	3,4	BS in PE	
Boston School of Physical Education, Boston, Mass.	1913	3		Boston University
Columbia Normal School of Physical Education, Chicago, Ill.	1913	(3 mo., 2-6 mo., 9 mo.)		
Newark School of Hygiene and Physical Education, Newark, N. J.	1917	2,3		
Central School of Hygiene and Physical Education, New York, N. Y.	1919	3		New York University
Marjorie Webster School Expression Physical Education, Washington, D. C.	1920	1,2	BPE	
Ithaca School of Physical Education, Ithaca, N. Y.	1923	3,4	BPE	
Bouve School of Physical Education, Boston, Mass.	1925	3		

*Elliot, Ruth: The organization of professional training in physical education in state universities, New York, 1927, Teachers College Contributions to Education, No. 268, Columbia University, p. 9.
†For college graduates only.

cerned with psychology, fundamental sciences, and methodology. The education of the physical education teacher became an important consideration.

With the advent of courses in physical education in some of the larger universities, leading to a bachelor's degree with a major in physical education, more and more of the graduates found their way into elementary schools and subsequently into the secondary field. An increasing number of teachers was being prepared, which brought forth a steady upgrading of requirements for teachers' certificates.

One by one the various states began to require 4 years of training with a degree, and it was not unusual to find minimum requirements in courses in education, psychology, and foundation sciences, as well as courses in physical education. More and more the schools began to ask for full-time specialists in physical education, and both men and women interested in this field rushed to the teacher-training institutions.

The rapid influx of prospective teachers in this area, together with the renewed emphasis upon teacher training, resulted in the abandonment of 2-year and 3-year training courses and the establishment of 4-year curriculums. Many normal schools became teachers' colleges with degree-granting privileges, and, in general, the quality of training improved. The period from 1920 to 1930, when institutions such as New York University, Teachers College, Columbia University, and Springfield College began to offer courses beyond the first 4 years of college, was a milestone in the advancement of the professional preparation of teachers of physical education.

A noticeable change took place in the field of education when in 1930 the financial depression began to be felt in the schools. The teaching of physical education was discontinued in many schools or combined with the teaching of other subjects. Few new teachers were hired, and this resulted in an oversupply of those trained in this field. Teacher-training institutions revised their programs and began to make a more careful selection of students, and some states raised the certification requirements to 5 years of study. The inevitable result was a decided improvement in the training of teachers in physical education.

Important in professional preparation programs after 1920 until the present was the initiation of more stringent admission requirements by teacher-training institutions. Selective admission, guidance, entrance examinations, and a more careful look at candidates became considerations at several institutions of higher learning.

Another point of concern was professional curriculums. More emphasis on general education, together with a closer examination of the professional education and specialization courses, became evident. The need for a broad training in all aspects of physical education, rather than just in coaching or other specialty, came into being. Furthermore, since 1926 there has been a definite trend away from medical training for specialists directing physical education programs in colleges.

The Cooperative Study in Teacher Education sponsored by the American Council on Education, 1938 to 1943; the reviving of the American Association for Health, Physical Education, and Recreation's Cooperative Study Committee, including representatives from many professional organizations; the Miami University, Oxford, Ohio, Conference in 1947; and the Report on Teacher Education by the American Association of Teachers Colleges in 1948 helped to raise professional standards in physical education.

A series of professional preparation conferences have been held in past years, starting with the Jackson's Mill Conference in 1948. One of the most important meetings was the Professional Preparing Conference held in January, 1962.* The pur-

---

*American Association for Health, Physical Education, and Recreation: Professional preparation in health education, physical education, and recreation education, Washington, D. C., 1962, the Association.

pose of the conference was to improve the training of teachers in health and safety education, physical education, and recreation and outdoor education, at the undergraduate level, and to give some direction to graduate study.

The complete report is available from the American Association for Health, Physical Education, and Recreation.

Another report, by James B. Conant,* also represented a milestone in the training of teachers. This report recommended some new departures from the traditional pattern of training and certifying teachers by suggesting such procedures as the following:

1. The university should assume the responsibility for endorsing and attesting that the student was properly trained for teaching, and that the president of the institution, on behalf of the faculty, certifies that the candidate is adequately prepared to teach.
2. The institution of higher learning should establish, in conjunction with a public school system, a state-approved, practice teaching arrangement.
3. An institution offering programs in art, music, or physical education should award a teaching diploma in these fields without grade distinction.
4. Graduate preparation in physical education was not necessary.
5. There should be an all-university approach to teacher training, with the liberal arts professors and departments sharing with the education professors the professional preparation of teachers.
6. Clinical professorships should be established where the professors would work with student teachers in the school internship program.
7. Physical education should not be given credit in elementary and secondary schools.

There were other recommendations in the Conant report in respect to the composition of accrediting agencies, certification reciprocity among states, revision of salary schedules by local boards of education, financial assistance to teachers for study in summer schools, and master's degree programs.

*Conant, James Bryant: The education of American teachers, New York, 1963, McGraw-Hill Book Co.

A conference on graduate education in health education, physical education, recreation education, dance, and safety was held in January, 1967. The purpose of this conference was to suggest principles and standards to improve graduate education in the special areas. The conference accomplished such tasks as the following:

1. Defined the nature of graduate education at the master's and doctoral levels, the functions of graduate education, and the competencies needed in research and other areas
2. Developed guidelines for the organization of graduate programs in respect to such things as student personnel, curriculum, instructional methodology, laboratory experiences, and facilities and materials
3. Explored new programs
4. Reviewed research completed in the area of professional preparation
5. Suggested new graduate program possibilities

Teacher education in physical education has continued to expand. After World War I and again after World War II, great eras of expanding teacher education programs developed in various colleges and universities. In 1918 there were twenty institutions preparing teachers of physical education; in 1929, 139; in 1944, 295; in 1946, approximately 361; and today, over 700.

Along with the growth of teacher education institutions in physical education, there has developed a growing concern as to the type of preparation needed for training potential physical education personnel. In the future a better selection and a better training of physical educators should be seen. This will be in keeping with the objectives of the physical education profession to serve society in the best way possible.

Status of professional preparation programs

More than half of the nearly 2,500 institutions of higher learning in the United States prepare teachers for the elementary and secondary schools. Approximately one-third of those teachers graduated each year are graduates of schools of education located in about 160 major universities. Another third of the graduating teachers are graduates of institutions of higher learning that have as their primary responsibility the preparation of teachers. The remaining third of graduating teachers are trained in departments of education in some 900 liberal arts colleges. A noticeable trend in those institutions primarily geared to training teachers is that they have become, and are becoming, liberal arts colleges with names and titles such as state colleges or even state universities.

It should also be noted that 2-year colleges are offering some courses for students who after their sophomore year transfer to a 4-year institution of higher learning where they take advanced work in physical education.

In respect to certification of teachers and the implications for professional preparing programs, forty-five states require 4 years of college for elementary teaching, and all states require at least 4 years for a teaching certificate at the secondary school level. Better than 90% of public school teachers have bachelor's degrees and approximately 25% have master's degrees. Some states issue temporary certificates for teaching.

A study conducted by the American Association for Health, Physical Education, and Recreation Professional Panel* identified 5,000 physical educators, health educators, and recreation education persons whose primary responsibility was in the area of professional preparation. Furthermore, more than 700 institutions of higher learning were identified that offer a major preparation program in one or more of the three special areas. The Identification Summary was as follows:

IDENTIFICATION SUMMARY

1. Number of institutions responding to the request — 680
2. Members of institutions identified and not responding to the request — 50
3. Number of professional preparation personnel by area of specialization:

---

*American Association for Health, Phyical Education, and Recreation: Professional preparation, Journal of Health, Physical Education, and Recreation **36:**71, 1965.

a. Administrative — 650
b. Health education, physical education, and recreation education — 350
c. Health education — 400
d. Physical education — 2,600
e. Recreation education — 175
f. Health education and physical education — 600
g. Physical education and recreation education — 225

Total professional persons identified — 5,000

In respect to qualifications for teaching in professional preparation programs, I conducted a survey of administrators who did the hiring in sixty-five institutions of higher learning. The survey revealed that, in respect to degrees attained, 76% of the administrators felt it was *very important,* 20% considered it *important,* and 4% *not very important* that staff members hold at least a master's degree. Fifty-six percent of the administrators felt it was *very important,* 42% felt it was *important,* and 2% felt it was *not very important* for professional preparation programs in physical education to have staff members who are specialists in a particular phase of the special field, such as adapted physical education. In respect to teacher qualifications, 56% of the administrators surveyed indicated that they felt it *very important,* 38% felt it was *important,* and 6% *not very important* for staff members to have knowledge of educational methods and psychological principles related to what they were teaching. Fifty percent of the hiring administrators felt it was *very important,* 40% felt it was *important,* and 10% felt it was *not very important* for staff members to have previous teaching experience in elementary and secondary schools. Thirty-two percent of the administrators wanted staff members to have previous college teaching. In respect to qualifications for coaches, 40% of the administrators felt it was *very important,* 38% felt it was *important,* and 22% felt it was *not very important* that the candidates have expert knowledge and experience in coaching a particular sport and the techniques involved.

I also participated in a survey of the professional preparation curriculums in physical education at ten selected colleges and universities throughout the United States. This survey considered the degree offered, undergraduate admission requirements, courses offered in the area of general education and educational theory, and specialized courses required in physical education.

All of the colleges and universities in the survey awarded the bachelor's degree to men, and nine of these schools also offered a bachelor's degree program for women. One school awarded a combined degree in health and physical education for men on both the bachelor's and the master's levels. Of the ten schools, nine also had graduate programs leading to the master's degree, and two had programs on the doctoral level.

All of the schools surveyed required a high school diploma for admission. Seven required that the applicant take the Scholastic Aptitude Test of the College Entrance Examination Board, and an additional school required this test for non-residents of the state only. One of the schools required applicants to take both a state admissions test and a test of physical skills but did not require the Scholastic Aptitude Test. High school units required for entrance totaled fifteen or sixteen units, depending on the college or university, and included such academic courses as English, social studies, mathematics, science, and foreign languages.

Courses required in general education during the undergraduate years by the colleges and universities in the survey included English and speech, mathematics and statistics, the humanities, art, music, philosophy, social sciences, psychology, sociology, history, foreign languages, natural and physical sciences, zoology, chemistry, physics, anatomy, bacteriology, and physiology.

All but one of the schools surveyed required three credits in educational psychology. Other educational theory courses included requirements ranging from two to six credits in such areas as adolescent psychology, educational sociology, history and philosophy of education, organization and administration of schools, and methods of teaching.

In the area of professional specialization, nine of the schools surveyed required from two to six credits in physical education methods, while eight schools required courses in physical education for the atypical child. All ten institutions required courses in the introduction to physical education, the organization and administration of physical education, tests and measurements in physical education, physical education skills courses, and a student teaching experience. Nine of the schools required from two to four credits in applied anatomy, and nine schools required from two to five credits in the foundations, philosophy, or history and principles of physical education. Other courses in the field of specialization required in the various schools were: the physical education curriculum, physiology of exercise, care and prevention of athletic injuries, methods of coaching, health courses, first aid, safety education, and courses in recreation and camping. Two schools included a twelve-credit teaching minor in its requirements, while one school included a thirty-credit teaching minor.

Of the ten colleges and universities surveyed, one school required a total of 120 points for graduation with a bachelor's degree in physical education, four schools required 124 credits, one school required 125 credits, one school listed 130 credits, and one listed 131 credits. Two of the schools required a total of 132 credits for graduation.

In a study of methods used by professors in teacher-training programs in physical education, the following methods were utilized: lecture method, group reports and discussions, problem-solving techniques, guest lecturers, laboratory experiences, and audiovisual aids.

The National Education Association Research Division surveyed a cross section of public school teachers to find out whether they thought teacher preparation programs were geared to actual teaching needs. The results are charted in the illustration on p. 596.

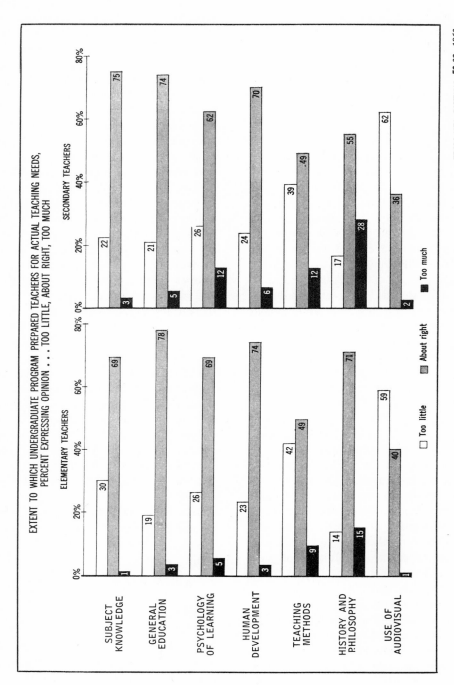

EXTENT TO WHICH UNDERGRADUATE PROGRAM PREPARED TEACHERS FOR ACTUAL TEACHING NEEDS, PERCENT EXPRESSING OPINION . . . TOO LITTLE, ABOUT RIGHT, TOO MUCH

FROM NEA JOURNAL **52**:32, 1963.

TWO-YEAR COLLEGES AND PROFESSIONAL PREPARATION

The 2-year college has become a very important factor on the American educational scene. This type of institution is expanding at a rapid rate and will continue to do so as the number of college-bound students rises. This means that more and more high school boys and girls will find their educational opportunities in this kind of college. Though there are exceptions, most junior colleges (and by this term the community college is included) have the following three functions:

1. *Two years of preprofessional training or general education.* A student may graduate with a degree of associate in the arts or sciences after 2 years or transfer to a 4-year institution for a bachelor's degree. This transfer program is sometimes called the university parallel curriculum. Most 4-year colleges and universities will accept transfer students from accredited junior colleges if the academic achievement of the student is high and if the subjects studied mesh with the curriculum of the higher institution.
2. *Provision for a complete program in a semiprofessional field such as secretarial work, home economics, medical laboratory techniques, and business education.*
3. *Provision for classes for adults who want more education to help them in their jobs, or who simply want to study subjects they never had a chance to study before.*

The type of curriculums offered by junior colleges is usually controlled by the needs and interests of the students they serve. Some junior college curriculums are planned almost entirely for students who want a general education and who plan to transfer to a 4-year institution. Other junior colleges enroll the majority of students in semiprofessional courses.

Physical education service programs are being developed in most of the 2-year colleges. Most of these institutions require physical education for 2 hours each week for 2 years.

With more and more students taking their 2 years of higher education in the 2-year colleges and with many of these students vitally interested in sports and physical education, the question naturally arises: What part should the 2-year college play in the professional preparation of teachers of physical education? One guideline might be the one recommended by the National Conference on Professional Preparation in Health Education, Physical Education, and Recreation held by the American Association for Health, Physical Education, and Recreation in 1962, which stressed that the freshman and sophomore years should be viewed primarily as general education. However, several leaders in physical education have pointed out that the student who has made a vocational choice by the time he enters college should be offered some professional education during the first 2 years and that it is not realistic to insist that this vocational interest should be delayed until the junior year in college. These leaders agree that a major share of the program should be devoted to general education, but at the same time, they point out, it is possible in the remaining time to orient the student to the whole field of specialization by providing such experiences as an introductory course in his professional field and, in addition, to strengthen the basic skill background of the student. These leaders, however, point out that a prerequisite to such experience should be a qualified staff and adequate facilities, in order to do the job properly.

Some 2-year colleges are preparing paraprofessionals for work in educational systems. Such colleges as Miami-Dade in Florida and Garland Junior College in Boston, Massachusetts, are two such institutions. Garland Junior College, for example, has a program preparing students who will be qualified as assistant teachers. Other colleges are preparing paraprofessionals for work in physical eduaction, recreation, police, and fire prevention programs.

The 2-year college should help each student in accordance with his interests, abilities, and needs, so that he may become a mature citizen and contribute to his own happiness and the welfare of his community.

SELECTED CURRENT DEVELOPMENTS IN TEACHER EDUCATION PROGRAMS

Selected current developments in teacher education that have strong implications for the training of physical education teachers are discussed in the following paragraphs.

Open admissions

The Carnegie Commission on Higher Education in 1970 in its report, *A Chance to Learn: An Action Agenda for Equal Opportunity in Higher Education,* proposed that by the year 2000 every American have the opportunity to attend college. Social and economic barriers should not prevent attendance at college. Instead, individual choice and ability should be the deciding factors. The commission stressed that the door to college should not be closed to blacks, Indians, or any other group of Americans. In other words, each of the fifty states should provide a place in college for every high school graduate, as California did in 1960 and New York City did in 1970. This does not mean, however, there should be "open admissions" to every university, since institutions of higher learning vary greatly in their nature and purpose. To achieve this goal, it was urged that elementary and secondary school education be upgraded and that students entering college be given remedial help where needed.

The *open admissions* program, which is expected to spread rapidly to every state in the union, means that teacher-training programs must provide staff members at all educational levels who are prepared to work effectively with students so that they can be successful in a program that fits their interests and needs and where they can progress in accordance with their own abilities.

The open admissions program also has another very significant implication for physical education. In some of these programs already inaugurated, it has been found that many of the students entering college who would have formerly been barred from admission are interested in sports. There has been a noticeable interest among some stu-dents to prepare for a career in physical education. Therefore, it can be anticipated that in the years ahead there will be more applicants trying to gain admission to our programs than ever before. Thus, a challenge is presented to professional preparation programs to provide a range of experiences for these students so that they can find a successful career in some phase of our program, whether it be in a school, college, agency, or some other institution and whether it be as a paraprofessional, coach, or full-fledged faculty member.

Teacher education—a campuswide concern

As a result of the Conant report and other reports, teacher education is becoming a campuswide concern. This is evidenced by faculty members in all departments of a college and university playing key roles in professional preparation programs. This is being accomplished by courses being taught by experts in the various disciplines throughout a college and university, rather than confining the staff to merely the school of education or to educationists. Professors and administrators in various departments and colleges are serving on planning committees, administrative councils, and other groups to advise and plan teacher education programs. All-university and all-college committees are evaluating teacher education programs and making recommendations for their upgrading. Admission requirements and professional standards that are collegewide and universitywide are being applied to those students who are preparing to be teachers, as well as to students in other departments, schools, and colleges. Students in professional teacher preparation programs are able and encouraged to take courses in general psychology, philosophy, and courses in other departments, schools, and colleges throughout the university.

By becoming a campuswide concern, teacher education in physical education should benefit. Majors in physical education should become better educated, have a broader background, be exposed to the teachings of outstanding professors, and have the backing and approval of a much larger segment of the academic community.

Internship gaining greater importance

Internship is one of the most important parts of the preparation of teachers. This period of training should be lengthened to a point where the prospective teacher is well oriented in the life of the school and the community.

The student teaching internship experience should be supervised by skilled and competent school and college personnel in a program that has been cooperatively worked out by the two. Supervising teachers should be the best teachers in the school. They should be given a reduced load in order to carry out their responsibilities in an efficient manner. The college supervisors should also be well qualified, both by preparation and experience, to assume this most important responsibility.

Although educators have recognized the need for such an experience, only in the last few years has there developed an emphasis on a longer period. Three reasons exist why a longer period in this phase of professional preparation is necessary. In the first place, a longer period is necessary so that the student may observe the total growth of the child. This means growth or progress, not only in academic subjects but also organically, socially, intellectually, and emotionally. Only if the student is allowed to be with the same children over a longer period of time will such an experience be possible. In the second place, a longer period is necessary because practice teaching is the core of the professional program and, as such, is necessary to develop the competence that will be needed when the teacher assumes complete responsibility in her first job after graduation. In the third place, a longer period is necessary so that the student may actually live in the community and participate in its various activities. Furthermore, he should feel a part of the school and become well acquainted with the children, the staff, and the total picture of school life.

Finally, there is the question of when the internship should take place in the training of the teacher and how much time should be allotted to it. The majority of educators favor placing this experience in the latter part of the training period, when the knowledge and experience that have been accumulated in the first few years of preparation may be put to good use. As to the length of time that should be allotted, there is wide variance of opinion. If the teacher is to adequately experience school and community life and is to observe the total growth of the child, the period of student teaching should be adequate to accomplish the realization of this objective.

Another recent emphasis in teacher education is the recommendation that an internship take place following the regular preservice program of teacher education, which includes student teaching. This internship would be planned by both the schools and colleges concerned. The need for continuity in preservice and in-service education is discussed in the following section.

Continuity of preservice and in-service education

The traditional arrangement whereby schools of education and other teacher-training institutions assign their practice teachers to school systems leaves much to be desired. In the usual arrangement the practice teacher gets his experience in schools largely determined by the local school administration and is then supervised by a critic-teacher and a representative of the college faculty. As a result, there has been much inconsistency and little continuity in respect to methods used and goals achieved.

Although there has been much discussion about the need for continuity between preservice and in-service education, there have been few instances where schools and colleges have united in a meaningful manner to accomplish this goal. There has been cooperation, but more than cooperation is needed. A strong bond of unity is necessary.

An example of what is needed is illustrated by a project where the New York

City Board of Education and Queens College of the City University of New York have established the School University Teacher Education Center, which uses a specific public school as a setting where undergraduate students receive their training. The curriculum and educational program of the school determine the teacher education program. The principal of the school and the college co-director perform such functions as making policy decisions, supervising and evaluating staff members, and establishing curriculum guidelines. Assistant principals work with college staff members in such areas as curriculum development and coordinating student teaching assignments.

The need for in-service education for teachers is being stressed more and more with the many educational changes that are constantly taking place. This in-service education again should take place through a uniting of school and college resources. An example of such an arrangement is in Atlanta, Georgia, where the Atlanta Public Schools have joint appointments with three of the local universities. In-service courses are planned and taught as a result of such a coalition. Institutes are planned, colleges supply instructors for courses at the request of schools, there is joint supervision of practice teachers, and other similar arrangements are made to provide a meaningful in-service program.

Physical education, as a part of the total school and college teacher education programs, needs continuity of preservice and in-service education. When such arrangements as have been illustrated here are made, better physical education programs will result with greater contributions being made to the students and community alike.

Stress on general education

Teachers need a broad cultural background instead of the limited educational background. If they are to be leaders in a society that desperately needs good leadership, they must not only have a knowledge of the total educative process but also a broad view and mastery of such things as the achievements of the human race; the fine arts; the English language; current political, social, and economic factors; the physical environment; and human institutions in general.

A broad, general educational background is especially necessary in our society because of the American way of life. A democracy such as ours provides for the election of public officials and leaders by the public. The teacher can do much toward laying the foundations for an informed citizenry. Through such a medium, our form of government will better serve the welfare of the constituents for which it has been established.

Second, a broad, general background will help the teacher to recognize his responsibility as a worker, a parent, a citizen, and a human being.

Third, a broad, general education can enrich the meaning of life and the social service of the individual. It aids in promoting an understanding of one's fellowmen that is based on human ideals. It aims at an understanding of the individual in relation to contemporary institutions and problems of American and world life. Finally, it emphasizes an appreciation of selective fields of cultural material that makes life more satisfying and enjoyable.

Although it has been previously indicated that teachers in general need a broad educational background, evidence points to the fact that this is especially true for the teacher of physical education. The nature of his work, his close personal contact with students, his place of leadership in the community, and the necessity for the coordination of his field with other phases of the school program have implications that in many ways do not exist for the general classroom or subject-matter teacher. Such training will make provisions for such things as a mastery of the English language, both oral and written, the social studies, the biological and physical sciences, and the fine arts.

If those who carry on the physical education program are to be leaders in society, they must possess a cultural training that will gain them the respect of the students, faculty, administration, and the community. The individual who has secured his position primarily because he was an outstanding athlete on some college team, despite the fact that he may have language difficulties and lack breadth of knowledge, must become a thing of the past if the profession is to continue growing. Teacher education should guarantee a physical education teacher who is enlightened, purposeful, and productive of good results. This is an age when a man must be an expert in the performance of his duties as an intelligent citizen as well as in some particular vocation.

Need for a 5-year program

The Professional Preparing Conference of 1962, sponsored by the American Association for Health, Physical Education, and Recreation, reaffirmed the need for increasing the preparation of physical education,

health and recreation leaders to a period of 5 years. Teaching is as complex as the medical profession, and therefore members of the teaching profession need many years of intensive preparation. Some states, such as California and New York, require 5 years of preparation in certain subjects before they can be taught on the high school level.

The 5-year program of teacher education will result in a much broader and more intensive preparation. It will enable teacher-training institutions to offer programs that take into consideration more adequately the general education of teachers by providing more preparation in the areas of the fine and practical arts, English, social sciences, physical sciences, biological sciences, and mathematics. It will make possible a more thorough background in various subject-matter fields. It will make provision for more preparation in the professional education area by making it possible to extend the internship period, by providing for more direct experiences with children, and by de-

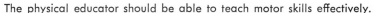

The physical educator should be able to teach motor skills effectively.

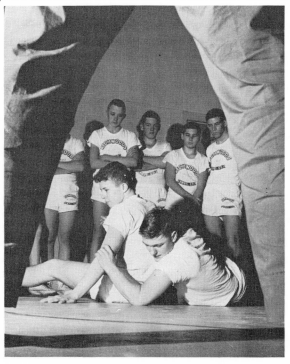

RICHWOODS COMMUNITY HIGH SCHOOL,
PEORIA HEIGHTS, ILL.

veloping a broader understanding of child growth and development and how children learn.

Importance of knowing how children learn

At no time in our educational history has there been so much talk about "knowing the child" as there is at present. Therefore, there is a feeling among leaders in teacher education that more emphasis should be placed upon how children learn in the training of future teachers. Teachers should know and understand the children with whom they spend so much time. Teachers should know why children behave in certain ways and under what conditions they learn best. A teacher cannot be successful in her job unless she is acquainted with this basic knowledge. Many of the faults of schools today come from the fact that teachers have been appointed to positions on school faculties because of their knowledge of subject matter and without reference to their knowledge of how children learn and develop.

In physical education, there is stress today on the scientific foundations area and in particular on motor learning. It is felt that teachers in physical education need to know more about how human beings learn physical skills, the most effective techniques that can be used in teaching these skills, the length of practice periods and how far apart they should be spaced, the role of mental activity in the learning of skills, and many other aspects of motor learning. (See Chapter 17 for more information.)

Teaching the disadvantaged

The Teacher Corps has been called by many observers the most radical experiment in teacher education that has ever been tried in this country. It grew out of dissatisfaction with the type of educational programs being provided for children in the ghettos and poverty pockets of our cities. It takes college graduates, gives them some training, and then assigns them to serve a 2-year internship in a school in a poverty area. After the 2-year period these students meet certification requirements and receive their Master's degree.

There is much interest today in teaching the disadvantaged. Physical education is playing an important role in many inner-city educational programs. In the years ahead there needs to be more attention to this segment of the nation's population and the most effective role that physical education can play in the educational process. (See Chapter 2 for more information on this subject.)

PROFESSIONAL CURRICULUM

The professional preparation given in the various institutions of higher learning should prepare the physical educator adequately for the duties he will assume after graduation.

Competencies to be developed

Professional competencies are important to all physical educators. The essential professional competencies needed are: a knowledge of the school and community, including their growth and structure; a knowledge and understanding of child growth and development; a sound knowledge of the process and theories of learning; the knowledge of and ability to use pertinent resource materials; the ability to apply proper teaching techniques; a knowledge of capable leadership; the ability to objectively evaluate the progress of each student; the ability to meet the needs and interests of each student; and the ability to cooperate and work with colleagues, administrators, parents, students, and the community at large for the good of all concerned.

In respect to competencies needed in physical education, Roundy* conducted a study in which he obtained the judgments of 456 educators regarding twenty-one problems identified by teachers of boys' physical education at the secondary level and the

---

*Roundy, Elmo Smith: Problems of and competencies needed by men physical education teachers at the secondary level, Research Quarterly **38**:274, 1967.

Table 21-2. Judgments of the 456 educators regarding the twenty-one problems and the most significant competencies needed to deal more effectively with each problem*

Problem and related competencies†	Percent indicating problem of:		
	Major concern	Minor concern	Mean ratio
Dealing with classes which have large enrollment: 1. Skill in grouping and organizing pupils for optimum control and learning. 72%‡ 2. Proficiency in getting student to accept responsibility for their own learning. 70.3% 3. Skill in improvising and using activities which are suited for large classes and limited facilities. 68.7% 4. Competence to improvise and use teaching techniques in the various activities which are adapted for large classes. 61.9%	54.29	35.82	1.4471
Working with limited facilities and equipment: 1. Proficiency in scheduling and organizing facilities for maximum use. 71.1%	48.24	37.89	1.3436
Grading and reporting pupil progress: 1. Ability to develop an over-all valid and objective system of grading. 76% 2. Competence to communicate effectively with parents regarding the progress and growth of students. 58.1%	47.14	34.14	1.2841
Working in the area of adaptive physical education: 1. Ability to recognize pupils who should be given a referral examination by a physician for placement in an adaptive program. 63% 2. Competence to select and set up the equipment needed for an adaptive program. 58.8% 3. Ability to work with students in implementing an adaptive program under the supervision of a physician. 57%	44.71	38.11	1.2753
Evaluating the program: 1. Ability to summarize and organize evaluational data for meaningful interpretation. 65.2% 2. Ability to use a variety of techniques and devices for gathering evaluational information. 64.5% 3. Skill in the use of sound research and statistical procedures for gathering and analyzing evaluational data. 58.4%	41.63	41.41	1.2467
Dealing with the small percentage of students who do not cooperate: 1. Ability to counsel effectively with these students in helping them meet their needs and adjust to their problems. 70.3% 2. Proficiency in impartially and consistently enforcing the standard of conduct. 63.9%	41.41	39.87	1.2269
Providing effective and continuous motivation: 1. Ability to help student develop correct concepts and good attitudes toward physical activity. 66.7% 2. Skill in using teaching techniques and planning instruction so that students can be given a maximum amount of individual instruction and reinforcement as they perform. 62.8%	38.11	40.31	1.1652

*Roundy, Elmo Smith: Problems of and competencies needed by men physical education teachers at the secondary level, Research Quarterly **38**:277-280, 1967.

†Problems are in boldface; competencies are listed below the problems to which they apply.

‡Percent indicates respondents signifying that this competency was needed to deal more effectively with the respective problem.

Table 21-2. Judgments of the 456 educators regarding the twenty-one problems and the most significant competencies needed to deal more effectively with each problem—cont'd

	Percent indicating problem of:		
Problem and related competencies	*Major concern*	*Minor concern*	*Mean ratio*
Providing effective and continuous motivation—cont'd			
3. Competence to select activities and to teach them in a manner so that each student can experience a measure of success. 60.1%			
4. Proficiency in using procedures and techniques which will keep the students continually informed of their progress. 59.3%			
5. Knowledge of a variety of instructional techniques, drills, games and materials. 54.6%			
6. Ability to provide for continuity of learning experience through developing the proper sequence of activities and the proper progression of movement patterns within an activity. 50.9%			
Developing a broad enough curriculum to meet the needs and interests of the students:	35.68	38.55	1.0991
1. Competence to teach a wide variety of activities. 61.9%			
Maintaining an orderly atmosphere without using overly rigid and militaristic methods of organization and control:	35.68	38.33	1.0969
1. Skill in helping class members develop a sense of responsibility to the group. 63.9%			
2. Sincere interest in helping each individual student. 55.3%			
Helping students who are having learning difficulties in class activities:	33.63	41.10	1.0837
1. Skill in motivating the low achievers. 76.9%			
2. Ability to develop and implement a program suited to the abilities and achievement level of the student. 65.2%			
Using tests and other devices to measure progress:	35.24	36.78	1.0727
1. Ability to motivate pupils to assume an important role in evaluating their own achievement and development. 69.6%			
2. Ability to devise and construct valid and objective skill tests. 68.5%			
3. Knowledge of standard skill tests. 60.6%			
4. Ability to devise and construct valid physical (organic) fitness tests. 60.1%			
5. Skill in setting up local norms for tests. 59%			
6. Knowledge of standard physical (organic) fitness tests. 58.8%			
7. Proficiency in evaluating pupil progress in general attitudes and social behavior. 57.7%			
8. Competence to administer tests in a valid manner. 54.8%			
Adapting instruction to the variation in growth and maturation:	30.31	39.34	1.0419
1. Proficiency in teaching students of varying abilities and capacities from the slow to the gifted. 69.2%			
Teaching physical education activities to students:	33.41	36.92	1.0396
1. Knowledge of proper teaching methods and drills in gymnastics. 72.9%			
2. Ability to demonstrate performance skills in gymnastics. 69.6%			
3. Ability to break down an activity or skill into basic movement patterns and to teach these patterns in the most effective sequence. 62.3%			
4. Competence to develop effective unit and daily instructional plans. 62.3%			

Table 21-2. Judgments of the 456 educators regarding the twenty-one problems and the most significant competencies needed to deal more effectively with each problem—cont'd

Problem and related competencies	Percent indicating problem of:		
	Major concern	Minor concern	Mean ratio
Teaching physical education activities to students—cont'd 5. Knowledge of proper teaching methods and drills in dance and rhythm activities. 60.4% 6. Ability to demonstrate performance skills in dance and rhythm activities. 59% 7. Knowledge of proper teaching methods and progression drills in individual and dual sports. 54.6% 8. Knowledge of the principles of physical (organic) fitness and conditioning. 52%			
Helping students with their social and personal problems: 1. Skill in identifying students who have significant problems in this area. 61.9% 2. Proficiency in using procedures in class that will aid students in acquiring the special skills of effective group membership and leadership. 60.6%	29.74	44.49	1.0396
Helping students to apply knowledge and skill in non-class situations: 1. Proficiency in helping students to understand the value of physical activities. 65.9% 2. Competence to teach activities with high transfer value. 55.1%	32.38	38.77	1.0352
Providing successful coeducational activities: 1. Knowledge of activities which are most successful with coeducational groups. 67.4% 2. Skill in teaching and handling coeducational groups. 67.4%	32.38	33.33	1.0308
Using good classroom teaching methodology: 1. Proficiency in using a variety of instructional materials and visual aids effectively. 61.9%	32.60	36.78	1.0198
Obtaining sufficient time for teaching and coaching: 1. Realization that teaching physical education must be given priority over coaching duties. 57% 2. Skill in planning and using time and energy more effectively. 55.7%	30.84	39.21	1.0088
Selecting activities and experiences suited to the needs and interests of the students: 1. Competence in choosing activities that are suited to the needs, interests, growth and maturation level of the pupils. 59.3% 2. Knowledge of individual differences, needs, and interests of the students at this particular age level. 56.4%	32.38	35.02	0.9978
Adjusting to the many interruptions due to excusing and taking students from physical education classes: 1. Ability to implement a stringent and equitable policy regarding the acceptance of excuses for medical reasons. 66.7%	24.67	42.95	0.9229
Providing opportunities for creative experiences: 1. Skill in developing the attitude and confidence necessary for students' creative expression. 61.9% 2. Knowledge of the opportunities for creative expression in physical education. 60.4%	25.11	39.65	0.8987

competencies needed to deal more effectively with each problem (see Table 21-2).

Training experiences

Those students who successfully meet the entrance requirements should pursue a curriculum that includes work in the academic area, foundation science area, professional education area, and specialized area of physical education.

In order to ensure that each prospective teacher receives the preparation that is best suited to his needs, it is necessary to recognize that the curriculum should be flexible to the extent that individual differences are taken into consideration. A blanket requirement for all students should not be listed. Some individuals, for example, may need more work in the academic area and less in the foundation science area, whereas others may need more in the specialized area and less in the academic area. A prospective teacher's capacity, educational background, and interests should be given careful consideration before his program is prescribed. Furthermore, the student should participate in the evaluation of his record and help in planning the prescribed work. The amount of preparation prescribed for each individual should be determined as a result of a study of school records, which takes into consideration the extent and quality of his previous preparation; conferences with the prospective teacher; and standardized tests that meet accepted test criteria and that should be selected by the admissions committee of the college.

EXPERIENCES IN ACADEMIC AREA

Each prospective teacher of physical education should, upon completion of his period of preparation, have a mastery of fundamental elements in the fields of English, fine and practical arts, social sciences, and mathematics.

EXPERIENCES IN FOUNDATION SCIENCE AREA

The content of the foundation science area should be concerned with providing the student with a general education, other than that included in the academic area, and with the basic knowledge in science needed for this specialized field of physical education.

Each prospective teacher of physical education should, upon completion of his period of preparation, have a mastery of certain elements in the fields of physical and biological sciences. In respect to the physical sciences, the prospective teacher of physical education should have a general knowledge of the fields of astronomy, geology, physics, and chemistry. Furthermore, such knowledge should include the development and appreciation of the contributions and limitations of science with a realization that increased knowledge is needed. In respect to the biological sciences, the student should have an appreciation of the principles fundamental to an understanding of the structure, function, and behavior of living things and the relationship and interdependence between plant and animal life. The student should receive a meaningful orientation to the field and discover how closely related and basic it is to the specialized area of physical education.

For those students whose interests, educational background, and time permit, more experiences should be provided in the fields of biology, zoology, and botany.

The biological sciences are basic and closely related to the specialized field of physical education. For this reason certain specified fields of knowledge should be included in this area such as personal and community health, mental health, bacteriology, human anatomy and physiology, and nutrition.

EXPERIENCES IN PROFESSIONAL EDUCATION AREA

The professional education area should be selected in view of the preparation that is needed to instill in the prospective teacher sound educational principles and practices in regard to teaching and learning. It should stress such areas as the following: behavioral sciences, evaluation, internship, and methodology.

EXPERIENCES IN AREA OF SPECIALIZATION

The content of the physical education area should provide the prospective teacher with that specialized knowledge that will be essential for the successful performance of his duties after graduation. These experiences should include work in such areas as philosophy, measurement and evaluation, education and care of the handicapped, applied anatomy and physiology, organization and administration, prevention and emergency care of injuries, health services, and methods and materials for teaching physical education activities.

The experiences just listed represent many of the essential needs of the student training for the physical education profession. Such experiences in a professional curriculum should hopefully help in equipping the physical educator with the necessary knowledge, skill, and competencies to successfully cope with the problems that will arise when he gets on the job and also help him to make an outstanding contribution to the welfare of children and youth.

PROFESSIONAL PHYSICAL EDUCATION CURRICULUMS

Examples of physical education professional curriculums are listed.

Curriculum for men and women

Two professional preparation programs are listed in this section. The first is a curriculum for both men and women desiring to teach at any educational level. The second is designed to prepare for teaching physical education in secondary schools.

FIRST YEAR

	Semester hours
Biology: Introductory Zoology and Botany	8
Oral English	4
Written English	4
Personal and Community Hygiene	2

FIRST YEAR

	Semester hours
Introduction to Psychology	4
Introduction to Camp Leadership	2
Man in Society: The Western Tradition	4
Introduction to Physical Education	2
Music in Physical Education (women)	1

SECOND YEAR

	Semester hours
Mammalian Anatomy and Physiology	8
Introductory Chemistry or Introductory Physics	8
Introduction to Religion and Philosophy	4
Expressive Arts	2 (women) 4 (men)
Community Service Experience	2
Social Science Electives (men)	4
Literature (women)	4
Physical Education in Elementary Schools (women)	2

THIRD YEAR

	Semester hours
Foundation of Education	4
Social Science Electives (women)	4
Educational Psychology	2
First Aid and Safety	2
Analysis of Motion	2
Tests and Measurements in Health Education and Physical Education	4
Physiology of Exercise	2
Administration of the Secondary School Physical Education Curriculum (women)	2
Methods and Materials in Sports (women)	3
Physical Education Methods and Materials (men)	6
Rhythmic Activities (women)	2

THIRD YEAR

	Semester hours
Teaching and Coaching Swimming and Diving (women)	1
Gymnastics Coaching (women)	1
Literature (men)	4
Nonrestricted Elective	2

FOURTH YEAR

	Semester hours
Supervised Student Teaching	10
Physical and Health Inspection	2
Physical Education for Atypical Children	3
Organization and Administration of Physical Education	3
Philosophy and Principles of Physical Education	2
Contemporary Problems	3
Expressive Arts (women)	2
Prevention and Care of Athletic Injuries (men)	2
Organization and Administration of Community Recreation (men)	3
Nonrestricted Elective	3 (women)
	2 (men)

Note: In addition to the above requirements, a total of 16 semester hours of Skills and Techniques courses is required.

Physical education major for teaching in secondary schools

FIRST YEAR

	Semester hours
English	6
Biology	4
Social Science	6
Mathematics	3
Physics	4
Physical Education	2
History and Introduction to Health and Physical Education	2
Team Sports Skills and Techniques	2
Practical Instruction in First Aid Methods	1

SECOND YEAR

	Semester hours
English	2
Social Science	3
Humanities	6
Minor	8
Physical Education	5
Team Sports Skills and Techniques	2
Fundamentals of Dance	2
Electives in Area of Concentration	6

THIRD YEAR

	Semester hours
Humanities	3
Psychology	6
Minor	3
School Health Education	3
Physical Education	6
Anatomy	3
Kinesiology	3
Organization and Administration of Health and Physical Education	2
Programs in Health and Physical Education	2
Introduction to Tests and Measurements in Health and Physical Education	2

FOURTH YEAR

	Semester hours
General Education Courses	19
Adapted and Developmental Physical Education	2
Minor	7
Electives in Area of Concentration	4

ACCREDITATION

Accreditation in the area of professional preparation is a system or evaluation procedure that certifies that certain colleges and universities have approved programs for training physical education teachers. Three ways in which accreditation can take place is by governmental agencies such as state departments of education, regional accrediting agencies such as the Northcentral Association for Colleges and Secondary Schools, and professional associations such as the AAHPER. The American Association for Health, Physical Education, and Recreation has long been interested in accreditation and has tried to develop an effective system. However, it was not until the representative assembly and the board of directors of this association approved recommendations for accreditation that strength was put into the process. The official action provides for such important regulations as the following:

1. The National Council for Accreditation of Teacher Education (NCATE) is the official accrediting organization for physical education, health education, and recreation, and AAHPER recognizes programs approved by NCATE.

2. State departments of education are encouraged to grant teacher certification only to graduates of institutions accredited by NCATE.

3. Professional organizations, such as the American Association of School Administrators, are urged by AAHPER to hire only teachers of health, physical education, and recreation who graduate from institutions accredited by NCATE.

4. Professional membership in AAHPER is contingent upon evidence of an earned bachelor's degree or advanced degrees from institutions accredited by NCATE. Student professional membership is contingent upon attending such institutions. Furthermore, state associations are urged to follow the example set by the national association.

These requirements represent a major stride forward in preparing leaders for physical education who are qualified and adequately prepared for their work.

What does NCATE accreditation mean to the graduate of an accredited school? This is a question that every student should ask. First of all, school and college administrators will be very hesitant to hire any person who has not graduated from an accredited school. Second, it helps in moving from one state to another and taking a position in another section of the country. In fact, some states do not require the applicant to meet all the detailed state certification regulations if he has graduated from a college that has NCATE endorsement. Third, NCATE-endorsed programs are better planned, have higher standards of admission and retention,

better staff, higher professional requirements in general, and render more outstanding professional services to their students and graduates. These are a few reasons why each student and teacher has a personal stake in, and responsibility for, the accreditation of teacher education programs.

CONSIDERATIONS IN SELECTING A COLLEGE PROFESSIONAL PREPARATION PROGRAM IN PHYSICAL EDUCATION

There are many factors that should be taken into consideration when selecting a teacher-training institution to prepare for work in physical education. The institution of higher learning should meet desirable standards as established by the profession. The physical educator's chances for employment and for success on the job will depend, to a great extent, on the experiences and opportunities that are provided during this training period. In order to make an informed decision, some of the factors to be considered when evaluating the training institution are discussed in the following sections.

Selecting teacher-training institution

There are many teacher-training institutions throughout the United States that prepare students for the profession of physical education. However, all the institutions that prepare teachers for this specialized work do not adhere to the highest standards of the profession. A careful analysis of various institutions will acquaint the prospective physical educator with their qualifications for preparing teachers of physical education. Such items as faculty, library facilities, purposes, quality and length of curriculums, accreditation, reputation, and placement are a few of the factors that should be taken into consideration.

Reviewing college entrance requirements

As a general rule, a person desiring to prepare for the teaching of physical education is required to meet college entrance requirements. The standard college preparatory course should be taken by all high school students who want to prepare for this work. Usually this means a minimum of fifteen to sixteen high school units of credit, as defined by the particular state. Frequently, five to ten units of the total number required should be in academic subjects, including English, mathematics, natural science, and social science. Foreign languages are required by an increasing number of teacher-training institutions. There are also general requirements as to character, physical fitness, and personality. Entrance requirements vary from state to state, and interested individuals should consult the institution or institutions in which they are interested.

Analyzing the cost

The cost of preparing for the teaching of physical education varies with the institution. Usually the cost is lower in tax-supported institutions such as state colleges and state universities. The expenses incurred by the student of physical education are similar to those of students preparing in other fields. In most teacher-training institutions it would be wise for the student to set aside approximately $4,000 per year to allow for tuition, board, room, and fees. The actual tuition fee varies from $50 to $100 in some tax-supported institutions to $500 to $3,000 or more in some privately endowed colleges and universities. The student with limited financial resources may supplement his income through scholarships, fellowships, loan funds, and part-time employment. To obtain further information on financial aid, interested persons should contact such places as the college or university of their choice, the U. S. Office of Education, the State Department of Education where the person is a resident, and the American Association for Health, Physical Education, and Recreation.

Recognizing the need for college preparation

A college degree should be held by all who plan to make a career of physical edu-

cation. Without this minimum preparation there will be few opportunities for employment. At the present time most college and university courses are 4 years in length, but in some states, such as New York and California, the period is equal to 5 years for high school teaching. Furthermore, the trend is more and more in the direction of an extended period of training. The degree usually granted at the end of the 4-year period is that of Bachelor of Science, Bachelor of Science in Education, or Bachelor of Arts. The Master of Education or Master of Arts degree is frequently granted at the end of the fifth year of training.

GRADUATE WORK

Graduate work in all areas of education is receiving increased emphasis. Some of the developments in this area stress that graduate students should be very carefully selected on the basis of their educational backgrounds, degree of motivation, intellectual competence, and maturity. In most cases, the student should be prepared for advanced study by having a good grounding in his specialty. Graduate courses normally extend beyond the undergraduate experiences and are concerned with experiences concerned with principles, history, philosophy, and research, rather than skills and techniques. A feature that should be common to all graduate courses is the emphasis upon mature thinking, extensive reading, and original work. Also, graduate courses should be research oriented. They should examine the research in various fields of study and critically evaluate its worth to the program.

Professional preparation is a continuous process. It does not end with commencement and the conferring of the bachelor's degree. It continues throughout one's professional career. The next step in improving qualifications for physical education work after leaving the undergraduate ranks is graduate study toward advanced degrees. In order, these usually are the master's degree, sixth-year or professional certificate, and doctor's degree. The master's degree usually requires the equivalent of 1 full year's work above the bachelor's degree; the sixth-year or professional certificate requires 1 full year beyond the master's; and the doctor's degree varies usually from 2 to 3 years beyond the sixth-year or professional certificate. Frequently, physical educators omit the sixth-year or professional certificate and work directly on the doctor's degree following the conferring of the master's degree.

Graduate work offers opportunities such as getting help in solving many practical problems that exist in the field, increasing one's knowledge and skills as a teacher, doing research, studying under some leader in the field, specializing in some facet of the physical education program in which one is interested, improving one's general education, and obtaining a better understanding of the total educational picture.

In addition to the educational improvement that accrues to the graduate student, there are also material benefits. Some states grant provisional certificates after graduation from undergraduate programs and then permanent certification after a certain number of graduate credit hours have been taken. Most school systems recognize graduate work in their salary schedules so that, with additional professional preparation, there is increased income.

The student who finds that additional financial aid is needed to pursue graduate work should investigate four kinds of financial aid:

FELLOWSHIPS. Many graduate schools in physical education offer grants of money for further study. This grant may include teaching some activity in a college service physical education program or doing some form of work as a means of obtaining aid.

SCHOLARSHIPS. An outright grant of money for graduate work not requiring service or repayment is termed a scholarship. These are awarded to outstanding physical educators who have demonstrated merit and leadership qualities and who require financial assistance to pursue graduate study.

GRANT-IN-AID. A grant-in-aid is usually thought of as an outright grant of money for a specialized purpose. For example, it could be given to a graduate student to work on a specific research project in physical education.

LOANS. Colleges, universities, state governments, banks, and the national government offer loans to students at moderately low interest rates to pay for educational needs.

A person going into physical education work and desiring to have a successful career should take some graduate work in his special field. It will assist him in his personal growth and in rendering a greater service.

QUESTIONS AND EXERCISES

1. Prepare a list of criteria that you would recommends as a means of selecting a teacher-training institution in preparing for physical education work.
2. Draw up a list of training experiences that you feel are essential in preparing for work in physical education.
3. How is it possible for a student with limited financial resources to go to college?
4. What is meant by the academic, foundation science, professional education, and specialized areas of preparation?
5. Prepare a chart showing the essential preparation that should take place in each of the academic, foundation science, professional education, and specialized areas.
6. Why is it important for the physical educator to have preparation in each of the following areas: English, fine and practical arts, social sciences, mathematics, modern languages, and physical sciences?
7. What are some of the subdivisions of biological science that are especially important for the teacher of physical education?
8. Why are many experiences needed in the professional education area?
9. Show how training in the following will be of help to you out on the job: measurement and evaluation, education and care of the handicapped, applied anatomy and physiology, organization and administration, prevention and emergency care of injuries, methods and materials, and school health problems.
10. What are the current developments in teacher education especially applicable to the teacher of physical education?
11. Make a list of as many reasons as possible to show the need for a general education.
12. Write an essay on the implications of the statement, "Those who can, do; those who can't, teach," in regard to physical education skills.

13. How will a knowledge of the community help you to perform a better job in teaching physical education?

Reading assignment

Bucher, Charles A., and Goldman, Myra: Dimensions of physical education, St. Louis, 1969, The C. V. Mosby Co., Reading selections 62 and 70.

SELECTED REFERENCES

American Association for Health, Physical Education, and Recreation: Professional preparation of the elementary school physical education teacher, Washington, D. C., 1969, The Association.

American Association for Health, Physical Education, and Recreation: Professional preparation in health education, physical education, and recreation education, Washington, D. C., 1962, The Association.

American Association for Health, Physical Education, and Recreation: Self-evaluation check list for graduate programs, Washington, D. C., 1969, The Association.

Astin, Alexander W.: Folklore of selectivity, the challenge to open admissions, Saturday Review, December 20, 1969.

Beggs, Walter K.: The education of teachers, New York, 1965, The Library of Education, The Center for Applied Research in Education, Inc.

Bucher, Charles A.: Administration of health and physical education programs including athletics, St. Louis, 1971, The C. V. Mosby Co.

Bucher, Charles A.: A professional curriculum in health and physical education for the State Teachers College at New Haven, Connecticut, doctoral thesis, 1948, New York University.

Bucher, Charles A., and Reade, Evelyn M.: Physical education and health in the elementary school, New York, 1971, The Macmillan Co.

Campbell, Ronald F.: Tomorrow's teacher, Saturday Review, January 14, 1967.

Conant, James Bryant: The education of American teachers, New York, 1963, McGraw-Hill Book Co.

Esslinger, Arthur A.: Professional preparation, Journal of Health, Physical Education, and Recreation 37:63, 1966.

Harvard Committee: Report. General education in a free society, Cambridge, 1945, Harvard University Press.

Hetherington, Clark W.: Professional education in physical education, Journal of Health and Physical Education 5:3, 1934.

National Conference on Undergraduate, Professional Preparation in Physical Education, Health Education, and Recreation, Jackson's Mill, Weston, West Virginia, May 16-27, 1948: Report, Chicago, 1948, The Athletic Institute.

Pearson, George B.: Trends in professional preparation for physical education in three districts of the AAHPER, Proceedings, National College Physical Education Association, 1964.

Professional preparation for health, physical education, and recreation, a special journal feature prepared by the AAHPER Professional Preparation Panel, Journal of Health, Physical Education, and Recreation 35:31, 1964.

Richardson, Deane E.: Professional preparation, Journal of Health, Physical Education, and Recreation 36:71, 1965.

Teacher education; special feature, NEA Journal 57:14, 1968.

Teeple, Janet: Graduate study in physcial education, Quest (Monograph XII), Spring issue, May, 1969, p. 66.

PART SEVEN

The profession

22/Professional organizations

23/Certification requirements for employment in physical education

24/Employment opportunities

25/Challenges facing physical education

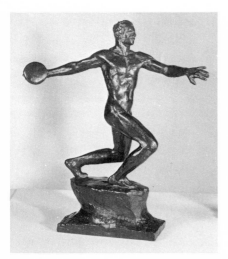

WORK OF R. TAIT
MCKENZIE. COURTESY
JOSEPH BROWN, SCHOOL OF
ARCHITECTURE, PRINCETON
UNIVERSITY.

22 / Professional organizations*

A survey of the field of physical education indicates the prevalence of many professional organizations. Such an imposing list of associations shows the field to be wide in scope and important in nature. These societies exist for specific purposes, and these purposes have a bearing on the work, welfare, and public appraisal of the physical educator. All physical educators should belong to their state and national associations and to others, as far as it is practical and possible. The fact that many physical educators do not belong to their national association, for example, is indicated by statistics that show there are probably more than 200,000 persons in the field today and approximately 50,000 members of the national association. Yet the thousands who are not members accept, experience, and participate in the advances, better working conditions, and benefits that the association has accomplished. This should not be the case. If all physical educators belonged to and worked for their professional organizations, the concerted effort of such a large professional group would result in greater benefits and more prestige for the profession.

The physical educator should become familiar with the role of professional organizations in his work. He should realize that these associations promote professional ethics, scholarship, leadership, and high educational standards. They are interested in doing more than just improving a member's personal welfare, although this is definitely

accomplished. Professional organizations such as the American Association for Health, Physical Education, and Recreation are also interested in developing a healthier, more physically fit, more democratic, and more intelligent citizenry. They seek to enrich the lives of people everywhere. They need help in accomplishing these noble purposes. If all practitioners unite and work together, there is a great future for physical education.

WHY BELONG TO A PROFESSIONAL ASSOCIATION?

There are many advantages in belonging to a professional organization. This is especially true of associations that give their strength and support to worthwhile programs of education. The publications, meetings, workshops, seminars, and social occasions represent a few of the benefits that can be derived. Factors that every physical educator should recognize about membership in professional associations include the following:

1. *They provide opportunities for service.* Through the many offices, committee responsibilities, and program functions that professional associations provide, the individual has an opportunity to render a service for the betterment of his field of work.

2. *They provide a channel of communication.* Communication in a profession is essential in order that members may know about what is going on, the latest developments in teaching techniques, new emphases in program content, and many other trends

---

*International professional organizations are discussed in Chapter 14.

that are happening continuously in a growing profession. Through associations, an effective channel of communication exists via the publications, meetings, and announcements that are periodically made.

3. *They provide a means for interpreting the profession.* There is a need to interpret one's profession to the public on national, state, and local levels. This interpretation is essential if public support is to be achieved for the services rendered by the professional practitioner. The professional association provides an opportunity for the best thinking and ideas to be articulately interpreted far and wide. Through such endeavors, recognition, respect, prestige, and cooperation with other areas of education, professions, and the public in general can be achieved.

4. *They provide a source of help in solving one's professional and personal problems.* Each physical educator has problems, both professional and personal. Through their officers, members, conferences, and other media, professional associations, can play an important role in solving these problems. If a person is a member of an association he does not "go it alone" but, instead, is surrounded by professional help on all sides. These groups are interested in helping and rendering a service. The associations can be of assistance, for example, in solving a professional problem involving the administration of an adapted program or a personal problem of life insurance.

5. *They provide an opportunity for fellowship.* Through association conferences and meetings the physical educator gets to know others doing similar work, and this common denominator results in friendships and many enjoyable professional and social occasions. A person literally gets a "shot in the arm" by associating with other persons dedicated to the same field of endeavor.

6. *They provide an organ for research.* Professions must continually conduct research to determine how effective their programs are, how many contributions they are rendering to human beings, how valid their techniques are, and the answers to many other questions that must be known if the

profession is to move ahead and render an increasingly larger service.

7. *They yield a feeling of belonging.* A basic psychological need is to have a feeling of being part of a group and accomplishing work that is recognized and important. A professional association can contribute much in meeting this human need.

8. *They provide a means for distributing costs.* The work accomplished by a professional association is designed to help the members who belong to the association. The work accomplished requires financial means. By joining a professional association, a physical educator helps to share the expenses that he rightfully has the responsibility to share. If he participates in the benefits, he should also want to share in the costs of achieving these benefits.

PROFESSIONAL ORGANIZATIONS

It would be difficult to discuss all of the organizations that pertain to the physical education profession. However, some of these organizations with which the physical educator should be familiar are discussed. Items concerned with the history, purpose, membership, organization, and publications of these organizations are considered in order to give the reader a brief description of these associations.

Amateur athletic union*

The Amateur Athletic Union (AAU) was founded in 1888. Its principal aim at that time was to protect amateur sports from being corrupted by unscrupulous athletes who, by such means as "fixed" games, side betting, and competing for money, were using amateur sports as a medium of profit. The leaders of the newly founded AAU proceeded to set down a clear definition of amateurism and established clear-cut standards that outlawed unscrupulous practices. Today, the AAU is the largest and most influential organization governing amateur

*Some of the following information is taken from You and the AAU, leaflet published by the Amateur Athletic Union, Indianapolis, Indiana.

sports in the world. It serves as the governing body in the United States for seventeen amateur sports: basketball, baton twirling, bobsledding, boxing, gymnastics, handball, horseshoe pitching, judo, luge, skibobbing, swimming and diving, synchronized swimming, trampoline, water polo, weight lifting, and wrestling.

The objectives of the AAU include:

1. The encouragement and development of amateur sport and physical fitness
2. Maintaining integrity in competition
3. Making facilities and opportunities available to all
4. Providing the best possible contestants to represent America in international competition

The AAU is composed of fifty-six associations serving 206,000 registered athletes. Its program of athletics reaches 12 million people under the supervision of 100,000 volunteers throughout the country.

The activities of the AAU are many and varied. It sponsors many adult programs, including fitness classes, and has developed an isometric fitness development program as well as a physical fitness and proficiency test. The AAU conducts pre-Olympic trials to aid with the selection of competitors. Today, as in the past, the AAU is involved in raising funds for the participation of American athletes in the Olympics. The AAU is the official representative of the United States in many international sports federations. Since 1949, it has sponsored an annual Junior Olympics for boys and girls between the ages of 9 and 17.

The AAU is directed by a Board of Governors elected from delegates representing the fifty-six associations. These officers serve without compensation. The paid employees of the AAU are the Executive Director and a staff of twenty-two administrators, clerks, and secretaries.

The list of AAU publications includes *Amateur Athlete,* a monthly magazine; *Directory of the AAU,* published annually; *Official AAU Handbook;* various sports guides and records; as well as rule books for the sports it governs.

Headquarters are at 3400 West 86th Street, Indianapolis, Indiana 46268.

American Academy of Physical Education

The American Academy of Physical Education was established "to advance knowledge, raise standards, and bestow honors in the field of physical education, health education, and recreation." This Association was established in 1930, and Clark W. Hetherington, R. Tait McKenzie, Thomas Storey, William Burdick, and Jay B. Nash were the first members.

Individuals are elected to membership in this Association as a result of such qualifications as making significant contributions to these specialized fields through research, writing, or exceptional service, providing trust funds for research purposes, recruiting promising students, making awards for outstanding contribution to these fields, sponsoring legislation, and spreading information of note from other countries. The principal types of fellows or memberships are designated active and associate fellows, fellows in memoriam, associate fellows (in the United States), and corresponding fellows (from other countries). The dues are $15 per year.

The Academy is committed to the function of furthering scholarship and excellence in the field of physical education. Through its meetings and work it provides an avenue of communication for new ideas and creative thinking, not only among leaders in the United States but throughout the world as well. It confers awards for excellent literary, administrative, and research contributions to individuals and citations to organizations or institutions.

In a publication entitled *Professional Contributions,* the Academy publishes, from time to time, papers presented by fellows, position statements, studies developed for and by the Academy, and the R. Tait McKenzie Memorial Lecture presented at its annual meetings.*

---

*Constitution and By-Laws, February, 1969.

For more information write to the Academy, care of Department of Physical Education, Sacramento State College, Sacramento, California 95819.

American Association for Health, Physical Education, and Recreation*

The American Association for Health, Physical Education, and Recreation (AAHPER) was established in 1885 under the title of American Association for Advancement of Physical Education. The leaders in this initial organization were some thirty-five physicians, educators, and other individuals. They were called together by Dr. William G. Anderson, then on the staff of Adelphi Academy. Other physical education leaders who were prominent in the early history of the Association were Dr. Hitchcock of Amherst, Dr. Sargent of Harvard, Dr. Gulick of the Young Men's Christian Association, Dr. Arnold of Arnold College, and Dr. Savage of Oberlin College. In 1903 the name of the Association was changed to American Physical Education Association. In 1937 the Departments of School Health and Physical Education of the National Education Association were combined to form the American Association for Health and Physical Education, a department of the National Education Association. In 1938 the term *recreation* was added to the title of the Association.

The six districts of the American Association for Health, Physical Education, and Recreation and the states or areas that come under each of these divisions are as follows:

Central district
- Colorado
- Iowa   Nebraska
- Kansas   North Dakota
- Minnesota   South Dakota
- Missouri   Wyoming

Eastern district
- Connecticut

---

*Some of the information in this section was taken from American Association for Health, Physical Education, and Recreation: This is AAHPER, Washington, D. C., 1969, The Association.

Eastern district—cont'd
- Delaware   New Jersey
- District of Columbia   New York
- Maine   Pennsylvania
- Maryland   Puerto Rico
- Massachusetts   Rhode Island
- New Hampshire   Vermont

Northwest district
- Alaska
- Idaho   Oregon
- Montana   Washington

Southern district
- Alabama
- Arkansas   North Carolina
- Florida   Oklahoma
- Georgia   South Carolina
- Kentucky   Tennessee
- Louisiana   Texas
- Mississippi   Virginia

Midwest district
- Illinois   Ohio
- Indiana   West Virginia
- Michigan   Wisconsin

Southwest district
- Arizona   Nevada
- California   New Mexico
- Hawaii   Utah

The national office of the American Association for Health, Physical Education, and Recreation is located at 1201 16th Street N.W., Washington, D. C. 20036.

The publications of the Association are many and varied. Starting in 1896, the *American Physical Education Review* was the official publication. This was discontinued in 1929 when it was combined with the *Pentathlon,* the publication of the Middle West Society of Physical Education. Then, the new publication of the Association became known as the *Journal of Health and Physical Education.* This periodical is known at the present time as the *Journal of Health, Physical Education, and Recreation.* The Association also publishes the *Research Quarterly,* a magazine devoted to research in health, physical education, and recreation; *AAHPER Update,* which features news about the Association; and *School Health Review,* a quarterly periodical related to the needs of health educators. In addition, it publishes many other pamphlets, books and materials pertinent to the work of the Association.

The services performed by the Association are numerous. Some are listed here:

1. The American Association, with its membership of more than 50,000, the largest organization of its kind in the world, influences professional standards.
2. State, district, and national conventions are held periodically.
3. The Association serves as a clearinghouse for information on positions in health, physical education, and recreation.
4. Pamphlets, brochures, reprints, bibliographies, and conference and convention reports are made available.
5. Individual and group sports guides are published by the Association for the Division on Girls' and Women's Sports.
6. The American Association for Health, Physical Education, and Recreation, as a democratic organization, influences public opinion.
7. Field service is given on professional problems in health, physical education, and recreation.
8. The Association serves in a consulting capacity to the President's Council on Physical Fitness and Sports and cooperates with the Council in administering the Presidential Physical Fitness Awards to students who demonstrate exceptional physical performance.
9. AAHPER headquarters staff specialists provide consultation and field services in the various areas of Association concern.
10. Responsive to the new school and research support programs of the federal government, AAHPER is undertaking an increasingly vigorous legislative program, working with legislators as well as relaying information on the programs to members.

Location of AAHPER headquarters at the NEA Center in Washington, D. C., enables officers and staff to represent health, physical education, athletics, and recreation in the conferences and projects of general education and to cooperate with more than thirty other specialized NEA departments.

Members of the Association are designated as professional members, associate members, fellows, life members, life fellows, student members, honorary members, emeritus members, and contributing members.

Professional members are persons working actively in one of the specialized fields of the association; associate members are those persons not professionally engaged in one of the specialized fields. Fellows, life fellows, and life members are the same as professional members with the exception of dues payment and variety of publications received. Student members include students attending professional and teacher education institutions preparing for one or more of the specialized fields in the Association. Honorary members are persons outside of the professions but who, because of unusual interest and meritorious services, are nominated to membership. Emeritus membership is open to those who have reached a certain age and meet other criteria. A contributing member is one who has contributed the annual payment of $100 or more to the Association.

The annual dues for professional members are $25 and $15; associate members, $20 and $15; fellows, $20 and $15; and student members, $10 and $5.

American College of Sports Medicine

On April 23, 1954, a few outstanding leaders in the fields of medicine, physiology, and physical education met in New York City and founded the American College of Sports Medicine (ACSM). The purposes this group set forth for the association are as follows:

1. To promote and advance scientific studies dealing with the effect of sports and other motor activities on the health of human beings at various stages of life
2. To cooperate with other organizations concerned with various aspects of human fitness
3. To sponsor meetings of physicians, educators, and other scientists whose work is relevant to sports medicine
4. To make available postgraduate education in fields related to the objectives of the College
5. To initiate, encourage, and correlate research
6. To publish a journal dealing with scientific aspects of activity and their relationship to human fitness
7. To establish and maintain a sports medicine library

American Association for Health, Physical Education, and Recreation
More than 50,000 members
A national affiliate of the National Education Association
and member of the International Council on
Health, Physical Education, and Recreation

LOCAL ASSOCIATIONS

STATE ASSOCIATIONS
53 with Guam, Puerto Rico,
and District of Columbia

DISTRICT ASSOCIATIONS

Central	Eastern
Midwest	Northwest
Southern	Southwest

REPRESENTATIVE ASSEMBLY
(Approx. 364 members)

State association delegates (increases according to AAHPER members in each state)
Division representatives   District presidents
Board of directors
Affiliated organization representatives (nonvoting)

Affiliated
organizations
(24)

BOARD OF DIRECTORS

President
President-elect
Past President
District representatives (6)
Vice-Presidents and Division Chairmen (8)
Chairman, Finance Committee (nonvoting)
Parliamentarian (nonvoting)
Executive Secretary-Treasurer (nonvoting)

EXECUTIVE SECRETARY-TREASURER

COMMITTEES

Standing
President's
Continuing
Joint or
   representational

Professional preparation
panel

**ASSOCIATE EXECUTIVE SECRETARY
FOR ADMINISTRATION**

Coordinator of Office Services
Director of
   Business Operations
      Accounting
      Publications-Sales
Coordinator of Convention
   and Advertising
Director of Information
Director of Membership Records
Program Assistant
   for Promotion
      Membership
      Publications
Director of Publications
   JOHPER
   Research Quarterly
   School Health Review
   Books/pamphlets/others
Director of Archives and Records Center

**ASSOCIATE EXECUTIVE SECRETARY
FOR PROGRAM**

Assistant executive secretaries
   and consultants for:
      Dance and General Division
      Elementary Education
      International Development
      Physical Education and Girls' and
         Women's Sports
      Physical Education and
         Men's Athletics
      Programs for the Handicapped
      Recreation and Outdoor Education
      Research (Acting)
      School Health and Safety Education
      School Nurses
Consultant for Student Services
Eastern States Regional Coordinator
Western States Regional Coordinator
Directors of special projects:
      Lifetime Sports Education Project
      Man's Environment Project
      Outdoor Education Project
      Smoking and Health Education Project

DIVISIONS*

Dance Division
Division for Girls' and
   Women's Sports (DGWS)
Division of Men's Athletics
   (DMA)
General Division
Physical Education Division
Recreation Division
Safety Education Division
School Health Division
*Assistant executive
   secretaries serve as
   consultants to the
   divisions.

Organization chart of American Association for Health, Physical Education, and Recreation
(revised), November, 1969.

Current membership in the organization consisted of 1,638 persons on April 2, 1970. There are representatives of nearly every state in the Union, as well as of twenty-one foreign countries. Of the three membership categories (medicine, physiology, physical education), the most numerous is physical education, with medicine being a close second. This listing of specialties within the ACSM is a clear indication that the College is an organization of many disciplines and is concerned with the many facets of the science and medicine of sports.*

The College is affiliated with the Fédération Internationale de Médicine Sportive, an organization that has played an important role for many years in Europe and South America. The official publication of the International Federation of Sports Medicine and hence of the College is the *Journal of Sports Medicine and Physical Fitness,* which is published in Italy but printed in the English language with French, Italian, and English summaries.

In addition, in 1969, the ACSM published an important work, many years in preparation, the *Encyclopedia of Sports Medicine.* This is a comprehensive volume consisting of 1,300 manuscripts by experts in the field. Also in 1969, the College began publication of a periodical entitled *Science and Medicine in Sports.* Included in this publication are research articles on such topics as athletic medicine, biomechanics, clinical medicine, growth and development, physiology, psychology, and sociology.*

The activities of the College and the research papers cover such topics as the treatment and prevention of athletic injuries, the effects of physical activity on health, and the scientific aspects of training.

The constitution of the American College of Sports Medicine provides for various types of membership. They are listed with the annual dues for each as follows; fellows ($20), members ($20), student members ($10), fellows emeriti (no dues), and honorary fellows (no dues).*

The American College of Sports Medicine has its national office at the University of Wisconsin, 1440 Monroe Street, 3062 Stadium, Madison, Wisconsin 53706.

American Corrective Therapy Association

The American Corrective Therapy Association (ACTA), formerly the Association for Physical and Mental Rehabilitation, is a nationwide professional organization operated for educational and scientific purposes.

The Association was formally organized in October, 1946, by a group of corrective therapists attending a special course of instruction at the Veterans Administration Hospital, Topeka, Kansas.

In 1969, the name of the organization was changed to the American Corrective Therapy Association.†

The objectives, as listed in the Association's constitution, are:

1. To promote the use of medically prescribed exercise therapy and adapted physical education
2. To advance the professional standards of education and training in the field of medically prescribed exercise therapy and adapted physical education
3. To promote and sponsor medically prescribed exercise therapy programs of the highest scientific and professional character
4. To encourage research and publication of scientific articles dealing with medical rehabilitation
5. To engage in and encourage those activities related to medically prescribed activity that might prove advantageous to medical rehabilitation and/or the Association

Membership in the American Corrective Therapy Association is divided into four categories:

1. *Active* ($26)‡—for those actively engaged in corrective or exercise therapy working

---

*American College of Sports Medicine Newsletter, vol. 4, no. 3, July, 1969.

*Constitution and By-Laws, 1969.

†Information taken from a letter from Kermit Rhea, Executive Director.

‡Information taken from membership application.

under the supervision of a licensed physician, whether in hospitals, schools, rehabilitation clinics, or colleges, and who meet the standards set up by the Professional Standards Committee of the Association

2. *Professional* ($8.50)—for those persons working in allied professional fields who wish to share and contribute to the educational and scientific progress of the Association
3. *Associate* ($8.50)—for those persons interested in the work of corrective therapy and who wish to receive the *Journal* and other pertinent information relating to Association matters
4. *Student*—for students enrolled in accredited schools of health and physical education

Through its recruitment and placement committee, the Association has much to offer its membership in the following areas of rehabilitation employment:

1. *Active* ($26)‡—for those actively engaged public and private schools, colleges, and universities
2. Special schools and camps for handicapped and atypical children
3. Government, public, and private rehabilitation clinics and hospitals: general medicine and surgery, neuropsychiatric, and domiciliary
4. Armed services hospitals
5. Nursing homes
6. Recreational programs for the handicapped
7. Research

The Association publishes the *Journal of American Corrective Therapy,** formerly the *Journal of the Association for Physical and Mental Rehabilitation,* which is a bimonthly magazine that contains information on education and scientific research; an *Information Bulletin;* and the yearly *Association Brochure.*

The American Corrective Therapy Association is located at 1222 South Ridgeland Avenue, Berwyn, Illinois 60402.

American School Health Association

The American School Health Association (ASHA) is interested in improving health services, health instruction, and healthful living in the nation's schools. It was organized October 13, 1926,† as the American Association of School Physicians, and for some time only physicians were eligible to become members of that Association. The number of persons who belonged to the organization in its early years was small, but the Association grew very rapidly. In 1929 the membership was 494. In 1946 it was more than 2,000. Currently, it is approximately 20,000.*

In 1927 the Association's name was changed to the School Physicians Association and a journal was published called the *School Physicians' Bulletin.* In 1937 the name of the organization was changed again to the American School Health Association. The membership requirements were broadened to include not only physicians but also dentists, nurses, nutritionists, public health workers, and others whose professional training included the premedical sciences and who were engaged in school health work. During this transition period, the name of the official publication was changed from the *School Physicians' Bulletin* to the *Journal of School Health.*

The American School Health Association works very closely with the American Public Health Association. Annual meetings are held jointly, and ideas are exchanged at this time. Much of the work performed by the Association is done through committees.

The dues are $15 per year, which includes the *Journal of School Health.* This periodical is published ten times each year and contains professional activities pertinent to the medical health professions; reviews of books, reports, and studies; abstracts of current literature; queries and answers; editorials on matters pertinent to school health work; and other material of value to anyone interested in health. The annual dues also include the *ASHA Newsletter* a quarterly publication.

Membership in the Association, in addition to providing a subscription to the *Journal,* offers other advantages, including informational service and the opportunity to help in promoting higher standards for the

---

*Association brochure.

†Information taken from Program, November 13, 1968.

*ASHA Newsletter no. 2, April, 1970.

The American School Health Association
— Organization Chart —

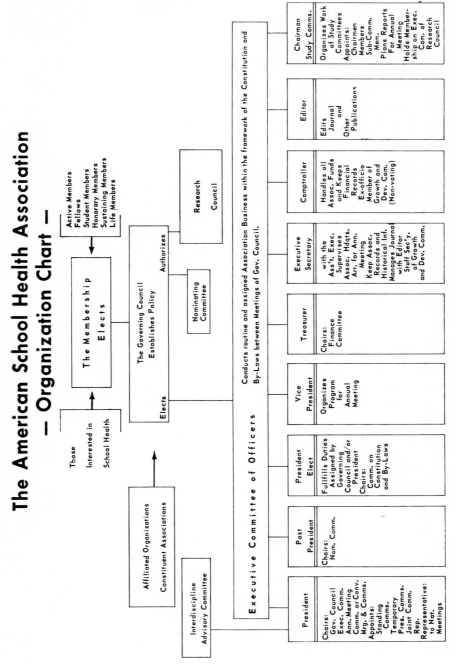

FROM JOURNAL OF SCHOOL HEALTH 39:282, 1969.

profession and to participate in other work to advance the profession. The address of the American School Health Association is ASHA Building, P.O. Box 416, Kent, Ohio 44240.*

Canadian Association for Health, Physical Education, and Recreation

The Canadian Association for Health, Physical Education, and Recreation (CAHPER) was organized originally as the Canadian Physical Education Association in 1933 through the joint efforts of the Quebec Physical Education Association and the Toronto Physical Education Association. The "father" of physical education in Canada was the late Dr. Arthur S. Lamb of McGill University, which was the alma mater of Dr. James Naismith and Dr. R. Tait McKenzie.

In 1948 the Association changed its name to the Canadian Association for Health, Physical Education, and Recreation. In 1951 it became an incorporated body, the original signing officers being John Lang, Iveagh Munro, and Gordon Wright, three outstanding Canadian physical educators. The constitution of the Association was given a major revision in 1960 under the chairmanship of Dr. M. L. Howell of Alberta, Canada.

The aims of the Association are as follows:

1. To encourage the improvement of the standards of those engaged in the furtherance of health education, physical education, and recreation
2. To provide such means of promotion as will service the establishment of adequate programs under the direction of approved leadership
3. To stimulate a wide, intelligent, and active interest in health education, physical education, and recreation
4. To acquire and disseminate accurate information concerning it
5. To cooperate with kindred interests and organizations in the furtherance of these aims

Yearly dues in the Canadian Association

for Health, Physical Education, and Recreation are $15 for a fellow membership, $10 for a professional membership, $10 for an associate membership, and $3 for student memberships. The address of CAHPER is 703 Spadina Avenue, Toronto 4, Ontario, Canada.

The publication of the CAHPER is the *Journal of the Canadian Association for Health, Physical Education, and Recreation.* It is published six times a year. The membership of the Association has increased to about 1,200 with each province of Canada having representation. The Association meets biennially.

College Sports Information Directors of America*

The College Sports Information Directors of America (SIDS) was formed in 1956 after separating from the American College Public Relations Association. The primary objectives of the organization include standardizing sport statistics, press box procedures and routines, and score books. The organization is composed of individuals in college and university sports information departments, public relations departments, and news bureaus.

Together with Football Writers Association of America, SIDS holds an annual workshop in Chicago in conjunction with the All-Stars football game. This organization also meets in January with the annual NCAA convention.

Some of the activities sponsored by SIDS include the sponsorship of university and college division and academic all-American football, basketball, and baseball teams. The SIDS gives the Jake Wade Award annually to a person associated with the communication media for outstanding work in covering or working with colleges. SIDS also supports the Helms Hall Foundation and Hall of Fame and annually makes awards to individuals named to the Helms Hall of Fame by SIDS.

---

*ASHA Newsletter no. 2, April, 1970.

*Information from a letter by Mr. Robert Culp, Secretary-Treasurer of SIDS.

In 1969, the organization together with the Spencer Advertising Company, published a Directory of College Sports Information Directors of America. SIDS also publishes a monthly *News-Digest.*

Presently, there are more than 600 members; included in this number are about fifty associate members. The dues of the active members are $5 per year and for associate members, $10 per year.

For more information write to Robert Culp, Western Michigan University, Kalamazoo, Michigan 49001.

Delta Psi Kappa

Delta Psi Kappa is a professional organization for women majors or minors in health, physical education, and recreation. The purpose of this organization is to stimulate fellowship among women in these specialized fields, to promote high educational standards, and to promote opportunities and mutual service among the women in these professions.

Delta Psi Kappa was founded in 1916 with thirteen members and was incorporated by the state of Indiana. Chapters have gradually been established in various colleges and universities throughout the United States, and alumnae organizations have been set up in some cities. Meetings of this fraternity are held biennially, and since all the work of this fraternity cannot be accomplished at these meetings, a great percentage of it is performed by the Grand Council of seven members.

Through various funds and wards, Delta Psi Kappa helps to stimulate high educational standards, and worthwhile projects. It supports an Educational Loan Fund for promising members who wish to use it for study. It also has a biennial Research Fellowship Fund that is used to make an award to a woman doing some outstanding research in health, physical education, and recreation.

Delta Psi Kappa promotes national and chapter projects. For example, in 1939 many pieces of equipment were presented to the Nashville, Tennessee, Home for Crippled Children. The various chapters of the organization also carry on worthwhile projects, such as sponsoring radio programs, maintaining hospital beds, and conducting playdays.

The official publication of Delta Psi Kappa is *The Foil,* which is published semiannually. *The Foil* contains news and articles from various chapters, contributions from outstanding leaders in the profession, and workshop and book reviews. The fraternity also publishes a newsletter semiannually entitled *The Psi Kap Shield.**

As stated previously, membership in Delta Psi Kappa is limited to women in major departments of health, physical education, and recreation. The school, however, must meet the standards established by the American Association for Health, Physical Education, and Recreation. These are as follows:

1. Be an accredited member of a recognized association of higher educational institutions
2. Be listed by the state department of education as approved for the training of health and physical education teachers for secondary schools
3. Have established an organized curriculum of health education and physical education
4. Have an efficient student health service program
5. Require a minimum of 4 years for completion of preparation for teaching in secondary schools
6. Conduct recreational activities including physical education programs

A minimum of ten women must constitute a group petitioning the national organization for membership. There are six kinds of membership: active, alumnae, inactive, honorary, alumnae associate, and active associate.

The address of Delta Psi Kappa is N. 70W, 1704 Faun Avenue, Menomonee Falls, Wisconsin 53051.

---

*Robsons, John, editor: Baird's manual of American college fraternities, ed. 18, Menash, Wisconsin, 1968, The Collegiate Press, George Banta Co. Inc., pp. 543-544.

National Association
of Intercollegiate Athletics

The National Association of Intercollegiate Athletics (NAIA) is a group of colleges and universities organized for the purpose of attacking cooperatively the problems that face them in the administration of a sound, challenging intercollegiate athletic program.

The organization has grown from a membership of approximately thirty institutions in 1940 to over 554 in 1970. The Association has thirty-four affiliated conferences. It is recognized as a "small college" organization. The enrollment of the institutions in this organization ranges from a few colleges, with under 200 students, to many institutions, with enrollment between 3,000 and 6,500 students. The average enrollment of the institutions with the NAIA, however, is approximately 1,172 students.

Within the membership are all types of institutions, from the private college and university, of which many are controlled and financed by religious denominations, to the state college and university.

Membership in the NAIA is based on the size of the undergraduate male enrollment of the member college and is on a sliding scale. Full membership is from $50 to $150, while associate membership ranges from $30 to $90.

The objectives of this Association as stated in its constitution are the following:

1. To establish a code of ethics and standards for the best interests of athletics
2. To establish uniform officiating and interpretation of rules
3. To establish uniformity of equipment
4. To issue a monthly bulletin throughout the school year devoted to furthering of NAIA and intercollegiate athletics
5. To cooperate with other national or state organizations in standardizing rules
6. To establish an eligibility code which is in conformity with the best interests of intercollegiate athletics
7. To take united and prompt action against any of the evils which may creep up to prevent the proper development of intercollegiate athletics and NAIA
8. To establish working committees and cooperate in the solution to problems for the improvement of intercollegiate athletics and NAIA. A few of these problems would include:
   A. Selection of officials for National Tournaments and Meets
   B. Establishing uniformity of procedures in districts throughout the organization
9. To publicize our national association throughout the United States by means of press, radio, motion picture, television, and any other medium which seems wise
10. To carry on research projects in athletics through the NAIA in order to assist in the over-all development of the athletic sports
11. To constantly seek to expand and enlarge the activities and the influence of NAIA
12. To set up committees for the purpose of carrying out any objectives deemed necessary by the Executive Committee and secretary to furtherance of NAIA
13. To establish strong and functioning district committees, aiding these districts in every way possible with respect to organization, and so far as practicable to determine the best method of carrying on the activities of the district and selecting the best team to represent the district at the National Championship Sports
14. To establish and use every means possible for the improvement of public relations between NAIA, the general public, and other sports groups
15. To establish a financial structure which will be sound for future growth, which will allow full expenses to all participating teams and an added amount of activities necessary to the development of NAIA and intercollegiate sports

The NAIA has a national office in the Aladdin Hotel, 106 West 12th Street, Kansas City, Missouri 64105.

National Association of Physical
Education for College Women

The National Association of Physical Education for College Women, although formally organized in 1924, had its beginning before this time. In 1909 Miss Amy Morris Homans issued an invitation to directors of physical education to meet at Wellesley College. This group continued to meet annually after this first meeting with Miss Homans and gradually grew into the Eastern Society, which was organized in 1915. Later, in 1917 and 1921 the Midwest and Western Societies, respectively, were organized. Then, in 1924 these three societies united and formed a national association at a meeting in Kansas City. At the present time the national Association represents five district associations: Eastern, Southern, Midwest, Central, and Western. Each district association is to a great extent autonomous in its own section.

The purpose of the National Association of Physical Education for College Women is to investigate and study problems that characterize departments of physical education for women in the various colleges and universities. Since its inception, this organization has concerned itself with such problems as establishing standards for policies, equipment, and programs; promoting research studies and making findings available to all; promoting sane athletic policies in institutions of higher learning; and developing an interest in women's health, skill development, and proper emotional adjustment.

Originally membership in this women's association was restricted to women directors of physical education. However, as physical education has grown, so has this organization, with a broadening of membership requirements. At the present time, membership is open to all women teachers of physical education in colleges and universities. This includes teachers' colleges and junior colleges. To be a member of the national organization, one must be a member of the district organization. Honorary members of the National Association of Physical Education for College Women pay no dues. Active and associate members pay $4 yearly.

The national Association holds meetings biennially, whereas the districts hold their meetings annually. The agenda for such meetings includes such items as discussion of topics pertinent to the profession, reports of research studies, leadership problems, and international problems. Once a year the Association sends newsletters to all its members, and after the biennial meeting a report is usually sent out concerning the meeting and important items that transpired at the conference.

For more information concerning this organization write to Association, Physical Education Department, Northeastern University, Boston, Massachusetts 02115.

National Collegiate Athletic Association

The history of the National Collegiate Athletic Association (NCAA) began in the early 1900's. Because of the alarming number of football injuries and the fact that there was no uniform or national control of the game of football, a conference of representatives of universities and colleges, primarily from the eastern section of the United States, was held on December 12, 1905. Preliminary plans were made for a national body to assist in the formulation of sound requirements for intercollegiate athletics, particularly football, and the name Intercollegiate Athletic Association was suggested. At a meeting March 31, 1906, a constitution and by-laws were adopted and issued. The first annual convention of the Intercollegiate Athletic Association was held at the Murray Hill Hotel, New York City, on December 29, 1906. On December 29, 1910, the name of the Association was changed to the National Collegiate Athletic Association.

The purposes of the NCAA are designed to uphold the principles of institutional control of all collegiate sports; to maintain a uniform code of amateurism in conjunction with sound eligibility rules, scholarship requirements, and good sportsmanship; to promote and assist in the expansion of intercollegiate and intramural sports; to formulate, copyright, and publish the official rules of play (in eleven sports); to sponsor and supervise regional and national meets and tournaments for member institutions (presently the NCAA conducts national meets and tournaments in many sports); to preserve collegiate athletic records; and to serve as headquarters for collegiate athletic matters of national import.

To achieve membership in the NCAA, a college must be accredited and compete in a minimum of four sports each year on an intercollegiate level. At least one sport must be engaged in during the normal three major sport seasons. Dues are scaled according to the enrollment of the college and range from $37.50 to $200.

The NCAA is a voluntary association of more than 700 members* institutions and affiliated associations. Its services include the following:

1. Serving as a discussion, legislative, and administrative body for college athletics
2. Maintaining a national headquarters staff
3. Publishing official guides in nine sports
4. Conducting national championship events in many sports
5. Participating in United States Olympic and Pan-American athletic events
6. Maintaining a central clearing and counseling agency in the field of college athletic administration
7. Providing a film library covering play in national meets and tournaments
8. Administering group travel and medical insurance programs for its member institutions

The NCAA has an office in the Midland Building, 1221 Baltimore Avenue, Kansas City, Missouri 64105.

National College Physical Education Association for Men

In 1897 the National College Physical Education Association for Men (NCPE-AM) was founded under the name of the Society of College Gymnasium Directors. In 1909 it became known as the Society of College Directors of Physical Education and in 1933 as the College Physical Education Association.

The men present at the organization in 1897 included Dr. Anderson of Yale, Dr. Sargent of Harvard, Dr. Seaver of Yale, Dr. Linhart of Ohio State, Dr. Savage of Columbia, Professor Goldie of Princeton, Mr. Marvel of Wesleyan, Mr. F. H. Cann of New York University, and Mr. Sharp of Yale.

The Association was formed for men performing health and physical education work in colleges. The purpose of the organization is the advancement of college health,

physical education, and recreation in institutions of higher learning. Many areas of these professions are represented and have sectional meetings, such as required physical education, adapted physical education, recreational activities, intercollegiate athletics, teacher education, and administration and supervision. The Association meets annually.

The work of the organization is largely carried on by committees. Some of the important committees that have been in operation at various times during the history of the Association are the following: Committee on Relationships of College Physical Education to National Preparedness, Committee on Constitution and Material Equipment, Committee on Curriculum Research, and Committees on Teacher Education, Research, and Physical Education and Athletics.

The National College Physical Education Association for Men has three types of members. First, there are active members, or those who are directly engaged in some phase of college health, physical education, or recreation; second, associate members, or those to whom the Association has extended membership by reason of work related to the fields of health, physical education, and recreation, but who are not teaching in a college; and, third, honorary members, or those who have been selected by the Association and who may be active or former active members. The dues for a member are $10 annually. Represented in the Association are more than 300 different colleges in five countries, with 1,041 members as of February, 1970.

The official publication of the NCPEAM is *The Proceedings of the College Physical Education Association*. This material is published once a year. Also available are such publications as *College Facilities for Health Education, Physical Education, and Recreation,* which sells for $2 a copy, and *Fit for College,* which sells for 50 cents. The NCPEAM also publishes the monograph *Quest* in conjunction with the Na-

---

*Brochure of the National Collegiate Athletic Association.

tional Association for Physical Education of College Women.

For more information write to the Association, Department of Physical Education, 203 Cooke Hall, University of Minnesota, Minneapolis, Minnesota 55145.

National Education Association

Every physical educator associated with the schools in this country should be familiar with the National Education Association (NEA). It has reportedly the greatest number of members of any professional organization in the world and is very active in promoting the cause of education. Its central offices are located at 1201 16th Street N.W., Washington, D. C. 20056.

T. W. Valentine and D. B. Hager were the two educators who were largely responsible for calling the first meeting of the National Teachers Association in 1857. This was the organization that later became known as the National Education Association. The first meeting of the National Teachers Association was on August 26, 1857, in Philadelphia. Forty-three educators, representing twelve states, were in attendance.

Some highlights in the history of the National Education Association have been the lecture delivered by Horace Mann in 1858, entitled "The Teacher's Motives"; President James Buchanan's recognition of the National Education Association and his attendance at one of its sessions; the incorporation of the National Education Association by a bill signed by President Theodore Roosevelt in 1906; the appointment of Willard E. Givens as executive secretary of the National Education Association in 1935; the establishment of the Education Policies Commission; and the establishment of the American Association for Health, Physical Education, and Recreation as a department of the National Education Association.

The purposes and services of the National Education Association are concerned with promoting education in this country. In doing so, it works toward the advancement of the interests of those in the teaching pro-

fession, helps to better care for the welfare of all American youth, and is interested in and strives to provide for the education of all individuals.

The services of the National Education Association are primarily to members only; however, indirectly it is of service to youth, to parents, and to the public and nation as a whole.

The National Education Association started with forty-three active members in 1857; today it consists of more than 1 million enrolled members and more than 2 million affiliated members. Annual membership dues are $25. In addition, there is a $225 life membership. Any student enrolled in a teacher education program in a college or university may become a student NEA member by joining a chapter of the student National Education Association. The dues are $1 per year. The membership year is from September 1 to August 31.

The publications of the National Education Association are too numerous to list in this chapter. However, the one that has the widest circulation and that is representative of the Association is *Today's Education*. It is published monthly, with the exception of June, July, and August, and is sent to all members of the Association.

National Intramural Association*

In the school year 1948-1949 William Wasson, an instructor at Dillard University in New Orleans, received a Carnegie grant-in-aid to study intramural programs in twenty-five colleges and universities. It was from this study that he conceived the idea of having the intramural directors meet annually and of developing a medium through which an exchange of information and ideas could take place.

The first meeting was held at Dillard University on February 22 and 23, 1950. At this meeting the National Intramural Association was formed.

---

*The information on the National Intramural Association was contributed by Ellis J. Mendelsohn.

The National Intramural Association is an affiliate member of the American Association for Health, Physical Education, and Recreation.

The objectives of the National Intramural Association are:

1. To provide a common meeting ground for intramural directors and members of their staff to discuss current problems and policies
2. To provide an opportunity to exchange ideas and thoughts for improvement in the operation of the intramural program
3. To determine policy, principles, and procedures to guide intramural directors in performance of their duties
4. To promote and encourage intramural and recreational programs
5. To serve as a medium for the publication of research papers on intramurals of both members and nonmembers
6. To work in close cooperation with the American Association for Health, Physical Education, and Recreation, the National Recreation and Park Association, and the Educational Policy Committee of our respective institutions

The official publication of the National Intramural Association is *The Proceedings of the Annual Intramural Conference.*

Membership in the National Intramural Association started with the eleven charter members who attended the first intramural conference held at Dillard University in New Orleans in 1950, rose to 250 by 1959, and has a much higher membership today. Membership in the Association, in addition to providing a subscription for a copy of the annual conference proceedings, offers other advantages, including information service and an opportunity to help in promoting higher stands for the profession.

National Junior College Athletic Association

The National Junior College Athletic Association (NJCAA) is an organization composed of the majority of junior colleges in the United States that sponsor intercollegiate athletic programs. The NJCAA was conceived in 1937 and became a functioning organization on May 14, 1938. The primary purpose of this organization is to promote

and supervise a national program of junior college sports and activities that would achieve the educational objectives of athletics.*

The association is organized into nineteen regions. The member colleges elect a Regional Director in each of the nineteen regions and conduct their regional affairs within the framework of NJCAA Constitution and By-laws. The Regional Directors hold their annual legislative assembly meeting at Hutchinson, Kansas, to determine the policies, procedures, and programs of the NJCAA. They also elect the President, Vice-President, Secretary, and Treasurer, who constitute the Executive Committee. This committee appoints the Commission of Eligibility, which is the final authority on all cases of individual eligibility.†

At present, the NJCAA conducts national championship events in football, cross-country, basketball, wrestling, golf, and tennis. In addition, the Association sponsors national invitational events in rifle, soccer, swimming, gymnastics, lacrosse, and skiing.†

The NJCAA has several official publications. The *JUCO Review* presents and interprets the program of the NJCAA to its members. This review also gives a list of articles on junior college athletics that have been written by outstanding junior college coaches. The *NJCAA Handbook* is a compilation of the constitution, by-laws, policies, procedures, programs, eligibility, rules, and history of the organization. This handbook is sent to each member college. In addition to these publications, the organization publishes numerous materials that keep its members informed of the latest developments within the organization.‡

The membership fee is $75 per year per college. Those colleges holding membership in the organization are entitled to all services

---

*National Junior College Athletic Association Handbook, 1969-1970, p. 49.

†National Junior College Athletic Association Brochure, 1969-1970.

‡National Junior College Athletic Association Brochure.

rendered by NJCAA, as well as the privilege of participating in all of its activities.* There were 454 member colleges of the NJCAA as of September 1, 1969.

Each member college of the NJCAA receives the following benefits:

1. All-American recognition
2. Consideration for NJCAA records and positions on the Honor Roll
3. An extremely reasonable intercollegiate insurance plan
4. Official handbook
5. National publicity releases from Service Bureau
6. The *JUCO Review* (official publication)
7. Eligibility casebook
8. Use of NJCAA film library
9. Participation in National and International athletic events sponsored by the NJCAA

The National Junior College Athletic Association is a nonprofit organization. The income received from its programs is turned back toward broadening the scope of the organization and bettering the program for the member colleges.†

The address of the Association is The Hilton Inn, Hilton Place, Hutchinson, Kansas 67501.

National Recreation and Park Association

The National Recreation and Park Association (NRPA) is an organization dedicated to the conservation and beautification of the environment and the development, improvement, and expansion of park and recreation programs, facilities, leadership and services. It is an independent, nonprofit organization whose primary goal is to continue the advance of environmental quality and an improved quality of life.‡

---

*National Junior College Athletic Association Handbook, p. 53.

†National Junior College Athletic Association Brochure, 1969-1970.

‡PROFILE of National Recreation and Park Association, p. 1.

The National Recreation and Park Association had at least part of its beginnings in 1906 when the Playground Association of America was organized. At the time of the founding of this Association, only forty-one cities reportedly had playgrounds with qualified leadership. One of the main objectives of this Association was to achieve the goal of having adequately trained men and women conducting play and recreation programs on a community basis. It also furthered the cause of spending leisure in a wholesome, profitable manner.

The National Recreation Association, as the Playground Association of America later came to be known, received support from such individuals as President Theodore Roosevelt, Jane Addams, Jacob Riis, Felix Warburg, Joseph Lee, and Luther Gulick. These persons helped the Association in achieving many of its aims. In 1965, the American Association of Zoological Parks and Aquariums, the American Institute of Park Executives, the American Recreation Society, the National Conference on State Parks, and the National Recreation Association united to form the National Recreation and Park Association.

The objectives of the NRPA are public policy formation, education, community service, citizen development service, and professional development services.

The Association has conducted an educational program that has brought to the attention of the public the necessity for playgrounds; the need for recreation, especially in a highly industrialized society; the need for conservation, beautification, and purification of water supplies; and the need for qualified leadership to conduct programs in such areas as sports, arts and crafts, drama, and dance.

The services rendered by the Association include leadership training, program planning and ideas, planning areas and facilities, recreation surveys, research, publishing a recreation magazine, and providing library conferences, and public information and education.

The Association is responsible for many

publications ranging from books to mimeographed bulletins. The content of the published material covers the entire field of recreation, including philosophy, administration, and operation; facilities, layout, and equipment; leadership and leadership training; public relations; parks; recreation for special groups; home play; and activities material covering the various fields of arts and crafts, camping and nature, drama, games, tests and special activities, holiday and special day material, music, radio dancing, and social recreation.

The national headquarters of the Association is at 1700 Pennsylvania Avenue N.W., Washington, D. C., where a professional staff of specialists in parks, recreation, conservation, and associated fields is carrying on the work of the Association.*

North American Society for the Psychology of Sports and Physical Activity

The North American Society for the Psychology of Sports and Physical Activity (NASPSPA) was founded in 1965 and became incorporated as a nonprofit corporation in 1967. NASPSPA is affiliated with the International Society for the Psychology of Sports (ISPS).†

The Association is composed of professional people (psychologists, psychiatrists, and physical educators) whose primary purpose is to promote scientific research and relations within the framework of sport psychology and physical activity, through meetings, investigations, publications, and other activities. Membership in NASPSPA is open to all people interested in the psychology of sports and physical activity. At present, there are approximately 300 members. Those persons requesting to be admitted to membership in the NASPSPA are required to pay $5 dues.

The Society publishes the *Sport Psychol-ogy Bulletin,* a quarterly bulletin, which keeps its members informed about affairs of the Society, as well as the field of sports psychology in general. The Society also publishes newsletters detailing the activities of the annual convention, which is usually held in the spring. For further information concerning the Society, contact the School of Health, Physical Education, and Recreation, Indiana University, Bloomington, Indiana 47401.

Phi Delta Pi

Phi Delta Pi is a national professional education fraternity for women. It was organized in 1916 at the Normal College of the American Gymnastic Union, Indianapolis, Indiana. The objects of Phi Delta Pi are listed here:

1. To provide a national physical education affiliation for women
2. To promote the progressive development of physical education
3. To emphasize and develop effective leadership*

This fraternity for women has a national convention every 2 years and a national council meeting every year. Sectional meetings are held in connection with the district meetings of the American Association for Health, Physical Education, and Recreation. Committees perform much of the work for this organization. Committees concerned with such problems as alumnae expansion, documents and rituals, history, necrology, scholarship loan, publicity, and professional standards have been established.

This association has sponsored many national projects. It has had a camp project as a service for underprivileged children. Camps for this purpose have been held at Elkhart Lake, Wisconsin; Johnstown, New York; Salt Lake City, Utah; Medford, New Jersey; and Cincinnati, Ohio. This fraternity has sponsored many projects in forms of symposiums. These have been held for a

---

*NRPA Fact Sheet.

†Encyclopedia of associations, Vol. III: New associations, Detroit, 1970, Gale Research Co. Booktower.

---

*Phi Delta Pi, national professional physical education fraternity for women: Phi Delta Pi, The Fraternity, p. 2.

discussion of such problems as posture and dysmenorrhea. Other projects include scholastic loans, magazine agency, professional standards, and round and square dances at the national convention of the American Association for Health, Physical Education, and Recreation.

Phi Delta Pi has four types of membership. The active membership is for majors in physical education in a school where a chapter of the fraternity exists. The alumnae membership exists when an active member graduates and becomes an alumna member. The honorary membership is for individuals who are outstanding in fields of health, physical education, or recreation. The special membership is for educators active in health, physical education, or recreation work. The membership in the fraternity is now approximately 5,200. Dues are $3.50.

The publications of Phi Delta Pi include *The Professional Physical Educator* and the *Handbook for Student Teachers.*

Active chapters in Phi Delta Pi may be installed in colleges or universities where there is a major course in physical education and upon approval of the National Council of Phi Delta Pi.

The address of Phi Delta Pi is 4595 East 4th Avenue, Hialeah, Florida 33012.

Phi Epsilon Kappa Fraternity*

Phi Epsilon Kappa Fraternity was founded on April 12, 1912, at the Normal College, American Gymnastics Union, Indianapolis, Indiana. In 1920, with the establishment of the Beta chapter at the American College of Physical Education, it became a national organization. At present there are sixty-two active collegiate chapters and twelve active alumni chapters.

The objectives of the Phi Epsilon Kappa Fraternity are as follows:

1. To further the individual welfare of its members

*All new information taken from a letter by R. R. Schreiber, Executive Secretary.

2. To foster scientific research in the fields of health education, physical education, recreation education, and safety education
3. To facilitate the exchange of information and experience gained in the various countries of the world concerning matters relating to the interdependent areas of health education, physical education, recreation education, and safety education, including programs, methods, techniques, material, training, and research
4. To promote sound community understanding leading to adequate support of these educational programs
5. To raise professional standards and ethics

The paid full-time staff consists of an executive secretary-treasurer and an office manager.

Membership in the fraternity is limited to males. Collegiate chapters must limit themselves to students and teachers of health education, physical education, recreation education, or safety education. To be eligible, a student must have completed at least one full semester of work with a "C" average. Alumni chapters may propose and accept men professionally engaged in health education, physical education, recreation education, or safety education within the territory of their jurisdiction.

Since 1913, the fraternity has initiated a total of more than 21,500 members and is initiating approximately 1,200 new members annually. There are four types of membership in the fraternity. The active membership in collegiate chapters is for students and teachers in colleges and universities where a chartered chapter has been installed and in alumni chapters for men in physical education work. The honorary membership is for prominent persons in physical education work who have received the approval of the Grand Chapter. The extraordinary membership is for individuals who have retired from active physical education work and have been approved by an alumni chapter. Life membership is for alumni members who pay a prescribed fee. Annual membership dues are $4.

The Phi Epsilon Kappa Fraternity publishes a professional magazine, *The Physical Educator,* which is available to nonmembers on a subscription basis. Members receive a copy without additional charge. Another publication is the *Index and Abstracts of Foreign Physical Education Literature,* which appears annually. They are available at $3 each. The fraternity has published four monographs, *Physical Education Around the World,* in 1966, 1968, 1969, and 1970. They are available at $1.50 each. It is currently in the process of publishing a series of five volumes of *Measurement in Physical Education.* Volume 1 is already published and Volumes 2, 3, 4, and 5 should be available by September, 1970. The *Black and Gold,* a bulletin of fraternal news, is published three times annually and is available to members only.

The central office of the Phi Epsilon Kappa Fraternity is at 400 Meadow Drive, Suite L-24, Indianapolis, Indiana 46205.

Physical Education Society of the Young Men's Christian Association of North America

The Physical Education Society of the Young Men's Christian Association of North America was founded in 1903. The purposes of this organization, as originally established, are as follows:

1. To unite in one body those professional workers in the Young Men's Christian Association who are related to physical education
2. To promote a fraternal spirit and fellowship among the members
3. To engage in original research
4. To study technical and professional problems
5. To cooperate with constituent or related bodies

The Society includes over 900 persons in the YMCA's of North America. There are seven chapters of the Society divided geographically throughout the nation, such as Southern Area and New England. The dues are $10 per year.*

The Society, through its program, attempts to help in the realization of the ob-

*Information obtained in interview with Mr. Arnold, National Director.

jectives of the Young Men's Christian Association. When the YMCA was founded in London in 1844, physical as well as spiritual, educational, and social needs were recognized as being an essential for youth. Consequently, gymnasiums, swimming pools, and recreational facilities are found in YMCA's, as well as provision for spiritual, educational, and social programs.

The first meeting of physical directors was held in Jamestown, New York, in 1902. In this same year the periodical *Physical Training* was published. This was later changed to the *Journal of Physical Education* and is published bimonthly.

For information about this Association write to the National YMCA Headquarters, 291 Broadway, New York, New York 10007.

Society of State Directors of Health, Physical Education, and Recreation

The idea and the initial impetus for the Society of State Directors of Health, Physical Education, and Recreation may be credited to James E. Rogers. The first meeting of the association was held in 1926, with Dr. Carl L. Schrader, State Director of Massachusetts, as the first president. James Rogers was elected secretary and served in this capacity for 15 years. The constitution for this organization was adopted in 1944 with Bernice Moss as chairman of the constitution committee. At first, the Society met twice a year—once with what is known as the American Association of School Administrators and once in conjunction with the council meeting of the American Physical Education Association. At present the meeting of the Society is held in conjunction with the American Association for Health, Physical Education, and Recreation.

The purposes of the Society have been described as follows:

1. To promote a more general understanding and a better appreciation of the importance of health, physical education, and recreation
2. To promote the establishment of a physical and health education program in each of the

states by legislative enactment or otherwise
3. To promote the development of physical and health education programs in states in which such programs have been established
4. To promote a closer and more cooperative relationship among persons engaged in physical and health educational service
5. To promote the adoption of wise policies and procedures in matters relating to state, interstate, and intersectional athletic contests
6. To promote the professional and official efficiency of members of the Society

Some of the accomplishments of the Society, since its inception in 1926, are as follows:

1. The Society has helped in the publication of the physical achievement standards for boys and girls.
2. It has worked with certification groups.
3. It has helped in campaigns for national legislation regarding health and physical education.
4. It has contributed to the upgrading of state legislation and standards.
5. It has made contributions to teacher-training programs, curriculums, and standards.
6. Widespread interest in the subjects of health and physical education has been developed.
7. Athletic ideals and practices in schools have been greatly elevated and improved.
8. Physical education activities for girls, taught and supervised by women teachers and directors and suited to their physiological social needs, have been promoted.
9. Intraschool programs rather than interschool contests have been encouraged.
10. Participation in physical education by all rather than by a minority of the pupils has greatly increased.
11. A closer relationship with other education organizations has been effected.

The Society has also passed many resolutions during its history that have been pertinent to programs of health, physical education, and recreation. Some of these were concerned with the supervision of state programs; the preparation of guides, manuals, and materials; the promotion of inservice training for teachers; the establishment of certification standards; the promotion of sports and playday programs; and the maintenance of library and reference files. The Society has also assisted in planning new facilities, written professional articles, and cooperated with various official and nonofficial agencies. The two main publications of the Society are *A Statement of Basic Beliefs* and *The Role of the State Department of Education in Recreation Today*.

An active membership in the Society of State Directors of Health, Physical Education, and Recreation is $5, while an associate member pays $2. There are approximately 180 members at the present time. The Society may be reached at the Office of Education, U. S. Department of Health, Education and Welfare, Washington, D. C.

U. S. Collegiate Sports Council*

The U. S. Collegiate Sports Council (USCSC), an affiliate of the International University Sports Federation (FISU), was founded in 1968. The Council has five members. They are the National Collegiate Athletic Association, National Intercollegiate Athletic Association, National Junior College Athletic Association, U. S. National Association, and American Association for Health, Physical Education, and Recreation.

The general purpose of the USCSC is to promote international understanding through collegiate athletics and physical education. The specific purpose of the Association is to encourage increased United States participation in the activities sponsored by the International University Sports Federation. The FISU is a confederation of fifty-six countries that sponsor biennial World Student Games in summer and winter sports.

The USCSC organizes the U. S. teams for competition in aquatics, basketball, fencing, figure skating, gymnastics, ice hockey, judo, skiing, tennis, track and field, volleyball, and water polo. Competition in these activities is sponsored by the International University Sports Federation. The address of the USCSC is 1725 K Street N. W., Suite 1212, Washington, D. C. 20006.

*Data taken from Encyclopedia of associations, Vol. III: New Associations, Detroit, 1968, Gale Research Co. Booktower, p. 121.

Table 22-1. Professional organizations

Name	Membership	Selected liaison organizations	Method of finance	Services
American Physical Therapy Association (APTA)	Graduates of accredited schools of physical therapy and others interested in the field	World Confederation for Physical Therapy National Health Council American Medical Association	Dues Sales of materials	Acts as a clearinghouse; gives assistance with programming, placement, and recruiting; sponsors research
American Youth Hostels, Inc.	Open to all willing to abide by hosteling customs	International Youth Hostel Federation	Memberships Program fees Contributions Income from special events	Promotes a spirit of friendship and understanding on an international basis
Boys' Clubs of America	Boys	American National Red Cross American Association for Health, Physical Education, and Recreation	Contributions Investments Endowments Fees and dues	Provides boys with a chance to put their leisure time to wholesome use
National Association of Jewish Center Workers	Professional workers in Jewish Community Centers, camps, and youth groups	National Conference of Jewish Communal Service National Jewish Welfare Board YMHA-YWHA	Dues Publications Interest on savings	Holds workshops, conferences, and promotes professional education in the field

Young Women's Christian Association

The Young Women's Christian Association was one of the first organizations for women to be founded in this country. It dates back to 1858, and since that time it has spread rapidly. Today, there are YWCA's in seventy-eight countries. In the United States alone, there are more than 6,700 locations where over 2.5 million persons participate as members of the YWCA. These locations include building-centered operations, decentralized units, residences, camps, colleges and university associations, and YWCA–USO Clubs.*

The Young Women's Christian Association has as its objectives the furtherance of democratic living and promoting educational and recreational programs to enrich the lives of girls and women. The activities program

*The story of the YWCA (leaflet) and interview with Ida Snyder, Association and News Director.

is designed in part to develop and maintain health and physical fitness so that routine tasks may be performed efficiently. Whereas the program of the YWCA was originally referred to as physical education, since 1920 it has been referred to as health education.

The YWCA works for community health through a program that improves the health and welfare of girls and women. Members may participate in activities designed to improve one's knowledge of body mechanics, sex education, nutrition, family life, various diseases, and other areas necessary for healthful living. It encourages health examinations as a prerequisite for participation in physical education activities, for health counseling purposes, and as a basis for educational programs. Through health education committees, it has done research in respect to girls and women. It furthers coeducational activities.

The regular publications of the YWCA

are *YWCA Magazine* (nine issues a year); *Y-Teen Scene* (four issues); *Interact* (student, five issues); *Staff-to-Staff Newsletter* (four issues); and *Public Affairs Newsletter* (six issues).*

The national headquarters of the YWCA is at 600 Lexington Avenue, New York, New York 10022.

Others

Four additional professional organizations with which physical educators should be familiar are listed in Table 22-1.

QUESTIONS AND EXERCISES

1. Prepare a chart listing all the organizations in this chapter, the physical education personnel that should belong to each, and essential factors about each association.
2. In an essay of around 250 words, discuss the reasons why physical educators should be members of their national association.
3. What is the National Education Association? What are some of the purposes for which it was founded?
4. Describe in detail the history, purposes, organization, and services of the American Association for Health, Physical Education, and Recreation.
5. What are some of the services available to members of the National Park and Recreation Association?
6. Why is membership in the American Academy of Physical Education a coveted goal of many physical educators?
7. Discuss the history of the American School Health Association.
8. Who is eligible for membership in the National College Physical Education Association for Men?
9. What is the purpose of the National Association of Physical Education for College Women?
10. What have been some of the accomplishments of the Society of State Directors of Health, Physical Education, and Recreation?
11. What are the objectives of the Young Women's Christian Association?
12. What are the purposes of the Physical Education Society of the Young Men's Christian Association of North America?
13. What are the services performed by the National Collegiate Athletic Association?

14. Describe the history of the Canadian Physical Education Association.
15. How do the following organizations contribute to physical education: Delta Psi Kappa, Phi Delta Pi, and Phi Epsilon Kappa?

SELECTED REFERENCES

Ainsworth, Dorothy S.: The National Association of Physical Education for College Women, Journal of Health and Physical Education **17:** 525, 1956.

Amateur Athletic Union: You and the AAU, 1969, The Union.

American Academy of Physical Education: Constitution and By-Laws, February, 1969.

American Association for Health, Physical Education, and Recreation: This is AAHPER, Washington, D. C., 1969, The Association.

American College of Sports Medicine: Constitution and By-Laws, 1969.

American College of Sports Medicine Newsletter, vol. 4, no. 3, July, 1969.

American Corrective Therapy Association Brochure.

American School Health Association: ASHA Newsletter, no. 2, April, 1970.

American Youth Hostels, Inc.: What is hosteling? 1970, The Association.

DeTurk, Wilbur C., and Foertsch, Fred E.: Phi Epsilon Kappa Fraternity, Journal of Health and Physical Education **18:**11, 1947.

Encyclopedia of associations, Vol. I: National organizations of the United States, ed. 5, Detroit, 1968, Gale Research Co. Booktower.

Encyclopedia of associations, Vol. III: New associations, Detroit, 1969-1970, Gale Research Co. Booktower.

Gable, Martha A., and Christaldi, Josephine: Phi Delta Pi, Journal of Health and Physical Education **17:**598, 1946.

Gilman, Estelle: Delta Psi Kappa, Journal of Health and Physical Education **17:**482, 1946.

Hostels—Guide and Handbook, 1970-1971, New York, American Youth Hostels, Inc.

Howell, Maxwell L.: The Canadian Association for Health, Physical Education, and Recreation, Inc., Journal of Health, Physical Education, and Recreation **36:**24, 1965.

Keene, Charles H.: The American School Health Association, Journal of Health and Physical Education **17:**147, 1946.

National Association of Intercollegiate Athletics: Constitution and by-laws, The Association.

National Collegiate Athletic Association: NCAA brochure, 1969, The Association.

National Education Association of the United States: NEA handbook, Washington, D. C., The Association.

National Junior College Athletic Association Handbook, 1969-1970.

*National Board YWCA—Annual Report, 1968-1969, p. 22.

National Recreation and Park Association: NRPA fact sheet, 1970, The Association.

National Recreation and Park Association: NRPA profile, 1970, The Association.

Palmer, Grace M.: The Young Women's Christian Association, Journal of Health and Physical Education **18**:150, 1947.

Phi Delta Pi: The Fraternity.

Phi Epsilon Kappa: Pledge manual, 1953, The Fraternity.

Plewes, Doris Willard: The Canadian Physical Education Association, Journal of Health and Physical Education **17**:273, 1946.

Robson, John, editor: Baird's manual of college fraternities, ed. 18, Menash, Wisconsin, 1968, The Collegiate Press, George Banta Co., Inc.

Rogers, James E.: History of the Society, 1945, The Society of State Directors of Health and Physical Education.

Young Women's Christian Association: The story of the YWCA, 1969, The Association.

Walters, M. L.: The Physical Education Society of the Young Men's Christian Associations of North America, Journal of Health and Physical Education **18**:311, 1947.

23/Certification requirements for employment in physical education

The teacher is the major factor in the educational process. Whatever happens in the school experience of a child is largely the result of the kind of teacher who has guided his destiny. If a child has a happy and profitable educational experience, the teachers with whom he has come in contact can be given a major share of the credit. On the other hand, if a child has an unhappy and unprofitable educational experience, the teachers with whom he has come in contact should assume a major share of the blame. Therefore, the teacher occupies a key position in the schools.

The educational process in which the teacher holds this key position has been a function of each state since the Tenth Amendment was made a part of the Constitution of the United States. If the state is responsible for education, it must establish certain minimum standards for those who desire to teach. Years ago teachers of physical education received little training and were required to meet very few standards for teaching. Gradually, however, as various states passed legislation incorporating physical education as part of the school programs, as the length of the preparatory period for teachers of physical education increased, and as the work of physical education became recognized as a vital experience in the education of the child, more stress was placed on the importance of having adequately trained teachers in physical education positions.

Certification requirements represent a first step in any system that attempts to fill positions on the basis of merit. The minimum requirements for teaching, which comprise the rules and regulations concerning state teachers' certificates, are designed primarily to secure teachers who are professionally and personally well equipped. They are designed to protect children from poorly prepared and inefficient teachers. They are designed to protect the teaching profession from unqualified teachers whose standards are so low that instruction suffers, and, finally, they are designed to protect administrators from local pressures urging the appointment of teachers who are not qualified for teaching positions.

There is a recognized need for certification requirements as a means of maintaining and ensuring the quality of physical education teachers in the various states. They are necessary to ensure that children in the schools will have well-prepared and effective teachers of physical education guiding their day-to-day activities. At the present time, teacher-training institutions have prospective teachers who are looking forward to obtaining positions. The certification standards that have been established determine, in some measure, the type of preparation that is offered in the various states, and thus, in the final analysis, these standards also determine to some degree whether or not teachers being prepared in physical education are qualified to guide the school activities of children.

An examination of the training of men

and women shows that the average male teacher has had more college education than the typical female teacher. About 43% of the men and about 24% of the women have two college degrees. Taking into account all public school teachers, it is found that slightly over 95% have a bachelor's degree or higher and over 30% a master's degree or higher.

A survey of the teacher certification requirements indicates a general lack of uniformity for the certification of teachers in general and physical education teachers in particular. At the same time there are some general conclusions and trends that may be drawn from a survey of the various requirements. The teacher may be able to obtain a clearer picture of the requirements for the various states by examining Table 23-1, which lists basic and minimum requirements for authorization to teach a special field or subject.

In respect to minimum special requirements for certification of teachers of physical education, there are no uniform qualifications from state to state. Some require graduation from an approved 4-year teacher-training course, and others say all that is required is "blanket certification," meaning that any teacher who holds a regular certificate can also teach any special field for which he is qualified. Some states have only a major certification requirement, and others have major and minor listings.

According to a survey by Hess,* the specialization requirements for certification in physical education range from 47 semester hours to a low of 21 semester hours. Nine states—Alabama, Kansas, Massachusetts, Missouri, South Carolina, Tennessee, Texas, West Virginia, and Wyoming—require 24 semester hours in physical education courses for certification. Ten states —Hawaii, Louisiana, New Hampshire, New Mexico, New York, North Carolina, Pennsylvania, Rhode Island, Vermont, and Virginia—require 36 semester hours in physical education courses for certification. Other states and the number of credit hours they require for certification in physical educa-

---

*Hess, Roland: Teacher certification in physical education, Journal of Health, Physical Education, and Recreation **41**:79, 1970.

Certification requirements are designed to ensure that only qualified persons teach physical education.

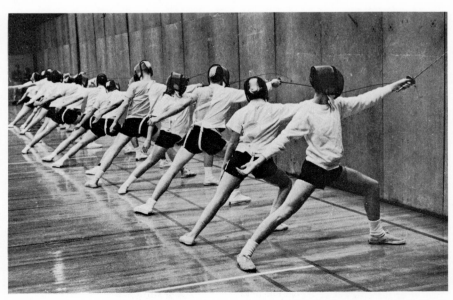

tion include: Arizona—30 SH,* Arkansas —21 SH, California—36 SH, Connecticut —28 SH, Delaware—40 SH, Georgia—45 QH, Idaho—30 SH, Illinois—32 SH, Indiana—40 SH, Kentucky—60 QH, Maryland—47 SH, Michigan—30 SH, Mississippi —30 SH, Montana—40 SH, Ohio—60 QH, Oklahoma—30 SH, and Oregon—47 QH.

Specific physical education courses that are required for certification vary from state to state. My survey identified some of the courses that are required in the various states: zoology, biology, anatomy, physiology, physiology of exercise, kinesiology, adapted physical education, first aid and safety, physical education activities, history and philosophy of physical education, administration of physical education, tests and measurements, health, and recreation.

An example of the certification requirements for one state (South Carolina) are shown on p. 646.

GENERAL AREAS FOR CERTIFICATION REQUIREMENTS

There are ten general areas in which states have governing regulations for teacher certification. Since states differ in their requirements, however, the prospective teacher should inquire directly of the state education department, division of teacher certification, for the exact requirements. To summarize these ten areas and the requirements presently established in the fifty states and the District of Columbia and Puerto Rico, the following information is presented.

CITIZENSHIP. Approximately thirty states, the District of Columbia, and Puerto Rico require United States citizenship or a declaration of intention clause. The teacher must be a citizen of the United States to qualify.

OATH OF ALLEGIANCE OF LOYALTY. Approximately twenty-four states, the District of Columbia, and Puerto Rico require a loyalty oath for teacher certification. The

others usually have a written statement that must be signed.

AGE. The age requirement varies among states. The lowest age limit is 17 years. In general, 18 or 19 years of age is acceptable in states specifying a particular age. Some states have no stipulation in this regard.

PROFESSIONAL PREPARATION. It is in this area that the greatest differences in state requirements may be found. Several states have specific courses that must be taken by candidates for certification. For example, in Illinois, teachers must have studied American government and/or history; in Texas, Texan and federal government; in Utah, school health education; in Wyoming, the United States and Wyoming Constitutions. Some of these special state requirements must be met before the first year of teaching, whereas others may be fulfilled within a certain period of time. For example, a course in Rhode Island education may be completed within 3 years of the first year of teaching in that state.

RECOMMENDATION. A large majority of the states require a teaching candidate to have a recommendation from college or from the last place of employment.

FEE. A fee for certification, ranging from $1 to $10, is required in a majority of the states.

HEALTH CERTIFICATE. Approximately twenty-one states, the District of Columbia, and Puerto Rico require a general health certificate, and twelve states, the District of Columbia, and Puerto Rico require a chest x-ray examination.

EMPLOYMENT. Candidates from other states may need to have secured employment to become certified within some states.

COURSE OF STUDY. Besides these general areas of state requirements, there are basic and minimum regulations regarding the course of study that must be followed to qualify for specific certification in physical education. Again, the states disagree in their differentiation of hours of study necessary within the subject of physical education.

---

*SH, Semester hours; QH, quarter hours.

Table 23-1. Basic and minimum requirements for authorization to teach a special field or subject*

State	Agriculture BR	MR	Art BR	MR	Commerce BR	MR	Home Economics BR	MR	Industrial Arts BR	MR	Journalism BR	MR	Library Science BR	MR	Music BR	MR	Phys. Ed.** (Men) BR	MR	Phys. Ed.** (Women) BR	MR	Speech BR	MR	Adult Education BR	MR	State
1	2		3		4		5		6		7		8		9		10		11		12		13		14
Alabama	50	18	24	18	34	18	45	18	24	18	24	18	24	18	24	18	24	18	24	18	24	18	–	–	Alabama
Alaska*	16	–	16	–	16	–	16	–	16	–	16	–	16	–	16	–	16	–	16	–	16	–	16	–	Alaska
Arizona	60	–	–	18	30	18	40	–	30	18	30	–	18	–	30	18	–	18	–	18	30	18	–	–	Arizona
Arkansas	VR[a]	VR	–	24	30	21	VR[a]	VR	VR[a]	VR	–	–	18	15	–	24	21	21	21	21	24	24	–	–	Arkansas
California[a]	AC	AC	AC	AC	AC	AC	AC	AC	AC	AC	AC	AC	15	AC	AC	AC	AC	AC	AC	AC	AC	AC	–[b]	–[b]	California
Colorado*	18	–	18	–	18	–[a]	AC	AC	18	–	18	–	12	–	18	–	18	–	18	–	AC	5	–[c]	–[c]	Colorado
Connecticut	35	35	35	35	42	42	35	35	35	35	30	30	18[b]	30	40[b]	40	40[a]	40	35	40	36[a]	24[d]	B[e]	B[e]	Connecticut
Delaware	30	30	40	40	30	30	30	30	30	30	30	30	30	30	30	30	30	30	30	30	24	24	–[c]	–[c]	Delaware
District of Col.	B[a]	–	30	30	36	36	42[a]	42	30	30	30	–	24	–	30	30	24	6	6	6	30	6	24	6	District of Col.
Florida	VR[b]	–	30	30	36	36	36	VR[b]	30	30	12[c]	–	24	–	36	M	M	M	M	M	M	M	24	M	Florida
Georgia[a]	30[a]	6	30	M	30	6	45[b]	24	30	6	M	20	6	M	30	20	24	20	24	20	30	20	–[b]	–	Georgia
Hawaii	46[a]	24	20	20	20	20	30[b]	24	24	24	30	20[a]	M	16	30	24	20	20	20	20	24[a]	24[a]	40	24	Hawaii
Idaho	24	24	20	20	24	24	24	24	40	24	24[a]	24	24	16	40	30	40	30	40	30	40	30	40	24	Idaho
Illinois	40	24	40	30	40	20	30[b]	20	30	30	10[d]	10	30[e]	15	30	24	30	24	30	24	10[d]	10	–[g]	–[g]	Illinois
Indiana	30[b]	20	30	30	30[c]	20	30[c]	20	30	30	24[d]	24	24	24	24[a]	18	24	18	24	18	24[f]	18	–[g]	–[g]	Indiana
Iowa**[a]	24[a]	18	48-..	–	48-	18	48-	18	48[f]	33	24[i]	18	24	18[g]	48-..	18	24	18	24	18	24[i]	18	B[b]	B[b]	Iowa
Kansas**[a]	60-	18	24[c]	39	24[d]	36	24[e]	42	48[f]	33	12	12	24	18	24[b]	62	33-	33-	33-	33-	18	18	B[b]	B[b]	Kansas
Kentucky[a]	24[d]	18	24[c]	39	36	36	24[e]	42	36	36	12	12	18	18	48-..	18	20[a]	20	20[a]	20	18	18	B[b]	B[b]	Kentucky
Louisiana	50	50	39	39	36	36	42	42	36	36	12	12	18	18	62	62	33-	33-	33-	33-	18	18	B[b]	B[b]	Louisiana
Maine*	B	B	30	30	B	B	B	B	B	B	–	–	–[a]	–	B	B	B	B	B	B	–	–	–	–	Maine
Maryland	45	45	30	30	36[a]	36	36	36	36	36	–[b]	–	18	18	30	30	B	B	B	B	24	24	–	–	Maryland
Massachusetts[a]	VR	–	18	9	18	18	18	15	18	9	NR	–	NR	15	18	18	18	9	18	9	18	9	–[b]	–[b]	Massachusetts
Michigan[a]	M	15	M	M	M	m	M	m	M	m	NR	24	–[b]	–	M	m	M	m	M	m	M	24	–	–	Michigan
Minnesota*[a]	M	M	M	M	M	M	M	M	M	m	–	–	–[b]	–	M	m	M	m	M	m	M	m	–	–	Minnesota
Mississippi	63	63	30	30	30	30	35	35	30	30	15	15	15	15	44	44	30	30	30	30	30[c]	30	–	–	Mississippi
Missouri	30[a]	30	30	30	30	30	30	30	30	30	30[a]	30	15	15	40	40	30	30	30	30	30[c]	30[b]	30	20	Missouri
Montana	30	20	30	20	30	20	30	20	30	20	20[a]	20	30	20	24	24	24	24	24	24	24	18	30	20	Montana
Nebraska**[a]	24	18[b]	24	12	24	18[b]	30	18[b]	24	18[b]	20[b]	16	20	16	24	12	30	12	30	12	10[b]	10[b]	VR	VR	Nebraska
Nevada	VR	–	M	–	M	M	VR-	–	M	M	M	–	M	16	M	12	M	12	M	12	M	16	VR	VR	Nevada
New Hampshire	AC	12	30[a]	12	30[b]	12[c]	30[b]	12[c]	30[b]	12[c]	M	6	24[d]	16	M	12	30[a]	12	30[a]	12	M	16	–	–	New Hampshire
New Jersey	40	40	40	40	40	40	39	39	40	40	–	–	30	30	40	40	40	40	40	40	18	18	–[a]	–[a]	New Jersey
New Mexico	60	–	36	36	36	36	36	36	36	36	36	6	18	18	36	36	36	36	36	36	36	36	–[a]	–[a]	New Mexico
New York	36	36	36	36	36	36	42	42	36	36	36[a]	–	36	36	36	36	36	36	36	36	36	36	–[b]	–[b]	New York
North Carolina	48	–	36	–	36	16	48	16	42	16	–	16	18	18	48	16	16	16	16	16	30	16	–	–	North Carolina
North Dakota**[a]	16	16	16	16	16	16	16	16	16	16	16	15	16	6	16	16	16	16[d]	16	16[d]	16	18[d]	NR	NR	North Dakota
Ohio[a]	24	18	36	18	30[a]	18	26	18	30	18	15	–	18[b,e]	18	36[b,f]	36	24[b,g]	24	15	24[b,g]	16	24	NR	NR	Ohio
Oklahoma	51	51	AC	AC	AC	AC	AC	AC	16	AC	AC	6	AC	18	46[b]	16	30	18	30	18	24	18	NR	NR	Oklahoma
Oregon	30	30	30	30	30	30	40	40	40	40	AC	–	14	6	16	16	24	24	24	24	AC	6	–	–[a]	Oregon
Pennsylvania	AC	AC	AC	AC	AC	AC	AC	AC	AC	AC	6	–	AC	AC	30	30	30	30	30	30	AC	AC	–	–[a]	Pennsylvania
Puerto Rico[a]	30	30	36	36	36	36	36	36	40	40	–	–	18	18	30	30	30	36	30	36	18	36	–	–[b]	Puerto Rico
Rhode Island	36	36	36	36	36	36	36	36	36	36	36	–	18	18	36	36	36	36	36	36	18	36	–	–[b]	Rhode Island
South Carolina	60	60	16	16	16	16	48	30	42	24	–	15	18	24	48	30	16	24	16	24	30	16	–	–[b]	South Carolina
South Dakota	24[a]	–	15	15	15	18[b]	15	16	15	16	15	–	15	6	15	16	15	16	15	16	15	16	24	15	South Dakota
Tennessee	–[a]	–	24[b]	18	18[b]	24	45[d]	48[c]	30[d]	18[c]	15	–	18[b]	18	36[b,f]	15	24[d,g]	24	24[d,g]	24	24[d]	10[b]	24	24	Tennessee
Texas	54[a]	54	42	24	42	24	42	48	42	30	26	24	6	18	42	48	42	24	42	24	24[f]	14	–	–	Texas
Utah*	42	42	42	24	24	15	42	42	42	15[a]	24	15	8	6	48	42	36	15	36	15	26	48	–	–[a]	Utah
Vermont*	36	36	15	15	24	12[d]	45[c]	45	30	30	15	–	30	12	42	15	42	15	42	15	12	15	–	–[a]	Vermont
Virginia	–[a]	–	30[b]	30	45[c]	–	M	m	30	24	12	12	18	18	36	36	36	36	36	36	12	12	–	–	Virginia
Washington**[a]	M	m	M	m	M	m	M	m	M	m	M	m	M	21	47[b]	24	34[b]	24	34[b]	24	M	m	–[b]	–[b]	Washington
West Virginia[a]	45	–	27[b]	–	M	24	34	34	52	28	M	18	21	21	M	24	39[b]	22	34[b]	22	M	24	–[c]	–[c]	West Virginia
Wisconsin	45	34	22	22	34	34	34	34	24	22	22	18	22	22	34	22	22	22	22	22	22	22	–	–	Wisconsin
Wyoming[a]	53	34	24	24	30	30	36	–	24	18	30	6[b]	24	–	36	18	22	18	22	18	30	6[b]	–	–	Wyoming

DEGREES. In approximately forty-four states and the District of Columbia the bachelor's degree is required for regular certification of beginning elementary school teachers. In Arizona, California, and the District of Columbia, 5 years of preparation are required for the regular certification of beginning secondary school teachers.

Because of the differences among states in regard to the ten general areas of certification that have been outlined, a certificate to teach in one state does not necessarily permit a teacher to teach in a different state. Reciprocity among states in the same region of the country is a growing reality, but it is not common at the present time.

A further problem in certification presents itself where localities within a state have specific regulations governing selection of teachers. These are often more rigid than the standards established by the state itself. Detroit, for example, has its own set of qualifications that must be met by its teachers. Local regulations usually involve such factors as teacher preparation or experience.

An applicant may also have to pass a written and oral examination for local licensing. Information regarding local teaching requirements may usually be secured by writing to the board of education of the city in question.

Applicants for teaching positions should try to determine state and local regulations far in advance, if possible. In so doing they may select courses of study in college to meet the requirements. They should submit their applications ahead of time in order to become certified before accepting a position.

TYPES OF CERTIFICATES

The type and value of certificates issued by the states vary nearly as much as do their regulations. In one state, for example, there may be two categories of certification, permanent and probationary, whereas in another state there may be many variations of certificates. The certificate to teach physical education is generally limited to this special field of work, but its validity may be for 1 year (probationary) or for life

---

*Stinnett, T. M.: A manual on certification requirements for school personnel in the United States, Washington, D. C., 1970, National Commission on Teacher Education and Professional Standards, National Education Association.

**Some states have separate certification for health education.

BR means the basic requirement for teaching a subject full time, for a major fraction of the school day, or in the highest classification of schools.

MR means the minimum requirement for teaching a subject part time, for a minor fraction of the school day, or in the lowest classification of schools.

Delaware: 40[a]—grades one to twelve.

Hawaii: *M* means a major and *m* means a minor.

Louisiana: 33-20[a]—gives authorization in health, physical, and safety education; 20—gives authorization only in physical education (including coaching).

Minnesota: *M* means a major and *m* means a minor.

Nevada: *M* means a major.

New Hampshire: 30[a]—plus 6 credits in methods of teaching the specialty on the elementary and secondary levels.

Ohio: 24[d]—40 credits for a special certificate.

Pennsylvania: AC—approved curriculum.

Tennessee: 24[b,g]—valid for grades one to twelve and including health (12 credits) and physical education (12 credits).

Washington: *M* means a major and *m* means a minor.

West Virginia: 39[b] and 34[b]—valid for grades one to twelve.

(permanent). Some states grant temporary or emergency certificates to teachers who do not fully meet all requirements, with the understanding that if certain courses are taken within a prescribed period of time the candidate may become fully qualified.

The value of the certificate again depends on state regulations. It may enable the holder to teach in any public school system within that state, except those where local standards require further qualifications. It may qualify the teacher to teach in neighboring states, depending on reciprocity agreements. It may also permit him to teach in private schools within the state.

The prospective teacher or the experienced teacher seeking employment in a different state should not let these differences in state requirements and qualifications become a hindrance. An inquiry sent to the state or local department of education will provide the necessary information regarding certification.

CERTIFICATION TRENDS

There are trends that are clearly noticeable throughout the country in the certification of teachers. One thing that is very obvious in studying certification requirements in the various states is that change is taking place. For example, in my survey of thirty-five states it was found that twenty-one of these states are initiating changes in their requirements. Four of the most significant changes taking place are approval of professional preparation programs by state departments of education, certification of coaches, separate certification of health and physical education teachers, and separate certification of elementary and secondary school teachers of physical education.

Approval of professional preparation programs by state departments of education

There is a trend toward placing the responsibility for certification upon the college or university where the prospective teacher receives his training. At least fifteen states have initiated such a certification program.

In such cases the state department of education approves an institution's teacher-training program and then the institution of higher learning recommends to the state department of education the students who have successfully completed the training program and who should be certified. States that have adopted this policy include, Alaska, Colorado, Florida, Iowa, Maine, Minnesota, Nebraska, Nevada, New Jersey, New York, North Dakota, South Dakota, Utah, Washington, and Wisconsin.*

Certification of coaches

There is a trend toward the certification of coaches of athletic teams at the secondary school level throughout the United States. The Coaching Certification Committee of the Illinois Association for Professional Preparation in Health, Physical Education, and Recreation conducted a status study on coaching certification in the fifty states† and reports that:

All fifty states require that coaching personnel be certified to teach.
Forty-one states have no specific certification requirements for coaching, although many of these states stress that coaching personnel be prepared in health and physical education. Also, several of these states including Arkansas, Kentucky, and Hawaii are considering the certification of coaches.
Some state departments of public instruction endorse collegiate playing experiences as desirable for coaching personnel.
Nine states have some type of certification requirement for coaching, of which the State of Minnesota has the strongest.

Some of the states that provide some type of certification requirements for coaching personnel and the nature of the requirements follows.

MINNESOTA. Head coach of football,

*Hess, Roland: Teacher certification in physical education, Journal of Health, Physical Education, and Recreation **41**:79, 1970.
†The Coaching Certification Committee of the Illinois Association for Professional Preparation in Health, Physical Education, and Recreation: A survey of special certification requirements for athletic coaches of high school interscholastic teams, Journal of Health, Physical Education, and Recreation **41**:14, 1970.

basketball, track, hockey, wrestling, or base-ball in a secondary or elementary school must be certified either in physical educa-tion or a special coaching requirement in physical education.

IOWA. Coaching personnel must be certi-fied to teach and must have completed an approved program of professional prepara-tion either in physical education or in the coaching of athletics.

SOUTH DAKOTA. At least 18 semester hours in the fields of health and physical education must be taken by coaching per-sonnel.

OKLAHOMA. Coaching as a major assign-ment (3 hours per day) requires a physical education certificate.

INDIANA. Varsity head football and bas-ketball coaches in senior high school are required to be licensed in the field of phys-ical education. All other coaches in grades seven to twelve must be licensed as a teacher and have a minimum of 8 semester hours of work in first aid and other courses related to the area of physical growth and develop-ment.

WYOMING. A coaching endorsement is entered on the teaching certificate after the applicant has taken one course in coaching that sport in which he is involved and also a course in first aid.

Separate certification for health and physical education teachers

With the continued emphasis upon school health education, there is a trend to sep-arate the certification of health education teachers from that of physical education teachers. Although there are many states that still certify health and physical educa-tion teachers with one certificate (my sur-vey of thirty-five states showed that eighteen of these states had one certificate for health and physical education teachers), according to Haag,* as of 1970, twenty-two states certify persons to teach secondary school

---

*Haag, Jessie Helen: Certification requirements in health education, 1949-1970, School Health Re-view **2:**11, 1971.

health education. The mean required num-ber of semester hours of health education required in these states is 25.4. These states are Arizona, California, Connecticut, Dela-ware, Florida, Indiana, Louisiana, Massa-chusetts, Minnesota, Montana, Nebraska, Nevada, New Jersey, New York, North Carolina, Ohio, Oregon, South Carolina, Tennessee, Texas, Utah, and Wisconsin.

Separate certification for elementary and secondary school teachers of physical education

The practice of certifying teachers in physical education for kindergarten to grade twelve is beginning to change with the current emphasis in physical education in the ele-mentary school. I surveyed thirty-five states and eight of these states reported separate certification requirements for elementary school teachers of physical education, and two more states indicated they were con-sidering such a certificate. The range of semester hours required for elementary school physical education certification was 18 to 30, and the range for secondary school physical education certification was 18 to 40 semester hours.

Other trends in teacher certification

There is a trend to increase the general education requirement. Many of the states are requiring as many as 30 or more semes-ter hours of work in this area. There is a trend toward requiring a bachelor's degree for the certification of a teacher; nearly all of the states now specify this require-ment. There is a trend toward requiring more work in the field of education with stress on the behavioral sciences and stu-dent teaching. Professional education re-quirements have been on the increase in many states. Some states require as many as 18 semester hours in this area. If James Conant's (former President of Harvard who has made many recommendations concern-ing the preparation and certification of teachers) recommendations are translated into practice, there may develop a trend to-

CERTIFICATION FOR HEALTH AND PHYSICAL EDUCATION–SOUTH CAROLINA

Professional preparation for secondary teachers

Eighteen semester hours of professional education are required. In adapting the professional work to a special teaching field, not more than 3 semester hours of the 18 may be devoted to special methods, the special methods courses to be taught in the education department as professional education. For candidates who are preparing to teach an academic subject in high school, a general methods course is suggested. Special methods courses are permitted and may be more appropriate for some special fields such as agriculture, commerce, home economics, and music.

The program of professional education courses must include the four areas on the secondary level as listed below:

A. Adolescent growth and development	12 semester hours
B. Principles and philosophy of education	
C. Principles of learning, materials, and methods	A, B, and C must be represented
D. Directed teaching in high school	6 semester hours
	18 semester hours

Health and physical education	**24***
History, principles, philosophy, organization, and administration	3
School health program	3†
Materials and applied techniques	15
Physiology and anatomy	3‡

Content to be included in each area

History, principles, philosophy, organization, and administration of health and physical education. This area should include the historical background of the health and physical education program as a basis for understanding the present program; the underlying principles, aims, and objectives; the problems relating to the setting up and conducting of the program including curriculum building, planning, and use of facilities.

School health. This work should cover the theory of the field of school health including the teaching materials to be used, presentation, problems relating to the healthful environment, the sources of materials and their uses, the principles and practice of first aid and safety as they may be used in the school program.

Materials and applied techniques. This area involves an understanding and mastery of the techniques of the various activities and their presentation and adaptation to the various age levels and groups. At least four of the following shall be included:

1. Games and activities of low organization
2. Rhythmical activities
3. Individual and dual sports
4. Team sports
5. Adaptive activities (exceptional or atypical children)
6. Gymnastics and self-testing activities
7. Intramural and interscholastic sports
8. Recreation activities and recreational leadership

English   12 semester hours

Composition, rhetoric, and literature are the usual courses in English. These include courses involving the satisfactory use of oral and written language and a background of general literature.

*Exclusive of all service courses.
†In addition to the 3 semester hours in the basic program.
‡In addition to the 12 semester hours of basic science requirements.

Biological and physical sciences   12 semester hours

Both biological and physical sciences are required. Laboratory or nonlaboratory courses in each field may be included. Any combination of hours in these sciences may be made provided the total amounts to 12.

Social studies   12 semester hours

The social studies, for certification, including history, political science, economics, geography (when taught as a social subject), sociology, religion, and philosophy. At least two fields must be represented, with 6 but not more than 6 semester hours in one field. The remaining 6 hours may be in any one or any combination of the remaining fields.

Health   from 2 to 3 semester hours

The course should include either personal or community health or both.

Art and music   from 4 to 6 semester hours

Appreciation or history of both art and music must be included, with not less than 2 semester hours in each.

---

ward having the college or university certify teachers that it trains.

There is a trend toward less discrimination against out-of-state applications. Such a trend makes it possible for qualified candidates to teach in various sections of the country. Furthermore, it makes possible the sharing of educational experiences in school systems that represent various geographical and economic sections. It also permits a qualified candidate to accept a promotion into a better position without being restricted by local requirements.

The trend toward certification reciprocity between the states will allow for the flow of qualified teachers across state boundaries, make for a better balance between supply and demand for teachers, increase a feeling of national unity, contribute to the breaking down of provincialism, and aid in teacher growth. Movements in the direction of certification reciprocity have been made by the Southern Association Study, the Ohio Valley Association, the North Central Association Studies, the Central States Conference, and the Compact of New England States, New York, and New Jersey.

Most states issue emergency teaching certificates in the absence of qualified candidates, although this practice is decreasing.

It seems logical that as the supply of teachers grows, the qualifications for teachers will be raised and emergency teaching certificates will be abolished.

All states have some type of certification system for teachers. Certificates for teaching are usually issued by the state departments of education or state school agency. It should be kept in mind, however, that although states have established certification requirements, many local school systems require more training than those listed as minimum requirements by the state certifying agency. Certification requirements pertain to teaching in the public schools. In most cases teachers in private schools are not required to meet state certification standards. However, these schools have their own requirements for teaching, which in many cases are similar to those that prevail for the public schools. College teachers are rarely certified. Some junior colleges must meet state certification requirements, which are very similar to secondary school requirements.

In the special certification requirements that prevail for the teaching of physical education, there is considerable difference in nomenclature and qualifications listed. The physical educator who desires to teach in a particular state selects courses that will qualify him for teaching in that particular state. It is practically an impossibility to prepare for the teaching of physical education in all of the fifty states. However, if a physical educator's work is planned with care, the certification requirements for many states may be met with only an additional summer session's training or less. A survey conducted several years ago showed that in order to be certified in all the states a candidate would have the following preparation:

135 semester hours of work in an accredited institution of higher learning
   Rank in upper four-fifths of class
   Bachelor's degree
   24 semester hours in the field of education
   42 semester hours of prerequisites including biology, anatomy, physiology, personal hygiene, community hygiene, English, American history and government, psychology, sociology, and child growth and development
   A minimum of 71 semester hours in physical education work including practice teaching, applied anatomy, applied physiology, kinesiology, correctives, physical inspection, first aid and safety, introduction to physical education, history of physical education, administration and supervision, methods and materials, coaching techniques, nature of play, recreational activities, leadership, and theory and practice of various types of games, rhythms, and dances*

Today a candidate would be required to meet even higher requirements than these that have been listed.

QUESTIONS AND EXERCISES

1. Why is it essential to have certification requirements?
2. A few educators are advocating national certification standards. What are the advantages and disadvantages of such a proposal?
3. What are the certification requirements for the state in which you desire to teach? To What extent does your present training program prepare you to meet these standards?
4. What are some of the requirements that are similar for the various states?
5. What are emergency teaching certificates? What are their advantages and disadvantages?
6. What are some of the common characteristics of the certification requirements in the states

of Alabama, Arizona, California, Illinois, Massachusetts, and New York?
7. What is the average semester-hour requirement in the specialized area of physical education for the fifty states?
8. What procedure should be followed by the student in order to make sure he understands thoroughly the certification requirements of a particular state?
9. Discuss the trends in regard to the certification of teachers in the various states.
10. Discuss the certification requirements for your state in the light of professional standards discussed in previous chapters.

Reading assignment
   Bucher, Charles A., and Goldman, Myra: Dimensions of physical education, St. Louis, 1969, The C. V. Mosby Co., Reading selection 69.

SELECTED REFERENCES

Armstrong, W. Earl, and Stinnett, T. M.: A manual on certification requirements for school personnel in the United States, Washington, D. C., current issue, National Education Association.

Bucher, Charles A.: Administration of school health and physical education programs, St. Louis, 1971, The C. V. Mosby Co.

Bucher, Charles A., Koening, Constance, and Barnhard, Milton: Methods and materials for secondary school physical education, St. Louis, 1970, The C. V. Mosby Co.

Coaching Certification Committee of the Illinois Association of Health, Physical Education, and Recreation: A survey of special certification requirements for athletic coaches of high school interscholastic teams, Journal of Health, Physical Education, and Recreation 41:14, 1970.

Conant, James Bryant: The education of American teachers, New York, 1963, McGraw-Hill Book Co.

Haag, Jessie Helen: Certification requirements in health education, 1949-1970, School Health Review 2:11, 1971.

Hess, Roland: Teacher certification in physical education, Journal of Health, Physical Education, and Recreation 41:79, 1970.

Meinhardt, Thomas: A rationale for certification of high school coaches in Illinois, Journal of Health, Physical Education, and Recreation 42:48, 1971.

Mueller, Frederick O.: Factors related to the certification of high school football coaches, Journal of Health, Physical Education, and Recreation 42:50, 1971.

Woellner, Elizabeth H., and Wood, M. Aurilla: Requirements for certification, Chicago, 1970-1971, The University of Chicago Press.

---

*Morehouse, Laurence E., and Schaaf, Oscar: Research Quarterly 13:293, 1942.

24/Employment opportunities

Teaching has more members than any other profession in existence today. The number of full-time men and women teachers in the United States is more than 2.5 million. Furthermore, no other profession offers so many employment opportunities for women. Approximately one-third of all teachers are women, more than twice as many as in the nursing profession. There are many more women than men teaching in the elementary schools of the nation. However, at the secondary level, in junior and senior high schools, the number of men and women in teaching is nearly equal, with a few more men than women. At the college and university level there are more male teachers. Men hold about four-fifths of all the college and university positions. However, the women's liberation movement is expected to eventually provide a better balance of men and women instructors.

Education is America's largest business. More than one out of every four individuals is in school. The proportion of young people getting more schooling, emphasis on quality education, and other factors indicate a bright future for this field of work. Total annual outlays for public elementary and secondary schools, excluding capital outlay and interest, is approximately $35 billion.

Educational construction costs approximately $4.5 billion a year. Expenditures on classroom equipment, such as books, audiovisual devices, and desks, amount to $1 billion a year. Certain leading corporations in the United States have linked themselves to the educational business in such areas as copying machines, microfilms, texts and other reading material, programmed instruction, electronics, language laboratories, and learning systems.

The growth of education during the last few years has been phenomenal. For example, expenditures in 1950 were about $9.3 billion. A rise to more than $50 billion has been projected by the middle 1970's. Ten years ago, school and college enrollments were under 40 million. The U. S. Office of Education foresees enrollments of approximately 65 million by the middle 1970's. Textbook sales have risen from about $200 million to $600 million annually in the past decade, or an annual growth of about 12%. Two-year college enrollments have jumped from less than 300,000 students in 1954 to nearly 1 million today.

PROFESSIONAL ADVANTAGES OFFERED BY TEACHING

Education is on the move. Those who decide to make a career in this field will be involved in a great adventure. Although the service that a teacher renders to human beings is a most attractive feature of this field of endeavor, other advantages exist.

Teaching salaries

The average salary for beginning teachers with a bachelor's degree on a national level in public schools, according to estimates by the National Education Association, is approximately $7,000. The national average beginning salary for the teacher with a

649

The following statistics are outlined by the U. S. Office of Education in a publication that projects the education of the present into the education of the future (1974-1975):

A 71% increase in students getting bachelor's degrees, up from 525,000 to 899,000.
Almost twice as many persons getting master's degrees, from 111,000 to 210,000.
Twice as many persons getting doctoral degrees, from 15,300 to 31,900.
An 89% increase in total spending by colleges and universities, from $11.9 billion to $22.5 billion.
A 74% increase in students seeking degrees at colleges and universities, up from 5 million in the fall of 1964 to 8.7 million in the fall of 1974.
A 13.5% increase in enrollment at public and private elementary and secondary schools, from 48.1 million in 1964 to 54.6 million in 1974.
A 25.9% increase in public and private high school graduates, from 2.7 million to 3.4 million.
An increase of 507,000 public and private elementary and secondary school teachers, from 1.9 million to 2.4 million.
A 47% increase in expenditures for elementary and secondary schools, from $26.1 billion to $38.4 billion in the 1974-1975 school year.
The projections indicate that in 1974 the number of high school students will have more than doubled, and the number of degree-seeking college students will have more than tripled the 1954 totals. A decade from now, an estimated 16.4 million students will be in high school.*

*Projections of educational statistics to 1974-1975, Washington, D. C., 1965 edition, U. S. Department of Health, Education and Welfare.

Average annual salaries of public school instructional staff.

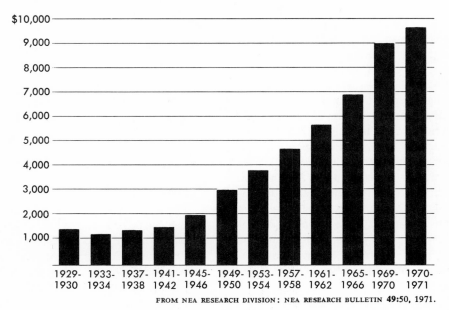

FROM NEA RESEARCH DIVISION: NEA RESEARCH BULLETIN **49:50**, 1971.

Median salaries paid college teachers, 1970-1971.

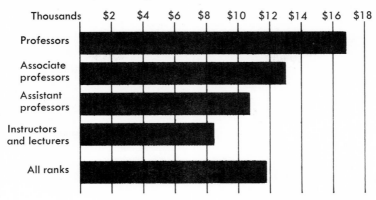

FROM NEA RESEARCH DIVISION: NEA RESEARCH BULLETIN **49**:55, 1971.

Median maximum annual supplements, 1969-1970, in selected pupil-participating activities (school systems enrolling 6,000 or more pupils).

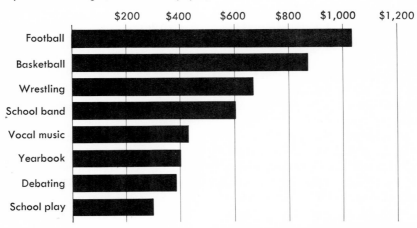

FROM NEA RESEARCH DIVISION: NEA RESEARCH BULLETIN **48**:42, 1970.

master's degree is nearly $8,000. On a regional basis the scheduled beginning salary for teachers with a bachelor's degree is as follows: New England—slightly more than $7,000; Mideast—nearly $7,500; Southeast—nearly $6,500; Great Lakes—nearly $7,500; Plains—about $7,000; Southwest—slightly more than $6,500; Rocky Mountain—nearly $6,500; Far West—slightly more than $7,000.

The average annual salaries for teachers in 4-year colleges and universities are in excess of $9,500 for 9 to 10 months' work. The approximate mean annual minimum salaries of full-time faculty members for 9 to 10 months' work in public and private institutions of higher education, by academic rank, are as follows: professors, $13,000; associate professors, $11,000; assistant professors, $9,000; and instructors, $7,500.

The mean scheduled minimum salaries for 2-year institutions according to academic preparation are as follows: bachelor's degree—slightly more than $7,000; master's degree—nearly $8,000; 6 years of study—slightly more than $8,500; and doctor's degree—nearly $10,000.

Other benefits for teachers

Teaching is a profession that has many benefits. Most importantly, it provides the opportunity to render a service in guiding the growth and learning of others, to become a member of a respected and growing profession, to further one's own self-development and personal growth, to travel, and to participate in unlimited exciting experiences with children, youth, and adults. Furthermore, in many school systems it offers tenure, sabbatical leaves, sick leaves, retirement benefits, and a strongly organized profession.

TENURE. Many school systems provide tenure for teachers who serve successful probationary periods of 3 or 5 years. This means that the teacher who has tenure cannot be dismissed, demoted, or suspended, except as prescribed by law and according to definitely prescribed procedures. This helps to provide security for the teacher.

SABBATICAL LEAVES. More school systems are adopting sabbatical leave schedules. Teachers, after a period of satisfactory service, say 7 years, may take 1 year or a semester with pay or partial pay to improve themselves, such as by pursuing graduate work, traveling, or performing research.

SICK LEAVES. Many school systems across the country are instituting sick leave provisions for the teacher and family. For example, during one school year (1967-1968 to 1968-1969) the percentage of negotiation agreements with family illness considerations increased from approximately 30% to 50%. The teacher is permitted to take time from his job when ill and still draw full salary. School systems usually designate the amount of time that may be used for such a purpose, frequently 5 to 10 days.

RETIREMENT BENEFITS. Most states have some provision for retirement benefits for teachers. After a stipulated period of service, usually from 25 to 35 years, and a minimum age, perhaps 55 to 65 years, the teacher may retire and draw a regular retirement benefit, which is usually computed on the amount of salary he earned. There is a trend toward using a fixed formula, which approaches 2% times a final average salary times the number of years a teacher has served, as a basis for determining a person's retirement benefits. In addition, about three-fourths of all the states are now covered by Social Security, which gives teachers additional benefits upon retirement.

A STRONGLY ORGANIZED PROFESSION. Teachers now have a voice in their own affairs. Teacher militancy, in combination with a recognition by parents that education should have a high priority in America, has had its impact on teachers as well as on the public in general. The teaching profession has gained a new respect and as a result it is a more attractive field in which to work.

SCHOOL AND COLLEGE ENROLLMENTS

The total enrollment in all types of schools and colleges is approximately 60 million. Increases are expected in most categories. For example, it is expected that in colleges the enrollments will jump to over 8 million by 1975. The growth of the 2-year college alone in recent years has been phenomenal. Nearly 1 million students are enrolled in approximately 900 junior colleges from coast to coast. Furthermore, it is projected that the enrollments will increase to approximately 1.5 million by the middle 1970's. Enrollment in regular public elementary and secondary schools is expected to be in excess of 47 million in the middle 1970's. Enrollment in kindergarten through eighth grade is expected to be in excess of 32 million in the middle 1970's. Enrollment rates at the elementary level will level off, but those at the high school and college levels will continue to increase.

The striking fact about education is that more of the population is going to school and more pupils are staying in school for

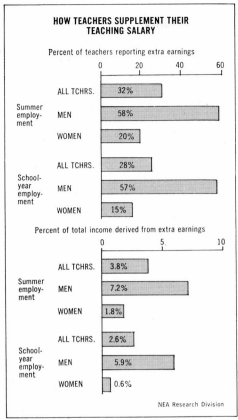

HOW TEACHERS SUPPLEMENT THEIR TEACHING SALARY

Percent of teachers reporting extra earnings

Summer employment
- ALL TCHRS. 32%
- MEN 58%
- WOMEN 20%

School-year employment
- ALL TCHRS. 28%
- MEN 57%
- WOMEN 15%

Percent of total income derived from extra earnings

Summer employment
- ALL TCHRS. 3.8%
- MEN 7.2%
- WOMEN 1.8%

School-year employment
- ALL TCHRS. 2.6%
- MEN 5.9%
- WOMEN 0.6%

NEA Research Division

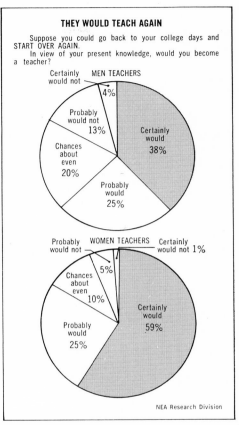

THEY WOULD TEACH AGAIN

Suppose you could go back to your college days and START OVER AGAIN.
In view of your present knowledge, would you become a teacher?

MEN TEACHERS
- Certainly would not 4%
- Probably would not 13%
- Chances about even 20%
- Probably would 25%
- Certainly would 38%

WOMEN TEACHERS
- Certainly would not 1%
- Probably would not 5%
- Chances about even 10%
- Probably would 25%
- Certainly would 59%

NEA Research Division

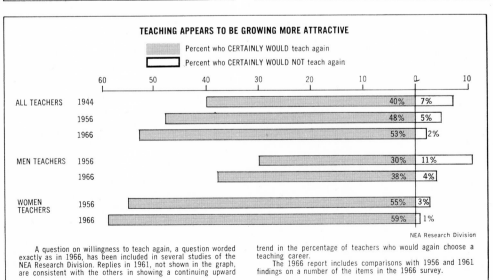

TEACHING APPEARS TO BE GROWING MORE ATTRACTIVE

Percent who CERTAINLY WOULD teach again
Percent who CERTAINLY WOULD NOT teach again

ALL TEACHERS
- 1944: 40% / 7%
- 1956: 48% / 5%
- 1966: 53% / 2%

MEN TEACHERS
- 1956: 30% / 11%
- 1966: 38% / 4%

WOMEN TEACHERS
- 1956: 55% / 3%
- 1966: 59% / 1%

NEA Research Division

A question on willingness to teach again, a question worded exactly as in 1966, has been included in several studies of the NEA Research Division. Replies in 1961, not shown in the graph, are consistent with the others in showing a continuing upward trend in the percentage of teachers who would again choose a teaching career.

The 1966 report includes comparisons with 1956 and 1961 findings on a number of the items in the 1966 survey.

FROM NEA JOURNAL **56:15, 1967.**

longer periods of time. More states also have compulsory attendance laws.

END OF THE TEACHER SHORTAGE

Thousands of qualified teachers are unable to find positions in the nation's schools and colleges. Taxpayer revolts against rising educational costs with some school districts reducing the size of their staffs, a leveling off of student enrollments, and an oversupply of teachers are some of the reasons for this dilemma. The oversupply is concentrated in such fields as English, foreign language (especially French), and social studies.

Shortages exist in such fields as preschool teaching, work with the handicapped, industrial arts, and women's physical education.

The reasons for the oversupply are many and varied, but the main one seems to be that the number of teachers is growing while student enrollments are declining. For example, the size of graduating classes preparing to enter teaching doubled between the years 1954 and 1964 and has been more than three times the 1954 levels since 1969.

In regard to student enrollments and number of teachers, the population trend changed greatly from the early 1950's until the middle 1960's, when the schools

Total teaching staff will expand by one-fifth to over 2.9 million during the 1968-1980 period. College enrollments will show the fastest growth rate between 1968 and 1980, rising to over 10 million.

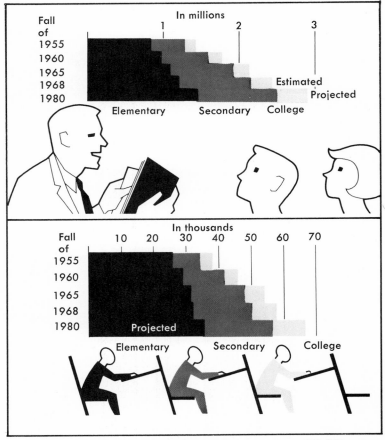

FROM OCCUPATIONAL OUTLOOK HANDBOOK, 1970-1971 EDITION,
U.S. DEPARTMENT OF LABOR, WASHINGTON, D.C., U.S. GOVERNMENT PRINTING OFFICE.

had large enrollments that began with the post–World War II baby boom. At the same time, these large enrollments were dependent upon a low supply of teachers who were born during the birth rate depression years. The situation has now reversed itself, with many of the post–World War II babies becoming teachers, thus increasing the supply. A further answer to the increased number of teachers is that many of the disadvantaged minorities, such as Negroes and Puerto Ricans, are now entering teaching at a much larger rate than before. One study has predicted a surplus of 55,000 teachers a year by the middle 1970's. The U. S. Department of Labor predicted that if the present trend continues, by 1980 there will be 4.2 million graduates of teacher-training institutions to fill only 2.4 million vacancies.

Another consideration is the nation's birth rate. The birth rate has declined from 4.1 million in 1963 to a little over 3 million annually at present.

Some specific statistics on the current employment situation for teachers, as furnished by the National Education Association, accents the problem. For example, 114,400 elementary school teachers, 167,800 secondary school teachers, and 8,300 teachers trained in special education completed their college preparation in anticipation of starting their teaching career in the fall of 1970. This represented an increase over the previous year of 6.3% at the elementary school level, 12.8% at the secondary school level, and 5.5% in special education. On the other hand, the estimated 35,000 additional positions needed for the fall of 1970, based on enrollment growth, was the smallest annual increase in a period of 16 years.

There are many bright spots to the current situation, however. The oversupply of teachers makes it possible for the selection, training, and appointment process to stress quality more than it has in past years. It will make it possible to eliminate the unsuited and incompetent teacher. Furthermore, it will enable school districts to replace an estimated 100,000 substandard teachers, many of whom hold emergency certificates. Finally, it will make it possible to have a lower student-teacher ratio, thus improving the learning climate of the classroom and gymnasium.

Those states that have reported an increased need for teachers list as the reasons

School-age population, 1958 to 1982.

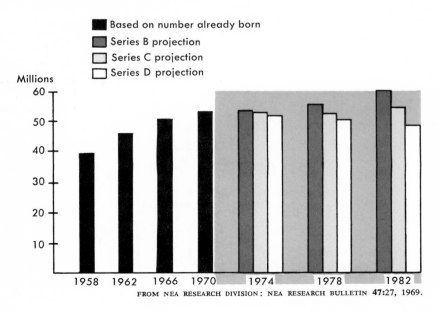

FROM NEA RESEARCH DIVISION: NEA RESEARCH BULLETIN **47:27**, 1969.

Growth in supply of beginning teachers.

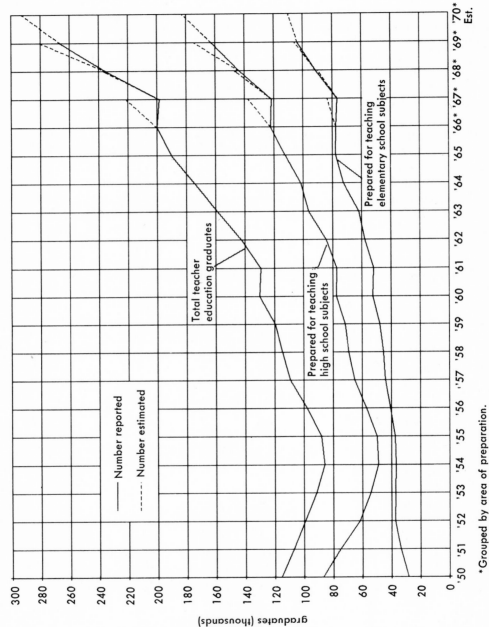

Number of teacher education graduates (thousands)

Number reported
Number estimated

Total teacher education graduates

Prepared for teaching high school subjects

Prepared for teaching elementary school subjects

*Grouped by area of preparation.

*A few institutions in four states did not respond in 1968, making the actual numbers reported for 1967 lower than the number that probably graduated that year.

FROM NEA RESEARCH DIVISION: TEACHER SUPPLY AND DEMAND IN PUBLIC SCHOOLS, 1970, P. 12.

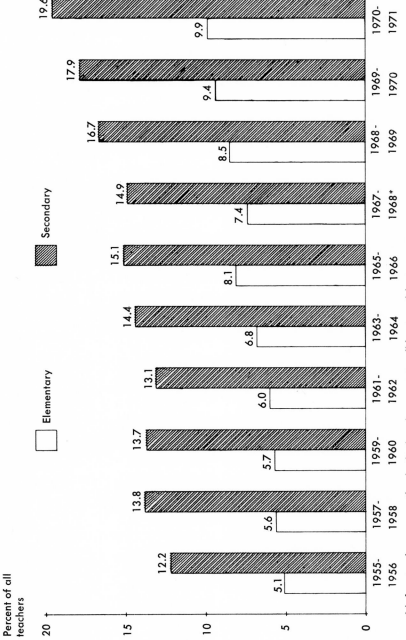

Teacher education graduates as percent of all teachers in the session following their graduation.

Percent of all teachers

Elementary

Secondary

	1955-1956	1957-1958	1959-1960	1961-1962	1963-1964	1965-1966	1967-1968*	1968-1969	1969-1970	1970-1971
Secondary	12.2	13.8	13.7	13.1	14.4	15.1	14.9	16.7	17.9	19.6
Elementary	5.1	5.6	5.7	6.0	6.8	8.1	7.4	8.5	9.4	9.9

*A few teacher preparation institutions in two states did not participate in the 1967-1968 study, making the estimated number of graduates in 1967 from 2% to 6% lower than the projected actual data.

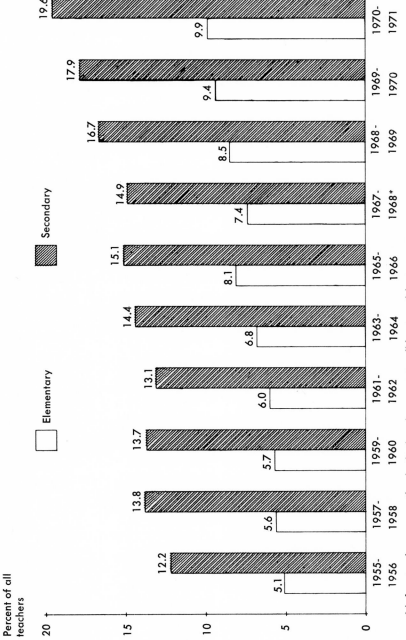

FROM NEA RESEARCH DIVISION: TEACHER SUPPLY AND DEMAND IN PUBLIC SCHOOLS, 1970, P. 41.

such factors as added curricular offerings, reduction in class size, and new positions resulting from federal legislation. Furthermore, the best prospects for employment in the next few years appear to be in rural areas and in large cities rather than in suburban areas of population.

Beginning teachers should not look upon the present teacher employment situation as unpromising, because many vacancies still exist for the well-qualified person. Teachers planning to teach at the elementary school level will find many vacancies. By 1980, about 1 million teachers will be needed to replace those who retire, die, or leave the profession for other reasons. Although enrollments will be at about the same level in 1980 as today, it is expected that about 40,000 new teachers will be needed to reduce the pupil-teacher ratio. In addition, it is expected that another 56,500 teachers will be needed to replace persons with substandard teaching certificates. Furthermore, increased emphasis upon the education of very young children, children in low-income areas, and the handicapped means that more teachers will be needed.

There will be a need for approximately 100,000 new secondary school teachers each year until the middle 1970's to take care of enrollment increases, to reflect some improvement in the pupil-teacher ratio, to replace teachers who retire, marry, or leave the field for other reasons, and to replace persons who do not meet certification requirements. Although some job openings for secondary school teachers will be created by rising enrollments, most of the job openings —about 70% of the total requirements— will come from the need to replace teachers who for various reasons may leave the field. Also, considerable additional demand for teachers may be generated by federal legislation that provides for supplementary educational centers and a national Teachers Corps (federally recruited teachers and teacher-interns for low-income areas). Furthermore, many teachers trained for secondary schools may qualify for junior college positions, where demand for teachers is expected to be especially great in the years to come.

College teaching opportunities in the years ahead are especially bright with increasing enrollments and the "open admissions" development. (See Chapter 21.) Furthermore, there will be many opportunities in junior colleges for persons who have master's degrees or have taken further graduate work.

The U. S. Office of Education estimates that the full-time college teaching staff will increase to approximately 337,000 by the middle 1970's, an increase of about two-thirds. In addition to the teachers needed to take care of the enrollment growth, about 16,000 more teachers may be needed annually up to the middle 1970's to replace those who retire, die, or leave the profession for other reasons. Furthermore, the fact that new degree recipients may be drained from the college teaching ranks by better paying opportunities in industry, government, and nonprofit organizations may increase the critical need to meet the demand in many subject fields through the mid-1970's.

EMPLOYMENT IN PHYSICAL EDUCATION

The supply and demand situation in physical education reveals that the supply of men physical education teachers throughout the nation has surpassed the demand. On the other hand, the supply of women physical education teachers is inadequate, with extreme shortages existing in some states.

Women's physical education

A recent national survey of the Research Division of the National Education Association of the nation's sixty-seven largest school systems revealed that although several school systems were short on supply, five school systems reported extreme difficulty in filling teaching positions in women's physical education. In those five school systems, 228 positions had not been filled by late July.

Supply and demand for beginning teachers by type of assignment, adjusted trend criterion estimate, 1970.

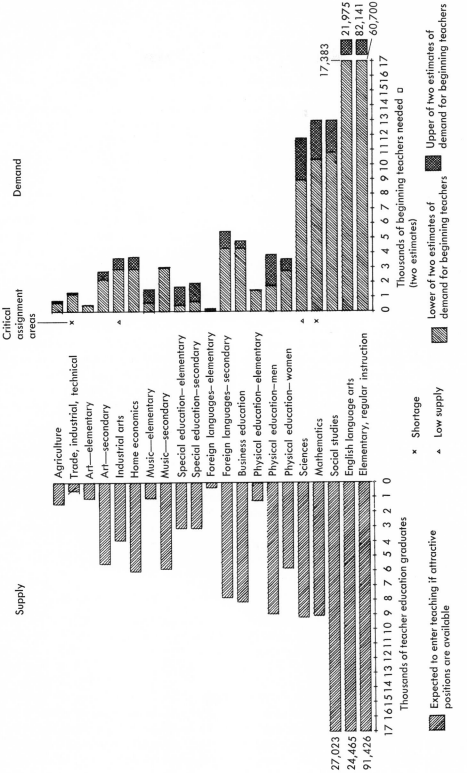
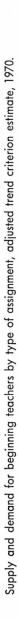

FROM NEA RESEARCH DIVISION: TEACHER SUPPLY AND DEMAND IN PUBLIC SCHOOLS, 1970, P. 46.

State	Demand in men's physical education	Demand in women's physical education
Alabama	Large demand (elementary) Little demand (secondary)	Large demand
Arizona	No demand	No demand
Colorado	No demand	Little demand
Indiana	Little demand (elementary) No demand (secondary)	Little demand
Kentucky	Little demand (elementary)	Little demand (elementary)
New Jersey	Little demand	Large demand
New York	Little demand	Large demand
Oklahoma	Little demand	Large demand
Washington	Little demand (elementary) No demand (secondary)	Little demand

Qualified women physical educators have been getting their choice of positions, high salaries, and other conditions that are attracting more women to the profession. Leaders in the profession, college admissions officers, and teacher-training institutions have stepped up their recruitment programs for women physical educators. High school girls are being better oriented in regard to the opportunities available in becoming a teacher of physical education. Young women are recognizing the important place that such programs have in the schools and colleges of our nation, and as a result more women want to become a part of it. They realize that it is not a profession pursued by a superathletic woman but, instead, is a field of endeavor in which the woman who is interested in developing a healthy, more beautiful female population has an important role to play.

Many women have achieved respected positions in schools, colleges, and professional associations. They have received many awards and tributes from the general public as well as their colleagues. They have provided excellent examples of the important role that girls and women can play in the field of physical education. As a result, more girls will try to emulate them.

Men's physical education

The oversupply of men physical education teachers may be similar to other teaching subjects where the same conditions exist. Factors that may be involved in the present supply-demand situation include more college graduates entering men's physical education field; fewer jobs available outside teaching because of the economic slowdown; fewer teachers retiring or leaving the profession unless absolutely necessary; and a reduction in teaching positions because of school financing problems.

A questionnaire sent to nine states asking about employment opportunities in the field of physical education provided the information given at the top of this page on the teacher supply-and-demand situation in the field of physical education.

The placement services of a large eastern university showed the following physical education vacancies for various sections of the nation that were reported for a recent year. Since approximately 70% of the vacancies were for women, it is somewhat indicative of the number of positions also open for men physical educators.

Area	Number of vacancies
Northeast	736
North Central	107
Northwest	8
Southeast	13
South Central	3
Southwest	109

This placement agency felt that although for the last 4 or 5 years there has been a more than adequate supply of men in physical education, the trend will soon change. They cited the fact that they believed fewer men will be entering the field, with the result that the supply will diminish.

Encouraging employment developments

Physical education is playing an increasing role in the total educational endeavor of the United States. The President's Council on Physical Fitness and Sports is one agency that has done much to encourage the promotion of physical education, not only among the youth of this nation but also among the adult population as well. Furthermore, the increased recognition of the contribution that physical activity can make to physical, mental, and social health is a factor. Today, there are many encouraging employment developments that augur well for the future of physical education.

ELEMENTARY SCHOOL PHYSICAL EDUCATION PROGRAMS. The elementary school offers an opportunity to specialize in physical education. The self-contained classroom, where the classroom teacher is the only person to conduct physical education classes, is now diminishing. The specialist in elementary school physical education is being hired in more and more elementary schools across the country. The surge in movement education is taking hold, with the need for more physical education personnel trained in this area. Specialists are particularly needed in grades 4, 5, and 6. These physical educators may work with classroom teachers or teach the physical education classes themselves. If this practice becomes nationwide, it will mean many more physical education teachers will be needed. The fact that there are about 84,000 public elementary schools as contrasted with about 26,000 high schools supports this premise.

STRESS ON THE HANDICAPPED. The emphasis upon the handicapped student including the mentally retarded and physically handicapped, together with the research that shows the contribution physical education can make to students who are so characterized, has opened up an entire new area for employment.

INNER-CITY PROGRAMS. The problems encountered by large cities with their ghettos and poverty pockets, together with the appeal of physical education and sports for inner-city children and youth, augurs well for the contribution that professionals can make to such important areas of the nation.

COACHES TRAINED IN PHYSICAL EDUCATION. The trend across the country to hire coaches who have been trained in the field of physical education should result in many new positions as more and more states adopt such a practice. It is common practice for states to permit anyone to coach who has a teaching certificate. As a result, a large percentage of coaches are teachers of subjects other than physical education. However, with the trend toward hiring coaches trained in the field of physical education, a new avenue of employment has opened up, since it means that more physical educators will be needed to work in school athletic programs.

TWO-YEAR COLLEGES, OPEN ADMISSIONS, AND RISING COLLEGE ENROLLMENTS. The trend toward more 2-year colleges, open admissions, and increased enrollments means that more physical educators will be needed to satisfy the requirements at this educational level. The baby boom is reaching colleges, and this, together with the fact that more high school graduates are going on to college, means a rise in college enrollments during the next decade. The spectacular rise of the 2-year college means there will be more opportunities for physical education personnel at this level in order to accommodate the students who will be attending these institutions. Furthermore, surveys show that most 2-year colleges are offering physical education service courses for each of the 2 years, some have started professional programs, and some also include a course in health for freshmen.

EMPHASIS UPON PHYSICAL FITNESS. With federal backing, the country is rapidly becoming fitness conscious. On all sides there is evidence of increased emphasis on physical education in order to enhance the well-being of our youth and adults. The emphasis on physical fitness has also carried over into industrial fitness. Many corporations are establishing physical fitness centers for their executives and other employees. These developments mean the need for more physical educators.

LOWER RATIO OF TEACHERS TO STUDENTS. Pressures are being exerted in some sections of the country to have smaller classes per teacher. Physical educators can do a better job with fewer students, as the English teacher does, and this is a goal that must be accomplished. This will mean that more teachers of physical education will be needed.

EXPANSION OF SPORTS. Sports are playing a more prominent role in the American culture. As a result, more leaders will be needed to teach and guide programs involved with various sports.

SUMMER SCHOOL PROGRAMS. New York and other states have experimented with summer school programs at the precollege level. The results have been highly satisfactory and should result in the need for more teachers.

TEACHING OPPORTUNITIES ABROAD. There are many opportunities for physical educators to teach in other countries of the world. (See Chapter 14.)

FEDERAL LEGISLATION. Such governmental legislation and innovations as the Elementary and Secondary Education Act, the Higher Education Act, Project Head Start, and the Teacher Corps will increase the need for teachers. These programs place special emphasis on groups of children and adults that need to have greater educational opportunities. These innovations in our culture will mean greater attention to all individuals in our society regardless of intellect, physical condition, economic status, race, and other factors that differentiate human beings. Consequently, this will mean a demand for more teachers of varying specialties in order to provide such programs.

EMPLOYMENT OF PHYSICAL EDUCATORS IN ALLIED AREAS. A significant development during recent years has been the increased emphasis on such allied areas as recreation, health education, camping, and physical therapy. Although these are distinct and separate fields of endeavor from physical education, nevertheless, some aspects of these specialties offer opportunities for physical educators. Furthermore, in some areas of the country shortages of trained personnel force these responsibilities upon physical educators, who in many cases shoulder them reluctantly.

According to the U. S. Department of Labor, at the present time a serious need exists for persons in the field of recreation. These opportunities are expected to increase rapidly, at least through the mid-1970's. Serious shortages presently exist in all parts of the country for trained recreation workers, particularly in local governments, hospitals, and youth-serving agencies. As a result of this shortage and the great demand for qualified persons, many physical educators will be able to obtain full- or part-time employment in these programs.

The Boys' Clubs of America are a rapidly growing national movement, with a new Boys' Club being started somewhere in the nation on the average of one every 8 days. The Boys' Clubs of America point out that they have great need for more people.

The American National Red Cross points out that college graduates with majors in health, physical education, and recreation can find employment with them if they are interested, motivated, have the right type of personality, and possess leadership potential. For example, they cite that they are seeking recreation aides and physical educators for their programs of service in military hospitals and clubmobile programs overseas. They also point out that graduates with a physical education major who have had teaching experience and possess a knowledge of community organization may be employed as safety service representatives on the national staff of Red Cross and as directors of safety services in many of the larger chapters.

The preceding represent only a sampling of employment opportunities for physical educators in allied fields. Others that might be explored, depending upon a person's qualifications and interests, are work in such voluntary youth agencies as the Young Women's and Young Men's Christian and Hebrew Associations, work with the physically handicapped in hospitals and other agencies, camping and outdoor education, churches, resort areas, and the armed forces. Many opportunities are available if one will take time to investigate them thoroughly.

TIPS FOR QUALIFIED TEACHER TO FOLLOW IN SECURING A POSITION IN PHYSICAL EDUCATION

Some advice that will help the qualified teacher in securing the right position is incorporated in the following five points:

START EARLY. Start looking well in advance of the time you want to begin to work. Administrators plan far ahead of their needs. "The early bird catches the worm" may be true in your case. Know what you want and start early to achieve your goal.

KNOW WHERE THE JOBS ARE. Do considerable research to find out what positions are available. Talk with your friends and alumni, register with the placement bureau, write school systems where you would like to work. Write the letter of inquiry with care. Give enough information about yourself to evoke interest, use good English and form, and have the letter typewritten.

HAVE YOUR CREDENTIALS UP TO DATE. Select with care and then contact the persons you would like to use for references. Ask if you may use their names. Prepare a list of your qualifications—personal, training, experience, and any other information in which a prospective employer might be interested. Fill out the forms required by the university placement bureau. Register with a commercial agency if you feel it will help, but be selective and use an agency that is particular about its candidates. A complete list is available from the National Association of Teachers Agencies, Room 400, 64 East Jackson Boulevard, Chicago, Illinois 60604.

Many state education associations and state departments of education also provide placement services for a small fee. Some education associations place nonmembers as well as members. The American Association for Health, Physical Education, and Recreation maintains a placement service for its members. It sends personal data forms of qualified applicants to employers, and then employers make all further contacts directly with applicants. Members of the Association who desire to enroll with this placement service should request personal data forms from the National Office, AAHPER Placement Service. An AAHPER placement booth is also maintained each year at the national convention to assist members who desire to seek new positions.

Other key sources of information are:

1. *The superintendent of schools or director of personnel in a particular school district.* Names and addresses of these officers are listed in the United States Office of Education's annual Education Directory, Part 2, Public school systems (available from the Superintendent of Documents, U. S. Government Printing Office, Washington, D. C. 20401).

2. *U. S. Employment Service.* Offices throughout the country list vacancies and help place educators without charge.

3. *NEA Search.* This is a computerized education locator service providing a nationwide clearinghouse to inform prospective employers and employees of available applicants and positions. The address is 1201 16th Street N.W., Washington, D. C. 20036.

4. *Association for School, College, and University Staffing.* This is a placement service located at the National Communication and Service Center, Inc., Box 166, Hershey, Pennsylvania 17033.

WRITE AN APPLICATION LETTER THAT WILL LAND THE JOB. In writing a letter of application, use good form, be sincere, appeal to the interest of the employer, offer a service rather than apply for a job, and be specific as to your qualifications.

LEAVE A FAVORABLE IMPRESSION DURING THE INTERVIEW. The interview is the culmination of the search. Dress conservatively, put on a smile, use a firm handshake, be on time, answer questions directly, speak so that you can be heard, volunteer any information you feel is important, and listen to what the employer says.

Good luck!

A CONCLUDING STATEMENT

The old adage that there is always a job for a well-qualified person is usually true in the field of physical education. Students who have the essential qualifications for this work and who conscientiously apply themselves should not have any difficulty in finding employment in a setting that will utilize their training and fulfill their ambitions.

The value of physical education to enriched living and its potentialities for building a better society are being increasingly recognized by the public. There is ample room for many qualified young men and women in this growing profession. There is no room for those who cannot meet the professional standards that have been established. Therefore the best advice that can be offered to a student who desires to find employment in physical education is, first, to make sure that he is equipped to do the job. If he is not, then he should seek other fields of endeavor where his talents can be more effectively utilized. If he is qualified, then he should feel confident of the future because he is a member of a profession that is just beginning to realize its potentialities.

QUESTIONS AND EXERCISES

1. What are the prospects for employment opportunities for physical educators during the next decade?
2. What are the implications for the recognition of the value of physical education in times of peace and in times of national emergency?
3. What are some of the advantages the physical education profession offers that other types of work do not offer?
4. Make a list of some laws and rules and regulations that have recently been enacted that point to an emphasis on physical education.
5. What are the predictions for school enrollments during the next decade?
6. What are the trends in higher education?
7. Make a bar graph that depicts school enrollments over the next 5 years.
8. Compare the predictions for school enrollments on the elementary school level with those on the secondary school level.
9. What advances have been made during the last 10 years in respect to teachers' salaries?
10. What is meant by the phrase "the teacher shortage has ended"?
11. How do the states in your particular section of the country rank as to the average annual salaries of teachers?

SELECTED REFERENCES

American Association for Health, Physical Education, and Recreation: Careers in physical education for girls, Washington, D. C., The Association.

American Association for Health, Physical Education, and Recreation: Health education as your career, Washington, D. C., The Association.

American Association for Health, Physical Education, and Recreation: Physical education and coaching as your career, Washington, D. C., The Association.

American Association for Health, Physical Education, and Recreation: Recreation—a new profession for our time, Washington, D. C., The Association.

Bureau of Labor Statistics, U. S. Department of Labor: Employment outlook for elementary and secondary school teachers, current year, Washington, D. C., U. S. Government Printing Office.

Marsh, Robert R.: How about recreation, New York, 1966, New York State Recreation Society.

National Education Association: Better staffing and expanded programs can result from larger teacher supply, NEA News, September, 1970.

National Education Association: Careers in education, National Commission on Teacher Education and Professional Standards, Washington, D. C., 1968, The Association.

National Education Association: A new era in teacher supply and demand, Today's Education **59:**51, 1970.

National Education Association: Salaries in higher education, NEA Research Bulletin, vol. 49, March, 1971.

National Education Association: Teacher supply and demand in public elementary and secondary schools, Washington, D. C., 1970, The Association.

National Education Association Research Division: Teacher supply and demand in universities, colleges, and junior colleges, Washington, D. C., 1970, NEA Publication.

Publications of the National Education Association concerned with the future of education.

Publications of the U. S. Office of Education on future school enrollments.

U. S. Department of Labor: Occupational outlook handbook, current edition, Washington, D. C., Department of Labor.

U. S. Office of Education: Digest of educational statistics, Washington, D. C., 1969, U. S. Government Printing Office.

U. S. Office of Education: What we need to know about educational manpower, Washington, D. C., 1968, U. S. Government Printing Office.

25/Challenges facing physical education

Physical education has great promise as an emerging profession if it faces up to the many challenges that are presenting themselves. Whether or not these potentialities are realized will be determined to a great extent by the professional student in teacher-training institutions at the present time. Professional students who have chosen physical education as a career can accept these challenges with firm resolve and strive to meet them, or they can sit idly by and allow their chosen field of endeavor to drift into ineffectiveness and aimlessness. They are the leaders of tomorrow. Upon their shoulders falls the responsibility of establishing their work as an essential need in today's society.

This book has attempted to show what a challenging field of endeavor physical education is for the student who has a sincere interest in this work. It has attempted to point out such things as an interpretation of the true meaning of physical education, the diversified types of work and settings where it takes place, its need in present-day living, its scientific bases, and the duties and requirements of its leadership. This book has attempted to impress upon the student's mind his part in raising the profession to lofty heights.

A national survey of recognized leaders in the field of physical education identified what are some of the greatest challenges facing physical education today. These include the following:

1. There is a need to recruit men and women into the field who will gain respect for physical education. These men and women should be scholars, dedicated, enthusiastic professionals, and motivated to help physical education gain greater stature and self-respect.
2. The need to develop programs of physical education that will be meaningful to students while they are in school and will also leave an imprint on their lives after they graduate.
3. The need to develop programs described by the term *physical education* rather than *physical training*. The need to develop a program of physical education for each educational level, elementary through college, that is meaningful, progressive, sequential, and identifies basic concepts that guide professionals in their day-to-day work.
4. The need to develop a research program that clarifies and develops a body of knowledge and support for the relationship of physical activity to the psychological, sociological, and intellectual development of human beings. Such knowledge would represent the foundation upon which a professional program is built. Furthermore, there should be more research in relation to the contribution that physical education can make to the physically handicapped, mentally retarded, and emotionally disturbed.
5. The need to find ways of interpreting to the various publics a more accurate and complete understanding of what physical educators are trying to do.
6. The need to better define the relationship of physical education, health education, and recreation and to determine how all can work together in a manner that helps each area to grow and prosper.
7. The need to bridge the gap between theory and research and practice, so that what has been pioneered through sound scientific research in our colleges and universities and by leaders in the field will be implemented and interpreted at the grass-roots level or the action level by our practitioners.
8. The need to place more stress on elementary school physical education, with men and

women trained as specialists for this responsibility.

As a closing chapter of this book, I would like to list and very briefly discuss what I consider to be some of the greatest challenges facing the physical education profession today. It is hoped that the student will keep these in mind and attempt to meet them wherever they may appear in his work. In so doing, physical education can be aided in realizing its potentialities.

NEED TO BE CREATIVE

Of all the challenges facing physical education today, the need for creativity is very important. Creativity as used here refers to the discovery of something in physical education that is truly new and that will be an achievement in its own right. Examples of creativity in the history of the world were the development of the theory of relativity and the invention of the telephone. In education, it was such things as the nongraded school and the teaching machine. An example in physical education might be the development of the game of basketball by Naismith. Each of these examples of creativity resulted in a novel work that was accepted as useful and satisfying to society.

Physical education has had very few exciting and dynamic creative ideas in its history. It desperately needs some at the present time to pull it out of its doldrums and help it to play a more dynamic role in education. More creative ideas are needed like Wood's "new physical education," Laban's "movement education," and Hetherington's "fundamental education."

Physical educators need to think more about the present status of their field of endeavor, including the problems they face and the goals they wish to achieve, and then come up with some creative ideas that will help to solve these problems and achieve these goals.

A review of the literature reveals some characteristics of the creative person. He will possess imagination, inner maturity, the ability to think and to analyze, a rich background of knowledge in his field, and flexibility in approaching problems. He will be skeptical of accepted ideas and less suspicious of new ones, persistent, sensitive to his environment, fluent in the production of ideas, and self-confident.

Charles Patrick, in his book entitled *What is Creative Thinking?,* points out that creative thinking proceeds through several distinct stages. For example, there is the *preparation stage,* where the individual becomes familiar with his field and the situation where it is desired to produce creative ideas. Intuition will not come without hard work, prior education, and a thorough understanding of the field. A second stage is *incubation,* where the problem is defined, various suggestions and solutions are considered, and much thought takes place. A third stage is *illumination,* where a specific idea is envisioned and the individual begins to explore and work toward a solution. Finally, there is the *verification* stage, where the idea is tested, altered, and eventually completed and utilized. These steps to creativity indicate that to be productive of new ideas requires much study, thought, and critical evaluation. It does not occur automatically.

Each physical educator should strive to be more creative. As a result, new ideas will be born and better physical education programs will develop. Major students in professional preparation institutions and young leaders in the field represent persons who have the potential for giving birth to new ideas that will make physical education more relevant to the rapidly changing world in which we live.

CLOSING THE GAP BETWEEN RESEARCH AND PRACTICE

Basically, there are three aspects of closing the gap between research and practice in physical education that constitute a challenge to all professionals.

The first part of this challenge is that physical education has available today valid research findings that are not being applied in programs across the country. For example, much is known about learning theory

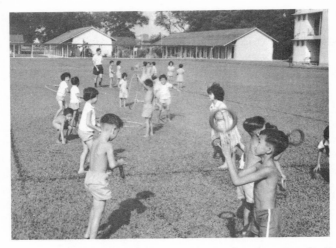

Physical educators need to be creative. Physical education class in Singapore.

in general and about motor learning in particular—but it is not applied. There are even some excellent articles in our professional literature and one or two books that have summarized the pertinent research findings in motor learning. However, much of the skill teaching that goes on today is still a hit-and-miss procedure based on traditional ways of doing things or upon an individual teacher's own unscientific opinion. In addition to learning theory, much is known but not applied in such areas as human behavior, physical fitness, activity and weight control, body image, and other important considerations in physical education. This gap between what we know to be right and what is practiced must be closed. This is indeed a major challenge, which requires the proper dissemination of research information and the desire and interest on the part of teachers to see that it becomes part of their programs.

A second phase of the problem is that more scholarly research is needed on many of the problems with which physical educators are faced today. For example, the profession needs to know such things as the value of selected physical education activities and programs for inner-city youth, the relation of coaching styles to the development of certain character traits in youth, the most desirable length and fre-

quency of practice periods for teaching badminton and other activities and skills, the kind of physical education program most beneficial for emotionally disturbed children, and the value of movement education as compared to traditional physical education in the development of skill in various team sports. These represent only a few examples of problems that, if the answers were known and applied, would produce physical education programs more scientifically based as well as contribute significantly more to the consumers of their services.

The third phase of this problem is that of interpreting the research findings. Many physical educators do not understand research terminology and how to interpret research findings. It is a language far beyond their grasp. As a result, research fails to be used in many cases. One answer to this problem is to have significant research studies interpreted in "lay" language that is meaningful to the physical educator on the job. It might be helpful for physical educators to read reports of technical subjects in such magazines as *Reader's Digest* and *Life*. Even the most technical details are spelled out so that the material and information is intelligible to a person with only a grade school education. Consequently, the material is read by great numbers of people, and the circulation of these magazines runs into millions of copies. Similarly, the physical education profession must also have someone perform this task who has communication skills for these classical studies that have implications for physical education programs. If this can be done, programs of physical education will be upgraded considerably.

The challenge of closing the gap between research and practice represents one that must be met if physical education is to become a respected, established profession.

CHALLENGE OF LEADERSHIP

In the first chapter, the qualities of leadership that are necessary if physical education is to become a profession were pointed out. The trends show us that future leaders in physical education must play certain roles, whether that of a teacher or practitioner, researcher, administrator, professor who specializes in history and philosophy, or some other role. Leaders are needed who are well prepared for their work and who are motivated in pursuing excellence in their position, whatever it is. In order to have such leadership, it means that physical education must be selective in the students it admits to such careers. All persons who apply will not be qualified to enter. Furthermore, it means that individuals who use the term *physical educator* for commercial reasons, such as strength builders, female slenderizers, and so-called phyical fitness experts, must be labeled for what they are. There must be a clear identification in the public's mind as to who is and who is not the professionally trained physical education person.

Physical education desperately needs qualified leadership. This is the key to the realization of many of the potentialities of physical education. Students going into this work as a career should realize that in order to be an asset to this emerging profession they should be enthusiastic and interested in their work; possess the competencies, knowledges, and attitudes necessary to do a good job; and accept the challenges and responsibilities that go with their positions. This type of leadership does not exist in sufficient amount at the present time. Standards must be established that allow only qualified individuals to become members of the profession. This challenge must be met if physical education is to be a respected profession and one in which the public has faith and can place its trust.

Methods by which more outstanding leaders may be attracted to physical education

MAKE PHYSICAL EDUCATION A RESPECTED PROFESSION SO THAT THE BEST HIGH SCHOOL STUDENTS WILL WANT TO JOIN THE RANKS. A person looks at the law or medical profession and finds respect for an intellectual discipline that has prestige in our society. This respect and prestige were developed only as it became recognized that the leaders in these professions were well qualified for their positions, guided by high ethical standards, and recognized as rendering an outstanding service to society. We must have scholarly individuals in physical education who possess the physical skills but, at the same time, who possess the mental capacity to understand the psychological, sociological, and biological foundations upon which their field rests.

RAISE THE STANDARDS OF ADMISSION TO THE PROFESSION. The American Association for Health, Physical Education, and Recreation's decision to allow only students to enter the profession who graduate from accredited colleges and universities was a very commendable step forward. It will help to raise admission standards in our institutions of higher learning. But it is only a beginning. We must be very selective in our choice of colleagues. Young people who are admitted should be required to struggle and work hard and then feel honored that they are permitted to join the ranks.

INITATE A CONCERTED RECRUITMENT DRIVE FOR OUTSTANDING STUDENTS. Science, business, and other vocations are exerting major pressures to find the best young people in the country. National Merit Scholarship winners are sought after as feverishly as potential All-American football players. Physical education must also seek with all its vigor and strength to interest and recruit the best young people for their field of work. We are not going to get these people by sitting back and wishing. It will be accomplished only through hard work and professional persuasiveness.

UPGRADE PROFESSIONAL PREPARATION PROGRAMS. Teacher-training institutions represent a key setting for improving the quality of leadership that comes into our professional field. The quality of the staff, number of books in the library, course offerings, facilities for research and laboratory work, and general education offering are a few of the essentials necessary for an excellent professional preparation program. Accrediting procedures must ensure that institutions meet acceptable standards and train professional leadership and that those that fail to meet the standards will not be permitted to offer work in our field.

AIM FOR MORE UNIFORMITY IN CERTIFICATION REQUIREMENTS AMONG THE VARIOUS STATES. The degree to which certification requirements vary from state to state is a factor that needs attention. Some states permit teaching of physical education with only a few semester hours of course work. Others require as many as 36 semester hours plus prerequisite science. There must be greater uniformity of stringent requirements for teaching physical education. Since education is a state responsibility, this is a difficult task. However, our associations can help considerably in urging our various states to upgrade their requirements in accordance with standards recommended by the profession.

HAVE EACH MEMBER OF THE PROFESSION BECOME AN AMBASSADOR. Each member of the profession must take it upon himself to build an image of physical education that is characterized by respect, scholarly endeavor, and a dedication to serving humanity. As each person attempts to improve his own qualities, academicians, educators, and the public in general will realize that physical eduction is an impor-

tant phase of total education and deserves their support.

CHALLENGE OF MAKING ATHLETICS MORE EDUCATIONAL

Educators have lost the battle for a sound sports program in many of our educational institutions. The commercial interests have reaped a bonanza from a gigantic sports boom; the sportswriters have found a gold mine in copy for their newspapers and radio and television programs; and parents have found pleasure in basking in the limelight of their children's athletic achievements. Educators must assume the leadership role just as they do in other aspects of the school program—in mathematics, history, science, and foreign languages. We need a *new athletics* in our schools and colleges today—athletics that we can rightfully label educational athletics, as contrasted with the highly competitive spectacular form where athletes are selected and trained to please the rabid customers in the stands, rather than using sports as a means of individual self-improvement.

In other areas and fields of specialization in the schools we seem very much concerned about having a sound educational program that uses the developmental aspects of child growth as guidelines, and we demand progression and sequential development of subject matter. Yet, when it comes to athletics, we become indifferent, bowing to community pressures and ignoring the way children grow and develop. For example, one can hardly recognize the sequential development of our athletic experiences from the grades to college. They should progress gradually and smoothly from the informal type of activity, the low intensity of competition, and the fundamental skills to the more highly organized activities, higher intensity of competition, and more complex skills. The way the athletic program is conducted in many schools, however, seems to follow an adult formula that is projected downward upon our children and youth, instead of being developmental and progressive in approach.

Do coaches always use the tools of their trade as forces for educational good? Evidently not, if the words of Dr. James Bryant Conant are any indication. The former president of Harvard refers to school sports as the "poison ivy" of education. Unfortunately, there are many educators who agree with him.

What should be our course of action? Should we roll with these lethal punches and refer to such academicians as ivory-towered educators who never had the guts to get in there and win for dear old State? Or should we recognize that at times it is difficult to see the relationship between football, basketball, or baseball and the objectives of education? I think most of us would agree there is some truth in the little verse:

Games are evil, games are good;
Oft are games misunderstood.

Each coach has his own ideas as to the place of athletics in the schools and colleges of this nation. He has seen the worth of sports as well as the abuses. And for this reason, those who have glimpsed athletics as an effective medium of education know what can be accomplished.

It should be made clear that physical educators are not for less but for more athletics, not for a deemphasis but a reemphasis along educational lines, not for fewer players but more players, and not for insecure coaches but ones who are regular members of the faculty with tenure and all the other privileges enjoyed by full-fledged teachers and professors. These goals can be reached if we make athletics more educational.

Ten ways that we might consider in making athletics more educational are as follows:

1. *Give the player more opportunities to think rather than usurping the privilege for ourselves.* Let us reverse the trend that seems to be for the coach to call the plays, plan the strategies, and do the thinking. Today, the coach sends in a substitute to call the pass play, yells from the sidelines for the change to a zone offense, and flashes the signal for the player to keep the bat on his shoulder. The player is a puppet to be manipulated by the man on the bench. In our desire to sip from the victory cup we may forget that the more thinking that is done by the players, the more educational the activity becomes.

2. *Have shorter practice sessions.* A famous coach once said that what cannot be accomplished in 1 or 1½ hours of practice is not worthwhile. Perhaps if we paid more attention to the organization of practices and carefully evaluated the worth of longer sessions, we might be able to arrange shorter periods. In turn, this would provide many more hours of study for the player. As a result, both the coach and the player would benefit. The student would have a better chance to be a success in his studies, and scholastic ineligibility would be less likely.

3. *Provide for brainstorming sessions.* The coach might be surprised at how creative some of his players are in thinking up new plays, new strategies, and new ideas for overwhelming the opposition. A regular brainstorming session would enable the players to get their intellectual machinery into action and the coach and team to be a better ball club.

4. *Furnish tutors out of the athletic treasury for those players who need special help in their studies.* Athletic monies are used to buy drinks for members of the press and better accommodations for the spectators. What better way can such money be used than to help players who are having scholastic difficulties? Tutoring for students who are delinquent in their studies would reap rich rewards.

5. *Develop an attitude of respect for scholarly endeavor.* Young people in school and college are passing through a formative period when attitudes are developed and values are stablized. The coach is in a position to help shape a boy's outlook by stressing the importance of sports and athletics as a *means to an end—not an end in themselves.* We all know examples of some coaches who have encouraged their

players to enroll in snap courses, sign up for the most lenient professors, and get by as easily as possible in order to stay eligible for varsity competition. In such cases a detrimental imprint is being left upon the boy for the rest of his life. Players should meet the same academic requirements as all students and should recognize that the player who is most valuable to the squad and the team is the one who is a good student.

6. *Make coaches recognized members of the faculty.* Athletics are *a part of* education and not *apart from it.* Similarly, the coach should be a member of the faculty and enjoy all rights and privileges attendant thereto, including tenure and retirement benefits. For such a condition to exist, the coach must assume his responsibility in seeing that athletics contribute to educational goals and that he himself is an active member of the staff. This means playing an active part in faculty meetings and other school activities where policy is formed and educational programs developed.

7. *Keep players on the squad—do not cut.* In our comprehensive system of American education, we do not deny any boy the right to take courses in English or history. Neither should we deny any student the right to engage in athletics. If a boy voluntarily desires to go out for a team and is willing to spend the time and energy involved, then the opportunity should be provided for this experience, even though he may not be highly skilled. The educational potentials are great when there is built-in self-propulsion. We should exploit such opportunities. It may be that the contributions we make to the less skilled boy are even greater than the ones we make to the gifted athlete. It is said that President Kennedy was not too skilled, but the fact that he was kept on the squad was not without its rewards.

8. *Allow players to take charge at times.* Part of the training at West Point is a requirement that each cadet must coach and organize a team. The military academy has found that this experience develops leadership and turns out better graduates.

The services of varsity players could be used in junior varsity, intramurals, and sports days at great advantage to both the player and the school. This also enables players to devise their own plays and strategies and then to see how they work under actual game situations.

9. *Hire coaches as much for their educational qualifications as for their win-loss record and file of newspaper clippings.* It is important to have coaches who have been great players themselves and who know sports inside and out. However, since they are in the business of education as much as the teacher or professor of mathematics, it is also important they have a cultural background as well. If they are to be regular members of the faculty, they should meet educational standards required for membership in such a distinguished group.

10. *Emphasize the player rather than the spectator.* The tackle, forward, or first baseman is the one attending school or college—not the rooter in the stands. Rule changes should be designed to improve the player's status instead of helping make the turnstiles click faster. The focus of attention at all times should be that of providing an athletic experience for the player that is safe, free from undesirable pressures, and educational in nature.

CHALLENGE PRESENTED BY PUBLIC MISUNDERSTANDING OF PHYSICAL EDUCATION

Physical education is one of the most misunderstood professions in the world today. The average person is not aware of what it can offer to him as an individual or to society as a whole. There is ample evidence that it is still regarded as a "frill," that people think of it as a good means of entertainment but not connected with successful living, and that it is something to be tolerated in education but has no value in realizing educational objectives. In many schools, physical education is the last activity to be scheduled and the first to be canceled for special activities. Credit in physical education is not required for graduation in some schools. Few, if any, colleges require a unit of physical education as an entrance requirement as they do in many of the so-called academic subjects. Insufficient time, space, facilities, and sixty to 100 students in each physical education class are characteristic of many schools. Furthermore, children are not classified homogeneously for classes because of administrative misunderstanding.

These are only a few of the examples that may be listed as evidence of misunderstanding on the part of the public. Such a condition must be corrected if physical education is to realize its potentialities. The student should realize that this is one major problem with which he is confronted and should utilize every opportunity to interpret physical education in its true perspective.

CHALLENGE OF PLACING PHYSICAL EDUCATION IN A DEFENSIBLE POSITION

Physical education is not in a desirable defensible position at the present time. Evidence of this is the lack of answers to the following questions. At what grade or age level should each of the activities that comprise the physical education program be introduced for optimum learning efficiency? What are the individual achievement standards in activities at various age and grade levels? What are the scientific evaluative instruments available for measuring the importance of physical education activities in developing good human relations? How effective is physical education in developing interpretive thinking? Why should physical education be required at all educational levels? What contribution does physical education make to general education? What subject-matter facts and knowledge do we have that justifies physical education's rightful place in education? What is the relationship of physical activity to physical, psychological, and sociological development?

These are a few of the many questions that physical education cannot answer satisfactorily. If the profession is to serve the

individual and society in the best way possible and if it is to be interpreted to the public in its correct light, the answers to these and many other questions should be secured. The scientific process of selection, evaluation, and adaptation of activities is the heart of the physical education profession and yet remains largely unsolved. Desired levels of accomplishment in organic skill, knowledge, and adaptation for each age and grade level should be clearly defined. Physical educators should be interested in and work toward placing physical education in a truly defensible position.

CHALLENGE OF A RELEVANT CURRICULUM

Physical education is being challenged to revise its curriculum. In too many schools the same activities are taught over and over again, there is a lack of organization and progression, and the standards vary from school to school and state to state. Physical education is one of the few areas that has failed to do a major curriculum revision during recent educational history. Although a few leaders are cognizant of this, many of our practitioners have been oblivious to the patterns of curriculum change that are emerging in other areas of the educational curriculum. Examples can be found where schools offer such sports as basketball, volleyball, and softball for as many as 6 years in a row. If such repetition were practiced in other curriculum areas, it would not be tolerated, and such practices must be seriously questioned for physical education in light of the many new advances that are taking place in education.

Any curriculum revision must also look carefully at the "movement" movement. We must ask the question. Does physical education have a body of knowledge, and, if so, what is it? Is it the science of human movement or not? What is the role of movement education as expressed in Chapter 13? If this is our discipline, how can we most effectively communicate a correct view of this subject to all concerned? Physical education has suffered from lack of identification of an adequate framework of knowledge and role in education. If the "movement" movement is the answer, it should be given much more attention by physical educators.

CHALLENGE OF REEVALUATING THE SCHOOL PROGRAM

The educational system, to a great degree, has failed to accomplish many of the objectives that it has established for itself: health, ethical character, worthy use of leisure time, worthy home membership, and citizenship. The increased number of cases of mental illness in this country, the drug abuse problem, student unrest, the evidence supplied on the extent of crime and immorality in the United States, the quest for material rather than spiritual values, public indifference to public administration, increased divorce rates, and juvenile delinquency are problems that show that the whole educational structure of this country needs reevaluating.

The belief that a knowledge of facts will result in successful living seems to have been the premise upon which the present educational structure rests, and this has proved to be a fallacy. Education should result in changed behavior and in social, physical, mental, and emotional betterment. The evidence, however, does not point to such an accomplishment. Therefore the reevaluation of the whole educational structure should be made to determine what is the best type of education for successful living.

In such a reevaluation it seems that consideration should be given to determining what the physical, mental, emotional, and social needs of individuals are and then to include experiences in the curriculum that will meet these needs. Through such a study it might be discovered that many of the present offerings do not contribute to meeting such needs. Perhaps some of those who are being slighted in many of our schools at the present time would be found to be of much more value than previously determined. Under existing conditions, although health is listed as the first objective, how many schools adequately provide the proper health service, healthful school living, and health instruction for their students? How many schools provide planned instruction in physical activities suited to the sex, grade, ability, and special needs of pupils? How many schools place the same high priority on the physical, mental, emotional, and social health of the individual as they do on his ability to acquire facts in such areas as mathematics, English, and history?

A thorough reevaluation should bring to light the important role that physical education can play in the educational process. Students should recognize this challenge and aggressively agitate for reevaluation of the educational system. In this way they will be helping physical education to realize its potentialities.

A CONCLUDING STATEMENT

Physical education has been effectively contributing to the betterment of society since ancient times. However, it can do a better job; it can be a greater profession; it can contribute more to enriched living for the total population. These achievements will be possible if the professional students of physical education in our schools take up the many challenges that confront their field of endeavor and, after careful thought and deliberation, devise plans that will result in physical education achieving its true potentialities. Physical education is proud of those qualified students now training for this specialized work. It has faith in them to do the job and knows they will accept the challenges facing their field of endeavor. It wishes them the best of success and the most of happiness in a field of endeavor that has no equal for satisfaction derived from conscientious efforts.

QUESTIONS AND EXERCISES

1. Survey ten leaders in the field of physical education and determine what they believe are the challenges facing the profession of physical education in the next 10 years.
2. Survey your own community to determine the challenges facing physical education in your community.

3. Read three books published on education in the past 5 years to determine the challenges facing physical education in the years ahead.

Reading assignment

Bucher, Charles A., and Goldman, Myra: Dimensions of physical education, St. Louis, 1969, The C. V. Mosby Co., Reading selections 71 to 74.

SELECTED REFERENCES

Read all copies of the Journal of Health, Physical Education, and Recreation for the past 2 years.

Index

A

Abernathy, Ruth, 24
Ability grouping, 509-510
Academic achievement and physical education, 499-502
Accreditation, 608-609
Achievement and worth, 123-124
ACTION, 364
Activities in other countries, 361-362
Activity, why, 502-504
Adams, Miller K., 152-153
Administration
    changes in the 1970's, 96-97
    of programs, 41-43
Administrative developments affecting learning process, 513-517
Adolescence, 420-421
Adult
    fitness of, 468-469
    schools for, 79
Agencies, recreation, 247-248
Ages of development, 418
Aides for teachers, 554-555
Alcohol, 223
    and fitness, 456
Alexander, William M., 181
Allen, James E., 261-262
Amateur Athletic Union, 326, 535, 538, 616-617
Amateur sports, international competitions in, 370-371
Amateurism, 336-338
American Academy of Physical Education, 617-618
American Academy of Political and Social Science, 246
American Association for the Advancement of Physical Education, 199, 314
American Association for Health, Physical Education, and Recreation, 5, 9, 16-17, 23-24, 26, 30, 40, 51, 53, 111, 145-146, 155, 199, 206, 209, 232, 241, 253, 263, 315, 324, 326, 328-332, 334, 335, 362, 364, 365, 423, 450, 464, 467, 470, 503, 527, 544, 546, 563, 568, 592-594, 597, 609, 615, 618-620, 663, 669

American Cancer Society, 472
American College of Sports Medicine, 619-621
American Corrective Therapy Association, 621-622
American culture and sport, 536-538
American Heart Association, 438
American history of physical education; *see* History of physical education in America
American Medical Association, 111, 206, 207, 212, 232, 434-435, 443, 445, 447, 454, 457
American National Red Cross, 79, 242, 662
American Physical Education Association, 145, 199, 314
American Physical Education Review, 10
American School Health Association, 206, 216-217, 622-624
American Youth Hostels, Inc., 83
Analysis of movement, 352
Anderson, Jackson M., 255-256
Anderson, William C., 589
Anderson, William Gilbert, 10, 314, 316, 618
Andrews, J. D., 314
Annarino, Anthony A., 154
Antiathletics, 338
Aristotle, 118, 126, 128, 245, 275, 285, 431
Armed forces, 365
    and United Service Organizations, 81-82
Arnold College of Hygiene and Physical Education, 589
Asceticism, 288
Asham, Roger, 291
Asian Games, 5, 367
Athens, 283
Athletic clubs and sport organizations, 85
Athletic heart, 448-450
Athletic programs, 101-103
Athletic records, 103
Athletics
    challenge to physical education, 670-672
    for children, 421-422
    definition of, 6
    girls' and women's, 423
    and personality development, 497-498
    sociological implications of, 538-547
        beneficial impact of, 541-543

Athletics—cont'd
sociological implications of—cont'd
conditions under which they become valuable, 545-547
harmful impact of, 543-545
influence of American society on, 538-541
Attica Prison, New York, 88
Atypical individual, 469-470
Australia, 376-377
Axiology, 119

B

Bancroft, Jessie, 317, 318
Barber, Bernard, 10
Basedow, Johann Bernhard, 298
Basic instruction program, 112
Battle Creek, Michigan, 334
Baynham, Dorsey, 510
Beck, Charles, 309
Beecher, Catherine E., 309
Beginning teacher, 568-571
of physical education, 585-586
Bennett, B. L., 11
Benson, David, 500-501
Beter, Thais R., 20
Biddulph, Lowell G., 543, 546
Binational center, 366
Biological development and human behavior, 47-48
Biological fitness, 428-476
adults and, 468-469
alcohol and, 456
atypical individual and, 469-470
components of, 435-436
drugs and, 456-457
education for, 428
exercise and, 436-447
fatigue and, 460-462
fitness sucess formula, 470-474
and health, 430-434
meaning for young people, 428-430
nation's youth and, 466-468
paths to, 434-435
President's Council for Physical Fitness and Sports and, 464-466
relaxation and recreation and, 462-463
role of school and community in, 474-475
and state of nation's health, 463-464
stress and, 460
tobacco and, 456
training and, 447-456
weight control and, 457-460
Biological makeup of man, 403-427
athletics and, 421-423
biological basis of life, 411
body mechanics, 425-426
body types, 424-425
health of the nation and, 409-411
heredity, impact of, 416-418

Biological makeup of man—cont'd
history of, 403-408
makeup of human body, 411-416
organic foundations, 411-426
physical and motor growth and development, 418-421
Bishop, Nathan, 314
Black athlete, 336
Bleier, T. J., 505
Blood and effects of training, 450-451
Bloom, Benjamin S., 45
Bobbit, Franklin, 323
Body mechanics, 425-426
Body image, 498-499
Body types, 424-425
Bookwalter, Karl W., 149
Boston Normal School of Gymnastics, 312
Botwin, Louis, 512
Boy Scouts, 242
Boys' Clubs of America, 560, 662
Brace, David K., 323
Branting, Lars Gabriel, 301
Brazil, 377-378
Briggs, Paul W., 186
British Empire and Commonwealth Games, 367
Briton, S. W., 406
Broudy, Harry S., 120-121, 122-123
Bruner, Jerome, 165-166, 530
Bukh, Niels, 305
Burchenal, Elizabeth, 317
Burnham, William, 323
Bushnell, David, 517
Butler, George D., 237
Buttonwood Farms Project, 335-336

C

Caillois' theory of play, 529
Calhoun High School, Port Lavaca, Texas, 245
California Heart Association, 447
Calish, Richard, 539
Calories and exercise; *see* Exercise
Calver, George W., 438
Camp, Walter, 321
Camping and outdoor education, 37-38, 261-272
environmental problems and, 261-265
history of, 263
objectives of, 265
physical education teachers and, 271-272
programs for, 266-268
settings for, 265-266
study units in, 269
worth of, 269-271
Camps, 86
Campus Martius, 287
Canada, 378-379
Canadian Association for Health, Physical Education, and Recreation, 624
Capacities in which physical education teachers serve, 578-580

Cardinal Principles of Education, 3, 513
Careers in health education, 235
Carlile, Forbes, 447-448
Carnegie Commission on Higher Education, 598
Carnegie Foundation, 324
Cassel, Russell N., 561
Cassidy, Rosalind, 41, 148, 323
Catholic Youth Organization, 87
Certification requirements for employment in physical education, 639-648
  for elementary schools, 645
  general areas for, 641-643
  reasons for, 639-641
  for secondary schools, 645
  in South Carolina, 646-647
  trends in, 644-648
  types of certificates, 643-644
Challenges facing physical education, 24-28, 666-675
  athletics, 670-672
  closing research and practice gap, 667-669
  educator, 24-26
  leadership, 669-670
  motives for participation, 28
  need to be creative, 667
  physical education in a defensible position, 673
  public misunderstanding of physical education, 672-673
  reevaluating school program, 674
  relevancy to today, 26-27
  relevant curriculum, 673-674
  survey of greatest challenges, 666-667
Change agent in physical education, 107-108
Changing concepts of physical education, 273-399
  from beginning of modern European period to present, 298-341
  from early times to modern European period, 275-297
  in international education, 357-399
  in movement education, 342-356
Charlemagne, 289
Charlesworth, James C., 246-247
Chautauqua Institute for Physical Education, 311, 316
China, 277-279
Christianity, 288
Chromosomes and genes, 417-418
Churches, 87
Cicero, 287
Circulatory system, 412-413
Circus Maximus, 287
Civic development and recreation, 240
Civic responsibility and physical education, 191-195
Civil War, 310-317
Clark, Norvel, 245
Clarke, H. Harrison, 446, 501
Class reorganization, 510
Clear Lake Camp, 269
Clein, Marvin I., 506, 507

Cleveland Heights, Ohio, schools, 265
Coaches
  certification of, 644-645
  and their professional preparation, 332-333
Coaching, 38-40, 583
Code of Ethics, 26, 109-110, 559
Cogan, Max, 28, 496-497
Cognitive development objective, 159-161
College
  entrance requirements for, 609-610
  and meaning of physical fitness, 430
  and university, 74-76
College Sports Information Directors of America, 624-625
Colonial period, 308-309
Colorado Springs, Colorado, schools, 455
Comenius, John, 275, 291, 357, 499
Commission on Goals for American Recreation, 237-239
Community and athletics, 538-539
Community duties of physical educator, 573-574, 585
Community-school cooperation in recreation, 257-258
Computer and education, 92-93
Conant, James Bryant, 47, 593, 671
Concepts
  and objectives of physical education, 165-169; *see also* Changing concepts of physical education
  of movement education, 346-352
Conceptual approach to health education, 207-209
Contiguity theory, 483-484
Cooper, Kenneth H., 456
Cooper, Samuel M., 538, 543
Corey, Arthur, 14
Counseling, 40-41
Cowell, C. C., 501
Cratty, Bryant J., 485, 497
Creativity, 508, 667
Critical health areas, 220-224
Cultural explosion and recreation, 258
Cultural values, 520-521
Culturally disadvantaged students, 51-54
Cureton, Thomas K., Jr., 170
Current attitude toward physical education, 18-22
Current developments
  having implications for physical education, 331-341
  in teacher education programs, 598-602
Curriculum
  new, 516
  professional, 602-608
  relevant, challenges of, 673-674
Curriculum reform movement, 334-336

D

da Feltra, Vittorino, 291
Damon, Walter E., 541

Dance, 33-35
Danford, Howard G., 249
Dark Ages, 287-289
Davenport, Iowa, schools, 7
Davis, Hazel, 65-66
De Mar, 450
de Montaigne, Michel, 291
Death, major causes of, 408
Definition of physical education, 3-8
DeKalb, Illinois, schools, 334, 353-354
Delsarte, François, 182, 312
Delta Psi Kappa, 625
Denmark, 304-305
Depression years, 324-325
Descartes, Rene, 117, 126, 128
Des Moines, Iowa, 334
Detroit, Michigan, schools, 68
Developments in teaching, 554-559
Dewey, John, 111, 131-132, 139-141, 174, 176, 317
Differentiated staffing, 554
Digestive system, 415-416
Division of Girls' and Women's Sports, 328, 423
Domination theory of play, 529
Douglas, Paul F., 244, 251
Dowell, Linus J., 214-215
Driver education, 43, 582
Drugs
    and drug addiction, 222-223
    and fitness, 456-457
Duggar, Benjamin C., 469
Dukelow, Donald A., 212
Durant, Henry (Mrs.), 313
Duties of physical education personnel, 573-587
    capacities in which to serve, 578-580
    coaching, 583
    community, 585
    expectations of beginning teachers, 585-586
    general responsibilities of, 574-578
    groups to whom responsible, 573-574
    health, safety, and driver education, 582
    measurement and evaluation, 583
    other duties, 583-584
    physical education activities, 581-582
    range of, 574
    school levels of instruction, 580-581
    second jobs, 584-585
    teaching loads, 584
    teaching other subjects, 582
    time devoted to physical education, 580-581

E

Ecology, 223-224
Economics and physical education, 188-191
Education
    changes in the 1970's, 93-97
    for fitness, 428
    in international relations, 358-359
    meaning of, 176-178
    physical education as applied to, 178-179

Education—cont'd
    responsibility for, 175-176
    and schools and colleges, 175
    for social change, 526-527
Educational athletics; *see* Athletics
Educational philosophies, 137-139
Educational Policies Commission, 177, 180, 230, 520-521, 540
Educational Research Information Center, 45
Educational research lines, 45-47
Educational television, 510-512
Eichhorn, Donald H., 69
Eisenhower, Dwight, 464
Elementary and Secondary Education Act, 517
Elementary school, 67-68, 420
    certification of physical educators in, 645
    and meaning of physical fitness, 428-429
    movement education program in, 352-354
    physical education programs, 661
Ellensburg, Washington, schools, 4, 19, 50, 334, 343
Elliot, Ruth, 591
Elyot, Sir Thomas, 291
Emotionally disturbed students, 58-59
Employment opportunities in physical education, 649-665
    advantages offered by teaching, 649-652
    employment in allied areas, 662-663
    encouraging developments in, 661-663
    end of teacher shortage, 654-658
    men's physical education, 660-661
    school and college enrollment, 652-654
    securing a position, 663-664
    women's physical education, 658-660
Endocrine system, 416
England, 344-345, 379-380
Enrollments, school and college, 652-654
Environment
    and recreation, 256-257
    and training and fitness, 453-454
Environmental problems and camping and outdoor education, 261-265
Epistemology, 119
Equipment in movement education, 352
Essex, Martin, 510
Esthetics, 120
Ethics, 119
Europe and outdoor education, 264
Evaluation of teachers, 556-559
Evergreen Park, Illinois, schools, 228, 506, 507
Evolution of man, 405-408
Excretory system, 416
Exercise
    and calorie intake and outgo, 436-438
    and daily program of physical education, 447
    effects of training, 448-453
    and general health, 440-441
    isotonic and isometric, 441-447
    and physical fitness, 436-447
    principles of training, 447-448

Existentialism, 135-137
Eyler, Marvin H., 307, 308

F

Facilities, 104-107, 339-340, 361
Family life education, 220
Fatigue, 460-462
Federal legislation, 662
Fédération Intérnationale de Médecine Sportive, 621
Feudalism, 289-290
Fitness; *see also* Biological fitness; Physical fitness
    definition of, 5-6
    state of the union, 463-464
    success formula, 470-474
Five-year program, 601-602
Flanagan, John C., 46
Flexible scheduling, 506-507
Flexner, Abraham, 10
Flint, Michigan, schools, 350, 589, 640
Follen, Charles, 309
Ford Foundation, 51
Fosdick, Raymond, 321
Frederick County, Maryland, schools, 266
Frederiksen, Norman, 46
Freeberg, William H., 265, 266
Fulbright Program, 358, 365
Functions of philosophy of physical education, 124-125

G

Gaito, John, 47
Galen, 285
Games, 33
    classification of, 530
Gardner, John W., 15-16, 174
Gary, M. J., 276
Gendel, Evelyn S., 423, 452
General areas for certification requirements, 641-643
General education
    meaning of, 179-180
    physical education as applied to, 180-195
    role of physical education in, 174-196
    stress on, 600-601
General philosophies, 125-137
Germany, 298-300
Gertler, Menard, 436
Gesell, Arnold, 499
Gestalt theory, 485
Girls' and women's athletics, 328, 423, 539-540
Good life, philosophy of, 121-124
Gould Academy, 327
Government
    and recreation, 257
    and welfare agencies, 86-87
Graduate work, 610-611

Great Britain, 6, 146, 305-306
Greece, 281-285, 286
Greek physical education, 1, 120, 126, 193
Greenberg, Hank, 10
Grieve, Andrew, 71-74
Griffiths, Daniel E., 45, 46, 47
Grinnell, John E., 525-526
Groups to whom physical educators are responsible, 573-574
Guidelines for international relations in physical education, 362-363
Guilford, J. P., 45
Gulick, Luther Halsey, 10, 241, 313, 318, 319, 321
Guthrie, E. P., 483-484
Guts Muths, Johann Christoph Friedrich, 298-299
Gymnastics, 4-5

H

Haag, Jessie Helen, 645
Hale, Creighton J., 542
Hall, G. Stanley, 317
Handicapped, 49-59, 330, 335-336, 661
Hanna, Delphine, 318
Harrison, Paul E., 268
Hartford Female Seminary, 309
Harvard Committee, 180
Harvard University, 309
Havighurst, Robert S., 524-525
Hayden, Frank J., 52
Head Start Project, 86-87, 225
Health
    careers in, 235
    critical areas of, 220-224
    definition of, 6, 203-205
    exercise and, 440-441
    and fitness, 430-434
    of nation, 409-411, 463-464
    and physical education around the world, 359-362
    professional preparation for, 232-235
    public, interrelationship, 230-232
    relation to physical education, 210-215
    and school living, 224-225
    school program in, 203-236
    teaching for, 35-37
    terminology in, 209-210
Health attitudes, 229-230
Health concepts, 207-209
Health development and recreation, 239-240
Health education, 582
    content areas in, 218
    teacher certification in, 645
Health knowledge, 228-229
Health personnel, 227
Health practices, 230
Health services, 225-227
Health skills, 230
Hein, Fred C., 212

Hemenway, Mary, 310-312, 590
Hemphill, John, 46
Henry, Charles D., 508
Heredity, impact of, 416-418
Hess, Roland, 640, 644
Hetherington, Clark, 5-7, 145, 146-148, 156, 318, 323
Hettinger, T., 442, 446
Hines, Vynce A., 181
Hippocrates, 285
History
    of camping and outdoor education, 263
    of early physical education, 275-297
        in age of feudalism, 289-290
        in ancient Near East, 279-281
        in ancient oriental nations, 277-281
        during Dark Ages, 287-289
        in Greece, 281-285
        during Renaissance, 290-292
        in Rome, 285-287
    and objectives, 144-145
    of physical education in America, 306-341
        from Civil War until 1900, 310-317
        colonial period, 308-309
        current developments, 331-341
        in early twentieth century, 317-325
        in mid–twentieth century, 325-331
        national period, 309-310
    of physical education in modern Europe, 298-306
        Denmark, 304-305
        Germany, 298-300
        Great Britain, 305-306
        Sweden, 300-304
    of professional preparation, 588-596
    of recreation, 241-243
    of school health program, 205-207
Hitchcock, Edward, 314
Hjelte, George, 244, 248-249
Hoh, Gunsun, 278, 359
Homans, Amy Morris, 310-312, 626
Homer, 430-431
Hospitals, 87-88
Howell, M. L., 624
Hubbard, Elbert, 15
Hughes, Everett C., 9, 15
Hughes, William Leonard, 39
Hull, Clark L., 484
Hull House, 241
Human behavior, 47-49
Human body, makeup of, 411-416
Human nature, 522-523
Human needs, 523-524
Human relations and recreation, 240
Human relationships and physical education, 185-188
Humphrey, James H., 501
Hunsicker, Paul A., 467
Hunt, Douglas W., 571
Hygiene, 3-4

I

Idealism, 125-128
Identification Summary, 594
India, 279, 280, 380, 381
Individual differences and learning, 480
Individual exploration and movement education, 346-348
Industrial concerns, 82-84
Infancy, growth in, 418-419
Inheritance or recapitulation theory of play, 528
Inner city
    and recreation, 257
    and youth, 336
Instinct or Groos theory of play, 528
Institute for Developmental Studies, 46
Institute of International Education, 365
Instrumentalism, 137-138
Integumentary system, 416
Intellectual self-realization and physical education, 180-185
Intelligence and learning, 480-481
International Amateur Athletic Federation, 373-374
International Association of Physical Education and Sports for Girls and Women, 375
International Bureau of Education, 374-375
International Congress in Physical Education, 329
International Council on Health, Physical Education, and Recreation, 330, 371-373
International Council of Sport and Physical Education, 374
International dates, 364
International Education Act, 358
International Federation of Physical Education, 374
International Federation of Sports Medicine, 375-376
International physical education
    competitions in, 366-371
    definition of, 357
    education and, 358-359
    guidelines for, 362-363
    health and physical education and, 359-362
    historical milestones in, 357-358
    opportunities for service in, 363-366
    organizations in, 371-376
    in selected countries, 376-398
        Australia, 376-377
        Brazil, 377-378
        Canada, 378-379
        England, 379-380
        India, 380-381
        Israel, 380-382
        Italy, 382-383
        Japan, 383-386
        Mexico, 386-387
        Netherlands, 387-388
        New Zealand, 388-389
        Philippines, 389-390, 391, 392

International physical education—cont'd
   in selected countries—cont'd
      Sweden, 390-392
      Thailand, 392-394
      Union of South Africa, 394-395
      Union of Soviet Socialist Republics, 395-396
      West Germany, 396-398
International Recreation Association, 374
International Sports Organization for the Disabled, 375
International University Sports Federation, 375
Internship, 599
Interscholastic athletics; *see* Athletics
Intramurals, 329
Ismail, A. H., 501
Isometric exercise; *see* Exercise
Isotonic exercise; *see* Exercise
Israel, 282, 380-382
Italy, 382-383

J

Jackson Prison, Michigan, 88
Jackson's Mill Conference, 592
Jacobson, Edmund, 463
Jahn, Friedrich Ludwig, 299-300, 309
James, William, 174, 275, 317
Japan, 115, 383-386
Jarman, Boyd O., 501
Jennings, Frank G., 479
Jennings, Herbert S., 275
Jersild, Arthur T., 419-420, 499
Job Corps, 86
Jogging and training and fitness, 455-456
Johns, Edward B., 234
Johns, W. Lloyd, 561
Johnson, Lyndon, 328, 464
Jones, Frank B., 540
Jousts and tournaments, 290
Junior high school, 70
   athletics in, 421-422
   and meaning of physical fitness, 429

K

Kansas City public school system, 554
Karpovich, Peter V., 450, 460, 461
Kasper, Robert N., 292
Kellogg Foundation, 263
Kelly, John B., 325, 326
Kelly, Susan E., 75
Kennedy, John F., 174, 328, 432, 464
Kennedy Foundation, 50, 330
Keogh, Jack, 500-501
Kephart, Newell C., 181, 499, 501
Kierkegaard, Søren, 135-136
Kinesiologists, 345
Kirk, Robert H., 229
Klaus, E. J., 452

Knight, 289-290
Kong Fu gymnastics, 279
Korea, 372
Kretschmer, E., 424

L

La Sierra, California, schools, 422, 435
Laban, Rudolf, 344
Lamb, Arthur S., 624
LaPorte, William R., 145, 325
Lareau, Jeanne Doyle, 542
Larson, Jordan L., 542
Larson, Leonard A., 435-436
Law
   of effect, 482-483
   of exercise, 482
   of readiness, 481-482
Lawrence, Indiana, schools, 226
Le Mars, Iowa, schools, 266
Leaders objectives of physical education, 146-149
Leadership
   challenge of, 669-670
   in other countries, 360-361
   in physical education, 108-109
      duties of, 573-587
      preparation of, 588-612
      teaching profession, 553-572
   for recreation programs, 252
Learning
   administrative developments affecting, 513-517
   definition of, 477
   elements of, 478-481
   motor, 485-495
   new developments affecting, 504-510
   social, 524
   theories of, 481-485
Learning curve, 489
Leisure, 245-247
   and education, 104
   and school program, 250-252
Lewis, Dio, 14, 310, 588
Lewis, Gertrude M., 539
Libicer, Stephen J., Jr., 470
Lieberman, Myron, 9, 10
Lifetime Sports Foundation, 329
Ling, Hjalmar Fredrik, 301-302
Ling, Per Henrik, 300-301
Little Leagues, 329
Livingstone, Mary, 561
Locke, John, 291, 431
Logic, 119
Long Beach, California, schools, 270-271
Loop films, 512-513
Loret, John, 527
Los Angeles, California, schools, 55, 257-258, 483, 491
Loy, John W., Jr., 533, 535
Luther, Martin, 291

M

Maccabiah Games, 367, 369
MacCarthy, Shane, 326
Macfadden, Bernarr, 4
MacKenzie, Jack, 264
Maclaren, Archibald, 306
Madison Square Garden, New York, 534
Marshall, Peter, 242
Marusak, F. M., 470
Maslow, A. H., 478
Maturation and learning, 478-480
Mayer, J., 457
Mayshark, Cyrus, 229
McCloy, Charles H., 446, 488
McCue attitude scale, 539
McCurdy, James H., 313, 318
McGraw, L. W., 541
McKee, Robert, 500
McKenzie, Robert Tait, 318, 321, 551, 617
McKenzie, Ronald F., 245
Mead, George H., 317
Mead, Margaret, 104
Measurement and evaluation techniques, 583
Membership in professional associations, 615-616
Menninger, William, 244, 439
Mental-emotional development, 48-49
Mentally retarded, 49-51
Merriman, J. J., 501-502
Metaphysics, 118-119
Metheny, Eleanor, 540
Mexico, 386-387
Meylan, George L., 10, 323-324
Michael, Ernest D., 460
Michigan public schools, 213, 218
Middle school, 68-69, 514-515
Milestones in international physical education, 357-358
Miller, A. T., Jr., 453
Miller, Peggy L., 107-108
Milton, John, 291
Minor program in health education, 234-235
Minority studies, 516
Modern philosophy of education, 139-141
Montgomery, Katherine W., 546
Morris, Van Cleve, 524
Morse, Horace T., 179
Moss, Bernice, 634
Motivation and learning, 478
Motor and movement development objective, 156-159
Motor growth and development, 418-421
Motor learning, 485-495
Mott Foundation, 257
Movement education, 143, 342-356
  concepts of, 346-352
  elementary school and, 352-354
  guidelines for, 354-355
  nature of, 342-343
  as an objective of physical education, 143

Movement education—cont'd
  origins of, 344-345
  schools of thought in, 345-346
  traditional approach versus, 346-347
Movement experiences, 31-33
Muller, A., 442, 446
Munroe, Richard A., 462
Muscular system and effects of training, 451
Musculature, 412

N

Nachtegall, Franz, 304-305
Nagel, John, 441-447
Naismith, James, 312
Nash, Jay B., 7, 110, 148, 252, 318
National Aeronautics and Space Administration, 100
National Association of Intercollegiate Athletics, 78, 320, 325, 626
National Association of Physical Education for College Women, 345, 626-627
National College Physical Education Association for Men, 28, 628-629
National Collegiate Athletic Association, 78, 192-193, 320, 532, 535, 537, 627-628
National Committee on School Health Policies, 232
National Conference of City and County Directors, 336
National Conference on Fitness for Secondary School Youth, 171
National Conference on Outdoor Education, 263
National Conference on School Recreation, 249-250
National Council for Accreditation of Teacher Education, 609
National Council on Education, 322-323
National Council of Secondary School Athletic Directors, 40
National Education Association, 3, 96, 138, 139, 206, 207, 362-364, 514, 555, 558-559, 584, 586, 596, 629, 650-651, 653, 655-657, 659
National Education Association of Secondary School Principals, 538
National Facilities Conference, 331
National Federation of High School Athletic Associations, 323
National Institute on Girls' Sports, 328
National Intramural Association, 329, 629-630
National Junior College Athletic Association, 630-631
National Nutrition Survey, 204
National Organization for Women, 339
National period, 309-310
National Recreation Association, 237, 241, 244
National Recreation and Park Association, 241, 252, 258, 259, 631-632
National Summer Youth Sports Program, 465
Naturalism, 133-135

Nature
  of man, 521-524
  and scope of physical education, 1-113
  of sport, 532-533
Near East, 279-281
Neo-humanism, 138
Nervous system, 414-415
  and motor learning, 487-488
Netherlands, 387-388
Neuberger, Tom, 454
New Orleans, Louisiana, 334
"New" physical education, 110
New Trier, Illinois, schools, 335
New York State Physical Fitness Screening Test, 467
New York University, 244, 304
New Zealand, 48, 175, 344, 388-389
Nissen, Hartvig, 310, 590
Nixon, Richard, 464
Nolte, Ann E., 205
Nongraded school, 513-514
Normal College of the American Gymnastic Union, 309
Normal Institute of Physical Education in Boston, 588
North American Society for the Psychology of Sports and Physical Activity, 632
North American Turnerbund, 588-589
Nyblaeus, Gustaf, 301

O

Oberteuffer, Delbert, 149, 203-204, 232
Objectives
  accomplishment of, 577-578
  of camping and outdoor education, 265
  cognitive development, 159-161
  definition of, 143
  excellence
    as a civic being, 191-195
    as an economic being, 188-191
    as an intellectual being, 180-185
    as a social being, 185-188
  historical analysis of, 144-145
  of leaders, 146-149
  motor and movement development, 156-159
  need for, 143-144
  physical development, 155-156
  of physical education, 143-173
  and physically educated boys and girls, 169-172
  plus factor and, 162-163
  priority of, 163-165
  of professional preparation, 588
  of recreation, 237-241
  social development, 161-162
  stated as concepts, 165-169
  in terms of scientific principles, 152-153
Ogilvie, Bruce C., 498
Oliver, James N., 502

Olympic games, 284, 328, 366-367, 454
Olympic ideal, 284
Open admissions, 598
Operant conditioning theory, 484-485
Opportunities
  and challenges in recreation, 256-258
  for placement in recreation, 258-260
Organic foundations, 411-426
Oriental nations, 277-281
Outdoor education; *see* Camping and outdoor education
Outdoor Recreation Resources Review Commission, 105
Oxendine, Joseph B., 75

P

Pan-American Games, 367
Pan American Health Organization, 366
Pangle, Roy, 470
Paraprofessionals, 332
Payne, Arlene, 208
Peace Corps, 12-13, 329, 364-365
Peck, Robert F., 524-525
Peik and Fitzgerald study, 15
Pelton, Barry Clifton, 22
Penal institutions, 88
People-to-People Sports Committees, 330, 376
Peoria Heights, Illinois, schools, 601
Personnel in school health programs, 227
Phi Delta Pi, 632-633
Phi Epsilon Kappa Fraternity, 633-634
Philanthropinum, 298
Philippines, 358, 389-390, 391, 392
Philosophy
  definition of, 118-120
  of education, 117-142
  educational, 137-139
    instrumentalism, 137-138
    neo-humanism, 138
    rationalism, 138-139
  general, 125-137
    existentialism, 135-137
    idealism, 125-128
    naturalism, 133-135
    pragmatism, 130-133
    realism, 128-130
  and good life, 121-124
  and levels of discussion, 120-121
  modern, of education, 139-141
  of physical education, 115-196
  and its functions, 124-125
Physical activity and public, parents, and education, 20-22
Physical culture, 4
Physical development objective, 155-156
Physical education
  and academic achievement, 499-502
  as applied to general education, 180-195
  definition of, 6-8

Physical education—cont'd
 an emerging profession, 9-18
 meaning of, 3-8
 professional status of, 8-28
 projected into the future, 90-113
  athletic programs and, 101-103
  athletic records and, 103
  change agent of, 107-108
  computer and, 92-93
  facilities and, 104-107
  general education and, 93-97
  leisure and, 104
  participants and spectators and, 103
  program in, 98-101
  teachers of, 97-98
  ten-point program for, 108-112
 teacher qualifications for, 559-568
 and teaching profession, 553-572
Physical educator
 and camping and outdoor education, 271-272
 capacities in which to serve, 578-580
 general responsibilities of, 574-578
 as health teachers, 212-215
 leadership of, 576-577
 and opportunities in international relations, 363-366
 and recreation, 256
 teaching duties of, 581-582
Physical fitness; *see also* Biological fitness
 academic performance and, 500
 and adults, 468-469
 and alcohol, 456
 and atypical individual, 469-470
 and body types, 425
 components of, 435-436
 current emphasis on, 661-662
 defined, 5-6
 and drugs, 456-457
 and exercise, 436-447
 formula for, 470-474
 history of, 326-328
 meaning for young people, 428-430
 and nation's youth, 466-468
 paths to, 434-435
 President's Council for, 464-466
 role of community and school in, 474-475
 tests of, 437
 and tobacco, 456
 training and, 447-456
Physically educated boys and girls, 169-172
Physically handicapped students, 54-56
Piaget, Jean, 46, 479-480, 499
Plamann's Boys School, 299
Plato, 125-126, 144, 275, 285
Play as a socializing force, 527-531
Playground Association of America, 10, 241, 631
Playground and Recreation Association, 320
Plus factor in physical education, 162-163
Pooley, Robert C., 138
Pope Pius II, 291

Positions in recreation, 253-254
Posse, Baron Nils, 315, 590
Posse Normal School of Gymnastics, 590
Pragmatism, 130-133
Preschool years, 419-420
President's Council for Physical Fitness and Sports, 165, 240, 328, 447, 464-466, 468, 475
Primitive gymnastics, 305
Profession
 of physical education, 9-18, 553-572, 613-675
  certification requirements in, 639-648
  challenges facing, 666-675
  definition of, 9
  employment opportunities in, 649-665
  professional organizations for, 615-638
  steps in making, 11-17
 and recreation, 252-253
Professional competencies, 602-606
Professional organizations, 615-638
 Amateur Athletic Union, 616-617
 American Academy of Physical Education, 617-618
 American Association for Health, Physical Education, and Recreation, 618-619
 American College of Sports Medicine, 619-621
 American Corrective Therapy Association, 621-622
 American School Health Association, 622-624
 Canadian Association for Health, Physical Education, and Recreation, 624
 College Sports Information Directors of America, 624-625
 Delta Psi Kappa, 625
 National Association of Intercollegiate Athletics, 626
 National Association of Physical Education for College Women, 626-627
 National College Physical Education Association for Men, 628-629
 National Collegiate Athletic Association, 627-628
 National Education Association, 629
 National Intramural Association, 629-630
 National Junior College Athletic Association, 630-631
 National Recreation and Park Association, 631-632
 North American Society for the Psychology of Sports and Physical Activity, 632
 Phi Delta Pi, 632-633
 Phi Epsilon Kappa Fraternity, 633-634
 Physical Education Society of the Young Men's Christian Association of North America, 634
 reasons for belonging to, 615-616
 Society of State Directors of Health, Physical Education, and Recreation, 634-635
 United States Collegiate Sports Council, 635
 Young Women's Christian Association, 636-637

Professional preparation, 328
  of health educators, 232-235
  of the physical education teacher, 588-612
    accreditation for, 608-609
    current developments in, 598-602
    curriculum for, 602-608
    at graduate level, 610-611
    history of, 588-596
    objectives of, 588
    selecting institution for, 609-610
    and 2-year colleges, 597
  of the recreator, 255-256
Professional preparation programs, 35
Professional Preparing Conference, 597
Professional status of physical education, 8-28
  challenge for, 24-28
  current attitude toward, 18-22
  as emerging profession, 9-18
  occupations and professional status, 22-24
Program
  for camping and outdoor education, 266-268
  for movement education, 354-355
  for recreation, 248
  for school health, 203-236
Program changes in physical education in the
  1970's, 98-101
Programmed instruction, 504-505
Project Life, 527
Project ME, 253
Project on Recreation and Fitness for the Mentally Retarded, 330
Project Talent, 46
Projections of educational statistics to 1974-1975,
  650
Psychological development and physical education,
  495-496
Psychological interpretations of physical education, 477-519
  developments affecting learning process, 504-
    510, 513-517
  educational instructional media, 510-513
  getting at the "why" of the activity, 502-504
  learning, elements of, 477-481
  motor learning, 485-495
  other psychological bases for physical educa-
    tion, 495-499
  physical education and academic achievement,
    499-502
  theories of learning, 481-485
Public health programs, 230-232
Public and private schools and colleges, settings
  for physical education, 63-79
Pullman, Washington, 335

Q

Qualifications
  for physical educators, 559-568
  for the recreator, 254-255
  for teachers, 559-562
Queens College, 266-267

R

Rabelais, François, 291
Radler, D. H., 499
Rarick, G. L., 500
Rationalism, 138-139
Ray, Harold L., 310, 311, 316
Raycroft, Joseph E., 321
Reade, Evelyn, 352, 354
Realism, 128-130
Reams, David, 505
Recreation, 54, 237-260
  agencies and settings sponsoring, 247-248
  areas of, 84-85
  definition of, 6, 237
  history of, 241-243
  leadership for, 252
  leisure and, 245-247
  need for, 244-245
  objectives of, 237-241
  opportunities and challenges in, 256-258
  physical educators and, 256
  placement in, 258-260
  positions in, 253-254
  profession and, 252-253
  professional preparation for, 255-256
  program for, 248
  qualifications for recreator, 254-255
  and relaxation, 462-463
  school and, 248-252
Recreation theory of play, 528
Reevaluating school program, 674
Reiff, Guy G., 467
Reinforcement theory, 484
Relationship of physical education to health, rec-
  reation, camping, and outdoor education,
  197-272
Relaxation theory of play, 528
Religion and recreation, 258
Renaissance, 290-292
Reproductive system, 416
Research, 43-47
Research Council, 330
Resources for international education, 364
Respiratory system, 413-414
Responsibilities of physical educator, 574-578
Retirement benefits, 652
Rewards of teaching, 553-554; *see also* Teaching
Rhea, Kermit, 621
Rickey, Branch, 526
Riis, Jacob A., 320
Roaring 20's, 323-324
Roberts, Robert J., 312-313
Robsons, John, 625
Rockefeller, Laurence S., 252
Rogers, Frederick Rand, 323
Rogers, James Edward, 10, 634
Roman Empire, 287-288
Rome, 285-287
Rook, Sir Alan, 438

Rosentswieg, Joel, 146, 163-164
Round Hill School, 309
Roundy, Elmo Smith, 602-605
Rousseau, Jean Jacques, 117, 134, 275, 291-292, 499
Royal Central Institute of Gymnastics, 301
Ruffer, William A., 75, 544
Russell, Bertrand, 122
Ryan, Allan J., 156
Ryans, David G., 562

S

Sabbatical leaves, 652
Safety and driver education program, 43
Safety education, 582
Salaries of teachers, 649-652
Salz, Art, 542
San Diego, California, schools, 262, 267-268
Sargent, Dudley Allen, 145, 314, 321, 589
Schneider, Edward C., 438, 450
Schnepfenthal Educational Institute, 299
Scholasticism, 289
School
  and colleges, role of physical education in, 175
  and community in fitness, 474-475
  levels of instruction in, 580-581
  and recreation, 248-252
School-age population, 655
School Health Education Study, 36, 168, 206, 207-209, 216
School health program, 203-236; *see also* Health
  areas of, 215-227
  history of, 205-207
  outcomes expected from, 227-230
  personnel in, 227
  and physical education, 210-215
  preparation of educators for, 232-235
  and public health program, 230-232
  terminology for, 209-210
School University Teacher Education Center, 600
Schopenhauer, 275
Schrader, Carl L., 634
Scientific foundations of physical education, 401-550
  biological, 403-476
  psychological, 477-519
  sociological, 520-550
Scientific principles and objectives, 152-153
Scott, M. Gladys, 495-496
Scott, Phebe Martha, 539
Seattle, Washington, schools, 55, 178
Second National Conference on School Recreation, 250
Secondary schools, 69-70
  certification of physical educators in, 645
  student health worries and interests, 214-215
Selective Service Act of 1917, 321
Self-development and recreation, 240-241
Self-expression theory of play, 529

Selye, Hans, 460
Sensitivity training, 508-509
Service organizations, 79-82
Services rendered by physical educators, 30-61
  administering programs, 41-43
  in camping and outdoor education, 37-38
  in coaching, 38-40
  conducting research, 43-47
  conducting safety and driver education, 43
  in counseling, 40-41
  in dance, 33-35
  in games, 33
  with handicapped and exceptional persons, 49-59
  human behavior and, 47-49
  interpreting the worth of physical education, 59-60
  in movement experiences, 31-33
  professional preparation programs, 35
  in recreation, 37
  specific examples of, 31
  Teacher Corps, 35
  teaching, 31-38
  teaching health, 35-37
  world service, 47
Settings
  for outdoor education, 265-266
  for physical education activities, 62-89
    athletic clubs, 85
    camps, 86
    churches, 87
    considerations for, 62-63
    government and welfare agencies, 86-87
    hospitals, 87-88
    industrial concerns, 82-84
    other countries, 357-400
    penal institutions, 88
    professional and commercial areas, 85-86
    public and private schools and colleges, 63-79
    recreational areas, 84-85
    service organizations, 79-82
    youth organizations, 83-84
  for recreation, 247-248
Settlement and neighborhood houses, 79-81
Shaker Heights, Ohio, schools, 176
Shane, Harold G., 92
Shane, June Grant, 92
Sharman, Jackson, 7
Sharp, L. B., 261
Sheldon, William H., 424, 425, 498
Sherwood, Colorado, schools, 106
Shivers, Jay S., 248-249, 264
Sick leaves, 652
Singer, Robert N., 498
Skills, learning of, 485-495
Skinner, B. F., 484-485, 504
Skinner, Elizabeth K., 547
Skubic, Elvera, 544
Sliepcevich, Elena, 207, 212-215

Smith, Julian W., 263, 271
Social change, 526-527
Social contact theory of play, 528
Social development, 49
Social development objective, 161-162
Socializing forces
    play, 527-531
    sport, 531-538
Sociological implications of educational athletics, 538-547
Sociological interpretations of physical education, 520-550
    building character in youth, 524-526
    cultural values, 520-521
    educating for social change, 526-527
    modes of social learning, 524
    nature of man, 521-524
    play as a socializing force, 527-531
    sociological implications of educational athletics, 538-547
    sport as a socializing force, 531-538
    youth problems in present decade, 547-548
Sokol, 85
Solomon, Amiel, 470
South Carolina certification, 646-647
South Pacific Games, 368
Sparta, 282
Spearman, Charles, 480
Special schools, 78
Spencer, Herbert, 275
Spiess, Adolph, 300
Sport
    as an institutionalized game, 533-535
    nature of, 532-533
    origin of, 292, 307-308
    as part of American culture, 536-538
    physical fitness ratings of, 462
    as a social institution, 535-536
    as a socializing force, 531-538
Sport medicine, 6
Springfield College, 10, 590
Stanford-Binet test, 481
State legal requirements for physical education, 71-74
Status of professional preparation programs, 593-596
Steinhaus, Arthur H., 462, 563
Stevens, S. S., 498
Stiles, Merrit H., 454
Still, Joseph W., 403-405
Stinnett, T. M., 642-643
Stoodley, Agnes, 145
Storey, Thomas D., 317
Strang, Ruth, 508
Stress, 460
Student
    and changes in the 1970's, 93-94
    impact of athletics upon, 541-547
Student Action Council, 333, 527
Student activism, 333-334

Student attitude toward physical education, 18-20
Student objectives in physical education, 149-152
Study units in outdoor education, 269
Summer school programs, 662
Suppes, Patrick, 46
Supreme Court, 537
Surplus-energy or Spencer-Schiller theory of play, 528
Sweden, 300-304, 390-392
Swedish gymnastics, 310
Swedish Movement Cure, 309-310, 588
Sweeney, John F., 466
Swengros, Glenn V., 469

T

Taiwan, 360, 440
Taylor, Harold, 137-138
Taylor, Loren E., 265, 266
Teacher
    beginning, 568-571
    changing role of, in the 1970's, 94-96
    end of shortage of, 654-658
    evaluation of, 556-559
    history of education programs for, 590-593
    of physical education and role in future, 97-98
    qualifications for, 559-562
        of physical educator, 562-568
    second jobs for, 584-585
    supply and demand of, 656-657, 659
Teacher accountability, 331, 556
Teacher aides, 554-555
Teacher Corps, 35, 365, 602
Teacher fatigue, 461-462
Teacher-Opinion Poll, 122
Teacher problems, 559
Teacher-training institution, 609-610
Teachers College, Columbia University, 315
Teaching
    advantages offered by, 649-652
    for health, 215-220
    new techniques for, 511
    of physical education, 31-38
    salaries for, 649-652
Teaching loads, 584
Teaching profession and physical education, 553-572
    beginning teacher, 568-571
    code of ethics, 559
    new developments in, 554-559
    qualifications for, 559-568
Teaching style, 555-556
Team teaching, 505-506
Ten-point program for the future of physical education, 108-112
Tenure, 652
Terman, Lewis, 501
Terminology
    for health programs, 209-210
    for physical education, origin of, 292-295
    synonymous with physical education, 3-8

Tests of fitness, 437
Teutonic barbarians, 288
Thailand, 392-394
Theodosius, 288
Theories
  of learning, 481-485
  of play
    Caillois, 529
    domination, 529
    inheritance or recapitulation, 528
    instinct or Groos, 528
    recreation, 528
    relaxation, 528
    self-expression, 529
    social contact, 528
    wish-fulfillment, 529
Thorndike, E. L., 317, 481-483
Thune, John B., 498
Thurstone, L. L., 480
Thwing, Edward, 314
Time allotment for physical education, 580-581
Tobacco and fitness, 220-222, 456
Tolbert, J. W., 541
Toledo, Ohio, schools, 392
Trade and vocational schools, 78
Training
  effects of, 448-453
  principles of, 447-448
Training experiences, 606-607
Tremble, Neal, 6
Trends in certification, 644
Trump, J. Lloyd, 510
Tunney, Gene, 10, 325
Turnverein, 85, 299, 309-310
Two-year college, 76-77, 597, 661
Tyler, John Mason, 317
Types of certificates, 643-644

U

Ulrich, Celeste, 149
Union of South Africa, 394-395
Union of Soviet Socialist Republics, 395-396
United Nations Educational, Scientific, and Cultural Organization, 358, 365
United States Collegiate Sports Council, 635
United States Military Academy, 81, 309
United States Office of Education, 650
University games, 367
University of Washington, 590

V

Values of camping and outdoor education, 269-271
VanDalen, Deobold B., 11
Verferio, Pietro, 291

Vermont–New Hampshire plan of cooperation, 257
Veterans Administration, 87
Visual aids, 510-513

W

Wasson, William, 629
Watson, Goodwin, 28, 502
Watts, Diana, 345
Webster, Randolph W., 118
Wegener, Charles, 139
Wegener, Frank C., 201
Weight control, 457-460
Wessel, Janet, 370
West Germany, 396-398
White, Paul Dudley, 275, 438-439
Whitehead, Alfred North, 9
Wilkinson, Charles B., 464
Willgoose, Carl E., 425
Williams, Jesse Feiring, 39, 145, 148-149, 152, 203, 323
Wilson, Clifford, 19-20
Winship, George Barker, 310
Wireman, Billy O., 169-172
Wish-fulfillment theory of play, 529
Women's Christian Temperance Union, 206, 321
Women's liberation movement, 338-339
Women's physical education, employment in, 658-660
Wood, Thomas Denison, 145, 148, 318, 323
Woodruff, Asahael D., 166
Woody, Thomas, 538
World Confederation of Organizations of the Teaching Profession, 329-330, 371
World Health Organization, 6, 365
World service, 47
Wundt, Wilhelm Max, 317
Wynne, J. P., 179

X

Xenophon, 285

Y

Year-round school, 515-516
Yocum, Rachael Dunaven, 435-436
Young Men's Christian Association, 79-80, 242, 312-313, 326, 469
Young Women's Christian Association, 79, 242, 313, 636-637
Youth
  building character in, 524-526
  problems of, in present decade, 547-548
Youth fitness, 466-468
Youth organizations, 83-84
Youth Services Section, Los Angeles schools, 55, 257-258, 483, 491